EPIDEMIOLOGY OF PAIN

Mission Statement of IASP Press®

The International Association for the Study of Pain (IASP) is a nonprofit, interdisciplinary organization devoted to understanding the mechanisms of pain and improving the care of patients with pain through research, education, and communication. The organization includes scientists and health care professionals dedicated to these goals. The IASP sponsors scientific meetings and publishes newsletters, technical bulletins, the journal *Pain*, and books.

The goal of IASP Press is to provide the IASP membership with timely, high-quality, low-cost publications relevant to the problem of pain. These publications are also intended to appeal to a wider audience of scientists and clinicians interested in the problem of pain.

Additional Publications from IASP Press

Assessment and Treatment of Cancer Pain, edited by Richard Payne, Richard B. Patt, and C. Stratton Hill, Jr.

Sickle Cell Pain, by Samir K. Ballas

Measurement of Pain in Infants and Children, edited by G. Allen Finley and Patrick J. McGrath

Molecular Neurobiology of Pain, edited by David Borsook

Proceedings of the 8th World Congress on Pain, edited by Troels S. Jensen, Judith A. Turner, and Zsuzsanna Wiesenfeld-Hallin

Pain Treatment Centers at a Crossroads: A Practical and Conceptual Reappraisal, edited by Mitchell J.M. Cohen and James N. Campbell

Reflex Sympathetic Dystrophy: A Reappraisal, edited by Wilfrid Jänig and Michael Stanton-Hicks

Pain in the Elderly, Task Force on Pain in the Elderly, edited by Betty R. Ferrell and Bruce A. Ferrell

Core Curriculum for Professional Education in Pain, Second Edition, Task Force on Professional Education, edited by Howard L. Fields

Back Pain in the Workplace: Management of Disability in Nonspecific Conditions, Task Force on Pain in the Workplace, edited by Wilbert E. Fordyce

Visceral Pain, edited by Gerald F. Gebhart

Temporomandibular Disorders and Related Pain Conditions, edited by Barry J. Sessle, Patricia S. Bryant, and Raymond A. Dionne

Touch, Temperature, and Pain in Health and Disease: Mechanisms and Assessments, edited by Jörgen Boivie, Per Hansson, and Ulf Lindblom

Classification of Chronic Pain: Descriptions of Chronic Pain Syndromes and Definitions of Pain Terms, Second Edition, Task Force on Taxonomy, edited by Harold Merskey and Nikolai Bogduk

Proceedings of the 7th World Congress on Pain, edited by Gerald F. Gebhart, Donna L. Hammond, and Troels S. Jensen

Pharmacological Approaches to the Treatment of Chronic Pain: New Concepts and Critical Issues, edited by Howard L. Fields and John C. Liebeskind

EPIDEMIOLOGY OF PAIN

a report of the

Task Force on Epidemiology
of the
International Association for the Study of Pain

Editors and Members of the Task Force on Epidemiology

Iain K. Crombie, PhD (Chair)
*Department of Epidemiology and Public Health, University of Dundee,
Ninewells Hospital and Medical School, Dundee, United Kingdom*

Peter R. Croft, MD, MRCGP
*Primary Care Sciences Research Centre,
School of Postgraduate Medicine, Keele University, Hartshill,
Stoke-on-Trent, United Kingdom*

Steven J. Linton, PhD
*Department of Occupational Medicine,
Örebro Medical Centre Hospital, Örebro, Sweden*

Linda LeResche, ScD
*Department of Oral Medicine, School of Dentistry,
University of Washington, Seattle, Washington, USA*

Michael Von Korff, ScD
*Center for Health Studies, Group Health Cooperative
of Puget Sound, Seattle, Washington, USA*

IASP PRESS • SEATTLE

Library of Congress Cataloging-in-Publication Data

International Association for the Study of Pain. Task Force on Epidemiology.
    Epidemiology of pain : a report of the Task Force on Epidemiology of the International Association for the Study of Pain / editors and members of the Task Force on Epidemiology, Iain K. Crombie, chair ... [et al.].
       p.   cm.
    Includes bibliographical references and index.
    ISBN 0-931092-25-6
    1. Pain—Epidemiology.   2. Chronic pain—Epidemiology.
I. Crombie, I. K.   II. Title.
    [DNLM: 1. Pain—epidemiology.   WL 704 I602e 1999]
RB127.I56   1999
616' .0472—dc21
DNLM/DLC
for Library of Congress

99-14319
CIP

IASP Press
International Association for the Study of Pain
909 NE 43rd St., Suite 306
Seattle, WA 98105 USA
Fax: 206-547-1703

Printed in the United States of America

Contents

Contributing Authors

Grethe Andersen, PhD, *Department of Neurology, Aarhus University Hospital, Aarhus, Denmark*

Geertje A.M. Ariëns, MSc, *Institute for Research in Extramural Medicine, Department of Social Medicine, Vrije Universiteit, Amsterdam, The Netherlands*

Jeroen A.J. Borghouts, MSc, *Institute for Research in Extramural Medicine, Department of Social Medicine, Vrije Universiteit, Amsterdam, The Netherlands*

Inger Brødsgaard, MD, *Department of Oral Medicine, University of Washington, Seattle, Washington, USA; and Social Medicine Division, Municipality of Aarhus, Aarhus, Denmark*

Peter R. Croft, MD, MRCGP, *Primary Care Sciences Research Centre, School of Postgraduate Medicine, Keele University, Hartshill, Stoke-on-Trent, United Kingdom*

Iain Kinloch Crombie, PhD, Hon MFPHM, *Department of Epidemiology and Public Health, University of Dundee, Ninewells Hospital and Medical School, Dundee, United Kingdom*

Huw Talfryn Oakley Davies, MA, MSc, PhD, Hon MFPHM, *Department of Management, University of St Andrews, St Katharine's West, The Scores, St Andrews, Fife, United Kingdom*

Clermont E. Dionne, PhD, *Department of Rehabilitation, Faculty of Medicine, Laval University, Sainte-Foy, Quebec, Canada*

Mark Drangsholt, DDS, MPH, *Departments of Oral Medicine and Dental Public Health Services, School of Dentistry, and Department of Epidemiology, School of Public Health and Community Medicine, University of Washington, Seattle, Washington, USA*

Stephen J. Gibson, BBSC (Hons), PhD, MAPsS, *National Ageing Research Institute, Parkville, Victoria, Australia*

Peter J. Hamlyn, MD, FRCS, FISM, *Department Neurological Surgery, St. Bartholomew's and the Royal London Hospital, London, United Kingdom*

Robert D. Helme, MBBS, PhD, FRACP, *National Ageing Research Institute, Parkville, Victoria, Australia*

Troels S. Jensen, PhD, *Department of Neurology, Aarhus University Hospital, Aarhus, Denmark*

Donna A. K. Kalauokalani, MD, *Department of Anesthesiology, Health Services, and Multidisciplinary Pain Services, University of Washington, Seattle, Washington, USA*

Bart W. Koes, PhD, *Institute for Research in Extramural Medicine, Department of Social Medicine, Vrije Universiteit, Amsterdam, The Netherlands*

Linda LeResche, ScD, *Department of Oral Medicine, School of Dentistry, University of Washington, Seattle, Washington, USA*

Steven J. Linton, PhD, *Department of Occupational and Environmental Medicine, Örebro Medical Center Hospital, Örebro, Sweden*

Richard B. Lipton, MD, *Departments of Neurology, Epidemiology, and Social Medicine, Albert Einstein College of Medicine, Bronx, New York, USA; Headache Unit, Montefiore Medical Center, Bronx, New York, USA; and Innovative Medical Research, Stamford, Connecticut, USA*

John D. Loeser, MD, *Departments of Anaesthesiology and Neurological Surgery and Multidisciplinary Pain Center, University of Washington, Seattle, Washington, USA*

Gary J. Macfarlane, PhD, *School of Epidemiology and Health Services, University of Manchester, Manchester, United Kingdom*

William Andrew Macrae, MB ChB, FRCA, *Department of Anaesthesia, University of Dundee, Ninewells Hospital and Medical School, Dundee, United Kingdom*

Robert McCarney, MPhil, *Primary Care Sciences Research Centre, Keele University, Keele, United Kingdom*

Patricia A. McGrath, PhD, *Department of Paediatrics, The University of Western Ontario, Canada; and Paediatric Pain Program, Child Health Research Institute, London, Ontario, Canada*

Rod Moore, DDS, PhD, *Department of Oral Medicine, University of Washington, Seattle, Washington, USA; and Department of Oral Epidemiology and Public Health, Royal Dental College, Aarhus University, Denmark*

Ann I. Scher, MS, *Department of Epidemiology, The Johns Hopkins University, Baltimore, Maryland, USA; and Neuroepidemiology Branch, National Institute for Neurological Disorders and Stroke, National Institutes of Health, Bethesda, Maryland, USA*

Suzanne M. Skevington, PhD, *Department of Psychology, University of Bath, Bath, United Kingdom; and Royal National Hospital for Rheumatic Diseases, Bath, United Kingdom.*

Walter F. Stewart, PhD, MPH, *Department of Epidemiology, The Johns Hopkins University, Baltimore, Maryland, USA; and Innovative Medical Research, Towson, Maryland, USA*

Daniëlle van der Windt, PhD, *Institute for Research in Extramural Medicine, Vrije Universiteit, Amsterdam, The Netherlands*

Karsten Vestergaard, MD, *Department of Neurology, Aalborg Hospital, Aalborg, Denmark*

Michael Von Korff, ScD, *Center for Health Studies, Group Health Cooperative of Puget Sound, Seattle, Washington, USA*

Joanna M. Zakrzewska, MD, FDSRCS, FFDRCSI, *Department of Oral Medicine, St. Bartholomew's and Royal London School of Medicine and Dentistry, London, United Kingdom*

Foreword

At the First International Symposium on Pain in Issaquah, Washington, in 1973, many of the participants noted the paucity of information on the incidence and prevalence of pain throughout the world. When the International Association for the Study of Pain (IASP) was launched following this meeting, one of the goals of the new association was to promulgate research on the epidemiology of painful conditions, both acute and chronic. Unfortunately, those who pursued epidemiology as a discipline were often not interested in pain, and those who cared for patients with painful conditions rarely understood the materials and methods of epidemiology. This book links these two perspectives.

Epidemiology provides information that is critical to an understanding of the causes of diseases, their natural history, and their impact upon societies. It also allows us to identify where a disease occurs and how it is transmitted from person to person. It is one of the critical sciences basic to an understanding of human disease and illness.

Although an increase in publications concerning the occurrence of painful conditions can be documented in the past 25 years, far too many of these studies are flawed to the point that meaningful extrapolations to the population at large cannot be made. It became obvious to the leadership of IASP that redoubled efforts were necessary to improve the quality of epide-

miological studies relevant to pain. With this in mind, the IASP Task Force on Epidemiology was established in 1994, chaired by Professor Iain Crombie, to address this issue and prepare a publication that would call attention to the methods of epidemiology and assess available information about painful conditions. It was my pleasure to work with Dr. Crombie and his associates in developing this task force, whose members represent different aspects of epidemiological sciences and who have prepared a report that will serve as a collation of available information and set the standards for future studies. Those who read this book will, I am sure, agree that the goals for this task force have been met.

On behalf of the IASP, I would like to thank Dr. Crombie and all of the other contributors to this wonderful source book. The field of pain management will take a giant step forward with its publication.

John D. Loeser, MD
Past-President, International Association
    for the Study of Pain
Departments of Neurological Surgery and
    Anesthesiology, and
Multidisciplinary Pain Center
University of Washington
Seattle, Washington, USA

Preface

Pain is a major public health problem. In their seminal book, *The Challenge of Pain,* Melzack and Wall give this compelling description: "Pain is one of the most challenging problems in medicine and biology. It is a challenge to the sufferer who must learn how to live with pain for which no therapy has been found. It is a challenge to the physician or other health professional who seeks every possible means to help the suffering patient. It is a challenge to the scientist who tries to understand the biological mechanisms that can cause such terrible suffering. It is also a challenge to society, which must find the medical, scientific and financial resources to relieve or prevent pain and suffering as much as possible" (Melzack, R., and Wall, P.D. *The Challenge of Pain.* London: Penguin, 1988).

A number of questions arise from Melzack and Wall's outline. Exactly what is the scale of the problem? How many individuals suffer from pain, and what proportion do not receive adequate therapy? What can and should be done to relieve and prevent pain? These questions fall within the realm of epidemiology. Epidemiological surveys can investigate the amount of pain and the adequacy of its management. Other epidemiological techniques, described in the first three chapters of this book, can be used to explore the possible causes of pain. The motivation for this is clear. If we understand the causes of pain, we can develop and test strategies to prevent it. Studies on the epidemiology of pain are a relatively new phenomenon. Moreover, these studies are published in a diverse array of journals. Many appear in the recognized pain journals and some appear in psychological journals, but the majority have been published in a host of general and specialist medical journals. This explains the reason for the publication of the present volume—the need to assemble in one volume current knowledge on the epidemiology of pain. But this book is not simply a series of reports from a team of experts. It was recognized just over 10 years ago that the traditional narrative review, often based on an incomplete set of reports, was inadequate (Mulrow, C.D. The medical review article: state of the science. *Annals of Internal Medicine* 1987; 106:485–488). It is now recommended that a much more systematic approach be adopted in reviewing the literature (Mulrow, C.D. Rationale for systematic reviews. *British Medical Journal* 1994; 309:597–599). This approach was adopted for this book. To facilitate a consistently high standard, the authors of each chapter were encouraged to perform systematic literature reviews, for example by using MEDLINE searches. The studies identified were to be graded into major (i.e., high-quality) studies and other studies. The major studies would be identified as those that met certain criteria: well-defined purpose, definition of the pain, appropriate study design, adequacy of sample size, appropriateness of the analyses, and validity of the interpretation of findings. The authors have complied with this approach, producing chapters of very high quality.

The book's three main aims were to provide a repository of epidemiological information on chronic pain syndromes, to review the problems and pitfalls in epidemiological studies of pain, and to identify high-priority areas for future research. In my view it has exceeded its expectations.

IAIN K. CROMBIE, PHD

Epidemiology of Pain, edited by
I.K. Crombie, IASP Press, Seattle, © 1999.

1

The Potential of Epidemiology

Iain Kinloch Crombie

*Department of Epidemiology and Public Health, University of Dundee,
Ninewells Hospital and Medical School, Dundee, United Kingdom*

Clinical medicine is concerned with the health and well-being of individual patients. In contrast, epidemiology studies disease as it occurs in groups of people or even whole populations. As with many other medical specialties, the origins of epidemiology can be traced to the writings of Hippocrates. The term *epidemiology* derives from the Greek and means the formal study of the health of the community (*epi* means on, *demos* the people, and *logos* word or reason). The Hippocratic book *Airs, Waters and Places* describes how environmental factors such as climate, soil, and water, as well as mode of life and nutrition, influence the occurrence of disease in communities (Rosen 1993).

Despite its promising start in ancient Greece, epidemiology did not advance significantly until the 19th century. Studies at that time were concerned with epidemics of infectious disease. The first epidemiological association, the London Epidemiological Society, was formed in 1850 to investigate the causes of the cholera epidemic that raged at that time (Lilienfeld and Lilienfeld 1980). The society quickly expanded its scope to embrace other infectious diseases such as smallpox and typhoid. The unifying characteristic of these early studies was the use of medical statistics to uncover the causes of diseases.

The role of medical statistics and the epidemiological approach to disease can be illustrated by the work of the Hungarian Ignaz Semmelweis. Semmelweis worked in a maternity hospital in mid-19th-century Vienna and was concerned with the high rate of mortality from puerperal fever. He was intrigued by the fact that the mortality rate from puerperal fever was much higher in the division in which medical students were trained than in the division where mid-wives were trained. In 1846 the medical division had a mortality rate of 11.4%, compared to 2.7% in the midwife division (Sinclair 1909). Semmelweis hypothesized that the medical students were carrying cadaverous matter from autopsies to their examinations of women in childbirth (midwives performed far fewer autopsies). He tested his idea by insisting, at the end of May 1847, that all staff and students wash their hands in chlorinated lime before clinical examinations. The mortality rate in the medical division immediately fell from 12.2% in May to 2.4% in June (Gortvay and Zoltan 1968). Careful research and the testing of an idea had identified the mechanism of disease transmission and allowed the disease to be brought under control.

THE DEVELOPMENT OF EPIDEMIOLOGY IN THE 20TH CENTURY

Although the origins of epidemiology lie in the study of infectious diseases, the 20th century has witnessed the development of epidemiological techniques to study chronic diseases. Some epidemiological studies were so successful that it is difficult to imagine our previous ignorance of their findings. For example, studies were undertaken in the late 1940s to determine the cause of the lung cancer epidemic, which was unknown at that time (Peto 1994). Evidence for the role of tobacco smoke was first obtained in the 1950s, and its causative role has now been confirmed in many studies throughout the world. Epidemiology has successfully contributed to our understanding of many diseases, including dietary deficiency diseases (goiter and pellagra), coronary heart disease, stroke, many cancers, and many diseases associated with industrial processes. More recently, epidemiology has helped identify the cause of AIDS and has enhanced our understanding of the natural history of this disease.

The emergence of the epidemiology of coronary heart disease illustrates the power of this approach. Clinical studies dating back to the 18th century describe the nature of atherosclerotic plaques (Stamler 1992). Subsequent clinical and animal studies led to the hypothesis that a diet rich in cholesterol and fat was responsible for the development of plaques. Comparisons among populations confirmed that atherosclerosis was much more common when consumption of cholesterol and fat was high. These observations led to formal investigations that related the risk factor levels of individuals to the subsequent development of coronary heart disease. These studies confirmed the role of elevated serum cholesterol and documented that smoking and high blood pressure were also important causes of heart attacks. The final stage was to test these findings by conducting intervention studies to determine the effect of lowering the risk factors. Expectations were confirmed: controlling the risk factors does reduce the frequency of the disease.

The cardiovascular example provides a model for the development of the epidemiology of a chronic disease. Insights from clinical and animal studies stimulate comparisons among populations and among different groups within a society. This research may suggest potential risk factors that can be investigated in detailed epidemiological studies. The most promising risk factors can then be tested in intervention studies to identify those which most strongly influence the development of disease. Progress will not always move in a strictly linear fashion through these stages, since new insights from one stage can have implications for the others. The important point is that a combination of these approaches will lead to the control of the disease.

THE ROLE OF EPIDEMIOLOGY

Epidemiology studies the occurrence of disease and illness in the community. This is put more formally in the accepted definition: "epidemiology is the study of the distribution and determinants of health related states or events in a specified population and the application of this study to the control of health problems" (Last 1988). This definition has several facets that are worth pursuing. For example, the phrase "health related states or events" has been deliberately chosen to embrace a wide range of types of illness. In early versions of the definition, the term "disease" was used, but this was later considered to be too narrow. The revised definition is particularly helpful for the study of chronic pain, where the concept of disease, with clearly defined diagnostic criteria and well-established treatment protocols, is not always helpful.

Last's definition indicates that epidemiological studies have two distinct aims: to study the distribution of disease and to discover its determinants. The study of the distribution of illness traditionally asks how many people get the disease and what types of people fall ill. Many studies have addressed the question of how many people develop chronic pain; estimates vary from 7% to over 50% (Crombie 1997). Explanations for this discrepancy are considered in Chapter 3. Less attention has been paid to the distribution of chronic pain among different groups in society. This is unfortunate, because diseases are seldom distributed uniformly throughout society. Often the frequency of disease varies with age and gender. Many diseases show marked variation by social class or occupational group, and diseases can certainly be more common in one geographical region than another. It is the purpose of epidemiology to find out how common the disease is overall and how its prevalence varies across the different groups in society.

Studying the determinants of illness simply means asking the question, Why do some people fall ill? There are many potential causes of pain, and studies have addressed such diverse questions as: Does obesity lead to low back pain? (Garzillo and Garzillo 1994); Does depression increase the risk of chronic pain? (Magni et al. 1993); Is sexual abuse associated with chronic pelvic pain in women? (Rapkin et al. 1990); and, Is there a genetic component to chronic tension headache? (Ostergaard et al. 1997). One of the interesting features of the occurrence of disease is that of all those who live in circumstances in which the disease occurs, only a small number usually go on to develop the disease. For example, it is well known that nurses are at high risk of developing low back pain, but only a proportion of them suffer from it. Similarly, of all the patients who experience a herpes zoster infection, only about 20% go on to develop post-herpetic neuralgia (Dworkin and Portenoy 1996). Epidemiology investigates the associations between potential risk factors and the development of pain to try to identify which factors are truly causal. The complexity of the task facing epidemiology has meant using special research methods.

EPIDEMIOLOGICAL RESEARCH METHODS

Epidemiology employs a variety of research designs, which are described in detail in Chapter 2. A brief outline of the main features of three principal methods—surveys, cohort studies, and case-control studies—is provided here to help clarify the uses of epidemiology.

Surveys are one of the most commonly used methods. They can describe how much pain is out there, or technically speaking, they can provide estimates of the prevalence of pain. One such survey showed how the frequency of pain can vary across different body sites (Von Korff et al. 1988), and also documented how the pain had affected the lives of individuals and their families (Von Korff et al. 1990).

Cohort studies involve following patients over time to determine how their pain changes. For example, to determine the effect of rectal amputation, Boas and colleagues (1993) followed patients from the time of their operation for a 5-year period. They found that 11.5% experienced persistent perineal pain, which in most patients developed within weeks of the operation. Cohort studies can also be used to investigate how pain changes over time. When Crook and colleagues (1989) followed up chronic pain patients for 2 years, they found that 13% no longer reported pain as a problem. Improvements may continue to occur over a longer period—one study found that over an 8-year follow-up, 32.5% of chronic pain sufferers had become pain free (Magni et al. 1993).

Case-control studies compare the characteristics of patients who have pain against a suitable control group. The goal is to determine the factors that distinguish those who have pain from those who do not. As might be imagined, one of the main difficulties lies in selecting a suitable control group (Marbach et al. 1992). Nonetheless, many interesting studies have been carried out. For example, Rapkin and colleagues (1990) investigated the contribution of physical and sexual abuse in chronic pelvic pain among women.They concluded that "the pernicious nature of abuse, whether physical or sexual, may promote the chronicity of painful conditions."

APPLICATIONS OF EPIDEMIOLOGY

HEALTH SERVICE PLANNING

Surveys of the prevalence of pain in the community are used to help decide what kind and level of health service provision may be required. Many surveys have tried to estimate the extent of specific pain conditions in the community. The unequivocal answer is that pain is common (Crombie 1993). However, equally important issues, which are often missed, are the way the pain is being managed and the extent to which effective services are not being provided to those who might benefit from them. Estimates of the amount of pain in the community and particularly the extent of untreated or poorly treated pain are essential for planning the amount of health care required and for improving its delivery.

WORKING OF THE HEALTH CARE SERVICE

A health care service may be well planned, but that is no guarantee that it will run effectively and efficiently. Epidemiological techniques are well suited for investigating the effectiveness of the health care service. Surveys can be conducted to assess whether services are available and accessible to patients, and to ascertain the level of patient satisfaction with services. Cohort studies can follow patients over time to determine how well they are being managed and whether the outcome of care is as good as it should be.

IDENTIFICATION OF SYNDROMES

Many syndromes have been identified by astute clinicians whose names they now bear: However, defining syndromes in chronic pain is often a challenging task. The constellation of signs and symptoms that define the syndrome can be difficult to identify. Thus, some groups have conducted empirical studies to try to define homogeneous groupings of pain patients (Costello et al. 1987; Rudy et al. 1990). Although these studies are at an early stage of development, the systematic investigation of pain patients is the only approach that is likely to lead to the establishment of valid diagnostic groups.

NATURAL HISTORY OF PAINFUL SYNDROMES

One of the key questions for chronic pain is how

the condition changes over time. There are many ways in which this question may be asked. For example, the patient suffering from an acute episode of low back pain might well ask: How quickly will I recover? Will I suffer a further attack? When might this occur? What will bring it on? Will future attacks get successively more severe or last longer? What can I do to prevent further attacks? These questions are not just relevant to low back pain; they also apply to other episodic pains such as trigeminal neuralgia. An equivalent set of questions applies to patients who have nonfluctuating pain. The answers to all these questions can be obtained from cohort studies that follow patients over time, often for several years.

PREVENTION OF DISEASE

The major aim of epidemiology is to uncover the causes of pain so that appropriate preventive measures can be instituted. This is why epidemiology places such emphasis on identifying the causes of disease. Epidemiological perspectives and methods can be applied to the investigation of pathophysiological and behavioral mechanisms that interact throughout the course of chronic pain, and can help elucidate how dysfunctional pain states develop, how they are perpetuated, and how they might be prevented (Dworkin et al. 1992). It is from this knowledge that preventive measures can be designed and targeted. Finding the causes of pain involves returning to the question of which factors differentiate those those who suffer from pain. Answering this question is not easy. It requires careful study design and will often involve the use of case-control and cohort studies. To date these methods have been little used to investigate the causes of pain, but it is hoped that the future will see their more widespread use.

Prevention is commonly thought of in terms of not catching a disease. For example, the way to avoid influenza is to avoid exposure to the virus or to be vaccinated against it. But there is much more to prevention than this. Three different types of prevention are recognized. Primary prevention focuses on stopping a pain condition from ever occurring. This is clearly the ideal, but ideals can be difficult to achieve. Even when the risk factors are known, prevention is not always possible. For example, riding motorcycles is a risk factor for avulsion lesions of the brachial plexus (Parry 1980); the method of prevention, restricting the use of motorcycles, is difficult to achieve.

Secondary prevention focuses on the early detection of disease with the aim of intervening to reduce subsequent ill-health. A good example is acute back pain, where the concern is to act promptly to prevent it from becoming chronic (Jayson 1997). An extension of this approach is illustrated by migraine, where the intention would be to understand what causes recurrences so that exposure can be avoided. The finding that occupational exposure of women to chemicals and fumes can cause migraine recurrence makes this chemical avoidance a potential strategy for secondary prevention (Rasmussen 1992).

Tertiary prevention seeks to minimize the impairments and disabilities that could arise from incurable disease, and to promote the patient's adjustment to his or her chronic condition (Last 1988). This is an area where substantial advances can be made. Pain affects all aspects of our lives: physical function (Polatin and Mayer 1992), psychosocial well-being (Philips and Jahanshahi 1985; Benedittis et al. 1990; Moffitt et al. 1991), and employment (Moffett ct al. 1995). Epidemiological studies are needed to identify the factors that contribute to the development of disabilities and the subgroups of patients who are most susceptible to them.

CONCLUSION

Epidemiology provides several research methods that can be used to answer a variety of research questions. Too often in the literature on pain the term epidemiology is used to refer solely to a prevalence survey. It is not true that epidemiology can only answer the question: How much pain is there? Instead, epidemiology provides a much richer set of perspectives and methods, which when pursued with vigor and imagination, can make substantial contributions to the control and prevention of chronic pain.

ACKNOWLEDGMENT

This work was supported by a grant from the National Institutes of Health: P01 DE08773, and by the Scottish Office Department of Health.

REFERENCES

Benedittis GD, Lorenzetti A, Pieri A. The role of stressful life events in the onset of chronic primary headache. *Pain* 1990; 40:65–75.

Boas RA, Schug SA, Acland RH. Perineal pain after rectal amputation: a five year follow up. *Pain* 1993; 52:67–70.

Costello RM, Hulsey TL, Schoenfeld LS, Ramamurthy S. P-A-I-N: a four-cluster MMPI typology for chronic pain. *Pain* 1987; 30:199–209.

Crombie IK. Epidemiological studies of pain. *J Pain Society* 1993; 11:30–32.

Crombie IK. Epidemiology of persistent pain. In: Jensen TS, Turner JA,Wiesenfeld-Hallin Z (Ed). *Proceedings of the 8th World Congress on Pain.* Seattle: IASP Press, 1997, pp 53–61.

Crook J, Weir R, Tunks E. An epidemiological follow-up survey of persistent pain sufferers in a group family practice and specialty pain clinic. *Pain* 1989; 36: 49–61.

Dworkin RH, Portenoy RK. Pain and its persistence in herpes zoster. *Pain* 1996; 67:241–251.

Dworkin S, Von Korff M, LeResche L. Epidemiologic studies of chronic pain: a dynamic-ecologic perspective. *Ann Behav Med* 1992; 14:3–11.

Garzillo MJD, Garzillo TAF. Does obesity cause low back pain? *J Manipulative Physiol Ther* 1994; 17:601–604.

Gortvay G, Zoltan I. *Semmelweis: His Life and Work.* Budapest: Akademiai Kiado, 1968.

Jayson IV. Why does acute back pain become chronic? *BMJ* 1997; 314:1639–1640.

Last JM. A Dictionary of Epidemiology. *Int J Epidemiol,* Oxford, 1988.

Lilienfeld AM, Lilienfeld DE. *Foundations of Epidemiology.* New York: Oxford University Press, 1980.

Magni G, Marchetti M, Moreschi C, Merskey H, Rigatti-Luchini S. Chronic musculoskeletal pain and depressive symptoms in the National Health and Nutrition Examination. I. Epidemiologic follow-up study. *Pain* 1993; 53:163–168.

Marbach JJ, Schwartz S, Link BG. The control group conundrum in chronic pain case/control studies. *Clin J Pain* 1992; 8:39–43.

Moffett JK, Richardson G, Sheldon TA, Maynard A. *Back Pain: Its Management and Cost to Society,* Discussion Paper 129, York, 1995.

Moffitt PF, Kalucy EC, Kalucy RS, Baum FE, Cooke RD. Sleep difficulties, pain and other correlates. *J Intern Med* 1991; 230:245–249.

Ostergaard S, Russell MB, Bendtsen L, Olesen J. Comparison of first degree relatives and spouses of people with chronic tension headache. *BMJ* 1997; 314:1092–1093.

Parry C. Pain in avulsion lesions of the brachial plexus. *Pain* 1980; 9:41–53.

Peto R. Smoking and death: the past 40 years and the next 40. *BMJ* 1994; 309:937–939.

Philips HC, Jahanshahi M. The effects of persistent pain: the chronic headache sufferer. *Pain* 1985; 21:163–176.

Polatin PB, Mayer TG. Quantification of function in chronic low back pain. In: Turk DC, Melzack R (Eds). *Handbook of Pain Assessment.* New York: Guilford Press 1992; pp 37–48.

Rapkin AJ, Kames LD, Darke LL, Stampler FM, Naliboff BD. History of physical and sexual abuse in women with chronic pelvic pain. *Obstet Gynecol* 1990; 76:92–96.

Rasmussen BH. Migraine and tension-type headache in a general population: psychosocial factors. *Int J Epidemiol* 1992; 21:1138–1143.

Rosen G. *A History of Public Health.* Baltimore: Johns Hopkins University Press, 1993.

Rudy T, Turk D, Brena S, Stieg R, Brody M. Quantification of biomedical findings of chronic pain patients: development of an index of pathology. *Pain* 1990; 42:167–182.

Sinclair WJ. *Semmelweis: His Life and His Doctrine.* Manchester: University of Manchester Publications, 1909.

Stamler J. Established major coronary risk factors. In: Marmot M, Elliot P (Eds). *Coronary Heart Disease Epidemiology.* Oxford: Oxford University Press, 1992.

Von Korff M, Dworkin SF, Le Resche L, Kruger A. An epidemiologic comparison of pain complaints. *Pain* 1988; 32:173–183.

Von Korff M, Dworkin SF, Le Resche L. Graded chronic pain status: an epidemiologic evaluation. *Pain* 1990; 40:279–291.

Correspondence to: Iain Kinloch Crombie, PhD, Hon MFPHM, Department of Epidemiology and Public Health, University of Dundee, Ninewells Hospital and Medical School, Dundee, DD1 9SY, United Kingdom. Fax: 44-1382-644-197; email: i.k.crombie@dundee.ac.uk.

Epidemiology of Pain, edited by
I.K. Crombie, IASP Press, Seattle, © 1999.

2

Epidemiological Methods

Michael Von Korff

Center for Health Studies, Group Health Cooperative of Puget Sound, Seattle, Washington, USA

Epidemiology is the study of the distribution and determinants of health states in populations (Lilienfeld and Lilienfeld 1980). It provides a scientific basis for preventing or ameliorating disease and disability on a population basis, and includes a range of scientific and public health research activities, including: (1) establishing the dimensions of morbidity and mortality as a function of person, place, and time; (2) quantifying risks of developing morbidity as a function of host, agent, and environmental factors; (3) identifying and defining syndromes; (4) describing the full clinical spectrum of disease and illness; (5) describing the natural history of disease in terms of onset, duration, recurrence, complications, disability, and mortality; (6) identifying factors that influence or predict clinical course; (7) identifying causes of disease, disability, and mortality; and (8) evaluating methods of disease prevention and control (Morris 1975; Von Korff 1992). The application of these uses of epidemiology to the study of pain was considered in Chapter 1. This chapter describes epidemiological methods that can be applied to accomplish these aims.

EPIDEMIOLOGICAL RESEARCH METHODS

THREE PERSPECTIVES ON PAIN RESEARCH

Epidemiological study of pain involves the application of three general perspectives (Dworkin et al. 1992; Von Korff 1992)—the population, developmental, and ecological perspectives.

When pain is studied on a *population* basis, a wide spectrum of severity emerges (Dworkin et al. 1992; Von Korff et al. 1992b, 1994). Most adults experience some form of recurrent pain condition, and a significant minority experience severe chronic pain, although relatively few experience major disability (Von Korff et al. 1990). Epidemiology provides methods for studying this variation in the occurrence and severity of pain conditions in populations. The population perspective does not mean that epidemiological studies always employ random samples drawn from defined populations, but it implies that the ultimate objective is to understand the distribution and determinants of illness on a population basis.

The *developmental* perspective recognizes that pain (like most illness and disease) is changing and dynamic rather than fixed and static. Studies of the pattern of development and variation of a pain condition across time provide a basis for learning about the nature, determinants, and sequelae of the condition.

Pain and related activity limitations are the result of integrated actions of agent, host, and environmental factors. From the *ecological* perspective, factors that initiate pain are analogous to disease agents. An agent is a proximal and necessary (but usually not sufficient) cause of disease or illness. A host factor is a characteristic intrinsic to an organism that influences susceptibility. For example, modulation of nociception and pain perception, as well as appraisal and emotional response to pain, are influenced by host factors. An environmental factor is an extrinsic circumstance that influences exposure to agents or that modifies host susceptibility. Social processes that influence the learning of cognitive and behavioral responses to noxious stimulation and social norms that govern pain behavior (e.g., the sick role) constitute environmental factors. Environmental factors may also include factors influencing the risk of injury or disease. Thus, the ecological model (like the biopsychosocial model) views pain as a dynamic and multifactorial process characterized by integrated action of agent, host, and environmental factors (Dworkin et al. 1992).

EPIDEMIOLOGICAL MEASURES

Epidemiological research seeks to study pain in populations as a dynamic process. Since pain is characterized more by change than by stability, transitions among different pain states (e.g., pain-free, acute, recurrent, and chronic pain) and changes in level of disability are to be expected. Epidemiology provides a framework for measuring the prevalence, incidence, and risks associated with changes in pain and disability status.

Measures of pain prevalence quantify the proportion of the population in a specified pain state (e.g., acute pain, chronic pain, or pain-related disability). Measures of incidence quantify the probability or rate of transition from a given pain state to a condition of increasing morbidity (e.g., onset of a pain condition, of chronic pain, or of disability related to a pain condition). Various clinical measures quantify the duration and severity of the condition and the likelihood of recovery or relapse or of death or disability. Kleinbaum and colleagues (1982) provide a thorough discussion of incidence and prevalence measures.

Risk factors for a pain condition control or predict the probabilities of onset or progression and may be classified as initiators (factors that set in motion a causal process), promoters (factors that enhance or potentiate a causal process already initiated) (Von Korff et al. 1990), and detection factors (factors that increase the likelihood of a case being identified) (Kleinbaum et al. 1982). Prognostic factors include variables that influence or predict clinical course. Several basic epidemiology texts develop these concepts (MacMahon and Pugh 1970; Lilienfeld and Lilienfeld 1980; Fletcher et al. 1982).

The clinical course of many pain conditions is episodic (Von Korff et al. 1990; Von Korff and Saunders 1996). For episodic conditions, prevalence is a function of incidence, episode duration, and number of episodes over the course of the illness (Von Korff and Parker 1980). This implies that differences in prevalence rates by risk factor status can be produced by differences in incidence rates, in episode duration, or in the probability of recurrence. Episode duration and

recurrence may, in turn, be influenced by rates of remission, relapse, or mortality. Because of the complexity of the factors that may influence prevalence rates, differences in prevalence rates by risk factor status should be interpreted with care.

CLASSIFICATION OF PAIN SYNDROMES

Pain is a multidimensional construct defined by subjective self-reported pain and by behaviors associated with the pain experience. Given the ambiguity in definitions of pain states, epidemiological study of pain is likely to be plagued by problems similar to those encountered in the study of other disorders defined by psychologic state and behavior, such as mental disorders. Classification of most pain syndromes is based on manifestational criteria (symptoms, signs, and behavior) rather than causal criteria (McMahon and Pugh 1970, pp 47–54). If epidemiological research on mental disorders can serve as a guide, research on chronic pain is likely to be enhanced by the development of consensus criteria for the classification of pain syndromes and by the development of standardized questionnaires for measuring pain syndromes in epidemiological research (Wing et al. 1981; Weissman et al. 1986; Last and Herson 1987). For example, diagnostic criteria that have been developed for classification of headache disorders (Headache Classification Committee 1988) and temporomandibular disorders (Dworkin and LeResche 1992) have enhanced the reproducibility and comparability of epidemiological studies for these pain conditions.

NATURAL HISTORY

The natural history of pain presents methodological difficulties for epidemiological research. Pain is often characterized by insidious onset, an episodic course, and a broad spectrum of severity. For chronic pain in particular, it is difficult to establish the initial point of onset, to differentiate initial episodes from recurrences, and to establish reliable methods of differentiating clinically significant from nonsignificant pain conditions. Since pain conditions have high prevalence (Sternbach 1986; Von Korff et al. 1990), it is critical to determine when epidemiological investigation should focus on only those cases meeting severity criteria and when the full spectrum of a pain condition should be studied. For example, should a prevalence survey of back pain count as cases all individuals who have experienced any back pain at all during the reporting period, or should the definition of a case be limited to individuals with more severe back pain or with activity limitations? Markedly different prevalence rates result from surveys with varying case definitions due to the broad spectrum of severity.

COMORBIDITY

A by-product of the high prevalence of specific pain conditions is that pain comorbidity is common (Dworkin et al. 1990). This raises methodological problems. Should cases with a comorbid pain condition be included or excluded from a study of an index pain condition? For example, should persons with migraine be included or excluded as control subjects in a study of back pain? Since epidemiologists have generally studied conditions that are relatively rare compared to pain conditions, they have often opted for exclusion of persons with comorbid conditions. This is unlikely to be a satisfactory solution in the epidemiological study of pain, because a large percentage of cases have comorbid pain problems, and these persons appear to be different from persons with only a single pain condition (Dworkin et al. 1990). For some purposes, it may be necessary to differentiate "pure" cases of the pain syndrome of interest from cases with comorbid pain conditions.

CAUSAL INFERENCE

The use of epidemiological methods to make inferences about the causes of particular pain syndromes faces difficulties. As in the case of many chronic diseases, causal processes are characterized by multifactorial etiology, multiplicity of effect (i.e., a single causal factor can produce different types of disease or dysfunction), and equifinality of effect (i.e., different causal paths can lead to the same outcome). In addition, causal mechanisms in pain can be "bi-directional." For example, an individual with severe back pain who limits activities may become dependent on others in the workplace and at home. This in turn may alter the person's pain perceptions and behaviors (Fordyce 1986). In this instance, there is a bi-directional relationship between pain behaviors and environmental factors influencing pain behaviors. The affected individual's behaviors may change the social environment and vice versa.

EPIDEMIOLOGICAL STUDY DESIGNS

With these methodological perspectives as background, the remainder of this chapter provides an overview of the different study designs that can be applied to the epidemiological study of pain. Lilienfeld and Lilienfeld (1980) classified epidemiological study designs as: (1) *observational* (relying on naturally occurring variation in risk factors) or *experimental* (introducing exposure to protective factors or treatments by design); (2) *individual* (the person is the unit of observation) or *ecological* (a social group, community, state, or nation is the unit of analysis); and (3) relying on *cross-sectional* (or retrospective) or *longitudinal* data collection.

Observational studies may be designed to draw samples from the total population without respect to disease or risk factor status, to compare cases and controls, or to compare persons exposed to a risk factor with persons not exposed. Experimental studies introduce, on a randomized basis, a protective factor to persons at risk of disease (a preventive trial) or treatment to persons with disease (a clinical trial). A community trial is a preventive trial conducted on an ecological basis in which a protective factor is introduced to all persons in a set of social units such as work sites or cities, with comparable social units serving as controls. An example of a community trial relevant to chronic pain would be a study comparing the effects of introducing new policies on disability compensation and return to work in one set of work sites to the effects of retaining existing policies in a second set of comparable work sites.

The following sections discuss each of these variations on individual level study design. This chapter does not consider ecological studies (e.g., community trials or analyses of morbidity data at the level of the social group, community, or other aggregation). Morgenstern (1982) has reviewed the use of ecological analysis in epidemiological research, while Von Korff et al. (1992a) have considered conceptual issues in epidemiological inference from ecological data.

CROSS-SECTIONAL SURVEYS

The methods of the sample survey have been well developed over the last 40 years. A sampling frame is established that enumerates individuals or sampling units in a defined population of interest. A probability sample is selected from the sampling frame using methods that may be relatively simple (e.g., a simple random sample) or complex (e.g., a multi-stage cluster sample). The methods of probability sampling are fully treated in a number of texts (e.g., Kish 1965; Cochran 1977).

Information to determine the presence or absence of chronic pain conditions and possible risk factors is collected by interview, usually either in person or by telephone. The interview typically follows a standardized questionnaire administered by a trained interviewer with precoded response categories. In some instances, a two-phase survey design can be used to permit clinical examination and diagnostic evaluation of a subsample of individuals (Cochran 1977; Eaton and Kessler 1985).

Selection of the subsample may be based on responses to the initial survey interview. An excellent example of the kinds of information that can be developed through morbidity surveys of pain syndromes is provided by a national survey of the prevalence of migraine conducted by Stewart et al. (1992). They collected data on migraine symptoms from a national sample of more than 20,000 persons aged 12–80 years. Migraine status was determined using a clinically validated algorithm based on the diagnostic criteria of the International Headache Association. They found that 17.6% of females and 5.7% of males had experienced a migraine headache in the prior year, and that migraine prevalence was higher among low-income groups and peaked in the 35–44-year age group.

Methodological considerations

In general, sample surveys are most useful for estimation of the prevalence of a condition and description of its distribution by sociodemographic characteristics. Survey-based analysis of the association of risk factors with a pain condition generally takes advantage of naturally occurring variation of risk factors in the sample, although a sample design may be devised to yield comparisons of special interest. The measurement of risk-factor status usually relies on self-reported information about the subject's current status, on his or her recollection of risk factor status in the past, or on simple objective measurements that can be made in the subject's home (e.g., weight or blood pressure). Sources of bias in health-survey research have been extensively studied (Cannell 1977; Converse and Traugott 1986; Bradburn et al. 1987) and include

measurement bias in questionnaires, a variety of reporting biases, and sampling biases such as undercoverage (persons missed by the sampling method) and nonresponse (persons refusing interview or not contacted).

Cross-sectional data provide a useful starting point for studies of risk factors, but they must be interpreted with caution. Common pain conditions typically have a long history of intermittent pain, so an association of pain with a putative risk factor may be due to factors affecting duration or recurrence rather than onset. The pain experience may also selectively influence recall of possible risk factors. Despite these (and other) limitations of survey methods, cross-sectional survey data can substantially advance understanding of pain by placing its occurrence in a population perspective. Eaton and Kessler (1985) and Rose et al. (1982) provide comprehensive reviews of how modern survey research methods can be applied in the study of specific chronic diseases. A useful review of the use of cross-sectional surveys in public health research is provided by Abramson (1985).

LONGITUDINAL STUDIES

Cook and Ware (1983) define a longitudinal study as research in which the same individuals are observed on more than one occasion. Longitudinal studies are useful for examining individual changes over time. In the epidemiological study of pain, longitudinal designs can help us understand the fluctuating course of pain and the extent to which pain syndromes go into remission, recur, or progress; they can also identify prognostic factors. Longitudinal designs are also useful for studying the development of pain syndromes, as the relationships among pain intensity, activity limitations, physical findings, and psychological variables can be investigated over time.

Following subjects over time can yield data that further explain associations found in cross-sectional studies. Von Korff and Simon (1996) used longitudinal data to shed light on the relationship between pain and depression. They found that among primary care pain patients, depressive symptoms were initially elevated around the time of the visit, but then improved to normal levels among patients with a favorable pain outcome. For patients who continued to have significant activity limitations, depressive symptoms remained elevated 1 year after their visit, but depressive symptom levels did not *increase* with time, even if pain dysfunction continued at moderate to severe levels. The fact that depressive symptoms did not increase with time suggests that continuing pain and activity limitation does not necessarily result in increased levels of depression, even though continued pain dysfunction is associated with continuing elevations in depressive symptoms. These kinds of longitudinal analyses can begin to shed light on the mechanisms that may produce associations between pain status and factors that may be either causes or consequences of pain dysfunction. Dionne et al. (1995) applied advanced methods of longitudinal data analysis, using general estimating equations, to the study of back pain outcomes, assessing the effect of educational status on the functional outcomes of back pain among primary care patients. This analytic approach handles the within-subject correlation of repeated observations. Cherkin et al. (1996) used a longitudinal design to clarify the outcomes of primary care back pain patients. They followed 219 patients making a primary care visit for back pain over a 1-year period. They found that only 67% were satisfied with their outcome after 7 weeks and only 71% were satisfied with their outcome after 1 year. They concluded that the proportion of primary care back-pain patients who have poor outcomes is higher than previously recognized. Information on outcomes of this nature can help physicians give more accurate prognostic information to patients, helping to make them aware that continuing back pain is a common outcome.

Methodological considerations

In theory, longitudinal designs permit analysis of three kinds of effects of time: aging effects, cohort or period effects, and time effects (Cook and Ware 1983). Aging effects represent change in the average measurement due to the natural aging process. Cohort and period effects represent the contribution of the past history or unique experience of a cohort to their series of measurements. A time effect represents the effect of the passage of time between measurements. For example, the decrease in headache prevalence with increasing age might be due to a beneficial impact of aging on the occurrence of headaches or it might be a result of younger cohorts experiencing conditions that increase the incidence, duration, or recurrence of headaches. Longitudinal designs can sometimes shed light on the relative merits of such alternative explanations. A longitudinal survey of headache might observe that some persons with persistent headaches at the first measurement were improved at time of follow-up. This improvement could be attributed to the aging process, to the passage of time, or to a combined effect. Analyses of time-dependent improvement with stratification by age might shed light on the relative contribution of different effects.

While they must take into account the sources of bias that affect cross-sectional surveys, investigators conducting longitudinal studies must also pay attention to loss to follow-up, missing data, and measurement biases. Missing data and losses to follow-up can substantially reduce sample size in a longitudinal survey, particularly if observations are made on more than two occasions. Such losses are generally not "at random," thus they may introduce an important source of bias. Measures that may be biased by repeat measurement or that may "drift" over time also present problems in longitudinal studies, as do unreliable observations. Measures that elicit a different response on repeat administration will provide a biased assessment of change, as the follow-up measurements are influenced by the same measure having been previously administered. Biased or unreliable measurements in longitudinal study designs can overwhelm the extent of true change in the phenomena being studied.

The analysis of data from longitudinal studies presents problems that are beyond the scope of this chapter. Analysts must take into account the intercorrelation of serial measurements and the specification of a plausible underlying statistical model, and must address special problems such as significant missing observations or individual variation in the timing of observations. Reviews of alternative approaches to analysis of longitudinal data are provided by Nessleroade and Baltes (1979), Ware (1985), Cook and Ware (1983), and Rose et al. (1982).

CASE-CONTROL STUDIES

In studies of the etiology of chronic disease, the case-control design has been the most extensively used epidemiological method over the last 20 years. It is a cost-efficient method of studying the association of a putative risk factor with disease onset. Because of a large number of threats to the validity of case-control studies, the use of this design has not been without controversy (Feinstein 1979). However, the successes of the case-control method in identifying causal processes later confirmed by more rigorous methods have been well documented. A thorough treatment of the methods of the case-control study is provided by Schlesselman (1982), and a useful synopsis of the methods is provided by Greenberg and Ibrahim (1985).

The elements of a case-control study include: (1) a sample of recent-onset cases of the condition of interest, (2) a sample of controls selected in a way that does not introduce sampling bias with respect to risk factors, and (3) measurements made on cases and controls using the same methods. The resulting data are analyzed via contingency table analysis. In the simplest case, a two by two table is constructed in which the columns represent persons with or without the condition under study. The rows represent persons with or without the risk factor of interest. Case-control studies are used to estimate the odds ratio for risk factors of interest. The odds ratio measures the risk of developing the disease or condition in a group with a particular factor relative to a group without the risk factor. Multivariate extensions of contingency table analysis have been developed to estimate odds ratios while controlling for other variables (Bishop et al. 1978).

Several excellent studies have applied the case-control method to studying risk factors for specific chronic pain syndromes. LeResche et al. (1997) found that exposure to exogeneous hormones, in the form of oral contraceptives and hormone replacement therapy, was associated with increased risk of seeking treatment for temporomandibular pain. Nuwayhid and colleagues (1993) used a case-control design to identify high-risk work activities among firefighters. They found that operating a charged hose inside a building, cutting structures, breaking windows, climbing ladders, and lifting objects of more than 18 kg placed firefighters at increased risk of first onset of back pain. Controlling for exposure to smoke (a surrogate for the severity of the fire) made the effects of the specific activities nonsignificant, which the authors interpreted as an indication of the combined role of the environmental circumstance and specific activities in the development of back pain. Despite difficulties in determining the order of causation, a well-designed and well-executed case-control study can still provide valuable data.

Methodological considerations

The case-control design has several important limitations as a method of studying risk factors for pain syndromes. These limitations derive from the potential sources of bias in case-control studies, as summarized by Sackett (1979). Among the most important are prevalence–incidence bias, introduced by studying prevalent rather than incident cases. In the case of chronic pain, this might cause factors affecting duration to be confused with those influencing risk. Admission rate (Berkson's) bias can occur in studies in which cases are identified in a treatment setting and the putative risk factor is associated with the probability of being treated in the facility where the cases are identified. This potential bias should be of concern to any investigator wishing to study etiological factors for chronic pain among cases ascertained in a pain clinic, because of the highly selected nature of persons utilizing such facilities. Recall bias may occur if the presence of the condition leads to selective recall of events possibly associated with onset. Persons with a chronic pain problem are likely to search for an explanation of their pain that may jog their memories about injuries or other possible risk factors that would be forgotten by a person without chronic pain. This potential bias might be overcome, in some instances, by using objective sources of information to assess risk-factor history, such as medical or employment records. Family information bias may occur in studies of familial aggregation of chronic pain. Persons with a pain condition may be more aware of the occurrence of similar conditions in relatives than persons without that pain condition.

The statistical basis of estimating relative risk using the odds ratio requires the assumption that the condition is rare in the population. Since the more common chronic pain conditions affect 10–50% of the adult population, this assumption is clearly not met. However, Davies et al. (1998) argue that qualitative judgments based on interpretation of odds ratios are unlikely to be seriously in error. Given the potential sources of bias affecting case-control studies, this approach should be used with appropriate caution. If attention is paid to unbiased selection of cases and controls, and to measuring risk-factor status in a manner not contaminated by the pain condition, useful information may be developed using this approach.

PROSPECTIVE DESIGNS

A prospective study is a longitudinal design that starts with cohorts not affected by the condition of interest if the goal is to study risk factors for onset of the condition, or persons in the early stages of illness if the goal is to study risk factors for chronicity. These cohorts are followed over time to identify onsets of the illness or other end points of the study (e.g., recurrence of the condition, chronicity, disability, or death). A prospective design requires surveillance of the cohorts to detect end points occurring over the follow-up period, and reasonably precise dating of the occurrence of the end point. Stratification of the cohorts by risk-factor status at the outset, or as the study progresses, provides a basis for inference about the relationship of the risk factor to the risk of subsequent occurrence of the end point. A retrospective (also referred to as nonconcurrent or historical) cohort study permits longitudinal investigation of a risk factor with disease experience by using historical records of exposure to a risk factor and subsequent disease experience. For example, records documenting the distance of survivors from the hypocenter of the atom bomb explosion in Hiroshima have been used to study the impact of differing levels of radiation exposure on the incidence of leukemia and the incubation period from exposure to onset of disease (Cobb et al. 1959).

Von Korff and colleagues (1993) used a prospective design to determine whether elevated levels of depressive symptoms placed individuals at risk of first onset of back pain, headache, temporomandibular pain, abdominal pain, or chest pain. They followed a sample of 803 persons initially interviewed in a pain prevalence survey. At a 3-year follow-up, they found that persons with elevated levels of depressive symptoms at baseline were more likely to report first onset of headache and chest pain, but were not at increased risk of first onset of back pain, abdominal pain, or temporomandibular pain. For chest pain and headache, first-onset rates were highest among the chronically depressed.

Methodological considerations

The analysis of data from a prospective (or retrospective) cohort study is based on comparison of the rates of occurrence of the end point (number of morbidity or mortality events in relation to person-years of experience) of persons with versus without exposure to a risk factor. Kleinbaum and colleagues (1982) provide a thorough discussion of the design of prospective studies. Feinlab and Detels (1985) review the different variations of cohort study designs used in epidemiological research. Methods used to analyze data

from prospective studies are outside the scope of this chapter (Gross and Clark 1975; Kalbfleisch and Prentice 1980; Cox and Oakes 1984). The methods of data analysis relevant to analysis of panel study data are also applicable in the analysis of data from prospective cohort studies.

Given the difficulties in interpreting cross-sectional and case-control studies of chronic pain, prospective and retrospective cohort study designs have an important role to play in understanding the onset of chronic pain, as well as factors producing disability. In order to facilitate the design of cohort studies, researchers should address the incidence rates of chronic pain conditions and disabling chronic pain. If incidence rates are low, larger cohorts and years of follow-up would be required to yield adequate statistical power to detect differences between persons exposed and unexposed to a putative risk factor. If incidence rates are higher, smaller cohorts would be required. A well-conducted cohort study not only provides a relatively strong base for inference about risk factors influencing the onset of pain or disability, it may also yield valuable information about the descriptive epidemiology of chronic pain (e.g., age-specific incidence rates or "incubation" periods between the onset of pain and the development of the chronic pain syndrome).

PREVENTIVE AND CLINICAL TRIALS

Epidemiology is a practical science whose fundamental objective is to produce knowledge relevant to disease prevention and control. Repeatedly, epidemiological methods have identified methods of disease prevention or control before the etiologic mechanisms were firmly established. The clinical trial is a rigorous means of evaluating methods of disease control, while the preventive trial provides methods of evaluating the effectiveness of presumed methods of disease prevention. Preventive and clinical trials are essentially prospective cohort studies in which exposure to a disease prevention or control measure is randomly allocated. Hill (1971) provides an excellent discussion of the need for randomization in the evaluation of interventions and describes the essential concepts of the randomized trial. An excellent text by Meinert (1986) provides a complete discussion of the methods of the clinical trial.

Daltroy and colleagues (1997) carried out a preventive trial among 4000 postal workers and their supervisors to determine whether an educational program designed to prevent low back injury would reduce work loss due to back pain. They randomly assigned 2534 postal workers and their supervisors to work units that would receive a two-session training program. Control workers and their supervisors did not receive training. Over a 5.5-year follow-up period, 21.2 back injuries occurred per 1000 person-years. The median time off work was 14 days per injury, and the median health care cost of an injury was $204. Workers receiving the educational program did not have lower injury rates than the control workers. There were also no differences in the median cost per injury, time off work per injury, or the rate of repeat injury after return to work. Only the worker's knowledge of safe behavior was increased by the training program.

CLINICAL EPIDEMIOLOGY

Clinical epidemiology has been defined as the application of epidemiological principles and methods to problems encountered in clinical medicine (Fletcher et al. 1982). The methods of epidemiology discussed in this chapter are directly relevant to the practice of clinical medicine. For example, primary care physicians frequently evaluate patients with a presenting complaint of pain. Evaluation of a pain condition should be influenced by an understanding of how common the complaint is in the general population (cross-sectional survey data). In order to make correct diagnostic decisions, the physician needs to have information on the probability that a particular presentation of pain is associated with specific somatic or psychiatric diseases (clinical diagnostic studies and two-phase survey data). Subsequent to evaluation, the physician needs to provide the patient with information on the likely course of the pain condition (longitudinal study data). In evaluating the condition, information on risk factors may influence both diagnostic and treatment decisions (case-control and prospective study data). The physician needs to identify differentials in risk for bad outcomes (e.g., disability, death) that may be quantified through prospective studies of the course of illness. Finally, the physician needs reliable information on how to treat presenting conditions (clinical trial), prevent major complications and recurrences (secondary prevention trial), and reduce the risks of developing chronic pain conditions (primary prevention trial).

This brief overview of the relevance of epidemiological methods to clinical practice indicates that epidemiology has a broader role to play than just quantification of incidence and prevalence rates of chronic pain. Used to their fullest potential, epidemiological methods can provide data that are essential to diagnostic and treatment decisions, and can provide a scientific basis for prevention of chronic pain and its major complications.

SUMMARY

Epidemiology has a vital role to play in improving our understanding of the causes of specific pain conditions, and in providing a firmer empirical basis for how the public health burden of pain conditions can be reduced on a population basis. Epidemiologists have a variety of methodological approaches that are directly applicable to the advancement of scientific knowledge about the causes and consequences of pain, its management, and its prevention.

ACKNOWLEDGMENT

This work was supported by a grant from the National Institutes of Health: P01 DE08773.

REFERENCES

Abramson JH. Cross-sectional studies. In: Holland WW, Detels R, Knox G (Eds). The Oxford Textbook of Public Health, Vol. 3: *Investigative Methods in Public Health*. Oxford: Oxford University Press, 1985, pp 89–100.

Bishop YMM, Fienberg SE, Holland PW. *Discrete Multivariate Analysis: Theory and Practice*. Cambridge, MA: MIT Press, 1978.

Bradburn NM, Rips LJ, Shevell SK. Answering autobiographical questions: the impact of memory and influence on surveys. *Science* 1987; 236:157–161.

Cannell CF. A summary of research studies of interviewing methodology, 1959–1970. *Vital and Health Statistics*. Series 2. Data evaluation and methods research; No. 69. DHEW Publ. No. (HRA)77–1343. Public Health Service. Washington, DC: U.S. Government Printing Office, 1977.

Cherkin DC, Deyo RA, Street JH, Barlow W. Predicting poor outcomes for back pain seen in primary care using patients' own criteria. *Spine* 1996; 21:2900–2907.

Cobb S, Miller M, Wald N. On the estimation of the incubation period in malignant disease. *J Chron Dis* 1959; 9:385–393.

Cochran WG. *Sampling Techniques*, 3rd ed. New York: John Wiley and Sons, 1977.

Converse PE, Traugott MW. Assessing the accuracy of polls and surveys. *Science* 1986; 234:1094–1098.

Cook NR, Ware JH. Design and analysis methods for longitudinal research. *Annu Rev Public Health* 1983; 4:1–23.

Cox DR, Oakes D. *Analysis of Survival Data.* London: Chapman and Hill, 1984.

Daltroy LH, Iversen MD, Larson MG, et al. A controlled trial of an educational program to prevent low back injuries. *N Engl J Med* 1997; 337:322–328.

Davies HTO, Crombie IK, Tavaakoli M. When can odds ratios mislead? *BMJ* 1998; 316:989–991.

Dionne C, Koepsell TD, Von Korff M, Deyo RA, Barlow WE, Checkoway H. Formal education and back-related disability: in search of an explanation. *Spine* 1995; 20:2721–2730.

Dworkin SF, LeResche L. Research diagnostic criteria for temporomandibular disorders: review, criteria, examinations and specification, critique. *J Craniomandibular Disorders Facial Oral Pain* 1992; 6:301–355.

Dworkin SF, Von Korff MR, LeResche L. Multiple pains and psychiatric disturbance: an epidemiologic investigation. *Arch Gen Psychiatry* 1990; 47:239–244.

Dworkin SF, Von Korff M, LeResche L. Epidemiologic studies of chronic pain: a dynamic-ecologic perspective. *Annals of Behavioral Medicine* 1992; 14:3–11.

Eaton WW, Kessler LG (Eds). *Epidemiologic Field Methods in Psychiatry: The NIHM Epidemiologic Catchment Area Program.* Orlando: Academic Press, 1985.

Feinlab, Detels R. Cohort studies. In: Holland WW, Detels R, Knox G (Eds). The Oxford Textbook of Public Health, Vol. 3: *Investigative Methods in Public Health.* Oxford: Oxford University Press, 1985, pp 101–112.

Feinstein AR. Methodologic problems and standards in case-control research. *J Chron Dis* 1979; 32:35–41.

Fletcher RH, Fletcher SW, Wagner EH. *Clinical Epidemiology: The Essentials.* Baltimore: Williams and Wilkins, 1982.

Fordyce WE. Learning processes in pain. In: Sternbach RA (Ed). *The Psychology of Pain,* 2nd ed. New York: Raven Press, 1986, pp 49–65.

Greenberg RS, Ibrahim MA. The case-control study. In: Holland WW, Detels R, Knox G (Eds). The Oxford Textbook of Public Health Vol. 3: *Investigative Methods in Public Health.* Oxford: Oxford University Press, 1985, pp 123–143.

Gross AJ, Clark VA. *Survival Distributions: Reliability Applications in the Biomedical Sciences.* New York: John Wiley and Sons, 1975.

Headache Classification Committee of the International Headache Society. Classification and diagnostic criteria for headache disorders, cranial neuralgias and facial pain. *Cephalalgia* 1988; 8(Suppl 7):1–96.

Hill AB. *Principles of Medical Statistics.* New York: Oxford University Press, 1971.

Kalbfleisch JD, Prentice RL. *The Statistical Analysis of Failure Time Data.* New York: John Wiley and Sons, 1980.

Kish L. *Survey Sampling.* New York: John Wiley and Sons, 1965.

Kleinbaum DG, Kupper LL, Morgenstern H. *Epidemiologic Research: Principles and Quantitative Methods.* California: Lifetime Learning Publications, 1982.

Last CG, Herson M. *Issues in Diagnostic Research.* New York: Plenum Press, 1987.

LeResche L, Saunders K, Von Korff M, Barlow W, Dworkin SF. Use of exogenous hormones and risk of temporomandibular disorder pain. *Pain* 1997; 69:153–160.

Lilienfeld AM, Lilienfeld DE. *Foundations of Epidemiology,* 2nd ed. New York: Oxford University Press, 1980.

MacMahon B, Pugh TF. *Epidemiology: Principles and Methods.* Boston: Little, Brown and Company, 1970.

Meinert CL. *Clinical Trials: Design, Conduct and Analysis.* New York: Oxford Press, 1986.

Morgenstern H. Uses of ecologic analysis in epidemiologic research. *Am J Public Health* 1982; 72:1336–1344.

Morris JN. *Uses of Epidemiology,* 3rd ed. Edinburgh: Churchill Livingstone, 1975.

Nessleroade JR, Baltes PB. *Longitudinal Research in the Study of Behavior and Development.* New York: Academic Press, 1979.

Nuwayhid IA, Stewart W, Johnson JV. Work activities and the onset of first-time low back pain among New York City fire fighters. *Am J Epidemiol* 1993; 137:539–548.

Rose GA, Blackburn H, Gillum RF, Prineas RJ. *Cardiovascular Survey Methods.* Geneva: World Health Organization, 1982.

Sackett DL. Bias in analytic research. *J Chron Dis* 1979; 32:51–63.

Sartwell PE, Merrel M. Influence of the dynamic character of chronic disease on the interpretation of morbidity rates. *Am J Public Health* 1952; 42:579–584.

Schlesselman JJ. *Case-control Studies: Design, Conduct, Analysis.* New York: Oxford University Press, 1982.

Sternbach RA. Survey of pain in the United States: the Nuprin Pain Report. *Clin J Pain* 1986; 2:49–53.

Stewart WF, Lipton RB, Celantano DD, Reed ML. Prevalence of migraine headache in the United States: relation to age, income, race and other sociodemographic factors. *JAMA* 1992; 267:64–69.

Von Korff M. Epidemiological and survey methods: chronic pain assessment. In: Turk DC, Melzack R (Eds). *Handbook of Pain Assessment.* New York: Guilford Press, 1992; pp 391–408.

Von Korff M, Parker RD. The dynamics of the prevalence of chronic episodic disease. *J Chron Dis* 1980; 33:79–85.

Von Korff M, Saunders K. The course of back pain in primary care. *Spine* 1996; 21:2833–2837.

Von Korff M, Simon G. The relationship of pain and depression. *Br J Psychiatry* 1996; 168 (Suppl 30):101–108.

Von Korff M, Dworkin SF, LeResche L, Kruger A. An epidemiologic comparison of pain complaints. *Pain* 1990; 40:279–291.

Von Korff M, Koepsell T, Curry S, Diehr P. Multilevel analysis in epidemiologic research on health behaviors and outcomes. *Am J Epidemiol* 1992a; 135:1077–1082.

Von Korff M, Ormel J, Keefe F, Dworkin SF. Grading the severity of chronic pain. *Pain* 1992b; 50:133–149.

Von Korff M, LeResche L, Dworkin SF. First onset of common pain symptoms: a prospective study of depression as a risk factor. *Pain* 1993; 55:251–258.

Von Korff M, Lipton R, Stewart WE. Assessing headache severity: new directions. *Neurology* 1994; 44(Suppl 6):S40–S46.

Ware JH. Linear models for the analysis of longitudinal data. *Am Statistician* 1985; 39:95–101.

Weissman MM, Myers JK, Ross CE. *Community Surveys of Psychiatric Disorders.* New Brunswick, NJ: Rutgers University Press, 1986.

Wing JK, Bebbington P, Robins LN. *What is a Case? The Problem of Case Definition in Psychiatric Community Surveys.* London: Grant McIntyre, 1981.

Correspondence to: Michael Von Korff, ScD, Center for Health Studies, Group Health Cooperative of Puget Sound, 1730 Minor Avenue, Suite 1600, Seattle, WA 98101-1448, USA.

Epidemiology of Pain, edited by
I.K. Crombie, IASP Press, Seattle, © 1999.

3

Requirements for Epidemiological Studies

Iain Kinloch Crombie[a] and Huw Talfryn Oakley Davies[b]

*[a]Department of Epidemiology and Public Health, University of Dundee, Ninewells Hospital and Medical School,
Dundee, United Kingdom; and [b]Department of Management, University of St Andrews, St Katharine's West,
The Scores, St Andrews, Fife, United Kingdom*

Epidemiological studies have a great potential to contribute to the control of chronic pain, but in practice this potential has yet to be fully realized. In part this is because the epidemiology of pain has been less well studied than have diseases such as cancer and cardiovascular disease. Only in recent years have large numbers of papers been published on the epidemiology of pain (Crombie 1997). In addition, many theoretical and methodological barriers impede research into the epidemiology of pain. The reasons lie in the nature of chronic pain: the complex psycho- and pathophysiology of pain, the diversity of pain conditions; and the practical problems of doing research on pain in health care settings and in the community. This chapter explores these facets of pain, identifying what is required to unravel the epidemiology of pain. It does so by contrasting advances made in understanding the epidemiology of cancer and cardiovascular disease with the problems faced by pain research.

CLEAR DISEASE DEFINITION

The investigation of the epidemiology of a disease requires a formal definition of a diagnostic group. Once a disease has been clearly defined, researchers can ascertain its frequency and investigate its association with risk factors. Patients grouped under the same diagnostic label must be homogeneous. Studies of the etiology of a chronic pain condition require a disease definition that specifies common causal pathways that are involved in the development of the disease. Likewise, studies of the natural history of a pain condition require a homogeneous set of underlying pathophysiological processes.

The need for homogeneity is well illustrated by the epidemiology of cancer. Cancer is a general term for many different diseases that afflict many sites in the body. Only by separating the cancers by the site of origin of the tumor can their epidemiology be usefully explored. Thus, early studies showed that soot was a cause of scrotal cancer among chimney sweeps, and that cancer of the cervix was uncommon among unmarried women and nuns, whereas breast cancer was less common among women who had given birth (Higginson et al. 1992). Classification by site of primary tumor is sometimes insufficient, and it may be necessary to subdivide the cancers at a site into different histological types to unravel their epidemiology. For example, skin cancer is divided into basal cell carcinoma, squamous cell carcinoma, and malignant melanoma. The three subtypes are markedly different in the way they are distributed in the population and in the risk factors associated with their development.

The development of the epidemiology of chronic pain is at a great disadvantage in comparison with many other diseases because of the complex and diverse nature of chronic pain. Many of these issues have been inadequately addressed in epidemiologic studies and are worth pursuing in some detail.

DEFINITION OF CHRONIC PAIN

Pain presents special problems to those seeking definitions to be used in epidemiologic studies. Pain has been defined as "an unpleasant sensory and emotional experience associated with actual or potential tissue damage or described in terms of such damage" (International Association for the Study of Pain Subcommittee on Taxonomy 1986). This definition clarifies that pain is a subjective experience, with consequent problems for measurement. Thus, research studies rely on patient self-reports for the duration and severity of the pain, its nature (e.g., dull, throbbing, or lancinating), and its temporal characteristics (e.g., continuous or recurrent).

MULTIDIMENSIONALITY OF PAIN

Chronic pain involves the interaction of psychosocial, behavioral, and pathophysiological processes (Rudy et al. 1990), which produce both a sensory experience and a behavioral response. One model distinguishes between the sensory experience (such as throbbing or lancinating), the associated suffering or emotional distress, and the resulting pain behavior (Raspe and Kohlmann 1994). Chronic pain is a multidimensional phenomenon. The challenge for epidemiology is that different sets of individual or environmental factors may influence different dimensions of pain. This has led one group to propose a biobehavioral model of chronic pain in which physiological, psychological, and social factors "interact in different ways at different stages in the development of pain and pain dysfunction" (Dworkin et al. 1992a). We need a set of clear definitions or diagnostic criteria by which to group chronic pain patients, or even better, a formal classification of chronic pain that is designed specifically for epidemiological research.

CLASSIFYING PAIN

Considerable attention has been paid to developing a classification for chronic pain with formal definitions for each taxonomic group. The requirement for the diagnostic process is "the assignment of a patient's illness to a category that links the symptoms with a pathological process, a known outcome, and—wherever possible—a cause" (McWhinney 1981). The most extensive classification of pain is that produced by the International Association for the Study of Pain (IASP) Subcommittee on Taxonomy, first published in 1986. This classification has been described as having "considerable potential and utility," although it is recognized to be only the first step (Turk and Rudy 1987). Others have been more critical of the classification

(Bowsher 1987; Vervest and Schimmel 1988). A revised version was published in 1994 (Merskey and Bogduk 1994); further research is needed to test its usefulness. A problem may arise through the use of body site as a key classification factor; a recent study has shown that grouping patients by body site can lead to heterogeneous groups (Davies et al. 1998).

The IASP classification was based largely on theoretical and clinical grounds, and other groups have used empirical approaches to develop classification schemes (Costello et al. 1987; Turk and Rudy 1990). As yet, their usefulness for epidemiological studies has not been fully assessed. Even when a formal classification has been developed, it may be difficult to use. For example, it can be difficult to arrive at a definitive diagnosis for many kinds of pain presenting at pain clinics (Crombie and Davies 1991). Progress is being made in developing classification systems for selected aspects of pain, as for example the work on headache by the International Headache Society (IHS) (Headache Classification Committee 1988). Further research needs to focus on the development of homogeneous disease entities, in which the dimensions of homogeneity are stated and are relevant to specific aspects of epidemiology (e.g., etiology, natural history, and population burden of morbidity).

DIVERSITY OF CHRONIC PAIN

The problem of classification is compounded by the diversity of complex syndromes that comprise chronic pain. Chronic pain is a common symptom of many diseases such as musculoskeletal disease, cancer, diabetes, and vascular disease, which are treated by different medical specialties. There may be a natural tendency for each specialty to focus on the underlying pathology most relevant to its own discipline (e.g., the inflammatory process in rheumatology, or control of glucose metabolism in diabetes), with the attendant danger that the pain is not accorded the attention it deserves.

Pain is the primary symptom of conditions such as migraine, trigeminal neuralgia, and abdominal pain of unknown origin, but pain is also associated with many other diseases. The second edition of the IASP classification (Merskey and Bogduk 1994) identified over 600 pain syndromes comprising 36 generalized syndromes; 66 syndromes affecting the head and neck; 35 the upper limbs; 154 the thoracic and cervical spine; 136 the lumbar, sacral, coccygeal, spinal, and radicular regions; 85 the trunk; and 18 the lower limb. Although there will be some overlap, each syndrome will have its unique epidemiology. For example, a comparative study has shown many differences between the two major neuralgias of the face, trigeminal (affecting the fifth cranial nerve) and glossopharyngeal (affecting the ninth cranial nerve) (Katusic et al. 1991). Trigeminal neuralgia has a much higher prevalence, is more likely to show recurrent episodes, has a preference for the right side of the face, and is less likely to be bilateral. If two similar conditions show such marked differences, there is little chance of discovering the epidemiology of chronic pain in an undifferentiated group of pain patients.

ONSET OF CHRONICITY

Chronic pain presents a further definitional problem, that of deciding when chronicity begins. Clearly a chronic pain is one that lasts, but how long must an acute pain last to be classed as chronic? The IASP Subcommittee on Taxonomy identifies three time categories: <1 month, 1–6 months, and >6 months. Published studies vary in the definition of chronic: some use pain over a 1-month period (Magni et al. 1990; McAlindon et al. 1992); others 3 months (Bowsher et al. 1991; Andersson et al. 1993), and others 6 months (Brattberg et al. 1989). This diversity needs to be resolved, and a suitable time period must be identified for each pain condition so that comparable findings can be obtained. But problems can persist even when a definition has been accepted. Meilman (1989) gives the example of back pain, where a patient may have a first acute attack that resolves within 3 weeks. A second attack occurs 1 year later and resolves within 3 months. Finally a third attack several years later leads to ongoing pain. When did chronicity set in? Was it the time at which pain became continuous, or was it the date of the first episode of what would become an ongoing condition? This problem is compounded by the emerging evidence that chronic back pain is not the same as long-lasting acute back pain (Jayson 1997). Again, we need to agree on consistent definitions. The challenge is to organize and encourage such a consensus.

RELIABLE ESTIMATES OF DISEASE FREQUENCY

One of the keys to the development of epidemiol-

ogy has been the provision of accurate estimates of the frequency of disease in order to determine its importance to public health. The extent of the morbidity and mortality attributable to a disease are important determinants of the health care resources allocated to it. The population burden of disease is one of the reasons why so much of our health service resources are devoted to cancer and heart disease, and helps to explain why they receive the major proportion of the available research funding.

Comparison of disease frequencies among communities also provides insights into potential risk factors. Thus, the substantial variation in the frequency of disease among countries (Higginson et al. 1992) has led to estimates that 80–90% of cancers may have an environmental cause (Doll and Peto 1981). In cardiovascular disease, international differences in the frequency of atherosclerotic disease suggested that the consumption of cholesterol and saturated fat could be an important causal factor (Stamler 1992). Descriptive epidemiological studies also allow rational planning of health care so that services can be provided to meet demonstrated needs. Unfortunately, current estimates of the frequency of chronic pain, far from serving to enlighten, lead largely to uncertainty (Crombie et al. 1994).

FREQUENCY OF CHRONIC PAIN

Many studies have investigated the overall frequency of chronic pain (reviewed by Crombie et al. 1994). However, their estimates of the prevalence of chronic pain vary across a wide range, between 7% (Bowsher et al. 1991) and 40% (Brattberg et al. 1989). This discrepancy may in part be explained by differences in the definitions of pain used (Crombie 1994). Some researchers (Sternbach 1986; James et al. 1991) include any type of pain, while others exclude "fleeting and minor" pain (Von Korff et al. 1988) or apply qualifying terms to the pain such as "obvious" (Brattberg et al. 1989) or "often troubled by" (Crook et al. 1984). The problem of diversity of estimates persists when specific pain conditions are investigated. Thus, prevalence estimates range from 8% to 45% for low back pain (Girolamo 1991) and from just under 2% to over 50% for migraine (Stewart et al. 1994).

The consequences of using differing definitions were highlighted in the careful study by Von Korff and colleagues (1990), which showed that while 37% of the population reported recurrent pain, only 8% had severe and persistent pain and less than 3% had severe and persistent pain lasting more than 6 days. Similarly, careful analysis showed that most of the variation in the frequency of low back pain and migraine could be attributed to differences in case definition (Girolamo 1991; Lipton and Stewart 1994). To solve this problem, standard definitions of chronic pain conditions need to be developed and used in epidemiological studies, following the lead of the IHS, whose definition of migraine has led to consistent findings in the prevalence of the condition, where previously there was considerable variation (Rasmussen and Olesen 1996).

PUTATIVE CAUSATIVE MECHANISMS

The search for the causes of disease requires theoretical models for possible causative mechanisms. In the development of cancer epidemiology, several theories were proposed for the etiology of cancer, including heredity, viruses, and environmental factors (Clemmesen 1965). The search for etiological factors is governed by the prevailing model of causality. Should an inappropriate or tangentially relevant model hold sway, the search for risk factors will be impeded. Thus, the emphasis given to the viral theory in the 1950s led researchers to play down the role of environmental factors to the extent that they were reluctant to accept the initial evidence that tobacco was the cause of lung cancer (Higginson et al. 1992). It took over 10 years until this was remedied and environmental factors were accorded a prominent place in the etiology of cancer.

Before considering the etiology of pain, we must emphasize that we do not need to fully understand causative processes for important advances to be made. Findings that cancer can be caused by X-rays, tobacco smoke, asbestos, benzidine, naphthylamine, nickel compounds, and many other chemicals led to efforts to minimize risks to humans, even before the exact processes by which these environmental agents cause cancer were known. Similarly, we do not need to understand the detailed pathophysiological development of chronic pain for risk factors to be identified and actions taken to minimize the risk of chronic pain.

CAUSES OF PAIN

The mechanisms underlying chronic pain are com-

plex, and the more they are investigated, the more complex they appear. A good example of this is sympathetically maintained pain, where suggestions for the underlying mechanisms include "ephaptic transmission, adrenergic receptors on sensory neurones, indirect coupling of sympathetic and sensory neurones, sensitization of nociceptive afferents, and, in the central nervous system, sensitization of dorsal horn neurones" (McMahon 1991). While a detailed treatment of the these pathophysiological processes is beyond the scope of this book, two key features are introduced here: the gate control theory and plasticity.

Without doubt the gate control theory has revolutionized our understanding of pain (Melzack and Wall 1988). It has led to the development of effective new treatments, and the abandonment of ineffective ones. It seems at first a little strange that this theory should pose a problem for epidemiology. But the central ideas behind it, the gate in the spinal column and the existence of descending control, indicate the complex nature of the development of chronic pain. Instead of simply looking for causative factors, researchers into the epidemiology of pain need to address the possibility of simultaneously acting causal, inhibitory, and excitatory factors.

Recent research has also helped clarify the role of central neuroplasticity in the development of chronic pain (Coderre et al. 1993). The theory holds that intense noxious stimulation can sensitize central neural structures involved in pain perception. Subsequent sensory stimuli can be interpreted quite differently, allowing innocent stimuli to induce severe pain. Thus when studying the causes of pain we must take into account not only events that led to the development of pain, but also preceding events.

IDENTIFYING RISK FACTORS FOR PAIN

Identifying risk factors for chronic pain presents special challenges. The combination of problems of diagnosis, the diversity of pain, and the complexity of causation makes it difficult to know where to start. For some pain conditions there are obvious clues to explore. For example, when studying pain following breast-cancer surgery it would seem reasonable to study both the details of the surgery as well as the characteristics of the illness that led to the surgery. But for many other pain conditions (e.g., trigeminal neuralgia or burning mouth syndrome), it is difficult to specify potential risk factors.

There has been an impressive expansion in our understanding of biological phenomena that influence the development and maintenance of chronic pain. A recent review has described a range of algogenic substances including protons, prostanoids, neurokinins, cytokines, and histamine, together with their known inhibitors (Johnson 1996). But at present there is little connection between the laboratory and clinical findings and the types of theories that can be investigated in epidemiological studies. We need insights that will foster research at the population level. The challenge is to synthesize the findings from basic research to provide causal mechanisms that can be tested in epidemiological studies.

ALLOWANCE FOR MEDIATING FACTORS

Epidemiological studies of disease recognize that in addition to external agents, e.g., chemical carcinogens in the case of cancer, other factors influence the development of disease. Risk factors are conventionally arranged under three headings: the agent (e.g., physical or chemical factor), the host (the individual characteristics of the person who develops the disease), and the environment (the physical and social context in which the individual lives). These three sets of factors are usually drawn as the apices of an equilateral triangle, and since they interact, are referred to as the web of causation (Lilienfeld and Lilienfeld 1980). Thus, although environmental factors are of major importance in the development of cancer, their impact is modulated by genetic and immunological factors (Bartsch 1992). In diseases associated with chronic pain, mediating factors are also important, possibly more so than in other diseases.

PSYCHOLOGICAL FACTORS

Psychological factors are recognized to be intimately involved in the development of chronic pain (see Chapter 4). Many studies have shown that psychological factors, in particular depression, are more common among chronic pain patients (Pilowsky et al. 1977; Benjamin et al. 1988; Tyrer et al. 1989; Main and Spanswick 1991). Depression has also been associated with specific pain conditions including back pain (Joukamaa 1994), chronic abdominal pain (Magni et al. 1992), and musculoskeletal pain (Magni et al. 1990). Demonstrating an association is comparatively straight-

forward; a greater challenge is to disentangle the role of psychological factors in the etiology of chronic pain. Specifically, do psychological factors predispose to the development of chronic pain, or is psychological disturbance a consequence of the pain? This issue is best approached via a cohort study in which pain-free persons with depression are followed over time to see if they are at an increased risk of developing pain compared to those without depression. This approach was followed by Von Korff and colleagues (1993), who followed a cohort of more than 800 subjects over a 3-year period. They found that subjects with depression were at a significantly increased risk for developing headache and chest pain but not for back pain or abdominal pain. As always, pain is a complex disease, and many more studies of this type are required to resolve this issue.

ENVIRONMENTAL FACTORS

The social and physical environment within which patients live can substantially affect the development and maintenance of chronic pain. Thus, stressful life events appear to be involved in the development of chronic primary headache (Benedittis et al. 1990). Work dissatisfaction has been repeatedly shown to be associated with the maintenance of chronic pain, particularly in the low back (Skovron 1992; Skovron et al. 1994) and the neck and shoulder (Linton and Kamwendo 1989). Patients even report that changes in the weather influence their pain, although the way this works is not fully understood (Jamison et al. 1995).

The existence of mediating factors in chronic pain greatly complicates the study of its epidemiology. They need to be measured in research studies so that their impact, and that of other risk factors, can be determined. Epidemiological studies need to employ rigorous methodology and sophisticated statistical techniques in order to estimate the independent contribution of each factor.

MECHANISMS FOR IDENTIFYING CASES

A classic approach in epidemiology is to identify a group of subjects thought to be at high risk of developing pain. For example, to study post-stroke pain, a cohort of stroke patients could be identified and followed through time to see which patients develop pain, and the characteristics of those in pain could be investigated. The identification of cases can be made through disease-specific registries; the international network of cancer registries has contributed substantially to cancer epidemiology (Stiller 1993).

When disease registries are not available, we may find hospital discharge records to be particularly useful, as they contain the principal diagnoses of all patients seen in hospital. Often these registers are computerized and can readily be searched to identify patients with defined conditions. Finally, patients with conditions such as peptic ulcers or thyroid disease, in which management is carried out as outpatients, can be identified by searching through records held in the appropriate outpatient clinic. However, the diversity of chronic pain conditions and the fact that pain may not be mentioned when associated with other diseases such as diabetes or rheumatoid arthritis make this approach unhelpful in chronic pain research.

IDENTIFYING CHRONIC PAIN PATIENTS

In theory it would be possible to set up a registry of chronic pain patients, but the difficulties of doing so would be immense. Pain patients are seldom hospitalized for their pain, and if they are seen at hospital they are likely to be cared for as outpatients. Some of these will be seen at specialist pain clinics, but they are likely to be a highly selected subgroup (Crombie and Davies 1998). Many other pain patients will be seen in the departments of rheumatology, orthopedics, neurology, or even gynecology, depending on the suspected pathology of their complaint. It would not be possible to search through the records of every department at which pain patients might be seen. It would therefore be difficult to recruit representative samples of pain patients through hospitals.

An alternative approach would be to use the records held by family practitioners, This approach has been used to estimate the frequency of conditions such as childhood asthma (Neville et al. 1992). Unfortunately, the very problems discussed above, which make it difficult to assign a specific diagnosis to many patients, make it difficult to identify them by case-note search.

IDENTIFYING SUFFICIENT PAIN PATIENTS FOR STUDY

Even when suitable sources of pain patients have been identified, there may be a problem of recruiting sufficient numbers for worthwhile research. Epidemiological studies tend to require substantial numbers of patients, and the instances in which modest numbers will suffice are few. While case-control studies can yield interesting results with 50–100 patients, more usually they require several hundred. Cohort studies are even more greedy for numbers: the classic cohort studies that revealed the causes of coronary heart disease required several thousand subjects. At first sight, this might suggest that epidemiological studies of pain conditions such as post-herpetic neuralgia or post-stroke pain can only be conducted in the very largest of centers. However, smaller centers could collaborate, pooling patients to achieve the required numbers. This might be most easily achieved if organizations such as IASP or its national chapters were to act as coordinating centers for this research.

MONITORING THE CONSEQUENCES OF DISEASE

Many of the classic studies that elucidated the epidemiology of coronary heart disease were cohort studies. These involved the long-term follow-up of subjects who had been screened to measure potential risk factors. The subjects were healthy at the time of screening and were followed up to determine how many subsequently suffered a heart attack. A key requirement of these studies was to be able to identify, after the elapse of some years, the occurrence of heart attacks. This could be achieved by restricting attention to fatal attacks: death certificates that record cause of death are legal documents that are stored. Bona fide researchers have access to these documents and can easily determine which subjects have had heart attacks. They can then relate the occurrence of these attacks to the screening data to identify potential risk factors.

THE OUTCOME OF CHRONIC PAIN

Cohort studies of chronic pain cannot take advantage of the convenience of death certificates because the condition is seldom fatal. Instead, patients have to be followed up individually by case-note reviews or by contacting the patient by telephone, postal questionnaire, or personal interview. Case-note reviews have been used to investigate such conditions as post-thoracotomy neuralgia (Conacher 1992). A potential problem with case-note reviews can occur if patients do not return for follow-up care, so other techniques may be needed. Pain after breast surgery was investigated by postal questionnaire (Wallace et al. 1996), telephone interviews were used to follow-up patients with post-herpetic neuralgia (Dworkin et al. 1992b), and face to face interviews have been used to study pain following rectal amputation (Boas et al. 1993). Long-term follow-up is possible, but it requires more effort for chronic nonterminal cases than for the study of diseases like cancer and heart disease.

CONCLUSION

This chapter has outlined the difficulties, some of them considerable, that hinder progress in the epidemiology of chronic pain. The conditions that are embraced by this heading are diverse and often difficult to classify. Pain is a multidimensional phenomenon and its risk factors may act in differing ways, in different dimensions, and at different times during the initiation, development, and maintenance of chronicity. The patients who suffer from these conditions can be difficult to identify and are difficult to track through time.

These obstacles have discouraged many epidemiologists from studying chronic pain. But such despair is unwarranted. The subsequent chapters of this book amply demonstrate that, although difficult, substantial progress can be made. We need enthusiasm, ingenuity, and attention to the pitfalls that beset the research. By establishing a clearer conceptual basis for the epidemiology of chronic pain, linked with international efforts at working definitions of pain syndromes, we can make progress in the epidemiology of pain.

REFERENCES

Andersson HI, Ejlertsson G, Leden I, Rosenberg C. Chronic pain in a geographically defined general population: study of differences in age, gender, social class and pain localization. *Clin J Pain* 1993; 9:174–182.

Bartsch H. Genetic and other host-factors. In: Higginson J, Muir C, Munoz N (Eds). *Human Cancer: Epidemiology and Environmental Causes.* Cambridge: Cambridge University Press, 1992, pp 189–208.

Benedittis GD, Lorenzetti A, Pieri A. The role of stressful life events in the onset of chronic primary headache. *Pain* 1990; 40:65–75.

Benjamin S, Barnes D, Berger S, Clarke I, Jeacock J. The relationship of chronic pain, mental illness and organic disorders. *Pain* 1988; 32:185–195.

Boas RA, Schug SA, Acland RH. Perineal pain after rectal amputation: a five year follow up. *Pain* 1993; 52:67–70.

Bowsher D. A camel is a horse designed by a committee. *J Pain Symptom Manage* 1987; 2:237–239.

Bowsher D, Rigge M, Sopp L. Prevalence of chronic pain in the British population: a telephone survey of 1037 households. *Pain Clinic* 1991; 4:223–230.

Brattberg G, Thorslund M, Wikman A. The prevalence of pain in a general population. The results of a postal survey in a county of Sweden. *Pain* 1989; 37:215–222.

Clemmesen J. *Statistical Studies in Malignant Neoplasms: Vol. 1. Review and Results.* Copenhagen: Munksgaard, 1965.

Coderre TJ, Katz J, Vaccarino AL, Melzack R. Contribution of central neuroplasticity to pathological pain: review of clinical and experimental evidence. *Pain* 1993; 52:259–285.

Conacher ID. Therapists and therapies for post-thoracotomy neuralgia. *Pain* 1992; 48:409–412.

Costello RM, Hulsey TL, Schoenfeld LS, Ramamurthy S. P-A-I-N: a four-cluster MMPI typology for chronic pain. *Pain* 1987; 30:199–209.

Crombie IK. Epidemiological studies of pain. *J Pain Society* 1994; 11:30–31.

Crombie IK. Epidemiology of persistent pain. In: Jensen TS, Turner JA, Wiesenfeld-Hallin Z (Eds). *Proceedings of the 8th World Congress on Pain.* Seattle: IASP Press, 1997, pp 53–61.

Crombie IK, Davies HTO. Audit of outpatients: entering the loop. *BMJ* 1991; 302:1437–1439.

Crombie IK, Davies HTO. Selection bias in pain research. *Pain* 1998; 74:1–3.

Crombie IK, Davies HTO, Macrae WA. The epidemiology of chronic pain: time for new directions. *Pain* 1994; 57:1–3.

Crook J, Rideout E, Browne G. The prevalence of pain complaints in a general population. *Pain* 1984; 18:299–314.

Davies HTO, Crombie IK, Macrae WA. Where does it hurt? Describing the body locations of chronic pain. *Euro J Pain* 1998; 2:69–80.

Doll R, Peto R. The causes of cancer. *J Natl Cancer Inst* 1981; 66:1191–1308.

Dworkin S, Von Korff M, LeResche L. Epidemiologic studies of chronic pain: a dynamic-ecologic perspective. *Ann Behav Med* 1992a; 14:3–11.

Dworkin S, Harstein G, Rosner HL. A high risk method for studying psychosocial antecedents of chronic pain: the prospective investigation of herpes zoster. *J Abnorm Psychol* 1992b; 101:200–205.

Girolamo GD. Epidemiology and social costs of low back pain and fibromyalgia. *Clin J Pain* 1991; 7(Suppl):S1–S7.

Headache Classification Committee of the International Headache Society, Classification and diagnostic criteria for headache disorders, cranial neuralgias and facial pain. *Cephalalgia* 1988; 8(Suppl):1–96.

Higginson J, Muir CS, Munoz N. *Human Cancer: Epidemiology and Environmental Causes.* Cambridge: Cambridge University Press, 1992.

International Association for the Study of Pain Subcommittee on Taxonomy. Classification of chronic pain. Descriptions of chronic pain syndromes and definitions of pain terms. *Pain* 1986; (Suppl):3S1–226.

James FR, Large RG, Bushnell JA, Wells JE. Epidemiology of pain in New Zealand. *Pain* 1991; 44:279–283.

Jamison R, Andersen K, Slater M. Weather changes and pain: perceived influence of local climate on pain complaint in chronic pain patients. *Pain* 1995; 61:309–315.

Jayson IV. Why does acute back pain become chronic? *BMJ* 1997;

314:1639–1640.

Johnson B. Tutorial 23: mechanisms of chronic pain. *Pain Digest* 1996; 6:97–108.

Joukamaa M. Depression and back pain. *Acta Psychiatr Scand* 1994 (Suppl); 377:83–86.

Katusic S, Williams DB, Beard CM, Bergstralh EJ, Kurland LT. Epidemiological and clinical features of idiopathic trigeminal neuralgia and glossopharyngeal neuralgia. *Neuroepidemiology* 1991; 10:276–281.

Lilienfeld AM, Lilienfeld DE. *Foundations of Epidemiology.* New York: Oxford University Press, 1980.

Linton S, Kamwendo K. Risk factors in the psychosocial work environment for neck and shoulder pain in secretaries. *J Occup Med* 1989; 31:609–613.

Lipton RB, Stewart WF. The epidemiology of migraine. *Eur Neurol* 1994; 34(Suppl)2:6–11.

Magni G, Caldieron C, Rigatti-Luchini S, Merskey H. Chronic musculoskeletal pain and depressive symptoms in the general population: an analysis of the 1st National Health and Nutrition Examination Survey data. *Pain* 1990; 43:299–307.

Magni G, Rossi MR, Rigatti-Luchini S, Merskey H. Chronic abdominal pain and depression: epidemiological findings in the United States. Hispanic Health and Nutrition Examination Survey. *Pain* 1992; 49:77–85.

Main CJ, Spanswick CC. Pain: psychological and psychiatric factors. *Br Med Bull* 1991; 47:732–742.

McAlindon TE, Cooper C, Kirwan JR, Dieppe PA. Knee pain and disability in the community. *Br J Rheumatol* 1992; 31:189–192.

McMahon SB. Mechanisms of sympathetic pain. *Br Med Bull* 1991; 47:584–600.

McWhinney J. *An Introduction to Family Medicine.* New York: Oxford University Press, 1981.

Meilman PW. On the difficulties of coding pain-related data [letter]. *Pain* 1989; 36:133–134.

Melzack R, Wall PD. *The Challenge of Pain.* London: Penguin, 1988.

Merskey H, Bogduk N. *Classification of Chronic Pain: Descriptions of Chronic Pain Syndromes and Definitions of Pain Terms.* Seattle: IASP Press, 1994.

Neville RG, Bryce FP, Robertson FM, Crombie IK, Clark RA. Diagnosis and treatment of asthma in children: usefulness of a review of medical records. *Br J Gen Pract* 1992; 42:501–503.

Pilowsky I, Chapman CR, Bonica JJ. Pain, depression, and illness behaviour in a pain clinic population. *Pain* 1977; 4:183–192.

Rasmussen BK, Olesen J. Epidemiology of headache. *IASP Newsletter,* March/April 1996, pp 3–6.

Raspe H, Kohlmann T. Disorders characterised by pain: a methodological review of population surveys. *J Epidemiol Community Health* 1994; 48:531–537.

Rudy T, Turk D, Brena S, Stieg R, Brody M. Quantification of biomedical findings of chronic pain patients: development of an index of pathology. *Pain* 1990; 42:167–182.

Skovron ML. Epidemiology of low back pain. *Baillieres Clin Rheumatol* 1992; 6:559–573.

Skovron M, Szpalski M, Nordin M, Melot C, Cukier D. Sociocultural factors and back pain: a population-based study in Belgian adults. *Spine* 1994; 19:129–137.

Stamler J. Established major coronary risk factors. In: Marmot M, Elliot P (Eds). *Coronary Heart Disease Epidemiology.* Oxford: Oxford University Press, 1992.

Sternbach RA. Survey of pain in the United States: the Nuprin Pain Report. *Clin J Pain* 1986; 2:49–53.

Stewart WF, Shechter A, Rasmussen BK. Migraine prevalence: a review of population-based studies. *Neurology* 1994; 44(Suppl 4): S17–S23.

Stiller C. Cancer registration: its uses in research and confidentiality in the EC. *J Epidemiol Community Health* 1993; 47:342–344.

Turk DC, Rudy TE. IASP taxonomy of chronic pain syndromes: preliminary assessment of reliability. *Pain* 1987; 30:177–189.

Turk DC, Rudy TE. The robustness of an empirically derived taxonomy of chronic pain patients. *Pain* 1990; 43:27–35.

Tyrer SP, Capon M, Peterson DM, Charlton JE, Thompson JW. The detection of psychiatric illness and psychological handicaps in a British pain clinic population. *Pain* 1989; 36:63–74.

Vervest ACM, Schimmel GH. Taxonomy of pain of the IASP [letter]. *Pain* 1988; 34:318–321.

Von Korff M, Dworkin SF, Le Resche L, Kruger A. An epidemiologic comparison of pain complaints. *Pain* 1988; 32:173–183.

Von Korff M, Dworkin SF, Le Resche L. Graded chronic pain status: an epidemiologic evaluation. *Pain* 1990; 40:279–291.

Von Korff M, Le Resche L, Dworkin SF. First onset of common pain symptoms: a prospective study of depression as a risk factor. *Pain* 1993; 55:251–258.

Wallace MS, Wallace AM, Lee J, Dobke MK. Pain after breast surgery: a survey of 282 women. *Pain* 1996; 66:195–205.

Correspondence to: Iain Kinloch Crombie, PhD, Hon MFPHM, Department of Epidemiology and Public Health, University of Dundee, Ninewells Hospital and Medical School, Dundee, DD1 9SY, United Kingdom. Fax: 44-1382-644-197; email: i.k.crombie@dundee.ac.uk.

Epidemiology of Pain, edited by
I.K. Crombie, IASP Press, Seattle, © 1999.

4

Psychological Factors

Steven J. Linton[a] and Suzanne M. Skevington[b]

[a]*Department of Occupational and Environmental Medicine, Örebro Medical Center Hospital, Örebro, Sweden; and* [b]*Department of Psychology, University of Bath, and Royal National Hospital for Rheumatic Diseases, Bath, United Kingdom*

THE PSYCHOLOGY OF PAIN

Imagine various painful events such as a dentist drilling your teeth without anesthesia, a bad abrasive scrape, cancer, or back strain. Each may bring to mind unpleasant memories and negative emotions. These mental and emotional reactions to pain are important psychological processes that contribute to the experience of pain, but they represent only one part of the psychology of pain. Psychological factors are viewed as important determinants in the entire span of pain perception and behavior. Indeed, psychological factors have been put forward to explain the increase in musculoskeletal pain and persistent pain of many types. Surely, our knowledge has expanded greatly since the days when pain with no apparent physical cause was cast to the realms of psychology as a last resort.

Today it is clear that psychological processes are instrumental in the complex process of attending to, interpreting, and reacting to noxious stimuli. The gate-control theory of pain was a landmark in that development as it underscored the complexity of pain and expanded pain from an entirely sensory phenomenon to a multidimensional one (Melzack and Wall 1982; Turk and Melzack 1992; Turk 1996). This theory identifies three main components of pain: the sensory (physiological), affective (emotional and motivational), and evaluative (cognitive) dimensions. By integrating physiological and psychological variables, this theory has altered our thinking about pain perception and has stimulated a great deal of research to discover how pain perception is modulated by psychological variables. The gate-control model of pain integrates peripheral stimuli with psychological states on the cortical level, such as depression or anxiety. It sees pain as an ongoing chain of events that can be modified by ascending and (above all) descending activity in the central nervous system. Consequently, psychological processes are not merely a reaction to pain but an integral part of pain perception. This process results in overt expressions of pain or behaviors such as grimacing that may be used to communicate or cope with the pain. At a pragmatic level, in the pain management clinic, the powerful imagery of the gating process is easy to convey and vividly recalled by those seeking to understand more about why they hurt (Skevington 1995).

Naturally, epidemiological studies of pain have attempted to explain specific aspects of pain problems in relation to various psychological factors to provide a richer, better understanding of painful illnesses. Although psychological factors have often been considered as mere correlates of a pain problem, the evidence indicates a more significant relationship. In some cases, psychological factors appear to be causative, and sometimes psychological processes may maintain chronic pain, while at other times they are a consequence of experiencing it. The task of untangling the relationship between psychological variables and pain has been tedious and remains incomplete. Epidemiological studies hold the promise of enhancing our understanding by illuminating this intricate relationship.

Understanding psychological processes in pain offers the hope of improved treatment and prevention programs. Identifying potent risk factors for a pain problem, for example, would provide valuable insight into how the illness might be managed or prevented.

Even if a psychological variable is not causally linked to a pain problem, it might be helpful in controlling or alleviating the pain. Relaxation training, for example, often provides pain relief, even though muscle tension may not be the cause of the pain. Regardless of the cause, psychological factors may be important in the management, treatment, and prevention of pain.

The aim of this chapter is to provide a better understanding of the role of psychological factors in pain so as to enhance the interpretation of current epidemiological studies and the design of future ones. We describe how psychological processes are believed to work and review many of the concepts used in the psychology of pain and their implications for interpreting epidemiological findings. Finally, we provide views on appropriate methods for conducting epidemiological research with psychological variables.

PAIN PERCEPTION AND BEHAVIOR

Various models of pain perception have evolved over the years, each stressing certain psychological aspects (Melzack and Wall 1965, 1982; Skevington 1995; Feuerstein and Zastowny 1996; Gatchel and Turk 1996; Turk 1996). We summarize current thought to provide a basic model of the role of psychological factors in pain perception, which is of course subject to change and debate.

Pain may be understood as an interaction of cognitive, emotional, motivational, behavioral, and physiological components. For example, a trauma may significantly influence cognitive appraisal and the emotional reaction of hurt, which in turn may be expressed in behaviors like a verbal complaint and the taking of medication. Likewise, cognitions such as the belief that movement may cause further injury may influence both behavior, perhaps through avoidance, and physiology, in a stress reaction.

Fig. 1 illustrates how psychological variables may intervene at several stages in pain perception and behavior. Some factors may *predispose* a person to be in pain, while others may *trigger* or initiate the problem. Psychological factors are often involved in *maintaining* or catalyzing the problem. Learning, for example,

may result in lifestyle changes that appear adaptive, but may maintain the problem in the long run. For example, resting may be reinforced by reductions in pain as well as by sympathy in the short term. However, although this learned behavior may become well established over time, resting may in the long term result in reduced mobility and poorer physical condition and may contribute to a negative outlook. Moreover, factors like depression may relate to *treatment prognosis*. Finally, *buffer* factors such as social support and active coping strategies may help people to withstand their pain problems. Certain factors, e.g., anxiety or depression, may be involved in several of these stages, but some factors will apply only to one stage. Unfortunately, few studies have explained which stage they are examining.

An important concept (detailed below) is the time perspective in the development of a pain problem. The length of suffering may be categorized as acute, subacute, recurrent, or persistent (chronic). Although this categorization is somewhat arbitrary, the length of suffering is crucial for understanding the psychological processes because cognitions and behavior are greatly influenced by the learning experience. Indeed, our understanding of the development of persistent pain is substantially enhanced by psychological models, both alone and in successful combination with methods from other disciplines. A prime example of this is psychoneuroimmunology.

Fig. 2 presents a cross-sectional view of pain perception that features cognitions and learning (Linton 1994). This model stresses the role of appraisal and beliefs, which complements those of coping and learning. As the figure illustrates, the first step is to attend to the noxious stimulus. This, in part, is controlled by psychological factors—for instance, whether a person's attention is focused inward or outward. In the second step, an appraisal of the stimulus is made, which is influenced by a host of psychological factors and previous experiences. The noxious stimulus is given meaning and evaluated to decide whether it is harmful, unusual, or irrelevant and not worth further attention. This in turn influences coping strategies—the way we "plan" to deal with the pain. These cognitive processes, according to the model, are im-

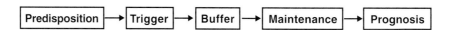

Fig. 1. Some examples of how psychological factors may influence pain in various ways. Based on Linton (1994).

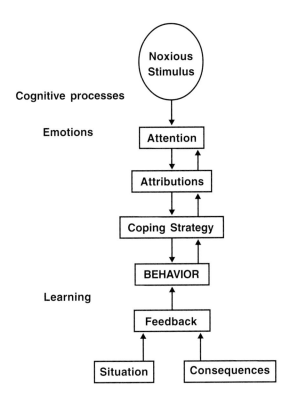

Fig. 2. A cross-sectional view of the psychological processes involved in pain perception including attributions, coping, and behavior. These may not be conscious processes. The consequences of the behavior affect the emotional, cognitive, and behavioral aspects. Based on Linton (1994).

portant prerequisites to the next step—behavior. However, these processes are not always conscious "thoughts" and may occur automatically.

Learning factors influence "pain" behaviors just as they do any other behaviors; behaviors that attempt to cope with a pain problem are influenced both by the situation in which they occur and by their consequences. Although the rules known to govern learning are very specific and intricate, behaviors that successfully reduce or eliminate pain will tend to increase in frequency in similar situations due to reinforcement. Similarly, behaviors that increase the pain will tend to decrease in frequency due to punishment. The avoidance paradigm is an example of how learning may affect pain behaviors. In the first stage, respondent conditioning occurs when stimuli such as a certain place, situation, or activity (e.g., heavy lifting) elicit a response such as increased anxiety, fear, and muscle tension. In the second stage, this stimulus is experienced as a threat: "Please help me lift this suitcase." This sets the stage for an avoidance response:

"I can't, I have back pain," which is reinforced by the consequences, such as a reduction of the anxiety, tension, and pain (Lethem et al. 1983; Linton et al. 1984). Once avoidance is learned, the person may never again come in contact with the threatening situation (heavy lifting). This paradigm is related to certain cognitive thought patterns, of which the most conspicuous is so-called catastrophizing, where the patient makes exaggerated and negative interpretations. The avoidance paradigm has recently received considerable attention as a partial explanation of how pain sufferers become disabled; researchers have coined the term "fear avoidance" to describe their behavior (Lethem et al. 1983; Waddell et al. 1993; Vlaeyen et al. 1995).

PSYCHOLOGICAL FACTORS IN THE TRANSITION FROM ACUTE TO CHRONIC PAIN

What happens to the psychology of individuals as they move from acute to chronic pain? Integrating the broad findings of the literature and drawing directly on clinical experience, Keefe and colleagues (1982) suggest that during the first 2 months of treatment for acute pain patients rely temporarily on medication, possibly seeking help from professionals and in some cases reducing their activities. Patients cope actively, believe that the pain is controllable through medication, and show heightened physiological arousal, often as anxiety. Muscle spasms are common at this stage. Keefe's team also identified a prechronic stage 2–6 months after an injury, when patients alternately increase and decrease their activities and test active and passive coping styles. They may withdraw from medication or become dependent on it. They may be working or trying to work, and may have limited contact with doctors. They become aware that medication cannot entirely control their pain and that their levels of pain are responsive to stress. Signs of depression are evident. Physiologically, this stage is similar to the first 2 months. A third phase develops at 6–24 months, when the likelihood of identifying organic pathology is diminishing. Patients' hope for a medical cure is diminishing, and they may "shop around" for doctors and may experience a permanent lowering of activity and addiction to pain medication. The belief that pain is uncontrollable and the use of passive coping strategies can lead to depression. Physiological arousal is reduced. Sufferers dwell on bodily complaints, and headaches and other psychophysiological disorders tend to increase. Chronic muscle spasms cause intense pain, while muscle strength and endurance have diminished.

This model summarizes trends that clinicians observe daily. Longitudinal studies to substantiate these insights have supported the model. In a prospective longitudinal study of outpatients with early synovitis, Skevington (1993) investigated their beliefs as to how well they would recover and monitored their pain and depression for 2 years. She found that affective pain, and to a lesser extent sensory pain, are consequences (rather than antecedents) of depression. A patient who believes on admission to the clinic that the pain will be uncontrollable and enduring is most likely to become depressed later.

Von Korff and Simon (1996) conducted longitudinal analyses of primary back care patients to investigate the relationship between pain and associated dysfunction. Patients followed up at 7 weeks showed improvements in depression, especially if their back pain had improved. In a 2-year follow up, those with pain dysfunction showed no increase in depressive symptoms associated with chronicity. Those with a more favorable back pain outcome showed reductions in depression to normal levels.

But who becomes the chronic pain patient? Not everyone seeks treatment for pain. In a complex social process, a person discusses symptoms with family, friends, and acquaintances to seek reassurance that complaints are legitimate before taking them into the consulting room (Telles and Pollack 1981). Egan and Beaton (1987) uncovered many courses of action that might be pursued for common symptoms like pain, coughing, and nausea. A common reaction is to work out a causal explanation for the symptom; coping strategies might include restricting social activities, scaling back work hours, informing one's supervisor or co-workers, staying at home, going to bed, resting more, and informing one's friends and family. Some individuals might ignore their symptoms, continue to work, take special nutrition, or treat themselves with nonprescription medication. Only a few are likely to follow the conventional routes of visiting a physician, taking prescribed drugs, going to a hospital emergency department, or calling emergency services.

A study of general practice in Canada has looked more closely at the reporting of pain. Surveying 372 families, Crook and colleagues (1984) found that in the 2 weeks prior to their survey, 36% of families had one or more members in pain. Eleven percent of these were in persistent pain, while for 5% the pain was temporary. However, 66% of those in pain had not used the health care system within this period, which shows that contrary to popular opinion, a substantial number of people continue to suffer rather than seek medical advice. Crook's study concludes that in 75% of cases, pain sufferers do not seek professional help. Those with sudden pain or severe disability are most likely to seek help (Twaddle 1980), probably because these features cause the most disruption to daily living. Others report that persistent back pain that limits activities creates the highest demand for health services (Engel et al. 1996). All these factors seem likely to play a role in decision-making about whether to visit a doctor. Furthermore, only a minority of people with chronic pain become high utilizers of back pain services. Personality variables also seem to be influential: anxiety (Ingham and Miller 1979) and depression (Magni et al. 1990) are related to seeking treatment. However, anxiety and depression are also interlinked with the severity and persistence of pain. Von Korff et al. (1991) attempted to study the effect of psychological distress more generally; they found that persistent pain and the degree of limitation of activity, rather than psychological factors, are the best predictors of seeking health care.

It might be expected that pain would be well controlled for patients in hospitals, where access to analgesics is relatively easy, but Abbot and colleagues (1992) show that this cannot be taken for granted. Interviewing 2415 randomly selected inpatients, they found that 50% were in pain and that 67% had been in pain the previous day. Although those in surgery during the past week were more likely to report pain, one-fifth of those who had not received surgery were also in pain. Furthermore, 6 months later, 20% of the 72% who were followed up remained in pain and were more distressed, although most had ceased treatment. These findings were broadly confirmed by Donovan and colleagues (1987), who found that only 49% of surgical in-patients had their postoperative pain charted, and that the average amount of analgesic received was less than a quarter of that prescribed.

Nonattendance for formal treatment may be associated with the availability of alternative sources of help. Greenley and Mechanic (1976) demonstrated the wide diversity of resources that students consulted for health problems. Although there are broad individual differences in the predisposition to seek health care, those in the community seek formal consultations relatively infrequently and appear to use a wide variety of alternative and informal resources. However, when they do seek care, they experience subtle, systematic differences in the way acute symptoms are interpreted and managed by the health care system. For example, in a study of 190 headache, neck pain, and back pain patients attended by 84 health professionals in an emergency department in Boston, USA, Raftery and colleagues (1995) found that providers described women as reporting more pain than men. However, women also experienced more pain, received more medication and more potent analgesics, and were less likely than men to receive no medication at all. Despite these differences, severity of pain correlated better with pain practices than did gender.

Other recent research shows how systematic biases may be perpetuated at different stages in the treatment process. Studying the management of acute chest pain in 1411 patients attending the emergency department of a U.S. hospital, Johnson and colleagues (1996) found that women were less likely than men to be admitted to a hospital or to take an exercise stress test within a month of their visit. Of those admitted to a hospital, the incidence of taking the stress test was the same for both gender groups, but the likelihood of receiving cardiac catheterization was significantly lower for women. These results show how social factors like gender may insidiously affect the way that treatment decisions are made, ultimately impacting the health of the patients. In secondary care, such judgments may determine which patients develop chronic pain and what styles of coping they may use. Johnson's study shows that the patients are not the only ones who drive this differential reporting and treatment process that fuels epidemiological statistics. Health professionals also have an active role in shaping the eventual population of chronic pain patients through their own biases and judgments, which may not be altogether conscious. The role of the health professional's beliefs and assumptions in delivering health care and forming the statistics has been clarified by Von Korff's (1994) investigation of physicians working in primary care. Despite evidence to the contrary, physicians tend to assume that back pain will be acute rather than recurrent or chronic. However, Von Korff reported that after 1 year, 34% of patients had experienced pain for 50% of the days in the previous 6 months and 21% had experienced pain every day, which provides a serious challenge to clinical assumptions.

This image of the pain coping mechanisms of those in the community who seek acute care contrasts starkly with statistical evidence that chronic pain patients are avid users of health care resources. How does the metamorphosis into a chronic pain patient affect their reporting behavior so dramatically? Can distinct categories of pain patient be defined by identifiable stages? Furthermore, is it safe to assume that patients with more than 6 months of continuous pain are homogeneous as a group thereafter? A comparative study investigated three groups of patients with recent, short, and long duration of pain (Zarkowska and Philips 1986). Patients with long duration (mean 14.3 years) reported more sensory and affective pain than the short-duration group, who had chronic pain for 2.2 years. This study demonstrates that changes in experience and reporting occur over time. Broadly similar findings are recorded by Swanson and Maruta (1980). Uncommon cases of "ancient" pain, defined as pain lasting 25 years or more, have also been identified (45 cases per 1000 consecutive admissions), but they seem to be largely confined to head and face pain patients (Swanson et al. 1986). They are a particularly difficult group to treat, so this category may be an artifact of the profession's inability to successfully relieve this specific type of intractable pain, rather than an inherent characteristic of long duration.

Despite the shortage of good prospective longitudinal studies in this area, assumptions about the homogeneity of chronic pain patients as a group do not seem to be justified. Interventions might be more successful if the developmental stages and their transition points in the pain sufferer's history were better understood. Long-term epidemiological studies to chart changing patterns for different styles of patient during a clinical lifetime could target the most efficacious time to introduce psychological intervention.

Some understanding of other variables that affect the psychological aspects of this process has just begun to emerge. An examination of sociodemographic variables reveals gender differences in the ways people adjust to chronic pain over time. In a cohort survey of 222 patients referred to a pain clinic, Weir and colleagues (1996) confirmed expected differential expenditures for health service use by gender. They also found that while there was a high overall incidence of poor adjustment to chronic pain, the higher utilization of health care services by women was partly explained by their psychological needs and the meaning of illness to them. In contrast, men's adjustment was better predicted by social variables such as level of social support; pain held a different set of meanings for men. Weir's team spells out the importance of social support and the role of different meanings of pain and illness in patients' ability to make psychosocial adjustments to chronic pain. They also point out some of the biases and barriers that may be at work in accessing and using health services. This work on adjustment and other studies of gender differences in response to cognitive behavioral treatments (e.g., Jensen et al. 1994) suggest that the profile of treatment and rehabilitation procedures at all stages in the transition from acute to chronic pain needs to be handled in gender-specific ways. Epidemiological studies on the psychology of pain may thus translate into distinctive changes in medical practice.

Time is also an important variable in epidemiological work, although the timing of interventions has not yet been systematically explored. When exactly is the best time to intervene to prevent a reoccurrence of back pain or to pre-empt chronicity? Linton and colleagues (1989) addressed this problem in an occupational study of working nurses. They provided a 5-week program of instruction, exercise, and education for nurses who had been absent from work with back pain during the two previous years. The results showed greater psychological improvements for the intervention group than for waiting-list controls for anxiety, tiredness, pain, sleep, satisfaction with daily activities, and relations with their spouse. More studies using this type of design are needed to explain changes in important psychological processes at the earliest stages of a range of painful conditions and to identify the most appropriate types of interventions.

THE ROLE OF LEARNING

Given that pain sufferers change their behavior over time, it seems plausible that learning plays a central role in creating these changes. A substantial body of evidence shows that the relearning approaches adopted in cognitive behavior therapy (CBT) can be influential in modifying the way chronic pain sufferers behave. Hence a great deal of emphasis has been placed on investigating various learning processes. Operant conditioning, with its principles of reinforcement, extinction, punishment, reward, and discriminative control, has been understood for more than 50

years, and behavior therapy based on these principles can be useful in modifying a range of pain behaviors. Many current methods also emphasize the importance of cognitive variables, and CBT has thus become the most frequently used term.

Claims for the success of operant conditioning as a rehabilitation technique for chronic pain patients (Fordyce 1976) arise from its efficacy in suppressing overt pain behaviors, such as moaning, grimacing, limping, rubbing, and taking medication, rather than reducing perceived pain intensity itself. The aims of CBT are to help patients manage beliefs about pain, and hence to solve problems in a resourceful manner. Patients are also assisted in monitoring their thoughts, emotions, and behaviors, and in identifying how these internal factors relate to events. The program helps patients to perform appropriate behaviors when they need to cope with distress and difficulties, and to develop and maintain adaptive ways of thinking, feeling, and responding that will help them to cope after treatment is completed (Holzman et al. 1986). To do this, CBT employs education, rehearsal of cognitive and behavioral strategies, skills training, and generalization and maintenance techniques (Bradley 1996). Results from CBT indicate that learning plays an important role in shaping the way pain sufferers look at their condition by showing them that their behavior can be changed through psychological methods. Of course, learning and relearning continue with or without psychological assistance, so we cannot assume that behaviors recorded at one time will continue unchanged during the entire period that a person is in pain. Learning processes may thus affect the results that are being monitored in some epidemiological studies.

Other ways of looking at learning have been to consider how experience and events affect those who are in pain. Changes in lifestyle occur as the patient moves from the acute to the chronic state, and epidemiologists must take these into account. These changes may be swift or slow and may result from positive or negative major life events, whether directly relevant to the current health state of those in pain, or indirectly, by impinging upon the way they interpret and respond to their condition. While a great deal of research has examined the impact of negative life events in the last 30 years, we still know remarkably little about how the patterning and timing of these events affect the lives of pain sufferers; further epidemiological studies could be instructive.

Alternatively, changes in lifestyle could be due

to the accumulated impact of minor, irritating happenings that have a gradual, insidious effect on the pain victim's perceptions, predisposition to report their health problems, and eventual coping methods. For some people, the hassles of daily living may have more damaging psychological consequences than major life events. In a major survey of pain and daily hassles in 1254 people in the United States (the Nuprin Pain Report), Sternbach (1986) found substantial evidence to support the widespread incidence and negative effect of hassles in pain sufferers. He reported that 5% were stressed on a daily basis, 38% several times a week, and 51% less than once a week. Furthermore, the greater the number of stressors in the course of the year, the greater the frequency and severity of reported pain. Information about the hassles that form the background to any study of negative life events must be integrated into long-term epidemiological studies.

THE ROLE OF SOCIALIZATION

Learning how to deal with a pain problem may start quite early in life, before any serious injury is experienced, as even healthy, pain-free children learn much from their parents about "appropriate" ways to behave when in pain. Subsequent injury may serve to activate this repertoire, assimilated many years earlier. One aspect is the predisposition to report pain and illness. Many psychological studies show that children are substantially influenced by their parent's attitudes in general, and so it is not particularly surprising to find that their attitudes to health and health care are also highly correlated with those of their parents. Quadrel and Lau (1990) surveyed 7000 teenagers and found that their decisions on whether or not to visit a doctor with influenza, fatigue, or a range of serious conditions such as lumps, or blood in the urine were heavily affected by the attitudes of their parents. Edwards and colleagues (1985) examined the proposal that pain behavior in children is modeled from other family members. They found that the number of current pains reported by college students corresponded to the number of family members who were in pain. This relationship was particularly strong for headaches and menstrual pain. This finding is supported by Violon and Giurgea (1984), who reported that 78% of acupuncture patients studied had family members who were also in pain, compared with only 44% of pain-free controls seeking ear, nose, and throat treatment.

Socialization has usually been used to denote the ways in which children learn from adults and refers to the processes of modeling and imitation. But socialization continues throughout the life-span, even though the most influential sources (initially parents) may change over time. Adult pain sufferers learn new cognitions, emotional reactions, and behavior from a number of sources, but a major source of influence is the behavior of those with whom they most closely come into contact—their family, friends, acquaintances, and colleagues.

Spouses have been identified as being particularly powerful in shaping pain behavior because as primary caregivers, they are usually a major source of reinforcement. Considerable evidence supports the view that when their spouses respond negatively to pain, married persons with painful illnesses experience more depression and distress (Kerns et al. 1990). Conversely, the more positive attention pain sufferers receive, the more pain they report (Block et al. 1980), the more pain behaviors they display (Romano et al. 1992), and the more disability they express (Flor et al. 1989). More recently, some researchers have suggested that the family may be the best place to teach therapeutic skills, because skills learned in the clinical environment may turn out to be difficult to put into practice in the home. Home-based therapy may prove to be the new frontier (Corey et al. 1987). However, in the search for problem families to research, it should be remembered that many families with pain sufferers cope surprisingly well (Turk et al. 1987). Despite the enthusiasm for family therapy arising from these findings, progress has been slow. Kerns and Payne (1996) recommend that family therapy should facilitate a flexible, problem-solving approach to coping with chronic pain. It should draw on the family's resources, teach new skills, and make patients aware of the most appropriate occasions to seek help from professionals. Reducing the stress and negative impact of pain and restoring family functioning are valuable additional goals. In a qualitative study that compared families with a pain sufferer with families that included persons with chronic, pain-free illnesses and those with no illnesses, Dura and Beck (1988) found that families where the mother was in good health were more cohesive and had less conflict than did those where the mother was ill. Although the direction of causality cannot be discerned from the cross-sectional nature of this work, the tentative conclusion is that family cohesion deteriorates and conflict increases as pain sufferers make the transition into chronicity. Such findings would bear further investigation using epidemiological designs.

DEVELOPMENT OF PSYCHOLOGICAL CONCEPTS

We discuss self-efficacy and fear avoidance to exemplify the way in which psychological ideas are developed and elaborated, how these concepts can be measured in a satisfactory manner, and how research data can be adapted to address clinical problems.

SELF-EFFICACY

The concept of self-efficacy provides a useful way to understand why people may or may not act in accordance with their beliefs about health (Bandura 1991). There are three dimensions to the concept of self-efficacy. The first concerns expectations about how difficult the chosen task will be; people are more likely to avoid difficult tasks than easy ones. Second, people may have quite different expectations about being able to carry out specific tasks e.g., to lose 2 pounds of body weight a week for 6 weeks, than much broader and more general plans of action, e.g., to lose weight. Third, to anticipate whether someone is likely to act or not, we need to know how confident he or she feels about being able to succeed. These ideas have been profitably applied to our understanding of pain. A 22-item scale known as the Chronic Pain Self-Efficacy Scale was validated in a multidisciplinary outpatient clinic (Anderson et al. 1995). Exploratory factor analysis was used to identify three important aspects of self–efficacy: pain management, coping with symptoms, and physical functioning. This measure promises to be useful in examining how well chronic pain patients feel able to cope with their pain.

Indicating three ways in which efficacy beliefs can bring relief from pain, Bandura (1991) shows that those who believe they can relieve their pain are more likely to search for skills and information that will enable them to do this and to persist with these newly learned self-help methods. In contrast, those who are less self-efficacious are more likely to give up quickly if their initial efforts are unsuccessful. Furthermore, feelings of self-efficacy reduce expectations of distress along with anxiety and physical tension, which

has positive ameliorating effects on pain. Lastly, those with strong self-efficacy beliefs tend to view unpleasant sensations as more benign and fear them less, which may lessen their pain levels.

Several studies have confirmed a relationship between strong beliefs in self-efficacy and less disability and point the way to interventions that may help us to better manage disability. Levin et al. (1996) found that 59 chronic low back pain patients with high levels of self-efficacy also had high activity levels, worked more hours, and had less psychological distress, less severe pain, and less pain behavior than those with low self-efficacy beliefs. But how good are self-efficacy expectations at predicting patients' physical functioning or their ability to perform activities such as essential jobs? A study of 85 chronic low back pain patients found that specific expectations about their physical capacity to do a particular job better explained the disability of these individuals than did their expectations about pain or possible reinjury related to that task (Lackner et al. 1996). Including information on gender and actual pain intensity improved this finding. A high level of self-efficacy beliefs has also been associated with lower self-reported pain and with less impairment in physical activities in fibromyalgia patients after controlling for age, education, symptom duration, and severity (Buckelew et al. 1995). Furthermore, self-efficacy is a better predictor of pain behaviors in patients with fibromyalgia than are personality indices like depression (Buckalew et al. 1994). Some of the most interesting work to emerge recently has studied the relationship among timing of pain, coping efficacy, and mood. In a longitudinal study, Keefe et al. (1997) looked at diaries completed by 53 rheumatoid arthritis patients over 30 consecutive days. They found that not only were high levels of coping efficacy related to decreases in pain and negative mood, but that these effects were time-lagged, so that high coping efficacy was followed the next day by less pain. Those who used pain reduction and relaxation strategies on a given day felt less pain and had a more positive mood the next day. This is a particularly good example of a study where the integration of epidemiological methods and design has served to enhance the understanding of psychological processes.

A notable application of the self-efficacy model is the Arthritis Self Management Program developed at Stanford by Lorig and colleagues (1993). This program teaches techniques originally designed for the daily management of arthritis, and which were later found to be applicable to the condition of a whole range of other nonmalignant chronic disorders (K. Lorig, personal communication). Various skills and techniques combine with education and social support in a package that encourages the self-care of chronic conditions over long periods of time (2 years). Well-being is developed and maintained on many dimensions. In a British program of six 2-hour weekly sessions designed for older rheumatoid and osteoarthritis patients, Barlow and colleagues (1997) reported some improvement in arthritis self-efficacy, especially in relation to pain. They also found small, but significant improvements in pain intensity, pain severity, depression, and positive affect. Participation in this course improved stretching and strengthening exercises, relaxation, and the use of cognitive behavioral techniques, with limited reductions in the number of visits to the general practitioner. However there was no change in social support. These findings are largely in line with those of the original studies from the United States published by Lorig and colleagues (Lorig et al. 1970, 1989, 1993; Lorig and Holman 1989), but the omission of a control group in the British study weakens the power of its results.

FEAR AVOIDANCE

Fear avoidance is of great interest conceptually because it is a powerful predictor of disability and days lost from work (Waddell et al. 1993). Since Fordyce's (1976) seminal work on the behavioral treatment of chronic pain, fear and avoidance have been key suspects in the role of maintaining pain in both positively and negatively reinforcing ways. A long tradition of experimental work in psychology dating from the 1930s has repeatedly shown how animals use avoidance to reduce their discomfort. The belief that certain activities will lead to pain is sometimes enough to initiate fear avoidance behavior as part of a vicious circle that involves reductions in beliefs about being self-efficacious (see discussion above), with increased fear and subsequent increases in avoidance and related disability (Asmundson et al. 1997). Avoiding undesirable activities lowers the anxiety of the pain sufferer, and this in turn serves to negatively reinforce the cycle. In acute pain, activities that are normally neutral or pleasant may elicit or aggra-

vate the pain and may subsequently become aversive and be avoided. This conditioned fear may be generalized and extended to many diverse and different situations, such as work, sexual activity, and leisure (Turk 1996). Avoidance behavior may become inextricably and cyclically linked to the anticipation of pain and the anxiety it generates. In turn, these processes affect the sympathetic nervous system and muscle tension levels (Flor et al. 1990).

A recent measure developed for use in the pain field is the Pain Anxiety Symptoms Scale (PASS), which assesses pain-related anxiety through four components: cognition, fear, escape/avoidance, and physiological response. Good internal consistency and acceptable convergent and divergent validity allow its use with outpatient referrals (Rose et al. 1992). Significant differences in fear avoidance have been reported when chronic pain groups with post-herpetic neuralgia, reflex sympathetic dystrophy, and low back pain were compared with recovered, pain-free comparison groups. This supports the theory that there is a psychological overlay common to chronic pain patients that is independent of their pathology (Rose et al. 1992).

Other interesting examples have been obtained in the primary care setting. In an English community study, Klenerman et al. (1995) assessed 300 acute low back pain patients on three occasions using psychosocial and physiological data. Seven percent had not recovered after 2 months and became chronic back pain patients after a year. Fear avoidance measures were the best predictors of outcome, correctly classifying 66% of the patients who would become chronic. A clinical implication of this finding is that confronting the intense fear of pain at the outset of treatment may be as important as treating the pain itself.

These examples of fear avoidance and self-efficacy show how psychological concepts can be developed in a clinical context to assist with patient care and management. At the same time, they further our understanding about the mechanisms and psychologically driven processes implicated in the etiology, expression, and maintenance of pain. Table I summarizes psychological factors implicated in the study of pain. Each is listed with a brief summary, together with a key reference to guide further reading on the subject. This is provided as a resource and is not intended to be a comprehensive review.

Table 1
Overview of some psychological variables believed to be important in the epidemiology of pain

Psychological Factor	Key Reference	Description
Pain Behaviors		
Overt	Keefe and Williams 1992	Various ways in which we communicate to others that we are in pain. Examples are grimacing, bracing, and rubbing.
Activity/Function		Low levels of daily activities and high levels of "down time" signify a problem, but not necessarily related to pain level.
Avoidance	Vlaeyen et al. 1995	A learning paradigm where certain activities, places, etc. are avoided. Behavior is maintained by reduction in fear, anxiety. Patients may avoid activity to reduce fear.
Cognitions		
Beliefs about pain	Kleinman 1988	Strongly held views about pain and illness containing both cognitive and affective components. Socially and culturally generated and modifiable. May include beliefs about pain control (locus of control), pain modification (self-efficacy), health professionals, and efficacy of treatments.
Catastrophizing	Sullivan et al. 1995	One of a number of maladaptive strategies for coping with pain, commonly related to the etiology of depression. Believed to be related to fear-avoidance vicious circle.
Cognitive distortion	DeGood and Shutty 1992	Systematic errors in thinking, particularly in the depressed. This may take the form of making arbitrary inferences or drawing mistaken conclusions in the absence of evidence. People may magnify the significance of an unpleasant event and minimize or discount a pleasant one. Commonly found in relation to pain and disability.
Locus of control	Skevington 1990	Beliefs concerning the place where the control of pain is based, e.g., personal responsibility for pain control, pain control by others (e.g., doctors), and pain control through chance happenings or misfortune. These beliefs may be the foundation for action to seek pain relief.
Coping strategies	Jensen et al. 1991	A number of ways of managing or deflecting unwanted stress or pain. These may include cognitive (distraction) and behavioral (take pill) aspects, and they may be passive (hoping) or active strategies (relaxation).
Control	Thompson 1981	Belief that it is possible to influence an aversive event. Desire to predict such an event. Control and predictability influence pain perception.
Attention	Suls and Fletcher 1985	A type of vigilance or monitoring activity that can be harnessed in coping strategies either to divert or distract from the source of stress or to focus directly on the pain, stress, or anxiety. Choice of strategy depends on the circumstances.
Helplessness	Skevington 1994	A style of beliefs predominantly used by those who are prone to depression, whereby negative events such as the onset of pain tend to be seen as likely to persist.
Emotions		
Mood	Gamsa 1990	Depression, anxiety, but also fear, sadness, anger, frustration are associated with pain and disability. More likely to be a consequence of pain than a precursor to it.
Anxiety/somatic anxiety	Main et al. 1992	Increased physiological arousal together with cognitive components like worry that enhance the detection of painful sensation and maintain perceived pain. Thus, a target for treatment. Somatic anxiety refers to distress and concurrent symptoms.

(continued)

Table I
Continued

Psychological Factor	Key Reference	Description
Social Factors		
Gender	Unruh 1996	Similarities and differences in the way women and men respond to, interpret, and report pain sensations and styles of obtaining treatment. Formed in part by social and cultural framework.
Social comparison	Blalock et al. 1989	Comparisons made with other people with different diseases or health states or with self (ideal self) at different times, defined by health events, within the lifespan.
Social support	Manne and Zautra 1989	Any input directly provided by another person or group that moves recipients toward the goals they desire, for pain may be positive or negative.
Spouse relations	Schwartz et al. 1996	The relationship between pain patient and spouse and the effect that this has on pain behaviors. A solicitous spouse may increase pain behaviors.
Work place	Bongers et al. 1993	Relationships at work with management as well as co-workers may influence perceptions of injury, pain, and disability.
Work management	Fordyce 1995	The way in which a workplace deals with pain problems and rehabilitation may influence pain perception and behavior.

PSYCHOLOGICAL METHODS IN EPIDEMIOLOGICAL PAIN RESEARCH

MEASURING PSYCHOLOGICAL VARIABLES

In this section we outline some of the challenges that psychological factors represent in epidemiological investigations. Psychological variables include a wide range of concepts that appear to enrich our potential for understanding pain, whether they involve observable behavior or subjective states. Thus it is important to consider how these concepts are defined and how they might best be measured (Karoly 1985; Palinkas 1985; Turk and Kerns 1985).

Psychological variables are subjective and can never be as accurate as the gradings on a thermometer, but precision is a shared concern throughout science, and psychologists have expended considerable research effort in developing their own methods for establishing the precision of their tools. Such tools include visual analogue scales, attitude measures, threshold estimations, behavior measures, checklists, and diaries. The very use of subjective measures has been debated, but let it suffice to say that such measures are useful when the research question demands them. If the psychological climate at work is relevant for a study, then measures of subjective experience such as job satisfaction and stress are necessary and probably more relevant than biological markers, for example stress hormones.

The definition and measurement of a variable natu-rally influence outcomes and may even render seemingly unequivocal results invalid or inconclusive. Measurement of psychological factors is complicated by their inaccessibility. Thus, measurements typically try to cover behavioral, physiological, and subjective aspects (Keefe et al. 1978; Keefe and Blumenthal 1982; Karoly 1985). Moreover, several types of assessment technique are available, which vary considerably on the objectivity scale. These include verbal reports in interviews, rating scales, self-monitoring, questionnaires, behavioral observation, and psychophysiological measures. Although all of these methods may be used in epidemiological studies, by far the most widely used technique is the survey or questionnaire, which will be the primary focus of this section (the references above address the specifics of working with other methods). Psychological factors may serve as both independent (exposure or risk factors) and dependent (outcome) variables, and it is vital to hold this difference in mind when designing or evaluating research.

Given the interrelationship between psychological concepts, the same entity may have more than one name, or concepts may overlap. "Fear avoidance," for example, is a term used to label beliefs about the consequences of activity on pain as well as the actual avoidance behavior (Waddell et al. 1993; Vlaeyen et al. 1995). "Helplessness" and "catastrophizing" are closely linked terms that relate to the interpretation of the effects of pain, and they are often included in inventories of coping strategies (Rosenstiel and Keefe

1983; Sullivan et al. 1995; Vlaeyen et al. 1995). "Self-efficacy" and "locus of control" are other terms used in overlapping ways to describe coping behaviors (Jensen et al. 1991). There is a conceptual as well as a methodological problem in that instruments developed to measure one concept may be surprisingly comparable to those developed to measure a similar concept. Thus, psychological factors may be interrelated, but the exact relationship often has not been established. Finally, to allow measurement, the definition must be operational. Although this is a basic principle, it may be difficult to fulfill as psychological concepts such as "sense of coherence" or "cognitive distortion" refer to unobservable conditions and are therefore only accessible by relying on subjective self-report measures. Subjective reports are not necessarily an unreliable method of tapping into a concept, as replies gathered to assess many of the newer psychological concepts (see Table I) are not subject to the same "social desirability" effects (the desire to appear in a good light) compared to many older personality tests. Therefore, their results can be taken much more at face value by the researcher who is anxious to ensure reliability.

Once a psychosocial variable has been operationally defined, the next stumbling block may be adequate measurement. Reliability and validity are essential here, as with any other type of variable (Dworkin and Whitney 1992). Several textbooks on the basic requirements are available (Nunnally 1970; Cronbach 1984; McDowell and Newell 1987; Anastasi 1988; Streiner and Norman 1996). However, for psychological variables, reliability and in particular validity may be a particular challenge (Anastasi 1988; Streiner and Norman 1996). Construct validity refers to how well an instrument actually measures the defined variable. As many psychological variables are not easily observed, determining construct or even content validity typically is troublesome. As a result, some instruments may not be tested for construct or content validity, while others are only tested for concurrent validity by comparing the instrument with other assessments said to measure the same entity (an indirect test of validity). Problems in firmly establishing validity have led to recommendations of broad-based, multiple measures for the proper assessment of most psychological variables (Keefe et al. 1978; Kazdin 1980; Keefe and Blumenthal 1982; Karoly 1985).

Reactivity is a special problem for psychological assessment methods. This refers to an inadvertent change (reaction) in the response being measured as a result of the assessment technique. Observing a patient's behavior or having them complete a questionnaire in the clinic may create particular changes that reduce the quality of the measurement. The patient may be self-conscious or may attempt to influence our conclusions. This is a particular problem when the reactivity is biased or systematic. For example, patients may systematically rate conditions at work as "poor" if they perceive the questionnaire as a measure of the "cause" of the problem.

Another aspect particular to psychological variables and pain perception is related to time. Many psychological factors vary considerably over relatively short periods of time. It is vital to consider this when evaluating psychosocial variables. Answers to questionnaires concerning pain, anxiety, depression, etc., may be different if they are completed *before* as compared to *after* meeting the doctor. One consequence is that single assessments are usually not as accurate as repeated measures of a psychological variable. Some researchers and clinicians attempt to compensate for this by phrasing the question to include a longer time frame, e.g., during the past month or year. However, ratings are generally influenced by the way the patient is currently feeling, and there is reason to question whether patients can accurately produce an "average" (Keefe et al. 1978; Kazdin 1980; Keefe and Blumenthal 1982; Karoly 1985; Streiner and Norman 1996). Thus, repeated measures may be advantageous. The rating scale used in gathering responses is also of interest in accurately measuring psychological parameters, but has been inadequately studied (Keefe et al. 1978; Kazdin 1980; Keefe and Blementhal 1982; Karoly 1985; McDowell and Newell 1987; Streiner and Norman 1996).

Given the difficulties in establishing distinct terms with operational definitions that may be measured with reliable and valid methods, broad-based assessment techniques are recommended. Usually it is advantageous to obtain repeated measures to gain an accurate estimate of the parameter. Psychological questionnaires that use the broad-based, multiple-criterion approach frequently have a relatively large number of items, and carefully conducted research typically employs several questionnaires. The probability of making "assessment" errors is reduced and reliability is enhanced by increasing the number of items that measure the psychological variable

(Streiner and Norman 1996). The goal of developing instruments with only a few items may be appropriate for some studies, but such measures need to be thoroughly tested as their reliability and validity may be questionable.

Measuring psychological entities with multiple instruments is a good strategy. Many psychological concepts have several distinct dimensions, each of which needs to be assessed. For example, depression includes such aspects as hope for the future, sense of failure, guilt feelings, suicidal wishes, crying, withdrawal, loss of libido, and distortion of body image (Steer and Beck 1988). As a result, depression inventories include items measuring these various aspects; the Beck Depression Inventory (Steer and Beck 1988) and the Zung Depression Measure (Becker 1988) have 21 and 20 items, respectively.

Since measurement is an essential part of epidemiological studies, we will provide another illustration of the difficulties in defining and measuring psychological terms. Depression is a well-known factor associated with pain, particularly with chronic pain (Romano and Turner 1985). Likewise, decreases in activity are common for patients with persistent pain. However, questionnaires designed to measure depression often contain items concerned with activity levels, as changes in activity level are a common complaint in depression. Similarly, activity assessments may focus on activity levels regardless of whether the decrease is related to pain or to depression. Consequently, instruments designed to measure depression may have inflated scores from questions concerning activity. In cross-sectional studies that employ multivariate data analyses and take intercorrelations into consideration, a relatively small number of variables typically provides the best solution. Burton and associates (1995) studied psychosocial risk factors that may predict the outcome of acute or subacute back pain. They used a relatively large number of psychosocial variables, but found that only five variables remained significant when a multivariate analysis was used. They also found that the variables associated with outcome differed according to whether the patients had acute or subacute pain upon entry into the study. Moreover, fear avoidance (as measured by the Fear-Avoidance Beliefs Questionnaire [FABQ]), which is a very significant risk factor, was *not* used in the multivariate analyses. Thus, fear avoidance appears to have overlapped with other psychosocial variables and did not increase predictive power.

INTERPRETING RESEARCH RESULTS

Although the results of many epidemiological studies into the relationship between psychological factors and pain may appear straightforward, we must take several precautions before drawing conclusions. Some are particular to psychological variables, while others hold true for the entire field of the epidemiology of pain. Since many clinicians and researchers who read and evaluate these studies are not psychologists, interpretations are sometimes clouded by unfamiliarity with the variables involved.

The results of epidemiological studies that use psychosocial variables should be interpreted with great consideration and caution. Several easily made errors may render the conclusion invalid. These errors are related to the issues described above such as overlap in terms, measurement issues, and study design. The likelihood of misinterpreting results may be reduced by considering the following points.

First, we must consider the purpose of the study in relation to the psychological variables employed. Some studies may have few or no measures of the subject under investigation. Caution is warranted if the purpose of the study is primarily to look at relationships other than psychosocial ones. Tagging psychological variables onto a study may be enticing, but it seldom yields clear results because of a lack of theoretical underpinnings, and an absence of high-quality measurements. Furthermore, researchers must specify the time the psychological variable is assessed in relation to the outcome (pain). For example, prospective or longitudinal studies measure the psychological variable and evaluate outcome at a specified follow-up time; these designs are stronger than cross-sectional studies. Some studies may combine several designs, and although this may be acceptable, it is vital for readers to be aware of the nature of the design when interpreting the results.

Second, we must analyze the definition of the psychological entity to determine if it is unique, clear, and operational. This is especially important in drawing conclusions and in the choice of terms used to describe any relationships found. Third, we must study the measurement methods. They should fulfill the basic requirements of reliability and validity so that the results are reproducible. Fourth, we must evaluate possible interrelationships, i.e., overlap in the variables assessed.

One particular caution, noted earlier, is the interrelationship among measures of different terms and concepts. As psychological factors often represent a type of exposure in the classic epidemiological study, errors in measurement may have undesirable consequences. For example, true differences in a psychological factor may not be detected if the measurement technique does not adequately isolate that factor. Moreover, the interrelationship may be misrepresented in the conclusions, because an instrument purporting to measure one entity in fact may also measure a related factor. One study may conclude that depression is important while the next concludes that catastrophizing is the main variable, when in fact these measures share considerable overlap. Studies with strong designs often have several measures and are prospective; they usually assist the reader in evaluating potential intercorrelations by presenting their data in the results section. Intercorrelations may influence the terms used in the conclusions section. Whether the entity is called anxiety, coping, or somatic distress may largely depend on the authors of the article, rather than on the data!

An especially important aspect, true for all research, is the design of the investigation. Psychosocial variables are often investigated in cross-sectional studies that are correlational in nature. This means that statements about causality are definitely premature. Results show a relationship or correlation but say little about why the relationship exists. Nevertheless, such findings may or may not support a given hypothesis; this is a far cry from proving the hypothesis or showing causality. Longitudinal and prospective studies follow developments over time, and are better able to isolate causal relationships. The design of the study is vital in determining what kinds of conclusions may be safely made, and we recommend making bold attempts and timid claims.

An important distinction concerns whether the relationship is correlational or causative. Certain designs such as cross-sectional studies cannot discern whether a relationship is causal, because the data may be correlational and the true cause may be a third variable that was not studied. Prospective designs shed light on causation, but may not be definitive. For example, job satisfaction was related to back pain injury reports in the Boeing study, where over 3000 workers took part in a comprehensive evaluation of workers and their work conditions and were then followed for about 4 years for reported back injuries (Bigos et al. 1991). The results show powerful evidence of job dissatis-

faction before any injury occurred, and reveal that job dissatisfaction may be related to the "causal" factor, for example repetitive work or poor self-efficacy, or multiple causes. Moreover, as back pain is recurrent, the pain may have been triggered by another variable before the measurement of job satisfaction. Thus, job satisfaction might be related to reporting an injury, but not necessarily to the pain.

Correlational data may be the cornerstone of epidemiological studies (especially those with cross-sectional designs), which raises the issue of interpreting the size of the correlation. Significance tests are of little help, since significance involves the reliability of the correlation and does not directly indicate its magnitude. If self-ratings are used to assess the psychological factor, we need to determine how the outcome variable, e.g., pain, was assessed. Bias introduced when the same person rates the risk variable and the outcome variable may inflate the size of the correlation. Similarly, the distinction between the risk variable and outcome should be considered, since an interrelationship may be built into the definitions. A high correlation between catastrophizing (risk variable) and depression (outcome) would be expected, for example, because catastrophizing is part of the definition of depression. The number of correlations calculated and the number of participants should be noted, as the probability of obtaining significant correlations increases with the number of participants. The most frequent error in interpreting correlations is to assume that a strong correlation means a causal relationship. Correlations are difficult to interpret, and the strength of correlation needed to be relevant is often greater than supposed.

Contrary to many traditional areas where epidemiological methods have been employed, identifying a psychological risk factor does not automatically lead to a treatment or prevention procedure. Identifying a chemical risk factor for cancer, for example, may result in direct interventions that are designed to reduce exposure levels. Psychological variables do not necessarily work in this way. Identifying anxiety as a risk factor does not mean that an intervention may be directly implemented. Although relaxation exercises might be attempted, there is no assurance that these will succeed, in part because the relationship may not be causal. Some psychological risk factors, furthermore, may not be readily changed, as in the case of IQ levels, trait anxiety, job satisfaction, self-efficacy, or personality disorders.

"Blaming the victim" is an easy trap to fall into. Observers may see the pain sufferer as having personal responsibility for the psychological "risk" variable, such as being depressed or having the belief that activity will increase pain, rather than seeing that variable as a consequence of some factor of environmental origin or the action of another person. Blaming the victim may be a convenient way of relegating the problem back to the patient, but appears to be harmful in that the cause of the "risk" factor may not be identified, not to mention the ill-will this attitude may create.

Both authors and readers are often tempted to draw conclusions or make implications not firmly supported by the data. Thus, it is wise to study the article carefully and draw your own conclusions rather than to rely on the face value of the author's conclusions.

SUMMARY

What then is the role of psychology in epidemiological pain research? This question might be answered by briefly reviewing some of the main contributions a psychological view may add to our understanding of pain. As epidemiology strives to study not only the prevalence of pain problems, but also their causes and remediation, we believe that the field of psychology offers a host of knowledge that may compliment, enrich, and expand our understanding of pain. We will outline some of the main areas where psychology may further contribute to the epidemiology of pain.

An important basic contribution is understanding the individual's pain perception and behavior. This is a pliable process where psychological variables are believed to influence the chain of events, from attending to the stimulus, to interpreting the meaning of the pain, to emotional and behavioral reactions. Learning principles enable us to understand how the setting or environment may affect pain responses and the cognitive processes involved. Thus, we may describe how patients with specified pain conditions react emotionally and behaviorally, and we may also obtain insight as to why they react that way. Moreover, this approach provides an understanding of the reciprocal action between psychological states and pain perception.

A second contribution is that a psychological view enhances a holistic conception of pain. For example, a psychological approach may help explain the relationship between physiological, behavioral, and cognitive and emotional aspects of pain. It emphasizes the reciprocal nature of the relationship, showing that pain may influence mood, but mood may also affect pain perception. Consequently, psychological theory helps us to capture the dynamics of pain perception and behavior, and such variables may provide new insights.

This contribution is closely related to a third, namely the relationship between the individual and his or her environment. Psychological factors appear to be instrumental in explaining how environmental factors affect pain perception and behavior, which helps us to determine how a given situation influences our perception of pain. For example, upon arrival at the emergency department, patients have been observed to experience considerable pain relief before any treatment has been provided (Melzack et al. 1982). We can better understand the effect of the environment by considering the social, cognitive, and emotional aspects of the situation together with the medical factors.

In a similar vein, a psychological perspective may explain the patient's reactions in specific contexts, particularly the doctor-patient relationship. In epidemiological studies, the relationship between the patient and his or her work and family situation may also be strongly related to the pain problem under study.

Indeed, psychology may offer a unique way to deal with categories like age, gender, and ethnicity, that are typically employed in epidemiological pain research. Rather than simply looking at the relationship between age and a given pain state, we might assess the process of aging in relation to pain perception. Thus, a decrease in reported pain among senior citizens would take on a different light if it were associated with general changes in perception due to "aging." In other words, a psychological approach may help us explain *why* a particular "category" responds in a specific way.

Turk (1997) maintains that a psychological perspective may help meet the challenge of explaining *why* and not just *who* suffers from a particular pain problem. Consequently, psychology may play an important role in epidemiological research, as it provides a model of pain perception and behavior. The model applied to modern research strategies may help find answers to the how and why of pain epidemiology.

REFERENCES

Abbott FV, Gray-Donald K, Sewitch MJ, et al. The prevalence of pain in hospitalized patients and resolution over six months. *Pain* 1992; 50:15–28.

Anastasi A. *Psychological Testing.* New York: McMillan, 1988.

Anderson KO, Dowds BN, Pelletz RE, Edwards WT, Peeters-Asdourian C. Development and initial validation of a scale to measure self-efficacy beliefs in patients with chronic pain. *Pain* 1995; 63:77–84.

Asmundson GJG, Kuperos JN, Norton GR. Do patients with chronic pain selectively attend to pain-related information? Preliminary evidence for the mediating role of fear. *Pain* 1997; 72:27–32.

Bandura A. Self-efficacy mechanisms in physiological activation and health promoting behavior. In: Madden J (Ed). Neurobiology of learning, emotion and affect. New York: Raven Press, 1991, pp 229–269.

Barlow JH, Williams B, Wright CC. Improving arthritis self-management among older adults: "Just what the doctor didn't order." *Br J Health Psychol* 1997; 2:175–186.

Becker RE. Zung Self-Rating Depression Scale. In: Hersen M, Bellack AS (Eds). Dictionary of behavioral assessment techniques. New York: Pergamon Press, 1988, pp 497–499.

Bigos SJ, Battié MC, Spengler DM, et al. A prospective study of work perceptions and psychosocial factors affecting the report of back injury. *Spine* 1991; 16:1–6.

Blalock SJ, De Vellis BMG, De Vellis RF. Social comparisons among individuals with Rheumatoid Arthritis. *J Appl Social Psychol* 1989; 19:665–680.

Block AR, Kremer EF, Gaylor M. Behavioral treatment of chronic pain: the spouse as a discriminative cue for pain. *Pain* 1980; 9:243–252.

Bongers PM, de Winter CR, Kompier MA, Hildebrandt VH. Psychosocial factors at work and musculoskeletal disease. *Scand J Work Environ Health* 1993; 19:297–312.

Bradley LA. Cognitive-behavioral therapy for chronic pain. In: Gatchel RJ, Turk DC (Eds). *Psychological Approaches to Pain Management: a Practitioner's Handbook.* New York: Guilford Press, 1996, pp 131–147.

Buckelew SP, Murray SE, Hewett JE, Johnson J, Huyser B. Self-efficacy, pain and physical activity among fibromyalgia subjects. *Arthritis Care and Research* 1995; 8:43–50.

Burton AK, Tillotson KM, Main CJ, Hollis S. Psychosocial predictors of outcome in acute and subchronic low back trouble. *Spine* 1995; 20:722–728.

Corey DT, Etlin D, Miller PC. A home-based pain management and rehabilitation program: an evaluation. *Pain* 1987; 29:218–229.

Cronbach LJ. *Essentials of Psychological Testing.* New York: Harper and Row, 1984.

Crook J, Rideout E, Browne G. The prevalence of pain complaints in a general population. *Pain* 1984; 18:299–314.

DeGood DE, Shutty MS. Assessment of pain beliefs, coping and self-efficacy. In: Turk DC, Melzack R (Eds). *Handbook of Pain Assessment.* New York: Guilford Press, 1992, pp 214–234.

Donovan M, Dillon P, McGuire L. Incidence and characteristics of pain in a sample of medical-surgical inpatients. *Pain* 1987; 30:69–78.

Dura JR, Beck SJ. A comparison of family functioning when mothers have chronic pain. *Pain* 1988; 35:79–89.

Dworkin SF, Whitney CW. Relying on objective and subjective measures of chronic pain: guidelines for use and interpretation. In: Turk DC, Melzack R (Eds). *Handbook of Pain Assessment.* New York: Guilford Press, 1992, pp 429–446.

Edwards PW, Zeichner A, Kuczmierczyk AR, Boczkowski J. Familial pain models: the relationship between family history and current pain experience. *Pain* 1985; 21:379–384.

Egan KJ, Beaton R. Responses to symptoms in healthy low utilizers of the health care system. *J Psychosom Res* 1987; 31:11–21.

Engel CC, Von Korff M, Katon WJ. Back pain in primary care: predictors of high health-care costs. *Pain* 1996; 65:197–204.

Feuerstein M, Zastowny TR. Occupational rehabilitation: multidisciplinary management of work-related musculoskeletal pain and disability. In: Gatchel R, Turk DC (Eds). *Psychological Approaches to Pain Management: a Practitioner's Handbook.* New York: Guilford Publications, 1996, pp 458–485.

Flor H, Turk DC, Rudy TE. Relationship of pain impact and significant other reinforcement of pain behaviors: the mediating role of gender, marital status and marital satisfaction. *Pain* 1989; 38:45–50.

Flor H, Birbaumer N, Turk DC. The psychobiology of chronic pain. *Advances in Behavioral Research and Therapy* 1990; 12:47–84.

Fordyce WE. *Behavioral Methods for Chronic Pain and Illness.* St. Louis, MO: Mosby, 1976.

Fordyce WE (Ed). *Back Pain in the Workplace: Management of Disability in Nonspecific Conditions.* A report of the Task Force on Pain in the Workplace of the IASP. Seattle: IASP Press, 1995.

Gamsa A. Is emotional disturbance a precipitator or a consequence of chronic pain? *Pain* 1990; 42:183–195.

Gatchel RJ, Turk DC. *Psychological Approaches to Pain Management: a Practitioner's Handbook.* New York: Guilford Press, 1996, p 519.

Greenley JR, Mechanic D. Social selection in seeking help for psychological problems. *J Health Soc Behav* 1976; 17:249–262.

Holzman AD, Turk DC, Kerns RD. The cognitive-behavioral approach to the management of chronic pain. In: Holzman AD, Turk DC (Eds). *Pain Management: a Handbook of Psychological Treatment Approaches.* New York: Pergamon, 1986, pp 31–50.

Ingham JG, Miller PM. Symptom prevalence and severity in a general practice population. *J Epidemiol Community Medicine* 1979; 33:191–198.

Jensen I, Nygren Å, Gamberale F, Goldie I, Westerholm P. Coping with long-term musculoskeletal pain and its consequences: is gender a factor? *Pain* 1994; 57:167–172.

Jensen MP, Turner JA, Romano JM, Karoly P. Coping with chronic pain: a critical review of the literature. *Pain* 1991; 47:249–283.

Johnson PA, Goldma L, Orav EJ, et al. Gender differences in the management of acute chest pain: support for the Yentl syndrome. *J Gen Intern Med* 1996; 11:209–217.

Karoly P. *Measurement Strategies in Health Psychology.* New York: John Wiley & Sons, 1985.

Kazdin AE. *Research Design in Clinical Psychology.* New York: Harper and Row, 1980.

Keefe FJ, Blumenthal JA. *Assessment Strategies in Behavioral Medicine.* New York: Grune and Stratton, 1982.

Keefe FJ, Williams DA. Pain behavior assessment. In: Turk DC, Melzack R (Eds). *Handbook of Pain Assessment.* New York: Guilford Press, 1992, pp 275–294.

Keefe FJ, Kopel S, Gordon SB. *A Practical Guide to Behavioral Assessment.* New York: Springer, 1978.

Keefe FJ, Brown C, Scott DS, Ziesat H. Behavioral assessment of chronic pain. In: Keefe FJ, Blumenthal JA (Eds). *Assessment Strategies in Behavioral Medicine.* New York: Grune and Stratton, 1982, pp 321–350.

Kerns RD, Haythornthwaire J, Sothwick S, Giller EL. The role of marital interaction in chronic pain and depressive symptom severity. *J Psychosom Res* 1990; 34:401–408.

Kerns RD, Payne A. Treating families of chronic pain patients. In: Gatchel RJ, Turk DC (Eds). *Psychological Approaches to Pain Management: A Practitioner's Handbook.* New York: Guilford Press, 1996, pp 283–304.

Kleinman AR. *The Illness Narratives: Suffering, Healing and the Human Condition.* New York: Basic Books, 1988.

Klenerman L, Slade PD, Stanley IM, et al. The prediction of chronicity in patients with an acute attack of low back pain in a general practice setting. *Spine* 1995; 20:478–484.

Lackner JM, Carosella AM, Feuerstein M. Pain expectancies, pain and functional self-efficacy expectancies as determinants of disability in patients with chronic low back disorders. *J Consult Clin Psychol* 1996; 64:212–220.

Lethem J, Slade PD, Troup JDG, Bentley G. Outline of a fear-avoidance model of exaggerated pain perceptions. *Behav Res Ther* 1983; 21:401–408.

Levin JB, Lofland KR, Cassisi JE, Poreh AM, Blonsky ER. The relationship between self-efficacy and disability in chronic low back pain patients. *Int J Rehab Health* 1996; 2:19–28.

Linton SJ. The role of psychological factors in back pain and its remediation. *Pain Reviews* 1994; 1:231–243.

Linton SJ, Melin L, Götestam KG. Behavioral analysis of chronic pain and its management. *Prog Behav Modif* 1984; 18:1–42.

Linton SJ, Bradley LA, Jensen I, Spangfort E, Sundell L. The secondary prevention of low back pain: a controlled study with follow-up. *Pain* 1989; 36:197–207.

Lorig K, Holman HR. Long-term outcomes of an arthritis self-management study: effects of reinforcement efforts. *Soc Sci Med* 1989; 29:221–224.

Lorig K, Konkol L, Gonzalez V. Arthritis patient education: a review of the literature. *Patient Education and Counselling* 1987; 10:207–252.

Lorig K, Seleznick M, Lubeck D, Ung E, Shoor S, Holman HR. The beneficial outcome of the arthritis self-management course are not adequately explained by behavior change. *Arthritis Rheum* 1989; 32:91–95.

Lorig K, Mazonson PD, Holman HR. Evidence suggesting that health education for self-management in patients with chronic arthritis has sustained health benefits while reducing health care costs. *Arthritis Rheum* 1993; 36:439–446.

Magni G, Caldieron C, Rigatti-Luchini S, Merskey H. Chronic musculoskeletal pain and depressive symptoms in the general population: an analysis of the First National Health Survey data. *Pain* 1990; 43:299–307.

Main CJ, Wood PLR, Hollis S, Spanswick CC, Waddell G. The distress and risk assessment method: a simple patient classification to identify distress and evaluate the risk of poor outcome. *Spine* 1992; 17:42–52.

Manne SL, Zautra AJ. Spouse criticism and support: their association with coping and psychological adjustment among women with rheumatoid arthritis. *J Pers Soc Psychol* 1989; 56:608–617.

McDowell I, Newell C. *Measuring Health: a Guide to Rating Scales and Questionnaires.* Oxford: Oxford University Press, 1987.

Melzack R, Wall PD. Pain mechanisms: a new theory. *Science* 1965; 150:971–979.

Melzack R, Wall PD. *The Challenge of Pain.* New York: Basic Books, 1982.

Melzack R, Wall PD, Ty TC. Acute pain in an emergency clinic: latency of onset and descriptor patterns related to different injuries. *Pain* 1982; 14:33–42.

Nunnally JC. *Introduction to Psychological Measurement.* New York: McGraw-Hill, 1970.

Palinkas, LA. Techniques of psychosocial epidemiology. In: Karoly P (Ed). *Measurement Strategies in Health Psychology.* New York: John Wiley & Sons, 1985, pp 49–114.

Quadrel MJ, Lau RR. A multivariate analysis of adolescents' orientations towards physician use. *Health Psychol* 1990; 9:750–773.

Raftery KA, Smith-Coggins R, Chen AH. Gender-associated differences in emergency department pain management. *Ann Emerg Med* 1995; 26:414–421.

Romano J, Turner JA, Friedman LS, et al. Sequential analysis of chronic pain behaviors and spouse responses. *J Consult Clin Psychol* 1992; 60:777–782.

Romano JM, Turner JA. Chronic pain and depression: does the evidence support a relationship. *Psychol Bull* 1985; 97:18–34.

Rose MJ, Klenerman L, Atchinson L, Slade PD. An application of the fear-avoidance model to three chronic pain problems. *Behav Res Ther* 1992; 30:359–365.

Rosenstiel AK, Keefe FJ. The use of coping strategies in chronic low back pain patients: relationships to patient characteristics and current adjustment. *Pain* 1983; 17:33–44.

Schwartz L, Slater MA, Birchler G, The role of pain behaviors in the modulation of marital conflict in chronic pain couples. *Pain* 1996; 65:227–233.

Skevington SM. A standardized scale to measure beliefs about controlling pain (BPCQ): a preliminary study. *Psychology and Health* 1990; 4:221–232.

Skevington, SM. Depression and causal attributions in the early stages of a chronic painful disease: a longitudinal study of early synovitis. *Psychology and Health* 1993; 8:51–64.

Skevington SM. The relationship between pain and depression: a longitudinal study of early synovitis. In: Gebhart GF, Hammond DL, Jensen TS (Eds). *Proceedings of the 7th World Congress on Pain.* Progress in Pain Research and Management, Vol. 2. Seattle: IASP Press, 1994, pp 201–210.

Skevington SM. *Psychology of Pain.* London: Wiley, 1995.

Steer RA, Beck AT. Beck Depression Inventory. In: Hersen M, Bellack AS (Eds). *Dictionary of Behavioral Assessment Techniques.* New York: Pergamon Press, 1988, pp 44–46.

Sternbach RA. Pain and hassles in the United States: findings of the Nuprin Pain Report. *Pain* 1986; 27:69–80.

Streiner DL, Norman GR. Health measurement scales: a practical guide to their development and use. Oxford: Oxford University Press, 1996.

Sullivan MJL, Bishop SR, Pivik J. The Pain Catastrophizing Scale: development and validation. *Psychological Assessment* 1995; 7:524–532.

Suls J, Fletcher B. The relative efficacy of avoidant and non-avoidant coping strategies: a meta-analysis. *Health Psychol* 1985; 4:249–288.

Swanson DW, Maruta T. Patients complaining of extreme pain. *Mayo Clin Proc* 1980; 55:563–566.

Swanson DW, Maruta T, Wolff VA. Ancient pain. *Pain* 1986; 25:383–387.

Telles JL, Pollack MH. Feeling sick: the experience and the legitimation of illness. *Soc Sci Med* 1981; 15a:243–251.

Thompson SC. Will it hurt less if I can control it? A complex answer to a simple question. *Psychol Bull* 1981; 90:89–101.

Turk DC. Biopsychosocial perspective on chronic pain. In: Gatchel RJ, Turk DC (Eds). *Psychological Approaches to Pain Management: a Practitioner's Handbook.* New York: Guilford Press, 1996, pp 3–32.

Turk DC. The role of demographic and psychosocial factors in transition from acute to chronic pain. In: Jensen TS, Turner JA, Wiesenfeld-Hallin Z (Eds). *Proceedings of the 8th World Congress on Pain,* Progress in Pain Research and Management, Vol. 8. Seattle: IASP Press, 1997, pp 185–213.

Turk DC, Kerns RD. Assessment in health psychology. In: Karoly P (Ed). *Measurement Strategies in Health Psychology.* New

York: John Wiley & Sons, 1985, pp 335–372.

Turk DC, Melzack R. *Handbook of Pain Assessment.* New York: Guilford Press, 1992.

Turk DC, Flor H, Rudy TE. Pain and families I: etiology, maintenance and psychosocial impact. *Pain* 1987; 30:3–27.

Twaddle AC. Sickness and sickness career: some implications. In: Eisenberg L, Kleinman A (Eds). *The Relevance of Social Science for Medicine.* Reidel Publications, 1980, pp 111–133.

Unruh A. Gender variations in clinical pain experience. *Pain* 1996; 65:123–167.

Violon A, Giurgea D. Familial models for chronic pain. *Pain* 1984; 18:199–203.

Vlaeyen JWS, Kole-Snijders AMJ, Boeren RGB, van Eek H. Fear of movement/(re)injury in chronic low back pain and its relation to behavioral performance. *Pain* 1995; 62:363–372.

Von Korff M. Perspectives on management of back pain in primary care. In: Gebhart GF, Hammond DL, Jensen TS (Eds). *Proceedings of the 7th World Congress on Pain*, Progress in Pain Research and Management, Vol. 2. Seattle: IASP Press, 1994, pp 97–110.

Von Korff M, Simon GE. The relationship between pain and depression. *Br J Psychiatry* 1996; 168:101–108.

Von Korff M, Wagner EH, Dworkin SF, Saunders KW. Chronic pain and use of ambulatory health care. *Psychosom Med* 1991; 53:61–79.

Waddell G, Newton M, Henderson I, Somerville D, Main CJ. A Fear-Avoidance Beliefs Questionnaire (FABQ) and the role of fear-avoidance beliefs in chronic low back pain and disability. *Pain* 1993; 52:157–168.

Weir R, Browne G, Tunks E, Gafni A, Roberts J. Gender differences in reports of chronic pain. *Clin J Pain* 1996; 12:277–290.

Zarkowska E, Philips HC. Recent onset vs persistent pain: evidence for a distinction. *Pain* 1986; 25:365–372.

Correspondence to: Steven J. Linton, PhD, Department of Occupational and Environmental Medicine, Örebro Medical Center Hospital, Örebro 70185, Sweden. Fax: 46-19-120-404; email: steven.linton@orebroll.se.

Epidemiology of Pain, edited by
I.K. Crombie, IASP Press, Seattle, © 1999.

5

Gender Considerations in the Epidemiology of Chronic Pain

Linda LeResche

Department of Oral Medicine, School of Dentistry, University of Washington, Seattle, Washington, USA

BASIC CONSIDERATIONS

This chapter reviews the epidemiological literature on age- and sex-specific rates of several of the most prevalent persistent pain conditions. Although some of these data appear in other chapters in this volume, this review evaluates whether the data support the notion of universal gender differences in the prevalence of pain, or whether gender differences are confined to particular pain conditions. Where age and gender differences are observed, we hope to stimulate thinking on possible reasons for these differences.

Much discussion has occurred concerning use of the terms "sex" and "gender," with some suggesting that "sex" be used to refer to biological aspects of the person (e.g., the presence of two X chromosomes vs. one X and one Y chromosome) and "gender" to refer to the person's psychosocial identity. Others suggest the use of more complex terms such as "gender-linked" and "sex-correlated" (Deaux 1985; Gentile 1993; Unger and Crawford 1993). Epidemiology has traditionally used terms like "sex ratio" and "sex-specific rates," although data identifying the respondent's sex are usually gathered by self-report (and arguably could be called data on gender by the strict definition stated above). Because we are interested in how both biological and psychosocial aspects of maleness and femaleness can affect pain, the terms "sex" and "gender" will be used interchangeably in this chapter.

Epidemiology, as traditionally defined, is the study of the distribution, determinants, and natural history of disease in populations (Lilienfeld and Lilienfeld 1980). Although epidemiology has traditionally fo- cused on well-defined diseases, the tools of epidemiology are being increasingly employed to study conditions such as pain and other symptomatic problems where the definition of who is a case is based on self-report, or a combination of self-report and clinical findings (Gordis 1988). While most pain researchers and clinicians are probably aware that epidemiology is useful for assessing the magnitude and burden on society of pain conditions, some may not be aware that epidemiological studies can also provide important clues concerning etiology (Morris 1975) and factors that contribute to the persistence of pain. As a case in point, the epidemiological data on patterns of chronic pain prevalence by gender suggest a number of hypotheses concerning possible reasons for gender differences that could be tested directly through basic and clinical research.

As we have discussed in a previous publication (Dworkin et al. 1992), three important perspectives are inherent in the definition of epidemiology: the population perspective, the developmental perspective, and the ecological perspective. In pain research, the population perspective implies that to understand the full spectrum of pain problems, pain conditions must be studied in entire populations, not only in persons seeking treatment. The relevance of the population perspective for understanding gender differences in pain is that for many conditions (including some pain problems) women with the condition are more likely to seek care than are men (Unruh 1996). For example, in secondary and tertiary care settings providing treatment for temporomandibular disorder (TMD) pain, the ratio of female to male patients ranges from about 5:1

to 9:1 (Bush et al. 1993), whereas in the community the ratio of prevalence in women versus men is only about 2:1 (LeResche 1997). Thus, treated patients represent a different fraction of cases in the population for each gender, and different factors may operate in women and men that influence the probability of seeking treatment. Data drawn only from clinic populations are thus likely to present an incomplete or even biased picture of gender factors related to pain.

The developmental perspective suggests that studying pain across the life cycle is essential because factors influencing a specific pain condition may vary with age. Thus, it is too simplistic to merely ask whether there are gender differences in the prevalence of a given pain condition, as the gender-specific prevalence may vary significantly with age (e.g., the probability of experiencing migraine headache may be similar for boys and girls at age 12, whereas a 30-year-old woman is much more likely than a 30-year-old man to experience this kind of pain). Data presented in this chapter will emphasize the importance of integrating the developmental perspective with a focus on gender factors in pain.

Finally, epidemiologists take an ecological approach toward the development and maintenance of a condition; disease agents, characteristics of the host, and environmental factors are all important in whether and how a condition manifests itself in a given person. This perspective is similar to the biopsychosocial perspective on pain (Engel 1960), which suggests that pain results from the dynamic interaction of biological, psychological, and social factors. Clearly, men and women not only differ in some aspects of biological and psychological processes, but also experience different socialization processes. Further, men and women are exposed to different risk factors for pain due to their differing occupational and social roles. When gender differences in pain are identified, the ecological perspective is heuristic for interpreting these differences and providing hypotheses for further study (e.g., of the range of possible associated risk factors).

This chapter will review population-based data concerning age- and gender-specific prevalence rates for a range of common chronic pain conditions. (Few studies address incidence of pain conditions.) We will discuss possible reasons for the observed differences from the developmental and ecological perspectives.

With gender-specific prevalence data, it is important to remember the fundamental relationships among prevalence, incidence, and duration in a steady-state population (prevalence = incidence × mean duration); that is, the number of cases in the population at any given time is a function not only of the rate at which new cases occur, but also how long the condition typically lasts. Most common pain conditions follow a chronic-recurrent course. For these types of conditions, the number of cases in the population at a given time (that is, prevalence) is a product of the incidence or onset rate, the number of episode recurrences, and the average episode duration (Von Korff and Parker 1980; Von Korff 1992). Thus, if we see a higher prevalence rate of a specific pain condition in one sex, that difference may be due to a higher onset rate, a higher probability of recurrence, a longer episode duration, or some combination of these components.

POSSIBLE SOURCES OF GENDER DIFFERENCES IN PAIN

What is it about being female, or about being male, that can influence the various components of prevalence? Because pain is a multidimensional experience, if we see sex differences in the prevalence or manifestations of chronic pain, differences could be occurring at several levels. Perhaps men and women have anatomical or physiological differences in the neural systems that transmit or modify pain signals (Gear et al. 1996; Berkley 1997). Men and women may differ in perceptual apparatus or perceptual styles (Fillingim and Maixner 1995), in their cognitive and emotional experiences of pain, and in their approaches to coping with pain, i.e., pain appraisal (Unruh 1996). The sexes may also vary in their pain behaviors. For epidemiological studies, the issues of willingness to report pain and how the differential socialization of males and females can influence pain report are especially important, as self-report is a primary source of data for the pain epidemiologist (LeResche 1995). Finally, the social and occupational roles of men and women differ, and those roles may present different risks for developing and maintaining pain. Societal expectations for the person in pain within the context of the family, the workplace, the welfare system, and the health care delivery system also differ by gender (e.g., Crook 1993). Most likely, differences operate simultaneously at several levels to influence the prevalence patterns of pain.

From a developmental perspective, it is clear that biological, psychological, and social factors may vary for both men and women at different points in the life cycle. Fig. 1 depicts just a few of the important biological, psychological, and social changes across the life cycle that may influence pain experience and pain behavior. Many of these life cycle changes may appear obvious, but all too frequently, gender differences are considered only in terms of biological differences, and not in a broader psychological and social context. For example, both boys and girls go through puberty, but after puberty women have monthly menstrual cycles that provide a set of physiological signals that are not experienced by men. These physiological signals (sometimes painful) could have a sensitizing effect on pain perception (Berkley 1997) or result in behavioral and social role responses (e.g., taking medication, staying in bed) that can generalize to other types of pain. To give another example, although not every woman bears children, this opportunity for pain experience is unique to women. In Western society both genders generally undergo similar phases of education followed by employment and retirement, but the specific types of educational and occupational experiences for men and women still differ to some degree. Fig. 1 could be elaborated with the addition of the social roles of parenthood, the changes in the perceptual system with age, and so on. The figure simply reinforces the point that when we think of a person of a particular age and sex, we are dealing with a whole range of biological, psychosocial, and environmental variables.

DATA ON AGE- AND SEX-SPECIFIC PAIN PREVALENCE PATTERNS

This section reviews sex-specific prevalence rates for selected pain conditions across the adult age span. In keeping with the epidemiological perspectives mentioned earlier, data are presented only for studies based on random samples of defined populations, rather than particular occupational groups or clinic attendees. Unruh (1996) has provided a more comprehensive review encompassing clinical as well as population studies. A similar analysis of the prevalence of specific pain conditions by age in children could be illuminating; see Goodman and McGrath (1991) for a review of the epidemiology of pain conditions in children and adolescents. The systematic format for presenting data from various studies is an attempt to make sense of the patterns of prevalence for men and women across

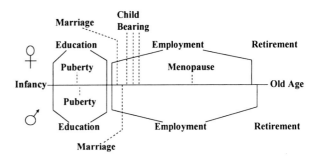

Fig. 1. Some major life cycle events that may affect the experience of pain in men and women.

the life cycle. Different authors have used different case definitions and sampling approaches and studied somewhat different age groups. For these methodological reasons, the absolute prevalence rates may differ. Presenting the classification of pain conditions by prevalence pattern is an attempt to encourage consideration of similarities and differences among pain conditions and to raise awareness of possible risk factors that may vary by age and gender. The classification of these prevalence patterns represents my own scheme and was not generally the initial intent of the authors of reviewed studies.

BACK PAIN

Back pain is one of the most common pain conditions in adults. Fig. 2 shows back pain prevalence data from four population-based studies. Data for men are designated by a solid line and those for women by a dashed line. In an epidemiological study of a health maintenance organization (HMO) population in Seattle (Von Korff et al. 1988), respondents were asked to report pains occurring in the last 6 months that had lasted at least a day and were not fleeting or minor. Fig. 2a shows that back pain prevalence in this population was higher among women at younger ages and increased steadily with age in men. For persons aged 45–64, the prevalence rate for men exceeded that of women, whereas rates for both sexes were similar after age 65.

In contrast, a study of 2667 persons aged 20–60 from small towns and rural areas in Great Britain (Walsh et al. 1992, Fig. 2b) found back pain prevalence rates to be higher in young men than in young women. Rates held steady or increased only very slightly for men with age, but fluctuated with age for women in the age group studied.

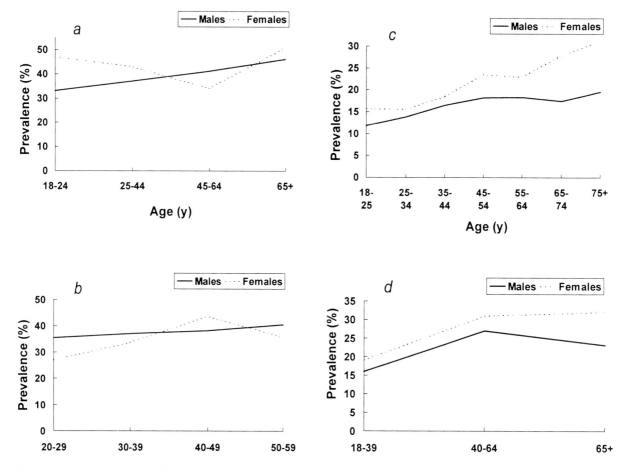

Fig. 2. Age- and sex-specific prevalence of back pain in adults. Data are from four population-based studies in North America and Great Britain. Note the different prevalence periods (1 month to 1 year) and age groupings used in the four studies. (a) Six-month prevalence of back pain in Seattle, Washington, USA ($n = 1016$); from Von Korff et al. (1988). (b) One-year prevalence of back pain in rural Great Britain ($n = 2667$); adapted from Walsh et al. (1992). (c) One-month prevalence of back pain in Great Britain ($n = 9003$); from Croft and Rigby (1994). (d) One-month prevalence of back pain in Great Britain ($n = 34,141$); from Wright et al. (1995).

Two other studies in Great Britain were consistent in finding slightly higher back pain prevalence rates in women than in men at all ages. One of these studies inquired into "problems with a bad back" in a household sample taken all over Great Britain, and found an increasing prevalence rate with age for both sexes up to age 64 (Croft and Rigby 1994, Fig. 2c). The other study (Wright et al. 1995, Fig. 2d) asked about the presence of "sciatica, lumbago, or recurring backache" in the past year. More than 34,000 persons in northwest England were surveyed. Rates rose in men from ages 18–39 to ages 40–64 and dropped slightly over age 65. For women, rates also increased from ages 18–39 to ages 40–64, but held steady thereafter.

A few epidemiological studies of back pain have

focused exclusively on the elderly. Although all these studies are consistent in finding higher rates of back pain among women than among men, the reported age-specific prevalence patterns differ from study to study. For example, in a study of rural elderly in Iowa (Lavsky-Shulan et al. 1985), prevalence showed a general decline with age, whereas a study of cohorts of 70-year-olds, 75-year-olds, and 79-year-olds in Göteborg, Sweden (Bergström et al. 1986) found the highest rates for women at age 75, but the lowest rates among men aged 75. An investigation of Hong Kong residents over age 70 (Woo et al. 1994) found stable rates for women and rising rates for men with age. Thus, it is interesting that, at least on first analysis, the data for the most prevalent and one of the most

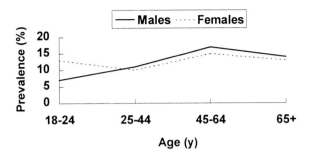

Fig. 3. Age- and sex-specific 6-month prevalence of chest pain in an HMO population in Seattle, Washington, USA (*n* = 1016). From Von Korff et al. (1988).

disabling pain conditions appear to be contradictory and to present no clear, consistent pattern across the studies reviewed. Urban-rural differences, socioeconomic, occupational, and cohort differences may be so powerful for back pain that the influences of age and gender on prevalence are difficult to discern (Walsh et al. 1992; Croft and Rigby 1994).

CHEST PAIN

There are few epidemiological studies of chest pain per se. Although there is some research on the prevalence of angina symptoms (Jensen 1984; Harris and Weissfeld 1991), these studies inquire into the experience of symptoms across the lifetime, rather than at a specific point in time. One investigation in an HMO population in Seattle (Von Korff et al. 1988) that inquired more broadly into the experience of chest pain in the past 6 months found that prevalence rates were higher in younger women and in older men, albeit only slightly (Fig. 3). Although this is only a single study, replication of this pattern would raise the interesting question of which factors might be operating in the lives of men and women at various ages to produce this pattern.

JOINT PAIN

Fig. 4a shows the age- and gender-specific pattern for knee joint pain from a large epidemiological study in the North of England (Lawrence et al. 1966); Fig. 4b presents data for finger joint pain from the same study. Although the patterns are not identical, both curves show a general increase in prevalence across the adult life span in both men and women;

after about age 50, the curves for women and men diverge, with higher prevalence in women.

ABDOMINAL PAIN

In contrast to the conditions so far reviewed, the prevalence of abdominal pain in both sexes appears to decrease with age. The data for abdominal pain shown in Fig. 5a come from a study of large cohorts of subjects aged 30, 40, 50, and 60 in Copenhagen County, Denmark (Kay et al. 1994). Subjects were asked to report only gastrointestinal pain; menstrual pain was excluded. The percentage of women with abdominal pain was higher than the percentage of men with abdominal pain for all the ages studied, but pain prevalence decreased with age in both sexes.

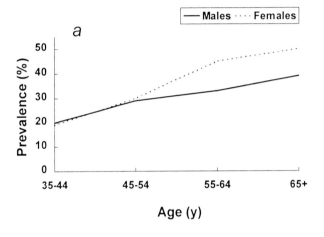

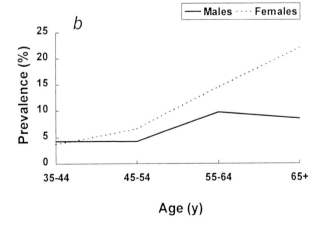

Fig. 4. Age- and sex-specific 1-week prevalence of pain, (a) in the knee joint and (b) in the finger joints in a large population-based study (*n* = 2292) in the North of England. From Lawrence et al. (1966).

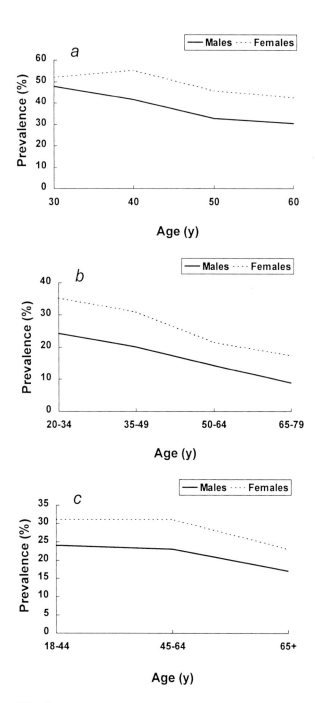

Fig. 5. Age- and sex-specific 1-year prevalence of abdominal pain in three population-based studies. Although the age groupings used are somewhat different, a similar pattern of higher rates for women and generally declining prevalence with age is found in all three studies. (a) Prevalence of abdominal pain in Copenhagen, Denmark (*n* = 3608); from Kay et al. (1994). (b) Prevalence of mid-abdominal pain in Östhammar, Sweden (*n* = 1290); from Agréus et al. (1994) . (c) Prevalence of abdominal pain in Howard City, Maryland, USA (*n* = 6199); from Adelman et al. (1995).

Another recent Scandinavian study conducted in rural areas and small towns in the municipality of Östhammar, Sweden, looked at pain by region of the abdomen (Agréus et al. 1994). The pattern for mid-abdominal pain (Fig. 5b) again shows a female predominance at all ages, but declining rates with age in both men and women. Prevalence rates for pain in the upper and lower abdomen, not presented here, showed similar patterns.

Finally, a study conducted in a large HMO population in Howard County, Maryland (Adelman et al. 1995, Fig. 5c) again resulted in prevalence rates showing the same pattern of higher rates in women, with declining prevalence with age. Thus, the available data on the prevalence of abdominal pain by age and sex appear highly consistent and show a higher prevalence for women than for men across the life span, with prevalence rates declining with age for both sexes.

HEADACHE AND MIGRAINE

Another common complaint that occurs at somewhat higher rates in women than in men, and appears to decline in prevalence with age, is headache. Chapter 13 presents a meta-analysis of numerous studies of the epidemiology of headache. Fig. 3 of that chapter includes an age- by sex-specific prevalence curve that suggests an almost unchanging prevalence rate across the adult life cycle for men (at about 60% of the population), and a curve for women that is relatively flat (with prevalence about 75–80%) until about age 45, when rates decline. By about age 60, prevalence rates for men and women appear similar. This curve summarizes studies using different definitions of headache; particularly for males, case definition explained much of the variability in prevalence rates. It is possible that prevalence curves based on studies that use different case definitions for specific types of non-migraine headaches (e.g., for tension-type headache) could show a somewhat different pattern (e.g., Rasmussen et al. 1991).

In contrast to the pattern for other types of headache, numerous epidemiological studies of migraine in a variety of cultures have replicated the finding of a clear bell-shaped curve for age-specific prevalence in both sexes, with rates rising over the reproductive years and declining after age 40 (see Stewart et al. 1994 for a review). As shown in Fig. 1 of Chapter 13, rates for women are substantially higher than for men at all adult ages.

TEMPOROMANDIBULAR DISORDER PAIN

Another set of pain conditions that follows the same age- by sex-specific prevalence pattern as migraine is pain in the muscles of mastication or the temporomandibular joint—TMD pain. Data from the Seattle study (Von Korff et al. 1988) shown in Fig. 6 indicate a peak in the 25–44 age range and a steep decline with age, again with higher prevalence in women across the entire adult life span. Other recent prevalence studies, including one in Toronto (Locker and Slade 1988) and one in Québec (Goulet et al. 1995), show a similar pattern.

CHRONIC WIDESPREAD PAIN AND FIBROMYALGIA

Chronic widespread pain is defined by the standardized criteria of the American College of Rheumatology (ACR) (Wolfe et al. 1990) as pain of longer than 3 months' duration in two contralateral quadrants of the body. Using these criteria Croft et al. (1993) surveyed a sample of persons enrolled in two general practices in Cheshire, England, in an area that included both a suburb of Manchester and a rural town. Prevalence data, based on the 1340 survey respondents, are shown in Fig. 7a. For men, rates of chronic widespread pain rose until about age 65, dropped in those 65–74 years of age, and then rose again in the very elderly. For women, the shape of the curve was similar, although the first prevalence peak appeared at a younger age for women than for men. For all the ages surveyed, except ages 55–64, prevalence rates were substantially higher for women than for men.

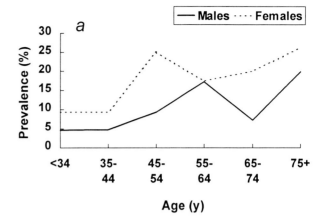

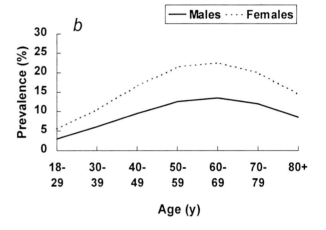

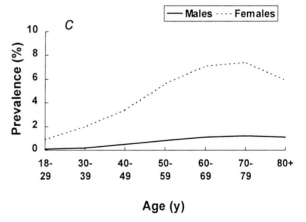

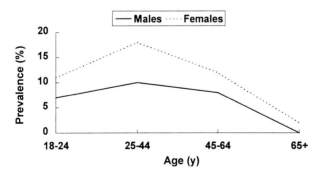

Fig. 6. Age- and sex-specific 6-month prevalence of temporomandibular pain in an HMO population in Seattle, Washington, USA (*n* = 1016). Rates for women peak in the 25–44-year-old age group. From Von Korff et al. (1988).

Fig. 7. Age- and sex-specific rates of chronic widespread pain and fibromyalgia from population studies in Britain and the United States. (a) Point prevalence of chronic widespread pain in Cheshire, United Kingdom (*n* = 1340); from Croft et al. (1993). (b) Point prevalence of chronic widespread pain in Wichita, Kansas, USA (logistic model, crude weighted rates, *n* = 3006); adapted from Wolfe et al. (1995). (c) Three-month prevalence of fibromyalgia in Wichita, Kansas (*n* = 3006); adapted from Wolfe et al. (1995).

Fig. 7b shows data from a community survey of 3006 persons from randomly selected households in Wichita, Kansas (Wolfe et al. 1995); this survey used the same case definition for chronic widespread pain as did the work by Croft et al. (1993). Unlike the data presented in the other figures in this chapter, which are strictly sample-based, the data in Fig. 7b represent weighted rates, based on the age-gender distribution of the Wichita population. The crude weighted rates were then smoothed using a logistic model. Fig. 7b shows prevalence rates that were consistently higher for women than for men, and rose across the adult life span through age 69, but dropped off in the very elderly. Thus, considering the difference in analytic methods, the age and gender patterns of chronic widespread pain for the two studies shown in Figs. 7a and 7b display some similarities. Rates in young adulthood are on the order of 5% in men and 10% in women. In middle age, the rates begin to rise fairly steeply, especially for women. However, the pattern found for the elderly differs in the two studies, with the British study showing rising rates after age 74 and the U.S. study showing falling rates. Nevertheless, both studies are consistent in finding higher rates in women than in men. Because neither study had a large sample in the very oldest age group, the discrepancy could be due to the unreliability of the estimates for persons over age 75.

In addition to studying chronic widespread pain, Wolfe et al. (1995) followed up a sample of respondents to assess how many met ACR examination criteria for fibromyalgia (i.e., the presence of pain on palpation in at least 11 of 18 designated body sites, and chronic widespread pain, as illustrated in Fig. 2 of Chapter 9). The resulting age- and sex-specific prevalence curve, weighted and smoothed, as in Fig. 7b, shows a pattern similar to Wolfe's prevalence data for chronic widespread pain, although the absolute rates are lower and the gender difference is more dramatic for fibromyalgia (Fig. 7c).

SUMMARY AND DISCUSSION

The data presented in this chapter suggest that there is not a simple relationship between gender and the occurrence of pain. Patterns differ from condition to condition, and gender-specific prevalence for most conditions varies across the life cycle. Although for most body sites women are more likely than men to report pain, this is not the case for every condition at every stage of life. For back pain, the available data are not consistent with regard to the prevalence by gender and age. Definitive information on chest pain is also lacking, not due to inconsistent results but to the paucity of epidemiological studies of chest pain per se.

For other pain conditions, however, the age- and sex-specific prevalence patterns are more clear. Joint pain, chronic widespread pain, and fibromyalgia all appear to *increase* in prevalence with age in both genders at least up to around age 65, and all show higher prevalence in women than in men. Abdominal pain also consistently shows higher prevalence in women than in men but *decreases* in prevalence with age. The prevalence of nonmigrainous headache also appears to decrease somewhat with age, at least in women. Finally, migraine headache and TMD are substantially more common in women than in men and appear to follow a bell-shaped curve, which peaks in the reproductive years.

Although there are clearly prevalence differences related to age, most of the common pain conditions reviewed here show a general pattern of at least somewhat higher prevalence in women than in men. These generally higher rates may be due to a higher biological sensitivity to stimuli; women may detect signals that men might not notice. At a cognitive level, the threshold for labeling stimuli as painful might be lower for women than for men. Another factor may be a social difference in the upbringing of boys and girls, which makes it more acceptable for women to report the experience of pain. There is some empirical support for all these hypothesized factors (Unruh 1996; Berkley 1997), and it is quite likely that biological, psychological, and social factors are all operating to some degree to produce the observed prevalence differences.

The pattern of increasing pain prevalence with age, such as that shown for joint pain, chronic widespread pain, and fibromyalgia, suggests either progressive, degenerative conditions (which are known to be relevant in at least some instances), or possibly the accumulation of cases in the population with age. Studies of pain incidence, in addition to pain prevalence, would be necessary to untangle the relative importance of these factors. Given that at least some data suggest a possible decline of these conditions among the very elderly (Bergström et al. 1986; Wolfe et al. 1995), it appears important to investigate whether persons with these conditions recover over time or are at increased risk for disability or even mortality, which removes them from community populations as they age.

In contrast, abdominal pain and headache (at least in women) show a consistent pattern of declining prevalence with age. It is intriguing to consider what biological or psychological changes associated with aging might be *protective* against the occurrence or continuation of these conditions. Likely candidates for investigation might be life stress or work-related factors. It is also possible that some abdominal pain is referred pain of gynecological origin (Giamberardino et al. 1997), which might be expected to diminish with age.

The pattern of prevalence for migraine and TMD pain suggests a possible relationship to factors that are present in young adulthood into middle age but are less common in the elderly. Hormonal factors have for some time been postulated as possible risk factors for migraine (e.g., Somerville 1972; Stewart et al. 1991), and recent evidence suggests the possible role of hormonal factors in TMD (LeResche et al. 1997; Dao et al. 1998). Interestingly, both the excellent incidence data available for migraine (Chapter 13) and the more limited data available for TMD suggest that both these conditions are rather uncommon in children and that incidence rates rise sharply beginning at puberty, further strengthening the possibility of a pain-hormone relationship. Of course, it is possible—even likely—that psychological as well as biological factors associated with life cycle changes also influence the onset and maintenance of these pain conditions (LeResche 1997). In any case, the unusual prevalence pattern of these pain problems raises a number of hypotheses regarding possible risk factors that could be further investigated not only with epidemiological methods, but also through basic and clinical research.

In conclusion, a review of the epidemiological literature indicates definite age by sex differences in the prevalence of many chronic pain conditions. Little information is available to shed light on whether these prevalence differences are due to different incidence rates, different probabilities of recurrence, or different durations of pain (or some combination of these factors) for women and men. However, a systematic examination of the epidemiological data may be an important step in helping pain researchers of all kinds to generate hypotheses in our search for a better understanding of chronic pain in both sexes.

ACKNOWLEDGMENTS

During the preparation of this chapter the author was supported in part by NIH Grant No. DE08773. Portions of this work have been previously presented at the NIH Office of Research on Women's Health Seminar Series (March 1998) and the NIH Conference on Gender and Pain (April 1998).

REFERENCES

Adelman AM, Revicki DA, Magaziner J, Hebel R. Abdominal pain in an HMO. *Fam Med* 1995; 27:321–325.

Agréus L, Svardsudd K, Nyren O, Tibblin G. The epidemiology of abdominal symptoms: prevalence and demographic characteristics in a Swedish adult population. *Scand J Gastroenterol* 1994; 29:102–109.

Bergström G, Bjelle A, Sundh V, Svanborg A. Joint disorders at ages 70, 75 and 79 years—a cross-sectional comparison. *Br J Rheumatol* 1986; 25:333–341.

Berkley KJ. Sex differences in pain. *Behav Brain Sciences* 1997; 20:371–380.

Bush FM, Harkins SW, Harrington WG, Price DD. Analysis of gender effects on pain perception and symptom presentation in temporomandibular pain. *Pain* 1993; 53:73–80.

Croft PR, Rigby AS. Socioeconomic influences on back problems in the community in Britain. *J Epidemiol Community Health* 1994; 48:166–170.

Croft PR, Rigby AS, Boswell R, Schollum J, Silman A. The prevalence of chronic widespread pain in the general population. *J Rheumatol* 1993; 20:710–713.

Crook J. Comparative experiences of men and women who have sustained a work related musculoskeletal injury. *Abstracts: 7th World Congress on Pain.* Seattle: IASP Publications, 1993, pp 293–294.

Dao TTT, Knight K, Ton-That V. Modulation of myofascial pain by reproductive hormones: a preliminary report. *J Prosthet Dent* 1998; 79:663–670.

Deaux K. Sex and gender. *Annu Rev Psychol* 1985; 36:49–81.

Dworkin SF, Von Korff M, LeResche L. Epidemiologic studies of chronic pain: a dynamic-ecologic perspective. *Ann Behav Med* 1992; 14:3–11.

Engel G. A unified concept of health and disease. *Perspect Biol Med* 1960; 3:459–485.

Fillingim RB, Maixner W. Gender differences in the responses to noxious stimuli. *Pain Forum* 1995; 4:209–221.

Gear RW, Miaskowski C, Gordon NC, et al. Kappa-opioids produce significantly greater analgesia in women than in men. *Nature Medicine* 1996; 2:1248–1250.

Gentile DA. Just what are sex and gender anyway? A call for a new terminological standard. *Psychological Science* 1993; 2:120–122.

Giamberardino MA Berkley KJ, Iezzi S, de Bigontina P, Vecchiet L. Pain threshold variations in somatic wall tissues as a function of menstrual cycle, segmental site and tissue depth in non-dysmenorrheic women, dysmenorrheic women and men. *Pain* 1997; 71:187–197.

Goodman JE, McGrath PJ. The epidemiology of pain in children and adolescents: a review. *Pain* 1991; 46:247–264.

Gordis L. Challenges to epidemiology in the next decade. *Am J Epidemiol* 1988; 128:1–9.

Goulet J-P, Lavigne GJ, Lund JP. Jaw pain prevalence among French-speaking Canadians in Quebec and related symptoms of temporomandibular disorders. *J Dent Res* 1995; 74:1738–1744.

Harris RB, Weissfeld LA. Gender differences in the reliability of reporting symptoms of angina pectoris. *J Clin Epidemiol* 1991; 44:1071–1078.

Jensen G. Epidemiology of chest pain and angina pectoris: with special reference to treatment needs. *Acta Med Scand* 1984; (Suppl) 682:1–120.

Kay L, Jorgensen T, Jensen KH. Epidemiology of abdominal symptoms in a random population: prevalence, incidence, and natural history. *Eur J Epidemiol* 1994; 10:559–566.

Lavsky-Shulan M, Wallace RB, Kohout FJ, et al. Prevalence and functional correlates of low back pain in the elderly. *J Am Geriatr Soc* 1985; 33:23–28.

Lawrence JS, Bremner JM, Bier F. Osteo-arthrosis: prevalence in the population and relationship between symptom and x-ray changes. *Ann Rheum Dis* 1966; 25:1–23.

LeResche L. Gender differences in pain: epidemiologic perspectives. *Pain Forum* 1995; 4:228–230.

LeResche L. Epidemiology of temporomandibular disorders: Implications for the investigation of etiologic factors. *Crit Rev Oral Biol Med* 1997; 8:291–305.

LeResche L, Saunders K, Von Korff M, Barlow W, Dworkin SF. Use of exogenous hormones and risk of temporomandibular disorder pain. *Pain* 1997; 69:153–160.

Lilienfeld AM, Lilienfeld DE. *Foundations of Epidemiology,* 2nd ed. New York: Oxford University Press, 1980.

Locker D, Slade G. Prevalence of symptoms associated with temporomandibular disorders in a Canadian population. *Community Dent Oral Epidemiol* 1988; 16:310–313.

Morris JN. *Uses of Epidemiology,* 3rd ed. Edinburgh: Churchill Livingstone, 1975.

Rasmussen BK, Jensen R, Schroll M, Olesen J. Epidemiology of headache in a general population—a prevalence study. *J Clin Epidemiol* 1991; 44:1147–1157.

Somerville BW. The influence of progesterone and estradiol upon migraine. *Headache* 1972; 12:93–102.

Stewart WF, Linet MS, Celentano DD, Van Natta M, Ziegler D. Age- and sex-specific incidence rates of migraine with and without visual aura. *Am J Epidemiol* 1991; 134:1111–1120.

Stewart WF, Shechter A, Rasmussen BK. Migraine prevalence: A review of population-based studies. *Neurology* 1994; 44(Suppl 4):S17–S23.

Unger RK, Crawford M. Sex and gender: the troubled relationship between terms and concepts. *Psychological Science* 1993; 2:122–124.

Unruh AM. Gender variations in clinical pain experience. *Pain* 1996; 65:123–167.

Von Korff M. Epidemiologic and survey methods: chronic pain assessment. In: Turk DC, Melzack R (Eds). *Handbook of Pain Assessment.* New York: Guilford Press, 1992, pp 391–408.

Von Korff M, Parker RD. The dynamics of the prevalence of chronic episodic disease. *J Chron Dis* 1980; 33:79–85.

Von Korff M, Dworkin SF, LeResche L, Kruger A. An epidemiologic comparison of pain complaints. *Pain* 1988; 32:173–183.

Walsh K, Cruddas M, Coggon D. Low back pain in eight areas of Britain. *J Epidemiol Community Health* 1992; 46:227–230.

Wolfe F, Smythe HA, Yunus MB, et al. The American College of Rheumatology 1990 criteria for the classification of fibromyalgia. *Arthritis Rheum* 1990; 33:160–172.

Wolfe F, Ross K, Anderson J, Russell IJ, Herbert L. The prevalence and characteristics of fibromyalgia in the general population. *Arthritis Rheum* 1995; 38:19–28.

Woo J, Ho SC, Lau J, Leung PC. Musculoskeletal complaints and associated consequences in elderly Chinese aged 70 years and over. *J Rheumatol* 1994; 21:1927–1931.

Wright D, Barrow S, Fisher AD, Horsley SD, Jayson MIV. Influence of physical, psychological and behavioural factors on consultations for back pain. *Br J Rheumatol* 1995; 34:156–161.

Correspondence to: Linda LeResche, ScD, Department of Oral Medicine, School of Dentistry, University of Washington, Seattle, WA 98195, USA. Fax: 206-685-8412; email: leresche@u.washington.edu.

Epidemiology of Pain, edited by
I.K. Crombie, IASP Press, Seattle, © 1999.

6

Cross-Cultural Investigations of Pain

Rod Moore[a,b] and Inger Brødsgaard[a,c]

[a]*Department of Oral Medicine, School of Dentistry, University of Washington, Seattle, Washington, USA;*
[b]*Department of Oral Epidemiology and Public Health, Aarhus University, Aarhus, Denmark; and*
[c]*Social Medicine Division, Municipality of Aarhus, Denmark.*

Cultural background or ethnicity has been investigated as to whether it is a predictive variable for descriptions of pain types, reactions to pain, coping strategies, and expected levels of suffering or disability related to pain. This chapter reviews the literature for studies that compare pain phenomena across different nations and cultural backgrounds, including meta-analytic reviews of some pain types.

Exchange of knowledge about diagnostic and therapeutic successes or failures can be facilitated by examining pain descriptions and normative coping strategies and treatments that are universal across cultural beliefs and health care systems. An example would be studying criteria for required or accepted dosage of narcotics for cancer pain, because practices for decreasing pain or improving the quality of life of cancer patients vary from nation to nation (Brasseur et al. 1993; Cleeland 1993a,b; Foley 1993; Zenz 1993). Also, by identifying unique, culture-specific pain and treatment phenomena, relevant case studies from that particular culture can provide a base of knowledge about similar symptoms or treatments that might be useful in other cultural contexts where the treatment concepts were previously unknown. An example of the latter is the "discovery" by Western medicine and proliferation of acupuncture and other paradigms of traditional Chinese medicine (Geiger 1975; Kleinman 1975, 1987; Kleinman and Kunstadter 1975; Koch-Weser 1975). Finally, from an epidemiological research perspective, cross-cultural population studies examining ethnic groups present a natural control situation due to variations in attitudes and beliefs about pain, coping, and suffering (Kleinman 1978;

Kleinman et al. 1978; Fabrega 1989; Moore 1996). Besides variations in pain beliefs, there are also variations in normative social values, such as child-raising practices, social welfare in welfare and nonwelfare states, differences in response of medical health care systems to acute or chronic ailments, and availability of health insurance or worker's compensation. In the past, some epidemiologists may have labeled such social factors as confounders. But in reality, they are all potential research variables that require careful consideration in any population studies involving measures of pain and suffering. To improve the validity and reliability of results, studies that make comparisons across cultural or national boundaries often call upon the expertise of social scientists skilled in the use of qualitative social science research methods.

This review describes studies that make direct cross-cultural comparisons within the same study protocol (Table I). This review of cross-cultural pain studies will also draw on results of major national epidemiological studies that appear to support or refute results of the cross-cultural studies; these national studies are not included in the table.

Finally, this chapter will review complex issues involving philosophy of science, pain semantics, diagnostic categories, and methodological problems. Opinions on these issues vary across cultures, as do the criteria and descriptive contexts within which pain, coping, treatment, and disability are defined. This discussion will form the basis for recommendations and methodological suggestions for future cross-cultural studies.

In exploring the literature, we did comprehensive

MEDLINE searches from 1966 to 1998. The literature described appeared in searches on the subject heading "Pain" and key word "epidemiology," the subject heading "Crosscultural-Comparison" and key word "pain," the subject heading "Ethnicity" and key word "pain," and country searches such as "China" or "Chinese" and key words "pain" and "epidemiology." Where possible, we used PubMed from the National Library of Medicine to conduct "related records" searches using important studies as a guide to other similar studies. PsychINFO searches were only productive under the subject heading "Crosscultural-Differences" and key word "pain." Key-word searches using "pain" were productive on the databases "Anthropological Literature 1984 to present" and "Sociofile 1974 to present." Bibliographies from literature derived from the above searches were also sources.

CROSS-CULTURAL COMPARISONS OF PAIN, PAIN REACTIONS, AND PAIN COPING

A steadily increasing number of studies are making direct attempts to compare pain prevalences, characteristics, or related phenomena across cultures or different nations. Almost none of these studies apply random sampling criteria, a common approach in epidemiological sampling for prevalence studies that hope to be representative. Some publications described below and in Table I are direct prospective comparisons and some are quasi-epidemiological or meta-analytic comparisons. Others are aggregate pain topic reviews that hint at meta-analysis. Clinical or anthropological studies are also presented if they relate thematically or heuristically to future possible representative studies. Most studies described below are summarized in Table I by article reference, kind of pain, sample, type of study, and critical summary of findings.

CANCER PAIN

Cleeland and colleagues in a prospective study (1996) investigated how cultural and linguistic backgrounds affect relationships among ratings reported by patients with metastatic cancer. They primarily studied the pain's interference with such functions as activity, mood, and sleep, which in turn can be related to pain severity and effective pain management. Mul-

tidimensional scaling (MDS) was used to analyze ratings of pain interference from a sample consisting of four culturally and linguistically different groups from the United States ($n = 1106$), France ($n = 324$), the Philippines ($n = 267$), and China ($n = 146$). Patients all completed the Brief Pain Inventory (BPI) (Cleeland and Ryan 1994), a self-report measure of pain severity, pain description, and pain interference. For each of these samples, MDS solutions consistently revealed two interpretable dimensions—affect and activity. These dimensions were also consistently interpretable across three levels of pain severity (mild, moderate, and severe) for all four samples. The dimensions were most prominent when pain was moderate, rather than mild (i.e., when little interference was produced) or severe (i.e., when highly affected by interference). Besides their utility in studying the epidemiology of pain and associated factors, the authors felt these dimensions would also be useful in clinical assessment to describe different patterns of pain interference that can predict effectiveness of pain management. The BPI has been translated from English to other languages, including Chinese (Wang et al. 1996), French, Filipino, Italian (Caraceni et al. 1996), Vietnamese (Cleeland et al. 1988), and Hindi.

Using an epidemiological process, given the sample sizes, Cleeland and colleagues have emphasized in their global assessment the need to find standard ways to evaluate difficult cancer pain management questions. However, local differences exist in attitudes toward pain, suffering, death, and dying, and their questionnaire may not have captured such differences when attempting to measure the subjective aspects of pain and its management. Although the authors claimed similarities across ethnic groups, an alternative explanation might be that the way item choices were translated from English may have led to the globally consistent but potentially artifactual results. Much as with translated versions of the McGill Pain Questionnaire (MPQ) (Melzack 1975) discussed below, the sections of the BPI requiring response to pain descriptors or activities translated from English may not include the most important and meaningful descriptors or activities from the native language of the respondent in non-English-speaking samples. We would expect more variation in responses from such diverse cultures with different customs, social traditions, and religions. Cleeland and colleagues (1996) were aware that "different item pools" could have been selected, depending on specific aims of a particular study. Another concern is that in the push to improve cancer pain management for standardization of cancer pain treatment outcomes, a cultural bias may favor North American values regarding criteria set as a standard for acceptable treatment. Certainly relief from the "total pain" of terminal cancer is an important humanitarian cause. But selection of variables and data collection aimed at specific universal outcomes for prescribed political solutions to cancer pain management problems could potentially contribute misinformation as to true needs as perceived by patients and affected family members within specific social contexts. For example, ethnospecific investigations might find that some patients and family members would prefer that the patient suffer more pain during the final days rather than to compromise social interaction because of drug-induced incoherent mental states.

In just such an anthropological qualitative study, Kodiath and Kodiath (1995) conducted an in-depth case comparative study of 10 Caucasian Americans and 10 natives of India with chronic malignant cancer pain. Unlike the survey study of Cleeland and colleagues (1996) that sought universal truths about cancer pain and pain behavior, this study used topic-focused, open-ended interviews in an effort to understand how ethnicity might affect cancer pain reactions and treatments. Patients studied in each culture experienced a noticeable difference in the degree of pain, which was mainly related to availability of treatment resources. However, the most important finding was that the report of pain quality or intensity was not proportional to the quality of life and the meaning found in the pain experience for each patient. While Indian patients lacked morphine or codeine, and by Western standards Indian physicians lacked knowledge about management of cancer pain, these patients appeared to handle suffering differently than American cancer patients. Indian patients experienced a spiritual dimension, a feeling of a higher good, and a belief in "life after death." With adequate morphine resources, although their physicians were often reluctant to prescribe them, American patients were more concerned with pain as the feared symbol of their demise and as punishment for circumstances that may have contributed to their terminal illness. An ethnospecific pain study by Pugh (1991) about the semantics of pain in Indian culture corroborates Kodiath and Kodiath's understanding of Indian concepts of suffering. Although results of such a small qualitative study raise questions as to generalizability from an epidemiological

perspective, the richness of nuance and sense of internal validity gained from such data indicate that other paradigms of "truth" may be worth considering in this kind of research, depending on the aims of the particular cross-cultural study.

Another qualitative study by Pfefferbaum and colleagues (1990) also sought to determine whether cultural heritage and acculturation influence the perception and expression of pain and anxiety in relation to cancer pain. The study was based on interviews, self-report scales, and observation of differences or similarities in reactions of 35 Anglo-American and 43 Hispanic children with cancer who were undergoing invasive procedures (spinal tap or bone marrow transplant). These patients, aged 3 to 15, were matched by age, gender, diagnosis, and duration of illness. Observations included evaluation of the pain and reactions by parents and care givers, although these groups were not described. A meaningful and significant inverse association between age and observed and reported distress was noted in both ethnic groups. The Anglo-American and Hispanic children had remarkably similar behavioral responses. Hispanic parents, however, reported significantly higher levels of anxiety than did Anglo-American parents. This study combined the best aspects of matched epidemiological design and qualitative descriptive method. However, generalizations to other ethnic groups or to types of pain may be limited given that the children were suffering from various forms and stages of cancer and that some were in remission and others were not.

Although based on widely divergent methodological approaches, the qualitative studies of Kodiath and Kodiath (1995) and Pfefferbaum and colleagues (1990) and the global cross-cultural cancer pain survey studies by Cleeland and colleagues (1994, 1996) all showed that health professionals and policy makers need to focus on the experience of pain and its effect on the quality of life in cancer patients and to consider patient beliefs about pain, suffering, and disability. A recent article reached a similar conclusion about the need for more research about ethnic influences on outcomes in nursing management of cancer pain (Gordon 1997). Although the qualitative studies lacked sufficient numbers for epidemiological representativeness, they provided evidence that understanding of the social factors allowed some generalization about reactions to cancer pain within the cultural contexts studied. These methodological issues will be further discussed at the end of the chapter.

Table I

Summarized descriptions of cross-cultural investigations of pain, pain reactions, and coping (see footnotes for explanation of abbreviations)

Reference	Kind of Pain	Samples Studied	Type of Study Design	Summary of Findings
Cancer Pain				
Cleeland et al. 1996	Cancer pain	USA $(n = 1106)$ France $(n = 324)$ Philippines $(n = 267)$ China $(n = 146)$ $N = 1843$	*Epidemiological:* Prospective global epidemiological study of psychosocial variables related to cancer pain using BPI (a self-report measure of pain and its interference with function). Samples not matched.	Nonconventional epidemiological methods to study pain interference among cancer populations. MDS revealed the scale to be sensitive to two dimensions, *affect* and *activity*, but only when pain was of moderate severity.
Kodiath and Kodiath 1995	Cancer pain	India $(n = 10)$ USA $(n = 10)$ $N = 20$	*Qualitative:* Focused open-ended interviews (qualitative case study research) using matched samples.	Significant difference in degree of pain experienced due to resource availability. Report of pain was not proportional to quality of life and meaning of pain.
Pfefferbaum et al. 1990	Cancer pain in children	Anglo-Americans $(n = 43)$ Hispanics $(n = 35)$ $N = 78$	*Qualitative/Epidemiological:* Self-report scales (STAI for anxiety), interviews, and observations. Matched samples by age, gender, diagnosis, and illness duration.	Looked at pain and reactions to pain of invasive procedures among child cancer patients and their parents. Found similar, universal reactions among children, but ethnospecific reactions among parents.
Headache				
Chen 1993	Headache	Adults versus children; reviewed studies including over 65,000 subjects from North and South America, Europe, Asia, and Africa	*Literature review:* Used "aggregate pain topic review" data tables (1937–1987) for comparison of headache studies. (No references listed.)	Migraine prevalence, children 7% to adults 11.5%. More than 60% of patients report severe headache consistently across nations, females reporting greater frequency and severity than males. Sensory descriptors and effective language describing headache were consistent across nations.
Ziegler 1990	Headache	Adults and children (aggregate subject number not tallied)	*Literature review:* Descriptive comparison (1947–1989); no aggregate tabling.	Western samples had similar prevalence rates that decreased with age; rates increased with age in Asian studies. More common in women in general and urban dwellers in Chinese studies. Concluded that comparisons were difficult due to lack of definition of headache syndromes and epidemiological methodologies.
Back Pain				
Lau et al. 1995	Low back pain (LBP)	Hong Kong ($n = 652$ Chinese: 364 women, 288 men) compared with Britain ($n = 2667$ English: 1495 women, 1172 men)	*Quasi-epidemiological:* Meta-analysis of prevalence and characteristics of LBP. Interview replication study of Walsh et al. (1992) for Chinese sample (4 y later). Walsh used a mailed epidemiological survey in eight areas of Britain.	Of Chinese subjects, 39% reported having LBP at some time compared to British 58%; 21% had LBP in the past 12 mo while British had 36%. Lower LBP prevalence in Hong Kong than Britain was partly explained by differences in stature and occupational lifting.
Walsh et al. 1992		$N = 3319$		

Table I
Continued

Reference	Kind of Pain	Samples Studied	Type of Study Design	Summary of Findings
Back Pain (continued)				
Carron et al. 1985	Chronic LBP	USA $(n = 198)$ New Zealand $(n = 117)$ $N = 315$	*Epidemiological:* Matched age and gender samples for comparison of impact of psychosocial factors on disability including economic compensation at 1 y follow-up.	Patients from both countries that received pretreatment compensation were less likely to return to full activity, esp. for U.S. patients (55% participation in follow-up). There is some evidence for differences in cultural beliefs about suffering and compensation.
Volinn (1997)	LBP	Countries with Low income $(n = 19,734)$ High income $(n = 13,583)$ $N = 33,317$	*Literature review:* Meta-analytical comparisons of LBP prevalences.	LBP is 2–4 times more prevalent in high-income countries (e.g., Sweden, Germany, Belgium) than low (Nigeria, south China, Indonesia, Philippines). Indications are that increasing rates are due to urbanization and rapid industrialization. Questions the methodologies behind disparity in rates within high/low categories of countries.
Volinn et al. 1996 (abstract)	Chronic LBP	Washington State (USA), Sweden, and Japan labor force statistics	*Epidemiological:* Meta-analytical study of LBP and rates of compensation claims. (Swedish rates were not limited to work-related claims.)	The rate of wage compensation claims for LBP for Washington State in 1992 was 45 times higher than for Japan and in 1991, 8 times lower than for Sweden.
Waluyo et al. 1996	Musculo-skeletal pain (mostly LBP)	Swedish workers $(n = 326)$ Indonesians $(n = 136)$ $N = 462$	*Epidemiological:* Prospective study on occupationally matched samples of industrial workers for comparison of impact of work environment factors on musculoskeletal symptoms, stress, and psychosomatic symptoms.	Musculoskeletal symptoms were high in frequency for both groups. Swedes rated working conditions worse and had higher prevalence of stress and psychosomatic symptoms. Indonesians were more satisfied with fewer symptoms.
Nelson et al. 1996	Chronic musculo-skeletal pain (mostly chronic LBP)	U.S. Caucasian $(n = 204)$ African Americans $(n = 55)$ Hispanic Americans $(n = 36)$ $N = 295$	*Epidemiological:* Prospective study using MMPI F scale and demographically matched ethnic samples (no controls).	Compared by MMPI basic validity and clinical scale patterns of subjects. Found that despite higher rates of pain among whites and Hispanics, African Americans tested with more psychologically disturbed functions from their chronic pain. Most differences were demographic or sample explanatory (years of education, duration of pain).
Strassberg et al. 1992	Chronic back pain	Australia $(n = 610$: 180 women; 430 men) USA $(n = 112)$ (from 1981) (74 women; 38 men) $N = 722$	*Quasi-epidemiological:* MMPI with previous U.S. MMPI data from Strassberg et al. (1981).	Australians' mean MMPI profiles corresponded closely to U.S. chronic pain patients. No data were tabled on the U.S. subjects; 11 y had elapsed.

(continued)

Table I
Continued

Reference	Kind of Pain	Samples Studied	Type of Study Design	Summary of Findings
Back Pain (continued)				
Brena et al. 1990	Chronic LBP	USA (pain $n = 10$, control $n = 10$) Japan (pain $n = 11$, control $n = 11$) $N = 42$	*Epidemiological:* SIP (Bergner et al. 1981) and a Medical Examination Protocol. Control subjects used in case-control matching study.	Both groups had similar medical-physical findings, but the Japanese were significantly less impaired in psychological, social, vocational, and avocational functioning.
Sanders et al. 1992	Chronic LBP	USA, Japan, Mexico, Colombia, Italy, New Zealand distributed equally ($N = 63$ chronic pain patients, $N = 63$ controls) $N = 126$	*Epidemiological:* SIP, standard Medical Examination and Diagnostic Information Coding system. Control subjects used in case-control matching study.	Patients from USA, New Zealand, and Italy reported significantly more self-perceived impairment in psychological, social, vocational, and avocational functioning, with Americans the most dysfunctional. Authors discuss possible cross-cultural differences in personal expectations, financial gains, and expectations about usage, type, and availability of health care.
Bates et al. 1995	Chronic LBP (majority), arthritis pain, neurological pain	Puerto Ricans mean age = 60 ($n = 100$) Anglo-Americans mean age = 44 ($n = 100$) $N = 200$	*Qualitative:* Focused open-ended interviews (qualitative case study research) using samples of 6 Anglo-Americans and 6 Puerto Ricans; no selection strategy reported. Quantitative data on all subjects using English and Spanish versions of MPQ.	Reported cultural differences in adaptation to chronic pain by beliefs, psychosocial support, age, SES, coping style, health care systems, economic compensation, and health insurance. Higher pain intensity, more emotion were reported in Puerto Ricans, but no differences between interference in daily activities.
Bates and Rankin 1994	Same as above	Same as above	*Qualitative:* Focused open-ended interviews plus LOC questionnaire.	Patients' LOC style and ethnicity affected reported chronic pain intensity. LOC style may vary at different stages in the chronic pain "career."
Childbirth Labor Pain				
Pesce 1987	Labor pain	Australians ($n = 22$) Italians ($n = 10$) Australians/Italians ($n = 8$) $N = 40$	*Epidemiological:* Prospective study with MPQ (Melzack 1975) PPI and Numbers of Words Chosen. English MPQ descriptors are translated into Italian (no validation).	No significant differences in pain description found among groups. Author concludes there are no pain differences.
Morse 1989	Labor pain	Births observed $N = 32$ Fiji Islanders ($n = 16$) Fijian Indians ($n = 16$) Questionnaires $N = 140$ Fiji Islanders ($n = 67$) Fijian Indians ($n = 73$)	*Qualitative:* Focused open-ended interviews with nurses or "wise women" in preparation for questionnaire construction. Observation of 32 live births. Questionnaires for samples of 140.	Fijians viewed traditional caring patterns as a valid replacement for hospital care, whereas the wish to conceal pregnancy delayed antenatal care among Fijian Indians, who showed exaggerated pain reactions. Results could be explained by lower "education" of Fijian Indians about pregnancy and labor, but the women were expected to be ignorant within their ethnic context.

Table I
Continued

Reference	Kind of Pain	Samples Studied		Type of Study Design	Summary of Findings
Childbirth Labor Pain (continued)					
Weisenberg and Caspi 1989	Labor pain	Middle Eastern Western	($n = 53$) ($n = 30$) $N = 83$	*Epidemiological:* Prospective study with VAS pain intensity scale, behavioral observation ratings, extroversion scale. Looked at pain beliefs and behaviors by education and ethnicity. Matched cases.	All rated pain as high, but Middle Eastern women rated pain higher and showed more pain behavior, especially if lower education level. Groups had same coping styles.
Dental Pain					
Moore et al. 1998b	Tooth-drilling and labor pain	Anglo-Americans Chinese Swedes Danes	($n = 122$) ($n = 123$) ($n = 49$) ($n = 46$) $N = 340$	*Epidemiological:* Prospective study with psychometric questionnaire on ethnic pain beliefs. Age-, occupation-, and gender-matched samples across cultures.	Ethnic descriptors for tooth-drilling and childbirth labor pains were significantly different. MDS of subject profiles showed higher intra-group agreement among Americans than Chinese. Estimates of informant reliability (consensus) within ethnic groups were provided.
Moore et al. 1998a	Tooth-drilling pain	Anglo-Americans Chinese Swedes Danes	($n = 163$) ($n = 195$) ($n = 55$) ($n = 122$) $N = 535$	*Qualitative/Epidemiological:* Interviews on age, gender, and occupation matched ethnic samples; specific information collected about patient pain or use of anesthetic from 129 dentists.	Ethnic descriptors for tooth-drilling pain and use of local anesthetic for drilling were significantly different. (Patients who used no anesthetic: Americans = 1%, Chinese = 90%, Scandinavians = 54%). Reasons varied by pain beliefs, health care systems (e.g., insurance), and dentist-patient relations.
Moore et al. 1996	Needle injection pain	Taiwanese Anglo-Americans	($n = 556$) ($n = 395$) $N = 951$	*Epidemiological:* Use of anesthetic items on prospective epidemiological survey; DAS (Corah 1969); fear of needle injections (pain); samples matched by age and gender.	Taiwanese used sig. less anesthetic than Americans. High dental anxiety (DAS • 12) correlated with high fear of injection pain. Despite similar fears about dental drilling, high-anxiety Taiwanese reported much less use of local anesthesia for routine treatments than did Americans.
Chapman et al. 1982	Dental pain	Japan U.S. Caucasians	($n = 20$) ($n = 20$) $N = 40$	*Quasi-experimental:* Measured effects of acupuncture on induced dental pain. No controls.	Significant reduction in pain perception for both groups. No significant differences between groups.
Weisenberg et al. 1975	Dental pain	African Americans U.S. Caucasians Puerto Ricans	($n = 25$) ($n = 24$) ($n = 26$) $N = 75$	*Quasi-experimental:* 8-item questionnaire (Zola 1966) measure of denial or willingness to deal with pain; STAI, palmar sweat prints, interviews about coping, DAS, posttreatment dentist rating.	No differences by ethnic and racial groups about pain or type of symptoms, but differences in coping. Puerto Ricans scored highest on denial, Caucasians lowest, with African Americans in between.

(continued)

Table I
Continued

Reference	Kind of Pain	Samples Studied	Type of Study Design	Summary of Findings
TMD Pain				
List and Dworkin 1996	TMD pain	Americans ($n = 247$) (nearly all Caucasian) Swedes ($n = 82$) $N = 329$	*Quasi-epidemiological (clinical):* Swedish study using RDC/TMD clinical criteria (Dworkin and LeResche 1992) compared with older U.S. data. Age, gender ratios matched.	Similar pain intensity, psychological profiles for Swedes and Americans, but lower Swedish dysfunction scores on Graded Chronic Pain scale (Von Korff et al. 1992). RDC/TMD definitions provided useful clinical classifications of TMD suitable for multicenter and cross-cultural comparisons.
Miscellaneous or Multiple Pains				
Moore et al. 1997	Common acute and chronic pains	Taiwan Chinese ($n = 62$) Anglo-Americans ($n = 329$) $N = 183$	*Epidemiological:* Prospective "Q-18" questionnaire survey based on interview results. Sample matched for age, gender, occupation.	Common descriptions of pains tested across cultures indicated that many descriptors thought to be universal were used ethnospecifically (e.g., Anglo menstrual cramping) and others were strictly ethnospecific (e.g., Chinese *suan*). Reliability (consensus) calculations demonstrated higher agreement about pain terms among Anglos than Chinese, but sample sizes were calculated to be adequate for theoretical generalizability, according to *cultural consensus theory* proponents (Romney et al. 1986).
Moore et al. 1986; Moore and Dworkin 1988; Moore 1990	Common acute and chronic pains	(U.S. immigrants) Chinese ($n = 25$) Anglo-Americans ($n = 25$) Scandinavians ($n = 35$) $N = 85$	*Qualitative/Epidemiological:* Prospective combination of interviews and matrix survey based on interview results. Sample matched for age, gender, occupation (pilot studies).	Interviews determined standard "kinds of pain" and "kinds of pain coping" for each ethnic group. Most were universal categories. Some were ethnospecific, e.g., real vs. imagined pains = Anglos; *suan* ("sourish") = Chinese. Matrix items showed overall significant MDS differences between ethnic groups. Ethnicity was best predictor of use of pain description, while professional or lay was best predictor of coping.
Calvillo and Flaskerud 1993	Cholecys-tectomy pain	Mexican Americans ($n = 30$) Anglo Americans ($n = 30$) $N = 60$ Nurse observers $= 32$	*Epidemiological:* MPQ PPI by nurses; patient matching study of amount of analgesics and physiology measures. Patients also evaluated their own pain on PPI.	No PPI differences by patient ethnicity. Nurses' ratings were significantly different from patients'; and they assigned significantly more pain to Anglo-American patients. No differences by nurse ethnicity were noted.

Table I
Continued

Miscellaneous or Multiple Pains (continued)

Reference	Kind of Pain	Samples Studied	Type of Study Design	Summary of Findings
Davitz 1976	Miscellaneous pain and suffering for 5 illnesses	Nurses equally distributed in USA, Japan, Taiwan, Thailand, Korea, and Puerto Rico $N = 554$	*Epidemiological:* Studied nurses' perceptions of patients' physical pain and psychological distress using a questionnaire of case studies to which nurses reacted. Nurses and patient cases were of same ethnicity. Authors state that the RNs were comparable in age, gender, and specialty across nations.	Results showed both similarities and differences. Asian nurses judged pain highest, Anglos and Puerto Ricans lowest; explained by Asian patient lack of pain expression and nurses' "needs" to second guess patients. Congruence was greater for Western nurses and patients. Puerto Rican nurses scored Puerto Rican patients low on physical pain, but high on emotional distress. In general, men and women were perceived to suffer the same psychological distress, but women were assigned more physical pain.
Ng et al. 1996	Postoperative pain	Caucasians $(n = 314)$ African Americans $(n = 30)$ Hispanic Americans $(n = 73)$ Asian Americans $(n = 37)$ $N = 454$	*Quasi-epidemiological:* Studied ethnicity influences on patient-controlled analgesia and prescriptions of physicians using hospital records. Statistical control for confounding was used since Hispanic ages were significantly higher.	Results indicated that patient ethnicity had a greater influence on the amount of narcotic prescribed than on the amount self-administered by patients.
Henriksson 1995	Fibromyalgia pain	Swedish women $(n = 20)$ American women $(n = 20)$ $N = 40$	*Qualitative:* Focused semistructured interviews with women in different health care and social welfare systems.	Noted that pain intensity and perceptions of dysfunction, as well as the social consequences, were about the same for both ethnic groups of women. However, system differences made life easier for Swedish patients.
Thomas and Rose 1991	Ear-piercing pain	Afro-West Indians $(n = 28)$ Anglo-Saxons $(n = 28)$ Asian-Americans $(n = 28)$ $N = 84$	*Qualitative/Epidemiological:* Prospective MPQ PRI questionnaire study. Sample matched by age, gender. Tried to relate childhood parental attitudes to coping differences.	Results showed that Afro-West Indians reported lowest pain scores, lowest ratings of parental concern in childhood, and highest coping ability. The design differentiated sensation-expectant vs. pain-expectant groups, also showing significant differences.
Gaston-Johansson 1990	Common acute and chronic pain terms	Caucasians $(n = 47)$ African Americans $(n = 32)$ American Indians $(n = 37)$ Hispanic Americans $(n = 37)$ $N = 153$	*Qualitative/Epidemiological:* Prospective MPQ–VAS study. Sample matched by age and gender. Examined relative intensity (VAS) and descriptions (MPQ) of the terms "pain," "hurt," and "ache."	VAS pain intensity ratings for the terms "pain," "hurt," and "ache" showed significant differences; "pain" was most intense, "hurt" next, and then "ache." Choice of MPQ descriptors varied by ethnicity.

(continued)

Table I
Continued

Reference	Kind of Pain	Samples Studied	Type of Study Design	Summary of Findings
Miscellaneous or Multiple Pains (continued)				
Zatzick and Dimsdale 1990	All experimental or laboratory cross-cultural pain studies	Covered 13 cross-cultural experimental studies $N = 42,933$	*Literature review:* Descriptive comparison (1944–1989); tabling is descriptive, and somewhat aggregate data analytic.	Authors concluded that few experimental studies have shown any ethnic differences by using pain threshold. Pain tolerance is recommended instead, as are cooperative efforts with social scientists to delineate variables by ethnicity (not race). Conclusions are similar to Wolff and Langley's review (1968), which also included experimental pain.
Morse and Morse 1988	Common pains (acute)	Anglo-Canadians $(n = 79)$ East Indians $(n = 22)$ Hutterites $(n = 41)$ Ukrainians $(n = 48)$ $N = 190$	*Qualitative/Epidemiological:* Prospective paired comparisons study. Sample not matched by age, gender. Examined relative pain intensity perceptions of common pains using English survey translations.	Intensity of common pains were perceived differently by ranks according to ethnicity. Labor pain showed most disagreement.
Abu-Saad 1984	Common pains (acute)	Arab Americans $(n = 24)$ Hispanic Americans $(n = 24)$ Asian Americans $(n = 24)$ $N = 72$	*Qualitative/Epidemiological:* Prospective interview study. Sample matched by age, gender. Examined relative pain intensity perceptions of common pains.	Children's perceptions of what hurt were about the same. But their emotional reactivity and coping varied by ethnicity.
Zborowski 1969	Common clinical pains (disk, back, other unspecified physical disabilities)	Irish Americans $(n = 31)$ Italian Americans $(n = 30)$ Jewish Americans $(n = 45)$ Old Americans $(n = 40)$ $N = 146$	*Qualitative:* Focused qualitative case studies with interviews and participant observations. Data collected in 1952 in a New York hospital setting. Men only. Samples not matched by strategy.	Findings showed that (1) similar reactions to pain by ethnicity don't always reflect similar attitudes or meanings, and (2) similar behavioral patterns to pain serve different functions in various cultures (e.g., sympathy seeking vs. beliefs in ability to rid self of pain).

Abbreviations: BPI = Brief Pain Inventory; DAS = Dental Anxiety Scale; LBP = low back pain; LOC = locus of control; MDS = multidimensional scaling; MMPI = Minnesota Multiphasic Personality Inventory; MPQ = McGill Pain Questionnaire; PPI = Present Pain Intensity; PRI = Pain Rating Index; RDC/TMD = Research Diagnostic Criteria for Temporomandibular Disorder; SES = socioeconomic status; SIP = Sickness Impact Profile; STAI = State Trait Anxiety Inventory; TMD = temporomandibular disorder; VAS = visual analogue scale.

HEADACHE

In a cross-cultural review of headache literature from 1937 to 1987, Chen (1993) examined age, gender, stress factors, headache characteristics, and modalities of pain control in adults and compared them with studies of headache prevalence in children. Although the author failed to list references at the end of the review, he provided tables with all available statistics for the above variables and noted the principal author, year, and country. Much of the data resulted from use of translated versions of the MPQ (Melzack 1975) for Korean, Chinese, Taiwanese, Italian, and French samples. A mix of epidemiological and other descriptive studies on North American, British, Belgian, Polish, Danish, Swedish, Norwegian, Austrian, Nigerian, Israeli, Brazilian, German, Russian, Dutch, Portuguese, Zimbabwean, New Zealand, and Ecuadorian samples were also tabled by sample size, gender, and prevalence among both children and adults for at total aggregate size of 65,000 subjects. The author reached five major conclusions: (1) The prevalence of migraine increased from approximately 7% in children to 11.5% in adults. Gender differences in prevalence were not apparent for migraine but were significant in general headaches during childhood with the female to male ratio up to 2.4:1 by adulthood. (2) More than 60% of patients report severe headache in a trend that was consistent across nations, with females reporting greater severity than males. (3) Physical and psychological stressors appeared to be the major precipitating factors of headache. (4) While medication is the most commonly used form of treatment, rest and relaxation also appeared to be important coping mechanisms for headache. (5) Sensory descriptors and affective language used to describe headache were generally consistent across nations.

In another cross-cultural review, Ziegler (1990) reported that headache in American and Western European societies affect high percentages of the population. In Finland in 1978, 73% of women and 57% of men in a population of 2811 reported headache in the previous year. These figures were similar to those of American studies of that time. Somewhat lower figures were reported for New Zealand (39% men, 60% women) in a 1985 study. Reports from various societies worldwide indicate that reports of headache, and specifically severe headache, are prevalent, although rates vary. While reported rates were very high in Western societies, they were very low, for example, in the People's Republic of China, where prevalence was reported to be 1.5–4% for men and 4–8% for women in two cited studies from 1986. Another Asian study from Thailand in 1986, however, reported that more than 10% of men and 35% of women had migraine. Whether prevalence varies with different socioeconomic groups remains uncertain, and evidence was conflicting about whether intellectuals experience more frequent headaches. In one Chinese study, "severe" and "incapacitating" headache were twice as prevalent in urban dwellers as in rural populations. Severe headache and specifically migraine are, for reasons still unknown, much more common in women. North American, British, and Scandinavian studies in the 1960s and 1970s reported a decrease in prevalence with older age. However, studies of a Chinese population published in 1986 and a Thai population in 1989 indicated an increase in prevalence with older age. Hormonal changes in women and family histories of headache are common associations, but the precise role of genetics or hormonal influence is unknown. Ziegler concluded that it was difficult to make comparisons because a major problem in epidemiological studies is the lack of uniform definition of headache syndromes and the methodological consequences of this issue. Ziegler's review did not provide tables with aggregate prevalence data, but it described existing studies with an emphasis on differences in headache prevalences and characteristics across cultures. Chen's (1993) primary aim in the preceding review was to emphasize universal aspects of headache across cultures.

BACK PAIN

Lau and colleagues (1995) reported results of a replication study of prevalence and characteristics of low back pain (LBP) in adults aged 20–59 years in a Hong Kong population of 652 Chinese in 1994–95. They compared them with a British study by Walsh et al. (1992) that used the same survey design to investigate LBP and disability in a 2667-person sample in eight regions of Great Britain in 1990–91. Thirty-nine percent of the Chinese subjects reported having had LBP at some time, and 21% had experienced it during the past 12 months. Rates were higher in women than men. Walsh and colleagues found that the lifetime and 1-year prevalences of LBP for British subjects were

58.3% and 36.1%, respectively. Rates in men and women were similar. In both Hong Kong and Britain, back pain (within 12 months) was most common in taller men and in both men and women with jobs requiring regular lifting of weights in excess of 25 kg. A study of 3159 Taiwanese nurses confirms this conclusion on a Chinese risk population (Chiou et al. 1994). A logistic regression model indicated a lower prevalence and lower risk for back pain symptoms in Hong Kong than in the British sample. The difference was partially explained by differences in stature and occupational lifting. Also, disability from LBP among the British appeared to be due largely to differences in patient behavior once symptoms had developed (Walsh et al. 1992). Lau and colleagues suggested that Hong Kong Chinese may have a higher threshold for reporting symptoms or may differ in their exposure to other unrecognized risk factors not covered in survey questioning.

A related British study (Croft and Rigby 1994) has explored at least some of the "other unrecognized risk factors" in Great Britain. The association between measures of socioeconomic status and reported back pain in a national survey of 9003 adults 18 years or older showed that of subjects reporting back pain compared with those who did not, women from households in the lowest income and educational levels reported pain nearly twice as often, while for men the only socioeconomic link with back pain seemed to be manual occupation. These associations were not explained by smoking, obesity, or coexistent depressive symptoms. The findings confirmed the higher burden of back pain in the socially disadvantaged among this Western population, but suggested yet other unreported risk factors, such as availability of worker's compensation or other benefits.

Carron and colleagues (1985) compared psychosocial and economic factors affecting severity of disability in Caucasians with LBP in the United States and New Zealand. They used a self-report questionnaire to assess physical, vocational, emotional, marital, familial, economic, and legal responses to chronic LBP on 198 U.S. patients (mean age 43 years) and 117 patients in New Zealand (mean age 48 years). One year later, approximately 55% of the sample from each country returned a follow-up questionnaire after participating in comparable outpatient treatment programs. Analyses of the results indicated that despite nearly similar between-country reports of pain frequency and intensity, U.S. subjects, both at pre- and

post-testing, reported greater emotional and behavioral disruption as a correlate of their pain. Subjects in the United States consistently used more medication, experienced more dysphoric mood states, and were more hampered in social, sexual, recreational, and vocational functioning. Subjects from both countries demonstrated a nearly equal degree of pre- to post-treatment improvement.

However, the relative initial differences favoring the New Zealand subjects remained constant across both questionnaire administrations. At the onset of treatment, 49% of the U.S. sample and only 17% of the New Zealand subjects were receiving pain-related financial compensation. At follow-up, subjects from both countries receiving pretreatment compensation were less likely to report a return to full activity, although the relationship appeared more pronounced in the U.S. subjects. Authors discussed differences in the systems of worker's compensation for the two countries. In New Zealand, worker's compensation is granted less often and for shorter durations than in the United States, and thus leads to less severe lifestyle disruption. The authors attributed these differences to attitudes toward compensation policy and cultural differences about wellness in the two countries; for example, New Zealanders were considered to be more health oriented and took fewer benefits for shorter periods. Despite the excellent design of this study, it produced somewhat questionable results in that only 55% of subjects participated in the follow-up. However, representative prevalence studies lend support to these conclusions comparing pain perceptions of New Zealanders and Americans. About 30% of New Zealanders reported back pain within their lifetime (James et al. 1991), while 41–56% of U.S. populations reported back pains within the last 6–12 months (Sternbach 1986; Von Korff et al. 1988), which may indicate differences in pain focus.

Volinn (1997; Volinn et al. 1996) has also studied low back pain phenomena across cultures using quasi-epidemiological reviews of aggregate data or meta-analysis where possible. In his provocative article entitled "The epidemiology of low back pain in the rest of the world: a review of surveys in low and middle income countries," Volinn (1997) pointed out that most studies are restricted to high-income countries, which comprise only 15% of the world's population. He also noted that little was known about the epidemiology of LBP in the rest of the world. He reviewed the few existing studies in developing nations and contrasted rates with selected high-income countries (Britain, Belgium, Germany, and Sweden). He reported that the rates of disability compensation in highly industrialized Western societies were much higher than in the less industrialized nations, even though industrial accidents were two to four times more frequent in the latter. He also found that hard physical labor itself was not necessarily related to LBP and that urban low-income populations (China, Indonesia) had higher rates than rural low-income populations (China, Indonesia, Nepal, India, Nigeria). These rates and sharply higher rates among workers in enclosed workshops of low income countries (India, China, Indonesia) suggested to Volinn that prevalence of LBP may be rising among vast numbers of workers as urbanization and rapid industrialization proceed. Volinn also called attention to the disparity in rates within categories of countries of both high and low income, which indicated that a high proportion of epidemiological studies used questionable methods. Volinn called for prospective studies that would develop standardized survey instruments to be used across cultures, which would provide more reliable and valid data for analysis of trends.

Volinn (1997) cited one well-designed cross-cultural study (Waluyo et al. 1996) that examined variance in work conditions among Swedish and Indonesian assembly workers and showed how these work environment factors influenced health and job satisfaction. Questionnaire data were collected on a sample of 326 Swedish and 136 Indonesian assembly industry workers. The prevalence of musculoskeletal symptoms was high in both groups. Stress and psychosomatic symptoms had higher prevalences in the Swedish group, which also rated their work conditions as worse in most respects. Work tasks were physically heavier in Indonesia, but less monotonous and with lower demands on productivity, and Indonesians were more satisfied with their jobs. Physical job demands were associated with musculoskeletal symptoms. Development of job competence was associated with increased job satisfaction. Conflicts and harassment at work were associated with stress and psychosomatic symptoms. Job pressure, especially deficient planning of the jobs, was associated with lower job satisfaction and with psychosomatic and stress symptoms in the Swedish group. The samples were well described and matched occupationally, but not for age or gender. Swedish workers were only described as younger and less concerned about family income than were the Indone-

sians. Thus, it is difficult to assess the influence of demographic confounders in this cross-cultural study.

Volinn et al. (1996) also examined cross-national disparities in rates of back pain disability, comparing U.S., Swedish, and Japanese workforce data. Given East-West cultural differences, socioeconomic factors were explored as explanatory variables. This study used the annual count of wage compensation claims for back pain in the numerator of the rate and the total number of persons eligible to file a claim in the relevant year as the denominator. According to the study, the 1992 Washington State rate of claims with greater than 3 days' work loss is 45 times higher than the Japanese rate, and the 1991 Swedish rate is nearly 8 times higher than the 1991 Washington State total claim rate. Despite possible problems in the composition of the rates by nation (e.g., due to coverage of nonwork-related claims in Sweden), Volinn concluded that the dramatic differences in rates of back pain disability warrant further investigation.

Nelson and colleagues (1996) compared the Minnesota Multiphasic Personality Inventory (MMPI) (Dahlstrom et al. 1972) clinical patterns of 295 white, African American, and Hispanic patients with chronic pain; 70% had pain of myofascial origin, while 8% had headache. This study also examined various highpoint, two-point, and other profile patterns about experience of pain, pain coping, and social and recreational activities and found notable gender/ethnic group differences. Most of the differences were demographic or sample explanatory, such as years of education and duration of pain, in which white and African Americans reported significantly higher rates. However, test results of African Americans, especially men, revealed more psychologically disturbed functions related to chronic pain, especially on MMPI scales indicating hypochondriasis, depression, and hysteria. White women were more inclined to verbal expressions of feelings about their pain experience compared with their black or Hispanic counterparts. The pattern of intercorrelations of the mean T scores with various demographic and clinical characteristics suggested that the MMPI is sensitive to group differences on certain correlates of the pain experience. However, it is doubtful that these differences are generalizable due to group differences in education and pain duration.

In a similar cross-cultural study using MMPI, Strassberg and colleagues (1992) compared scores of a sample of 610 Australian chronic back pain patients with MMPI data from the United States. Although it was not cited in the methods, the U.S. data were composed of mean scores for 112 U.S. chronic pain patients that the author had collected for a 1981 study (Strassberg 1981). Analysis revealed mean MMPI profiles (i.e., elevated hypochondriasis, hysteria, and depression clinical scales) and three profile types derived for the Australians by cluster analysis that corresponded closely to U.S. findings. Also, some of the same behavioral correlates associated with MMPI performance among U.S. pain patients were also found for Australian pain patients. However, it was not possible to verify that the sampling was comparable as described in this article, because the U.S. sample was collected 11 years prior to the Australian study, and although mean data were graphed, demographic data were not provided. No normal controls were used in the study. Nevertheless, the similarities in outcomes are interesting despite differences in time and sample origin.

Similarly, Brena and colleagues (1990) compared and contrasted medical, psychological, social, and general behavioral functioning of American (*n* = 10) and Japanese (*n* = 11) randomly selected LBP patients and the same numbers of normal controls. The Sickness Impact Profile (Bergner et al. 1981; Follick et al. 1985) and a standardized Medical Examination Protocol for Pain instrument were used to assess all subjects. Findings showed that the American and Japanese LBP patients had similar and significantly higher medical physical findings than their respective controls. Likewise, the American and Japanese LBP patients showed significantly greater psychological, social, and general behavioral dysfunction compared to control subjects. Finally, despite similar medical and physical findings, the Japanese LBP patients were significantly less impaired in psychological, social, vocational, and avocational functioning than were the American patients. The authors concluded that the American and Japanese patients showed significant cross-cultural differences, primarily in the psychosocial and behavioral areas for this small but controlled sample. The authors ventured possible explanations, such as cross-cultural differences in personal expectations, financial gains, and expectations about usage, type, and availability of health care, but did not provide any evidence. The use of controls in this design improves the sense of validity of these data, despite the small sample size.

Sanders and colleagues (1992) conducted a smaller study to investigate any significant cross-cultural differences in medical or physical findings, or in psychosocial, behavioral, vocational, or avocational social functioning for chronic LBP patients. This well-designed study used a partially double-blind and controlled but unmatched comparison of six different cultural groups selected primarily from ambulatory care facilities specializing in treating chronic LBP patients. Sixty-three chronic LBP patients and 63 healthy controls were randomly selected (demographically unmatched by nation) from American, Japanese, Mexican, Colombian, Italian, and New Zealand populations with 10–11 subjects per culture. The control subjects were healthy support staff. The Sickness Impact Profile and a Medical Examination and Diagnostic Information Coding system were used as primary outcome measures. Findings showed that (1) LBP subjects across all cultures had significantly more medical-physical findings and more impairment on psychosocial, behavioral, vocational, and avocational measures than controls did; (2) Mexican and New Zealand LBP subjects had significantly fewer physical findings than did other LBP groups; (3) the American, New Zealand, and Italian LBP patients reported significantly more impairment in psychosocial, recreational, or work areas, with the Americans the most dysfunctional; and (4) findings were not a function of working class, age, sex, pain intensity, pain duration, previous surgeries, or differences in medical and physical findings. The authors found important cross-cultural differences in chronic LBP patients' self-perceived level of dysfunction, with the American patients clearly the most dysfunctional. Possible explanations included cross-cultural differences in social expectation, attention, legal and administrative requirements, financial gains, attitudes and expectations about usage, type, and availability of health care, and self-perceived ability and willingness to cope.

Anglo-Americans were again chosen for a cross-cultural comparison with native Puerto Ricans in a study of adaptation to chronic pain by Bates and colleagues (1995). Using six case studies for each of the two ethnic groups and quantitative analyses of in all 100 native Puerto Ricans and 100 Anglo-Americans, this team documented that successful adaptation was associated with a reduction in depression, tension, and worry, and a realistic continuation of family, social, and work roles. The mean age of the Anglo-American sample was 44 years, compared with 60 years for the Puerto Ricans. Factors most often associated with adaptation were cultural meanings given to the pains, amount of psychosocial support, age, socioeconomic status, psychological coping style, the cultural context of care (providers' world views), and the political and economic circumstances under which compensation, health insurance, and rehabilitation were sought. Results showed significant inter and intracultural group differences in pain intensity and emotional responses to the pain. Despite higher reported pain intensity and more emotional responses among Puerto Ricans, there was no significant difference between the two groups regarding interference in daily activities. The two groups appeared to experience chronic pain differently. The researchers proposed that the difference was not positive or negative in itself, but simply a different reality. The report did not describe the selection strategy for the case studies. The samples were obviously not matched and may be biased, especially in regard to age, so there is some doubt about the comparative validity as well as generalizability of the case studies. Nevertheless, this study provides some understanding about the qualitative circumstances of suffering experienced by the ethnic chronic pain patients.

In another part of the same study, Bates and Rankin (1994) assessed the correlations between ethnic or cultural background and locus of control (LOC) style in the chronic pain of the Anglo-American and Puerto Rican chronic pain sufferers. They reported significant correlations between patients' LOC style and variations in reported chronic pain intensity and responses and an interaction between LOC style and cultural identity in reported pain intensity. The qualitative data also suggest that LOC style may not be a permanent, unchanging characteristic or cognitive interpretation. Instead, a person's LOC style may be altered by the chronic pain experience and may change at various stages in the chronic pain "career." The authors suggested that an increased sense of control may contribute to an increased ability to cope successfully with the chronic pain experience and that it may be possible to alter a patient's sense of control through the development of deliberate culturally appropriate and personally relevant programs designed to help the patients establish a sense of control over their lives and their pain.

CHILDBIRTH LABOR PAIN

Pesce (1987) used the Present Pain, Pain Rating, and Number of Words Chosen indexes of translations of the McGill Pain Questionnaire to evaluate reports of childbirth pain by 22 Australian mothers, 10 Italian mothers, and 8 mothers born in Australia of Italian parents. The lack of significant differences among the groups suggested that description of pain did not vary with ethnic background. However, the study did not include measures for pain reaction or coping, so these results may have limited clinical meaningfulness or utility. The English version of the MPQ was not designed to measure descriptors Italians would necessarily use in their native language. Furthermore, other cross-cultural studies (Moore et al. 1986, 1998b; Moore and Dworkin 1988) indicated East-West differences in use of descriptors for childbirth labor pain and perceived need for anesthesia, so perhaps even if the MPQ measures were valid, this particular cross-cultural sample may not have shown differences. Moore and colleagues (1998b) found that preferred descriptors for labor pains varied significantly by ethnicity among Anglo-Americans ($n = 122$), Chinese ($n = 123$), and Scandinavians ($n = 95$) when they compared labor pains and tooth-drilling pains across the groups matched by demographics.

Morse (1989) compared the culturally specific methods used during childbirth by 32 Fijians and Fijian Indians to control pain and reduce the risk of injury to the mother and infant. To ensure the cultural relevance of a paired comparisons questionnaire, the pain items included on the scale were obtained by asking Fijian and Fijian-Indian nurses and community members to list the 10 most painful conditions they could imagine. In addition, 32 live births were observed. Then, 67 Fijians and 73 Fijian Indians (about 50% men in both groups) used the paired comparisons scale to rate birth pain. Fijian women had significantly more pain before entering hospital care than did Fijian Indians. Fijians view their traditional social network as a valid replacement for hospital care, and women were reluctant to abandon the support and caring that they received in the village to travel to the hospital at labor onset. The wish to conceal pregnancy delayed antenatal care for the Fijian Indian women. They did not know the mechanics of delivery and transferred to the hospital at the first twinges of labor, often displaying panic behaviors during delivery, while Fijians often labored silently. Surprisingly, however, in comparing different types of pain, Fijians ranked childbirth pain higher than did Fijian Indians, and Fijian men ranked childbirth pain higher than did

Fijian women.

Weisenberg and Caspi (1989) investigated the effects of sociocultural origin and educational level on the verbal ratings of pain and pain behavior during childbirth for 83 women aged 19 to 38. They also measured coping style and extroversion, and found that all women rated the pain of childbirth as high. Overall, women from an Asian or Middle Eastern (North African, Mediterranean) background ($n = 53$) compared with a Western (North European, American) background ($n = 30$) gave higher ratings of pain and showed more pain behavior. This tendency was particularly strong for Middle Eastern women of a low educational background. For both groups, low education correlated with higher ratings of pain and more pain behavior. No trends were seen as a function of extroversion. Middle Eastern and Western women did not differ in coping style. However, women who had higher vigilance scores rated the pain as less, even though they showed no differences in pain behavior. Sociocultural group of origin and other relevant reference groups, such as educational level, were important in determining pain perception and behavior. The authors hoped that by combining this information with coping style they could promote an instructional intervention to better prepare women for childbirth. Generalizations about specific ethnic groups could not be made because the analysis did not delineate categories by specific ethnic groupings.

DENTAL PAIN

In a series of investigations on a cross-cultural population, Moore and colleagues (1986, 1997, 1998a,b; Moore and Dworkin 1988; Moore 1990) used a combination of qualitative and quantitative methods to compare descriptions of common pain and pain coping among samples of over 700 Anglo-Americans, Mandarin-speaking Chinese, and Scandinavians. The authors used quantitative instruments to validate qualitative findings and to provide a way to judge sample parameters such as intersubject agreement, accuracy, and thus reliability (Moore et al. 1997). From these calculations, they derived the probable sample size required to provide representative information. Moore and colleagues (1998b) studied differences in ethnic beliefs about perceived need for local anesthesia for tooth drilling and childbirth labor among Anglo-Americans (from Washington and Ohio), Mandarin-speaking Chinese (from Taiwan and People's Re-

public of China), and Scandinavians (89 dentists and 251 patients) matched for age, gender, and occupation. Subjects responded to questionnaire items selected from interview results to estimate (1) beliefs about possible use of anesthetic for tooth-drilling and labor pain compared with other possible remedies such as deep breathing, relaxing, and distraction, and (2) choice of pain descriptors associated with use or nonuse of anesthetic, including descriptions of injection pain. Unlike the one-way translations of existing MPQ English pain descriptors used for cross-cultural comparison in other studies, Moore's team took precautions to translate and back-translate item measures (Brislin 1973) and used a panel of expert judges for maximum semantic verification of terms. Frequency statistics and multidimensional scaling revealed that 77% of Anglo-American informants reported anesthetic as a possible remedy for drilling and 51% for labor pain compared with 34% of Chinese for drilling and 5% for labor pain, and 70% of Scandinavians for drilling and 35% for labor pain. Most Americans and Swedes described tooth-drilling sensations as sharp, Chinese as sharp and "sourish" (*suan*), and Danes as shooting (*jagende*). By rank, Americans described labor pain as cramping, sharp, and excruciating; Chinese as sharp, intermittent, and horrible; Danes as shooting, tiring, and sharp; and Swedes as tiring, "good," yet horrible. Preferred pain descriptors for drilling, birth, and injection pains varied significantly by ethnicity. Results corroborated conclusions of a qualitative study (Moore et al. 1998a) ($N = 525$) about pain beliefs in relation to perceived needs for anesthetic in tooth drilling. Descriptions of pains in that study revealed both some universal meanings across cultures and some ethnospecific or unique pain concepts. For example, the concept of *suan* or sourish to describe pain or a precursor thereof explained why the Chinese had expected that tooth drilling would not require local anesthesia. Anglo-Americans described the same tooth-drilling sensations as excruciating and requiring local anesthesia. Danes and Swedes were about equally divided as to whether local anesthesia was necessary, and most felt that the pain was not so bad and did not last long. Samples used to obtain the results were estimated to be generalizable for these ethnic groups using special reliability calculations.

In a more traditional epidemiological study, Moore and colleagues (1996) investigated the use of anesthetic injections for common tooth-drilling procedures and fear of injection pain among 951 adults from dental school clinics in Iowa City, Iowa, and Taipei, Taiwan. Subject samples were matched by age and gender across ethnic groups. Frequency and logistic regression analyses showed that use of dental anesthetics for routine treatment was significantly greater among Caucasian Americans than Taiwanese, as was fear of injection pain. Taiwanese and Americans with high dental anxiety had similar high fears of injections, but despite similar fears about dental drilling, high-anxiety Taiwanese reported using much less local anesthesia for routine treatments than did high-anxiety Americans. Moore and colleagues concluded that cultural differences in perceived need for local anesthesia are probably dependent on dental health care systems and associated dentist beliefs or patient expectations about injection pain. This epidemiological study supported some of the conclusions drawn from results in the studies (Moore et al. 1997, 1998a,b) described above.

In an experimental situation, Chapman and colleagues (1982) compared the effects of low-frequency electrical acupuncture stimulation on the perception of induced dental pain in two cultural settings. Twenty Japanese and 20 American adults (10 Caucasians and 10 second- or third-generation Japanese, aged 18–36 years) were tested in two functionally identical laboratories. Each subject had an acupuncture session and a control session on separate days with subjects counterbalanced for carry-over order effects. Sensory decision-theory analysis demonstrated a significant reduction in perceptual capability and an increased bias against reporting stimuli as painful following acupuncture treatment at traditional focal points. The results demonstrated no significant differences between groups in alteration of perceptual capability, bias, or pain threshold, which indicated that the cultural and racial differences studied did not influence responses to acupuncture in a laboratory setting.

In a 1975 quasi-experimental study of dental pain and anxiety among African American, Caucasian, and Puerto Rican ethnic groups ($N = 75$), Weisenberg and colleagues used an eight-item questionnaire developed by Zola (1966) for Italian American, Irish American, and Anglo-American samples to measure denial of pain or willingness to deal with pain. Puerto Ricans scored significantly higher on denial than did the other groups, but Weisenberg may not have been able to observe differences between black and the other groups because the survey instrument was designed for other ethnic group response categories.

TMD PAIN

The only reported cross-cultural investigation of TMD pain was a clinical diagnostic study by List and Dworkin (1996) in which they used "Research Diagnostic Criteria for Temporomandibular Disorders" (RDC/TMD) guidelines in classifying TMD patients on physical diagnosis (Axis I), pain-related disability, and psychological status (Axis II) (Dworkin and LeResche 1992). The authors used criteria originally developed in the United States to determine if a translated version was a clinically useful diagnostic research measure for cross-cultural comparisons. RDC/TMD profiles of 82 Swedish TMD patients (64 women; 18 men) participating in the study were compared with 247 American TMD patients who were matched by gender and age ratios. Pain intensity on a 10-point visual analogue scale (VAS) was 4.6 for Swedes and 4.0 for Americans. Axis II assessment of psychological status with an SCL-90-R scale (Derogatis 1983) showed that 18% of Swedish patients yielded severe depression scores, while 28% yielded high nonspecific physical symptom scores, which was similar to American results. Psychosocial dysfunction or pain interference was observed in 13% of Swedish patients based on graded chronic pain scores (Von Korff et al. 1992), which was lower than for Americans (20%). These initial results suggest that the RDC guidelines are a valuable diagnostic aid and that they can facilitate multicenter and cross-cultural comparisons of clinical findings. The investigators took precautions to translate and back-translate item measures (Brislin et al. 1973) for maximum semantic term verification.

Although no data are available for TMD prevalence in Sweden, American studies (Von Korff et al. 1988; LeResche 1997) have indicated that about 10% of the adult population has TMD and that it is most common among young and middle-aged adults. Female to male ratio was nearly 2:1. Shiau and Chang (1992) surveyed 2033 Chinese university students in Taiwan (mean age 20 years, range 17–32) for the prevalence of TMD and found that only 17% reported any awareness of pain. Women reported pain only slightly more frequently than did men. Scores on stress, general anxiety, emotion, and anger were higher in the TMD group. Severity and treatment demands were considered to be low. Deng and colleagues (1995) investigated TMD prevalence in a sample of 3015 mainland Chinese children and adolescents aged 3–19 years. Prevalence of TMD for the entire group was

18% with no significant gender difference. Prevalence was low from ages 3 to 6 but increased from age 6 to the early teens and then decreased in the late teens. Only 0.6% of subjects reported pain. Japanese longitudinal results (Onizawa 1996) for young adults indicated that TMD symptoms fluctuated with time and that 24% of a cohort of 275 university students reported discomfort over a 4-year period. Only 1% sought treatment for pain. The Asian studies appear to agree in regard to low rates of symptoms and that gender differences in prevalence are not as great as in Western samples, at least for younger age groups.

MISCELLANEOUS OR MULTIPLE PAINS

In another study, Moore and colleagues (1997) explored common pain descriptions among a sample of 183 Anglo-American and Mandarin-speaking Chinese patients and dentists matched by age and gender. They used a quantitative method to validate qualitative interview results and check sample parameters. Their methods were based on a cultural consensus theory described by Romney, Batchelder, and Weller (Romney et al. 1986; Batchelder and Romney 1988; Weller and Romney 1988). Basic assumptions for comparing subjects were that they were members of a sociocultural group (e.g., ethnic or professional versus lay) and answered questions independently about a monotonic domain (e.g., pain). Subjects answered 18 true/false items selected to reflect pain perceptions consistent with published and unpublished open interview data about "kinds of pains." Estimates of (1) consistency in use of descriptors within groups, (2) validity of description, (3) accuracy of subjects compared with others in their group, and (4) minimum required sample size were calculated using Cronbach's α, factor analysis, and Bayesian probability (Romney et al. 1986; Batchelder and Romney 1988; Weller and Romney 1988). Ethnic and professional differences within and across groups were also tested using multidimensional scaling (MDS) and hypothesis testing. Consensus (consistency of subject response by group) was 0.99 among Anglo-Americans and 0.97 among Chinese. Mean subject accuracy was 0.81 for Americans and 0.57 for Chinese, which indicated that the Chinese group needed more subjects to verify each others' statements than did the American group. However, more subjects were recruited than actually required for both ethnic groups at 95% CL. MDS showed similarities in use of descriptors within ethnic groups,

while there were differences ($P < 0.001$) between Chinese and American groups. Regarding scalable differences in descriptors of pain perceptions, 95% of the Americans described muscle pain as deep compared to 57% of Chinese. Americans (97%) perceived tooth-drilling pain as sharp compared with 79% of Chinese, while 82% of Chinese considered tooth drilling to be *suan* or "sourish" pain compared with 8% of Americans. Ninety percent of Americans said back pain could be shooting, compared with 60% of Chinese. For menstrual pains, 97% of Americans and 76% of Chinese described them as cramping, while 90% of Americans thought chest pains to be sharp compared with 53% of Chinese. More importantly perhaps, the authors provided methodological evidence that use of covalidating questionnaires that reflect results of qualitative interviews helps to improve internal and external validity of qualitative studies.

Moore and colleagues (1986; Moore and Dworkin 1988; Moore 1990) in earlier pilot studies used interviews and matrix questionnaire methods to gather and analyze data about verbal descriptors of pain and coping among 25 Chinese and 60 Western subjects (25 Anglo-Americans and 35 Scandinavians) in Seattle, Washington. The sample consisted of 54 patients and 31 dentists. Key pain descriptors from each cultural context were selected from initial "kinds of pains" and "kinds of coping" interviews for construction of matrix matching instruments that allowed MDS statistical analysis and production of other cross-cultural quantitative indices. Results revealed dimensions of pain that were universal in all cultures examined. These included time, intensity, location, quality, cause, and curability. More culture-specific dimensions included the Chinese concept *suan,* as described earlier. It was related to perceptions of bone, muscle, joint, tooth, and gingival pain. "Real" and "imagined" pains were contrasts described by Western subjects, especially dentists; "imagined pain" is the conversion of fear or anxiety into perceived pain. Anglo-American patients and all dentists preferred internally applied medicines (pills, injections, etc.) as a primary coping method. Chinese patients preferred external agents (salves, oils, massage, etc.) significantly more than did Chinese dentists or Western subjects. Some Swedish and nearly all Chinese patients preferred not to use local anesthesia for dental treatment. Other dimensions of coping were changes of body function (e.g., sleeping, deep breathing), psychosocial dimensions (e.g., touch, social presence), active pain coping (e.g., distraction, being prepared), passive coping (e.g., denial, waiting), ingestion of food or drink and nontraditional medicine (e.g., herbs, acupuncture). These pilot data indicated that the data gathering and data analytic methods were reliable and sensitive to cultural variables. Ethnicity played a stronger role in determining perceptions of pain description than did professional socialization. Professional socialization processes had more influence on remedy preferences than did ethnicity for this sample of Chinese and Western subjects.

Calvillo and Flaskerud (1993) examined the relationship between ethnicity and clinical pain behavior. The study looked at whether (1) responses of Mexican American women and Anglo-American women to cholecystectomy pain differed significantly, (2) nurses' attribution of pain to each of the two ethnic groups was comparable, and (3) patients' evaluations of the pain being experienced was comparable to nurses' evaluations of patient pain. The sample included 60 patient subjects and 60 nurse responses for those patients from 32 nurses, who were of mixed ethnicity (almost half Anglo-American and the rest African, Asian, and Mexican American). Patient data were collected at two major teaching hospitals in southern California and pain was measured using the MPQ, amount of analgesics used, and three physiological measures. Nurses assessed patient pain using the Present Pain Intensity scale of the MPQ. No significant differences were found between the two ethnic groups on any measures of pain. However, nurses judged the two ethnic groups' pain responses differently and assigned more pain to Anglo-Americans. Nurses' and patients' evaluations of pain also differed significantly; nurses judged patients' pain to be less severe than did patients. Nurses' judgments of higher pain experience in patients were not confounded by their own ethnicity and were significantly correlated with increased patient education level, blue-collar employment, birth within the United States, fluency in English, and Protestant religion.

In a similar, but older study, Davitz and colleagues (1976) investigated cross-cultural beliefs about patient suffering among nurses, using a 60-item questionnaire presented in six languages to 554 nurses (all women RNs) equally distributed in the United States, Japan, Taiwan, Thailand, Korea, and Puerto Rico. The items covered hypothetical patient case descriptions in which nurses were asked to judge the physical pain and psychological distress of patients of the same culture. Results revealed both similarities and differences. Korean and Japanese nurses gave the highest rating of overall suffering, U.S. and Puerto Rican nurses the lowest. Greater congruence between pain experience and pain expression of American patients was thought to affect the judgments of U.S. nurses, while less congruence in Japanese patients was a possible explanation for Japanese nurse judgments. Puerto Rican nurses tended to minimize physical pain while emphasizing psychological distress in their judgments. Similar responses were found among all the nurses in that (1) children suffer far less psychological distress than do adults, (2) psychological distress was greater than the physical pain, and (3) men and women suffered about the same amount of psychological distress but the physical pain inferred for women was greater than for men. The study, while quantitative in method, demonstrated qualitative, clinically meaningful differences and similarities, although it did not describe the samples of nurses in any detail.

Ng and colleagues (1996) studied whether ethnicity influenced patient-controlled analgesia (PCA) for the treatment of postoperative pain. Using a retrospective record review, they examined data from all patients treated with PCA for postoperative pain within a 6-month observation period. They excluded patients who would confound comparative results and included 454 subjects in the study. While they found no differences in the amount of self-administered narcotic, they reported significant differences in the amount of narcotic prescribed to Asian Americans, African Americans, Hispanics, and Caucasians. However, Hispanics differed significantly in age compared to the other groups, which was a possible confounder for ethnicity. (The authors insisted that ethnic differences in prescribed analgesics persisted after they statistically controlled for age, gender, preoperative use of narcotics, pain site, and insurance status.) They concluded that a patient's ethnicity had a greater effect on the amount of narcotic prescribed by the physician than on the amount of self-administered narcotic. Caucasians were prescribed most, African Americans second, followed by Asians, then Hispanics. Although the study came 20 years after the Davitz study (1976), it reconfirmed ethnic variations in perceptions by professional care providers about patient pain and possible clinical consequences. Similar conclusions were drawn from another recent study of ethnicity as a risk factor for inadequate emergency room analgesia (Todd et al. 1993).

Recently, Henriksson (1995) analyzed and described how women with fibromyalgia, living in two different cultural, health care, and social security settings, managed everyday life despite the limitations imposed by the condition. Data were collected through qualitative semi-structured interviews with 40 women, 20 in the United States and 20 in Sweden. The author identified the different strategies used by the women and proposed a preliminary typology of strategies for more specific quantitative studies. The qualitative approach provided rich contextual information about the women's own perceptions, interpretations, and experiences of how to deal with the problems that arose. Findings in the two groups were similar in terms of pain intensity, expression, and coping, but differences in the medico-legal compensation systems influenced the women's opportunities to reduce working hours and provided a main point of differentiation across the two ethnic groups. Changes of habits, roles, and lifestyle, and ergonomic considerations that were required for both groups were similar in description. These changes required time and continued support from the environment and the health care providers. The author called for more research into consequences of the condition so as to plan successful treatment and support programs.

Thomas and Rose (1991) studied ethnic differences in pain experience following ear piercing. After ear piercing, Afro-West Indian, Anglo-Saxon, and Asian adults in Britain ($n = 84$) completed a pain questionnaire and two rating scales about their parents' reactions to common painful incidences during their childhood. Half the subjects were told the study was about pain and half that it was concerned with sensation. The authors discussed the results in the context of subjects' ratings of their parents' attitudes to minor injury and their own ability to cope with pain. Ethnic differences in pain ratings were highly significant. The pain condition produced higher ratings than did the sensation condition, but results showed no significant sex differences. Afro-West Indians reported the lowest pain scores, lowest ratings of parental concern for childhood injuries, and highest coping ability. The authors argued that understanding factors in ethnic differences in pain experience is important to develop maximally efficient pain control regimes for all sections of the British population.

Gaston-Johansson and colleagues (1990) surveyed similarities in pain descriptions and identified terms commonly used by Hispanics, American Indians, African Americans, and Caucasians to describe painful experiences. Subjects ($N = 153$) were asked to rate the intensity of the terms pain, ache, and hurt on a visual analogue scale. Following this procedure, they were given three separate copies of the MPQ and asked to choose the words that represented pain, ache, and hurt, respectively. The results showed that all cultural groups rated pain as the most intense term, followed by hurt; ache was rated least intense. The intensity levels of the three terms differed significantly ($P < 0.001$). The group also identified adjective descriptors that distinguished pain from ache and hurt. However, the authors noted that these English scalings were different than Swedish scalings in which ache (*värk*) was ranked as more intense than hurt (*ont*). Authors also pointed out that semantics could be a problem, yet they do not raise an obvious caveat about their use of English scales for each of the ethnic groups. Perhaps they would have found differences in the meaning of Spanish terms, for example, had Spanish been used.

Zatzick and Dimsdale (1990) reviewed the literature on cultural differences in response to laboratory-induced pain and located 13 studies published between 1944 and 1989. The investigations were diverse with regard to racial and ethnic groups studied, methods of pain induction, and experimental outcome. There appeared to be no racial/ethnic differences in the ability to discriminate painful stimuli. The authors stated that it was more difficult to assess cultural variation in the response to laboratory-induced pain and suggested that age, sex, experimenter ethnicity, and the subjects' working conditions were possible confounders in response to painful stimuli. Given these confounders, there appeared to be no consistent experimental evidence to suggest cultural differences in pain response. They suggested, as did Wolff and Langley (1968) in their review of cross-cultural studies more than 20 years earlier, that perspectives derived from the social sciences could help future laboratory researchers better delineate cultural variations in the pain response. Zatzick and Dimsdale also felt that difficulties inherent in the translation of pain descriptors across cultural boundaries make pain tolerance, rather than pain threshold, the more relevant transcultural pain measure. They suggested that future studies focus on ethnic group differences rather than racial differences and presented specific guidelines so that future researchers might better operationalize culture in the laboratory setting.

Morse and Morse (1988) investigated cultural variation in pain inference, using Thurstone's techniques of paired item comparison surveys to quantify the amount of pain attributed to nine conditions. They selected 190 adults from English-speaking Anglo-Canadian, Ukrainian, East Indian, and Hutterite groups residing in western Canada. Intergroup differences in item choices were found both in rank ordering and quantitative evaluation of the painfulness of nine conditions (e.g., bad burn, heart attack, kidney stones, migraine, and toothache, with slight variation in that order). Childbirth pain showed the most disagreement. The authors concluded that the amount of pain inferred or attributed to these conditions is culturally learned. Although the authors did not attempt to identify ethnospecific descriptors, and the response items were only in English, comparisons of universal pain terms yielded ethnic differences. Significant age differences across groups and English "filtering" of pain meanings makes validity of comparisons dubious.

Abu-Saad (1984) examined how 24 Arab American, 24 Asian American, and 24 Hispanic American children (aged 9–12 years) perceived, described, and responded to common painful experiences. Subjects were interviewed over 6 months at home, in school, or at a recreational facility. The interview schedule was adapted from a pain questionnaire. Findings show that the range of physical and psychological causes of pain did not differ widely among the three groups, which suggests that causative factors of pain in children were universal. Arab American and Hispanic American subjects were more likely to use sensory words to describe pain, while Asian-American subjects tended to use more affective and evaluative words. The range and type of description of subjects' feelings varied by group, as did coping strategies. These results concurred with those of Pfefferbaum (1990) about Anglo-American and Hispanic-American children and parental reactions to invasive procedures in treatment of cancer pain.

Clark and Clark (1980) compared pain thresholds of six 23–42-year-old Nepalese porters to those of five 30–68-year-old Occidentals on a trek in the Himalayas. Responses to noxious transcutaneous electrical stimulation showed that the Nepalese subjects had much higher thresholds to electrical stimulation than did Occidentals. The ability to discriminate was the same for both groups, however, indicating a lack of neurosensory differences. Nepalese had higher (stoical) criteria for reporting pain but were not less sensitive to noxious stimulation. The battery of sensory measurement procedures described may be applied to any modality and are particularly applicable to difficult field conditions. Although the article appeared in the prestigious journal *Science,* the main purpose of the study was to validate sensory detection theory methods of pain measurement. The sample size, given this experimental condition, is of course too small for generalizations, and the study did not try to explain the ethnic differences in pain beliefs of the subjects using standard qualitative social science research methods.

Of course, some classical cross-cultural pain investigations using a variety of experimental and medical anthropological methods in clinical environments deserve attention. Wolff and Langley (1968) published a review about the effects of ethno-cultural factors on the response to pain that critically summarized the literature (32 references) from as early as 1944. They felt that studies at that time, primarily cross-cultural comparisons, revealed a paucity of information. The few experimental studies yielded equivocal results as to the significance of such factors, and in the authors' opinions suffered from anthropological naiveté. However, the authors reviewed some experimental evidence that attitudinal factors do influence the response to pain within cultural groups. They concluded that cultural or medical anthropologists need to combine forces with medical investigators in order to add to the body of knowledge about the pain response.

Wolff and Langley (1968) were most favorable to the classic study by Zborowski (1969), who in 1952 observed and interviewed subjects from four ethnic groups ($N = 146$) in a New York hospital to focus on reactions to different kinds of pain and coping strategies. He concluded that the Irish tended to be deniers and Americans optimistic belittlers of pain. Italians tended to be nonoptimistic expressers of pain, while Jewish patients were more optimistic and expressive. In general, he reported that (1) similar reactions to pain demonstrated by members of different ethnic groups do not always reflect similar attitudes about pain or the meaning of the pain experience, and (2) similar behavioral response patterns to pain may serve different functions in various cultures (e.g., sympathy seeking versus beliefs in ability to rid oneself of pain). Zborowski suggested that physicians use knowledge of these response patterns to facilitate patient coping within the patient's own context. Other empirical investigations of nearly the same ethnic groups have confirmed Zborowski's findings in descriptive (Koopman et al. 1984; Lipton and Marbach 1984) and experimental (Sternbach and Tursky 1965) studies. Although Zborowski's cross-cultural study of pain has probably been the one cited most frequently, his ethnic groups were not matched by age or education, and generalizations attributed to ethnicity were probably overstated because the sample was all men. However, Encandela (1993) has stated that not much new has been reported since Zborowski's book *People in Pain* (1969) showed that pain sufferers responded to pain with learned behaviors and attitudes and respond to health care givers' attitudes within the cultures in which they are socialized. Encandela called for research that would break down variables within ethnicity (e.g., gender, age, institutional relationships) to complete the understanding about how cultural contexts and expectations may affect the experience of pain.

CONCLUSIONS FROM CROSS-CULTURAL STUDY FINDINGS

The cross-cultural literature reveals a wide variety of pain perceptions, beliefs, and reactions and confirms that pain phenomena have universal and ethnospecific aspects. Most studies did not meet criteria for major high-quality epidemiological studies and were often qualitative in nature and of varying quality. Nearly all sampling was convenience sampling.

The most frequent cross-cultural differences reported in these studies related to gender characteristics and patterns of emotional meaning of pain, despite similar physical or sensory components of pain. Hispanic reactions to pain indicated patterns that were more emotional, especially in studies comparing them with Caucasian North American or English reactions (Zborowski 1969; Weisenberg et al. 1975; Davitz et al. 1976; Abu-Saad 1984; Pfefferbaum et al. 1990; Calvillo and Flaskerud 1993; Bates and Rankin 1994; Bates et al. 1995; Ng et al. 1996). Asians or Asian Americans were expected not to react to pain and reacted even less than did North Americans (Davitz et al. 1976; Chapman et al. 1982; Abu-Saad 1984; Brena et al. 1990; Sanders et al. 1992; Lau et al. 1995; Moore et al. 1997, 1998a,b). However, several studies reported that Americans were more dysfunctional than other ethnic or national groups in response to chronic pain (Brena et al. 1990; Sanders et al. 1992; List and

Dworkin 1996; Volinn et al. 1996). We could also conclude that emotional significance of pain is difficult to research in epidemiological studies without having identified the proper variables for a quantitative representative study. Thus, we consider a qualitative research focus to be important and offer further discussion below.

Studies and reviews on headache and low back pain especially indicated that diagnostic criteria or syndrome categories are often poorly defined and difficult to compare. Thus, some authors (Ziegler 1990; Chen 1993; Volinn 1997) called for standardized, easily replicable criteria that would improve the ability to compare prevalences and risks across nations or ethnic groups. These and other methodological issues will be discussed below.

METHODOLOGICAL ISSUES

The literature review points to a certain dissatisfaction by authors who have noted discrepancies in the pain prevalence data. Confusion also surrounds syndrome categorizations and assessment. Thus, it is important to keep the following interrelated methodological issues in mind, especially when designing cross-cultural pain research.

The choice of assessment criteria, including variable selection, must be carefully explored. Important questions in this regard should be: "Which criteria describe which category of any particular pain syndrome or symptomatology from within its social context? Do these need to apply universally across all social contexts?" The possibility for shifts in the social contexts of pain categories implies that a researcher must either choose to focus on and measure known universal pain concepts across cultures or focus on descriptions within ethnospecific contexts where categories may vary across cultures.

Issues about semantics of pain also affect categorization. Important questions are: "What do different ethnic groups expect to be painful or not painful? Do they expect a given pain to cause suffering or disability or to be accepted as a part of life?"

Confusion as to how to formulate aims and designs for cross-cultural investigations can result from these research and semantic issues. Thus, it becomes important to understand similarities and differences of content within the groups to be studied, including the context of institutions and social networks affecting the variables to be studied. These issues are discussed below.

ASSESSMENT CRITERIA AND THE "CATEGORY SHIFT"—"LOST IN A VARIETY OF PAIN UNIVERSES"

Choice of assessment criteria, as in the studies reviewed, is a major complication in efforts to assess what is standard or normal for any particular society. For example, there are at least 18 versions of the McGill Pain Questionnaire reported in the literature (Melzack 1975; Ketovuori and Pontinen 1981; Pontinen and Ketovuori 1983; Molina et al. 1984; Pakula 1984; Maiani and Sanavio 1985; Vanderiet et al. 1987; De Benedittis et al. 1988; Harrison 1988; Stein and Mendl 1988; Hui and Chen 1989; Satow et al. 1989; Strand and Wisnes 1991; Boureau et al. 1992; Drewes et al. 1993; Kim et al. 1995; Escalante et al. 1996; Pimenta and Teixeiro 1996). That so much attention has been paid to developing national versions of standardized pain questionnaires is in itself a statement of the need to understand the universal aspects of pain and social factors that could be influencing pain perception, reactions, and coping. In a thought-provoking article by Crombie and colleagues (1994) entitled "The epidemiology of chronic pain: time for new directions," the authors suggest that published studies on the epidemiology of chronic pain indicate little about the nature of the public health problem and that there is much more to the epidemiology of pain than describing its frequency. They called for development of standard definitions of pain to be used in studies that focus on specific syndromes, rather than aggregating diverse conditions. The problem has been that clinicians or patients often have different diagnoses or interpretations of the meaning of a diagnostic category for syndromes that would otherwise appear to be a standard or universal diagnosis, according to particular measures such as translated versions of the MPQ. Thus, response categories that researchers choose to study may not match those of other researchers or those preferred by their own research subjects. This factor was evident, especially across studies reported in the above literature reviews on cancer pain, headache, and low back pain. Those studies were much influenced by responses of the health care systems to a particular diagnosis, and include, for example, clinicians' knowledge base and their attitudes about diagnostic labeling in relation to disability compensation systems or considerations of patient's expectations or those of friends and families. These factors appear to vary from nation to nation and create social environments that reinforce or otherwise shape pain beliefs and behaviors (Fabrega and Tyma 1976), especially of chronic pain patients.

Thus, drawing guidelines for standard definitions of pain may not be the issue to address if we are to gain wisdom in comparisons across study samples or even across nations or cultures. Rather, a more productive basis for comparison (Kleinman 1987) in some studies might be to find the specific meaning of a pain or pain descriptor within the social context of its occurrence and how it manifests in pain behavior. Then perhaps a universal prospective comparison study based on key variables would yield results with richer clinical and health policy benefits.

Choosing the perspective from which to establish cross-cultural study aims should also become a conscious choice and effort. Recent use of the Brief Pain Inventory (Cleeland et al. 1996) for cancer pain offers an example of designing study aims in which all pains and coping or dysfunctions were regarded as standard or universal. This research perspective has many aspects that bear fruit in a cross-cultural design that looks for similarities in pain or interference variables. This is the so-called "etic" perspective of ethnocultural research as described in the sociolinguistic and anthropological literature (Brislin et al. 1973; Trimble et al. 1983). However, in other studies research aims will require identification of specific cultural factors (the "emic" perspective) (Trimble et al. 1983) that affect meaning and emotional significance, such as issues of religion or family involvements. An example of this perspective was the cancer pain study by Kodiath and Kodiath (1995) comparing Indians and Americans. Bates and Rankin (1995) also illustrated these sociolinguistic and anthropological principles in their study of 200 Puerto Rican and Anglo-American chronic pain patients. They noted that despite similarities in reports of pain intensity, differences in the ability to adapt to chronic pain conditions reflected the cultural context of health care and the availability of income compensation, health insurance, and rehabilitation. They also pointed out that the differences should be evaluated from the emic perspective, because of within-group differences of belief about availability and use of these versus other social network resources. Bates and Rankin (1995) reported that these intragroup analyses were essential because they could provide insight into standards, norms, and variations within specific cultural groups that transcend care provider or researcher preconceptions. Thus, the problem becomes one of variable selection that is based on careful observation and which includes the semantics of any particular variables or assessment criteria within or across the relevant social contexts of the populations that are sampled.

PAIN SEMANTICS—DESCRIPTIONS WITHIN THE CONTEXT OF CULTURAL UNDERSTANDING

The significance or emotional meaning of a pain is important in understanding the language of pain. Although one might ask as an example of the category problem described above—"Do Chinese feel the same kinds of pains as Americans do?"—perhaps an even tougher question is, "Even if an Anglo-American has a headache, is the meaning the same as when a Chinese person says he or she has a headache?" Thus, it is important in attempting to compare data across nations and cultures to understand that even a consensus or social definition of the experienced headache or backache may differ. This factor makes research comparisons across cultures more difficult, but not impossible. In an excellent article in *Pain,* Diller (1980) points out, "Pain experience undergoes cognitive sorting of different types, and it is important to be aware of how obligatory or optional imposed linguistic distinctions may be." He suggests that we "think of cognitive categorizations as exerting controls on affective perception itself through some type of neocortical monitoring or filtering of incoming neural messages." Diller concludes, "In view of the complexity of semantic issues involved, a general theoretical relationship between pain reporting and clinical measurement could hardly be determined on the basis of English speech behavior alone."

It is therefore important that investigators first find the subject response categories that are relevant. Unless investigations across cultures consider that definitions may limit the therapeutic usefulness of pain information to specific social contexts, difficulties may arise in using such epidemiological information in clinically meaningful ways. A useful approach is the idea of specific bits of comparable information that can be researched across the contexts of each of the nations surveyed, if the relevant variables have been carefully chosen for study. Examples of impor-

tant psychosocial variables would be existence of health insurance that covers medical expenses, worker's compensation or other public welfare benefits, attitudes within the culture as to work ethic and desire to work, attitudes toward community and family pride, beliefs in stoicism as normative pain response, and many more. It might be useful to think of a qualitative phase of "exploration and discovery of pertinent variables" as yet another one of the aims of a major epidemiological study of any particular pain topic. Then discovery is built into a research program and aims become more precise for a larger representative descriptive study or a small, but well-designed case-control comparative study. But even after having found the "correct" variables for cross-cultural survey comparison, the investigator must take precautions, such as to translate and back-translate item measures using bilingual judges (Brislin et al. 1973) for maximum semantic verification of terms.

Thus, issues of pain semantics and categories of pain experience are important to the study of pain within its ethno-social context and in guiding choice of research aims and variables. Most epidemiologists are concerned with universal perspectives, but they may find themselves needing specific emic information in order to select the important, most predictive variables for epidemiological surveys.

STUDY AIMS DICTATE THE DESIGN, SAMPLING, AND METHOD TYPE: SO WHAT ELSE IS NEW?

If we look at pain phenomena from this perspective of semantics or categories of meaningfulness, then we should want to integrate both the most relevant social and biological scientific aims into our epidemiological understanding of pain, pain reactions, and coping. These are the foundations of what psychiatrist Horacio Fabrega (1975) called an "ethnomedical science" in a 1975 *Science* article. Regarding research incentives for such a research paradigm, sociologist David Mechanic (1995) has noted that tensions are inevitable between funding agencies seeking to solve specific health care issues within existing frameworks as opposed to the perspective of many social scientists who see health and health care as reflections of societal stratification and processes of power and control. Many current and impending issues require deep scrutiny of values and meaning systems as they relate to class, gender, ethnicity, and other forms of social differentiation. But recategorizing contemporary sociomedical problems (e.g., chronic pain) in this way can help to clarify their roots and sources. Hahn et al. (1983; Hahn 1997) and others (Benson 1997; Spiegel 1997; Wynder 1997) have described our illness beliefs to be as deadly or as healing as drugs, and if we do not pay attention to the choices we face in our medical health care systems, we can allow ourselves to create as many problems as we solve. An example that comes to mind is worker's compensation policy and how it can affect chronic pain behaviors and reactions.

Most anthropologists and some sociologists are concerned with the emic or ethnospecific perspective, but need to know if there is any broader consensus or generalizability to a particular phenomenon or belief within its cultural context or if the data could be an isolated individual's pain beliefs. Representativity is inevitably linked to sampling and concepts of validity and reliability of the data regardless of the research paradigm. Numerical representativity is the most commonly employed paradigm in epidemiology. Thus, representativity is usually thought of as a quantitative research concept. But even the concept of reliability has become a part of the vocabulary of qualitative social scientists in what is now called "qualitative representativity" (Romney et al. 1986, 1987; Batchelder and Romney 1988; Weller and Romney 1988; Moore 1996).

Qualitative representativity is based on measures of how accurately subjects describe a given social phenomenon and the degree of agreement between subjects about such descriptions (Romney et al. 1986; Batchelder and Romney 1988) as described earlier, given careful sample selection (Johnson 1990; Moore 1996; Moore et al. 1997). Overall informant competency (accuracy in knowing the details about social phenomena related to pain) is mathematically equal to the square root of the mean agreement among all informants within a group (Batchelder and Romney 1988; Weller and Romney 1988), which is similar to the relationship between reliability and validity coefficients in psychometrics. So perhaps in the end, qualitative and quantitative research are much more closely related than earlier imagined, if they are considered in terms of concepts of probability and predictive validity. Emphasizing the strengths of both paradigms is important. Perhaps combining qualitative and quantitative methods to improve concurrent validity and reliability of results should become a goal in its own

right (Moore 1996).

The ultimate point in researching pain phenomena within and across cultural contexts is that one must choose the perspective that is most appropriate to the aims of any particular study and the sampling that makes it possible to accomplish those aims. As much as it may sound simple and a recurrent theme in research in general, it would not be overstated with respect to cross-cultural research of pain, to say that study designs, sampling, and method type are dependent on the specific aims of the intended study. Also needed in that regard is an increased focus on variable selection in epidemiology as part of the study aims.

OVERALL CONCLUSIONS

What can we deduce and induce from this review of cross-cultural pain studies? We offer concluding comments on two levels—substantive content and methods. Contrasting the differences in pain reactions and adaptation to pain, such as coping style and disability/dysfunction, seems to reflect the most variance across cultures. With the cross-cultural perspective we can gain an understanding of "the big picture" of the human condition in regard to pain and suffering. The incentives that drive or drag pain reactions, especially in nonspecific chronic back and headache pains, lead to the conclusion that agencies giving economic support to patients with those kinds of pain must operate within a family context. Support should include emotional and not just medical or financial help. For example, family counseling in how to support the suffering pain patient should be a prerequisite to expensive medical interventions or financial support.

In regard to the methodological issues raised in this review, we conclude that there are both qualitative and quantitative differences, especially in pain reactions and behaviors across sociocultural contexts. Universal pain conditions appear to be similar in regard to their social impact and can often be compared, given valid variables and a prescribed study aim. It is important for investigators to keep in mind that item selection in data collection phases and data reduction choices in the analysis phase should try to preserve the ethnic cultural and local situational characteristics of the populations surveyed so as to avoid systematic bias and invalid results. Again, depending on the study aims and the population to be studied, selection of the relevant variables is essential.

The advantages of looking cross-culturally at the human pain experience must outweigh the disadvantages. It is fascinating to observe that in the human condition there is something so personal yet so universal as pain and dealing with pain, and that in the end, these mirror aspects of human social experience. Exploring the social and psychological variables that govern pain perceptions, beliefs, and reactions, must, at least to some degree, be the task of every pain epidemiologist or clinical investigator who wants to attain a degree of success in understanding pain phenomena and their clinical implications.

ACKNOWLEDGMENTS

Supported by Grants 5 R29 DE09945-05 NIH/National Institutes of Dental Research, Bethesda, Maryland, Regional Center for Dental Research Clinic, University of Washington National Institute of Dental and Craniofacial Research P50-DE-08229-08, and Danish National Health Insurance Research Fund 11/215-93, Denmark.

REFERENCES

Abu-Saad H. Cultural group indicators of pain in children. *Matern Child Nurs J* 1984; 13:187–196.

Batchelder WH, Romney AK. Test theory without an answer key. *Psychometrika* 1988; 53:71–92.

Bates MS, Rankin HL. Control, culture and chronic pain. *Soc Sci Med* 1994; 39:629–645.

Bates MS, Rankin HL, Sanchez AM, Mendez BR. A cross-cultural comparison of adaptation to chronic pain among Anglo-Americans and native Puerto Ricans. *Med Anthropol* 1995; 16:141–173.

Benson H. The nocebo effect: history and physiology. *Prev Med* 1997; 26:612–615.

Bergner M, Bobbitt RA, Carter WB, Gilson BS. The Sickness Impact Profile: development and final revision of a health status measure. *Med Care* 1981; 19:787–805.

Boureau F, Luu M, Doubrere JF. Comparative study of the validity of four French McGill Pain Questionnaire (MPQ) versions. *Pain* 1992; 50:59–65.

Brasseur L, Larue F, Colleau SM, Cleeland CS. Cancer pain: barriers to effective care (France). In: *Refresher Course Syllabus.* Seattle: IASP Press, 1993, pp 191–192.

Brena SF, Sanders SH, Motoyama H. American and Japanese chronic low back pain patients: cross-cultural similarities and differences. *Clin J Pain* 1990; 6:118–124.

Brislin RW, Lonner WJ, Thorndike RM. *Cross-cultural Research Methods.* New York: Wiley and Sons, 1973.

Calvillo ER, Flaskerud JH. Evaluation of the pain response by Mexican American and Anglo American women and their nurses. *J Adv Nurs* 1993; 18:451–459.

Caraceni A, Mendoza TR, Mencaglia E, et al. A validation study of an Italian version of the Brief Pain Inventory (Breve Questionario per la Valutazione del Dolore). *Pain* 1996; 65:87–92.

Carron H, DeGood DE, Tait R. A comparison of low back pain patients in the United States and New Zealand: psychosocial and economic factors affecting severity of disability. *Pain* 1985; 21:77–89.

Chapman CR, Sato T, Martin RW, et al. Comparative effects of acupuncture in Japan and the United States on dental pain perception. *Pain* 1982; 12:319–328.

Chen ACN. Headache: contrast between childhood and adult pain. *International Journal of Adolescent Medicine and Health* 1993; 6:75–93.

Chiou WK, Wong MK, Lee YH. Epidemiology of low back pain in Chinese nurses. *Int J Nurs Stud* 1994; 31:361–368.

Clark WC, Clark SB. Pain responses in Nepalese porters. *Science* 1980; 209:410–411.

Cleeland CS. Barriers to cancer pain management: recent U.S. research. In: *Refresher Course Syllabus.* Seattle: IASP Publications, 1993a, pp 193–196.

Cleeland CS. Issues in cancer pain assessment. In: *Refresher Course Syllabus,* Seattle: IASP Publications, 1993b; p 209.

Cleeland CS, Ladinsky JL, Serlin RC, Thuy NC. Multidimensional measurement of cancer pain: comparisons of US and Vietnamese patients. *J Pain Symptom Manage* 1988; 3:23–27.

Cleeland CS, Ryan KM. Pain assessment: global use of the Brief Pain Inventory. *Ann Acad Med Singapore* 1994; 23:129–138.

Cleeland CS, Nakamura Y, Mendoza TR, et al. Dimensions of the impact of cancer pain in a four country sample: new information from multidimensional scaling. *Pain* 1996; 67:267–273.

Corah N. Development of a dental anxiety scale. *J Dent Res* 1969; 48:596.

Croft PR, Rigby AS. Socioeconomic influences on back problems in the community in Britain. *J Epidemiol Community Health* 1994; 48:166–170.

Crombie IK, Davies HTO, Macrae WA. The epidemiology of chronic pain: time for new directions. *Pain* 1994; 57:1–3.

Dahlstrom WG, Welsh GS, Dahlstrom LE. *An MMPI Handbook.* Minneapolis: University of Minnesota Press, 1972.

Davitz LJ, Sameshima Y, Davitz J. Suffering as viewed in six different cultures. *Am J Nurs* 1976; 76:1296–1297.

De Benedittis G, Massei R, Nobili R, Pieri A. The Italian Pain Questionnaire. *Pain* 1988; 33:53–62.

Deng YM, Fu MK, Hagg U. Prevalence of temporomandibular joint dysfunction (TMJD) in Chinese children and adolescents. A cross-sectional epidemiological study. *Eur J Orthod* 1995; 17:305–309.

Derogatis LR. SCL-90-R: Administration, Scoring and Procedures Manual II. Revised Version. *Clinical Psychometric Research,* Towson, MD, 1983.

Diller A. Cross-cultural pain semantics. *Pain* 1980; 9:9–26.

Drewes AM, Helweg LS, Petersen P, et al. McGill Pain Questionnaire translated into Danish: experimental and clinical findings. *Clin J Pain* 1993; 9:80–87.

Dworkin SF, LeResche L. Research diagnostic criteria for temporomandibular disorders: Review, criteria, examinations and specifications, critique. *J Craniomandib Disord Facial Oral Pain* 1992; 6:301–355.

Encandela JA. Social science and the study of pain since Zborowski: a need for a new agenda. *Soc Sci Med* 1993; 36:783–791.

Escalante A, Lichtenstein MJ, R'ios, N, Hazuda HP. Measuring chronic rheumatic pain in Mexican Americans: cross-cultural adaptation of the McGill Pain Questionnaire. *J Clin Epidemiol* 1996; 49:1389–1399.

Fabrega H, Jr. The need for an ethnomedical science. *Science*

1975; 189:969–975.

Fabrega H. Cultural relativism and psychiatric illness. *J Nerv Ment Dis* 1989; 177:415–425.

Fabrega H. Tyma S. Culture, language and the shaping of illness: An illustration based on pain. *J Psychosom Res* 1976; 20:323–337.

Foley KM. Changing concepts of tolerance to opioids—what the cancer patient has taught us. In: *Refresher Course Syllabus*. Seattle: IASP Publications, 1993, p 221.

Follick MJ, Smith TW, Ahern DK. The sickness impact profile: A global measure of disability in chronic low-back pain. *Pain* 1985; 21:67–76.

Gaston-Johansson F, Albert M, Fagan E, Zimmerman L. Similarities in pain descriptions of four different ethnic-culture groups. *J Pain Symptom Manage* 1990; 5:94–100.

Geiger HJ. Health care in the People's Republic of China: implications for the United States. In: Kleinman A, Kunstadter P, Alexander ER, Gale JL (Eds). *Medicine in Chinese Cultures: Comparative Studies of Health Care in Chinese and Other Societies*. Washington, DC: National Institutes of Health, 1975, pp 713–724.

Gordon C. The effect of cancer pain on quality of life in different ethnic groups: a literature review. *Nurse Pract Forum* 1997; 8:5–13.

Hahn RA. The nocebo phenomenon: concept, evidence, and implications for public health. *Prev Med* 1997; 26:607–611.

Hahn RA, Kleinman A. Belief as pathogen, belief as medicine: "Voodoo death" and the "placebo phenomenon" in anthropological perspective. *Med Anthropol Quarterly* 1983; 14:16–19.

Harrison A. Arabic pain words. *Pain* 1988; 32:239–250.

Henriksson CM. Living with continuous muscular pain—patient perspectives. Part II: Strategies for daily life. *Scand J Caring Sci* 1995; 9:77–86.

Hui YL, Chen AC. Analysis of headache in a Chinese patient population. *Ma Tsui Hsueh Tsa Chi* 1989; 27:13–18.

James FR, Large RG, Bushnell JA, Wells EJ. Epidemiology of pain in New Zealand. *Pain* 1991; 44:279–283.

Johnson JC. *Selecting Ethnographic Informants*. Newbury Park, CA: Sage, 1990.

Ketovuori H, Pontinen PJ. A pain vocabulary in Finnish: the Finnish pain questionnaire. *Pain* 1981; 11:247–253.

Kim HS, Schwartz BD, Holter IM, Lorensen M. Developing a translation of the McGill pain questionnaire for cross-cultural comparison: an example from Norway. *J Adv Nurs* 1995; 21:421–426.

Kleinman A. Clinical relevance of anthropological and cross-cultural research: concepts and strategies. *Am J Psychiatry* 1978; 135:427–431.

Kleinman A. Appendix to Chapter 36. In: Kleinman A, Kunstadter P, Alexander ER, Gale JL (Eds). *Medicine in Chinese Cultures: Comparative Studies of Health Care in Chinese and Other Societies*. Washington, DC: National Institutes of Health, 1975, pp 645–658.

Kleinman A. Anthropology and psychiatry. The role of culture in cross-cultural research on illness. *Br J Psychiatry* 1987; 151:447–454.

Kleinman A, Kunstadter P. Introduction. In: Kleinman A, Kunstadter P, Alexander ER, Gale JL (Eds). *Medicine in Chinese Cultures: Comparative Studies of Health Care in Chinese and Other Societies*. Washington, DC: National Institutes of Health, 1975, pp 1–18.

Kleinman A, Eisenberg L, Good B. Culture, illness, and care: clinical lessons from anthropologic and cross-cultural research. *Ann Intern Med* 1978; 88:251–258.

Koch-Weser, D. Comments on implication of the Chinese experience for developing countries and the United States. In:

Kleinman A, Kunstadter P, Alexander ER, JL Gale JL (Eds). *Medicine in Chinese Cultures: Comparative Studies of Health Care in Chinese and Other Societies*. Washington, DC: National Institutes of Health, 1975, pp 725–728.

Kodiath MF, Kodiath A. A comparative study of patients who experience chronic malignant pain in India and the United States. *Cancer Nurs* 1995; 18:189–196.

Koopman C, Eisenthal S, Stoeckle JD. Ethnicity in the reported pain, emotional distress and requests of medical outpatients. *Soc Sci Med* 1984; 18:487–490.

Lau EMC, Egger P, Coggon D, Cooper C, et al. Low back pain in Hong Kong: prevalence and characteristics compared with Britain. *J Epidemiol Community Health* 1995; 49:492–494.

LeResche L. Epidemiology of temporomandibular disorders: implications for the investigation of etiologic factors. *Crit Rev Oral Biol Med* 1997; 8:291–305.

Lipton JA, Marbach JJ. Ethnicity and the pain experience. *Soc Sci Med* 1984; 19:1279–1298.

List T, Dworkin SF. Comparing TMD diagnoses and clinical findings at Swedish and US TMD centers using research diagnostic criteria for temporomandibular disorders. *J Orofac Pain* 1996; 10:240–253.

Maiani G, Sanavio E. Semantics of pain in Italy: the Italian version of the McGill Pain Questionnaire. *Pain* 1985; 22:399–405.

Mechanic D. Emerging trends in the application of the social sciences to health and medicine. *Soc Sci Med* 1995; 40:1491–1496.

Melzack R. The McGill Pain Questionnaire: major properties and scoring methods. *Pain* 1975; 1:277–299.

Molina FJ, Molina BZ, Molina JC, Coppo C. The Argentine pain questionnaire. *Pain* 1984; 2(Suppl):S42, Abstract.

Moore R. Ethnographic assessment of pain coping perceptions. *Psychosom Med* 1990; 52:171–181.

Moore R. Combining qualitative and quantitative research approaches in understanding pain. *J Dent Educ* 1996; 60:709–715.

Moore R, Miller ML, Weinstein P, Dworkin SF, Liou HH. Cultural perceptions of pain and pain coping among patients and dentists. *Community Dent Oral Epidemiol* 1986; 14:327–333.

Moore R, Brødsgaard I, Mao T-K, et al. Fear of injections and report of negative dentist behavior among Caucasian American and Taiwanese adults from dental school clinics. *Community Dent Oral Epidemiol* 1996; 24:292–295.

Moore R, Brødsgaard I, Miller ML, Mao T-K, Dworkin SF. Consensus analysis: reliability, validity and informant accuracy in use of American and Mandarin Chinese pain descriptors. *Ann Beh Med* 1997; 19:295–300.

Moore R, Brødsgaard I, Mao T-K, Miller ML, Dworkin SF. Perceived need for local anesthesia in tooth drilling among AngloAmericans, Mandarin Chinese and Scandinavians. *Anesth Prog* 1998a; 45:22–28.

Moore R, Brødsgaard I, Mao T-K, Miller ML, Dworkin SF. Acute pain and use of local anesthesia: tooth drilling and childbirth labor pain beliefs among AngloAmericans, Mandarin Chinese and Scandinavians. *Anesth Prog* 1998b; 45:29–37.

Moore RA, Dworkin SF. Ethnographic methodologic assessment of pain perceptions by verbal description. *Pain* 1988; 34:195–204.

Morse JM. Cultural variation in behavioral response to parturition: Childbirth in Fiji. Special Issue: Cross-cultural nursing: anthropological approaches to nursing research. *Med Anthropol* 1989; 12:35–54.

Morse JM, Morse RM. Cultural variation in the inference of pain. *J Cross Cult Psychol* 1988; 19:232–242.

Nelson DV, Novy DM, Averill PM, Berry LA. Ethnic comparability of the MMPI in pain patients. *J Clin Psychol* 1996; 52:485–497.

Ng B, Dimsdale JE, Rollnik JD, Shapiro H. The effect of ethnicity on prescriptions for patient-controlled analgesia for postoperative pain. *Pain* 1996; 66:9–12.

Onizawa, KYH. Longitudinal changes of symptoms of temporomandibular disorders in Japanese young adults. *J Orofac Pain* 1996; 10:151–156.

Pakula A. Psychophysical validation of the Lithuanian pain questionnaire (LPQ) sensory scale: a clinical model. *Pain* 1984; 2(Suppl):S43 [Abstract].

Pesce G. Measurement of reported pain of childbirth: a comparison between Australian and Italian subjects. *Pain* 1987; 31:87–92.

Pfefferbaum B, Adams J, Aceves J. The influence of culture on pain in Anglo and Hispanic children with cancer. *J Am Acad Child Adolesc Psychiatry* 1990; 29:642–647.

Pimenta CA, Teixeiro MJ. [Proposal to adapt the McGill Pain Questionnaire into Portuguese], *Rev Esc Enferm USP* 1996; 30:473–483.

Pontinen PH, Ketovuori H. Verbal measurement in non-English language: the Finnish pain questionnaire. In: Melzack R (Ed). *Pain Measurement and Assessment.* New York: Raven Press, 1983, pp 85–93.

Pugh, JF. The semantics of pain in Indian culture and medicine. *Cult Med Psychiatry* 1991; 15:19–43.

Romney AK, Weller SC, Batchelder WH. Culture as consensus: a theory of cultural and informant accuracy. *Am Anthropologist* 1986; 88:313–338.

Romney AK, Weller SC, Batchelder WH. Interpreting consensus: a reply to Price. *Am Anthropologist* 1987; 90:161–163.

Sanders SH, Brena SF, Spier CJ, et al. Chronic low back pain patients around the world: cross-cultural similarities and differences. *Clin J Pain* 1992; 8:317–323.

Satow, A, Nakatani, K and Taniguchi, S. Japanese version of the MPQ and pentagon profile illustrated perceptual characteristics of pain [letter]. *Pain* 1989; 37:125–126.

Shiau YY, Chang C. An epidemiological study of temporomandibular disorders in university students of Taiwan. *Community Dent Oral Epidemiol* 1992; 20:43–47.

Spiegel H, Nocebo: The power of suggestibility. *Prev Med* 1997; 26:616–621.

Stein C, Mendl G. The German counterpart to McGill Pain Questionnaire. *Pain* 1988; 32:251–255.

Sternbach RA. Survey of pain in the United States: the Nuprin Pain Report. *Clin J Pain* 1986; 2:49–53.

Sternbach RA, Tursky B. Ethnic differences among housewives in psychophysiology and skin potential responses to electric shock. *Psychophysiology* 1965; 1:241–246.

Strand LI, Wisnes AR. The development of a Norwegian pain questionnaire. *Pain* 1991; 46:61–66.

Strassberg, DS. The MMPI and chronic pain. *J Consult Clin Psychol* 1981; 49:220–226.

Strassberg DS, Tilley D, Bristone S, Oei T. The MMPI and chronic pain: a crosscultural view. *Psychol Assess* 1992; 4:493–497.

Thomas VJ, Rose FD. Ethnic differences in the experience of pain. *Soc Sci Med* 1991; 32:1063–1066.

Todd KH, Samaroo N, Hoffman JR. Ethnicity as a risk factor for inadequate emergency department analgesia [see comments]. *JAMA* 1993; 269:1537–1539.

Trimble JE, Lonner WJ, Boucher JD. Stalking the wily emic: alternatives to cross-cultural measurement. In: Irvine SH, JW Berry JW (Eds). *Human Assessment and Cultural Factors.* Boston: Plenum Publishing, 1983, pp 259–273.

Vanderiet K, Adriaensen H, Carton H, Vertommen H. The McGill Pain Questionnaire constructed for the Dutch language (MPQ-DV). Preliminary data concerning reliability and validity. *Pain* 1987; 30:395–408.

Volinn E. The epidemiology of low back pain in the rest of the world: a review of surveys in low and middle income countries. *Spine* 1997; 22:1747–1754.

Volinn E, Kitahara M, Nachemson AL. A preliminary investigation of cross-national disparities in rates of back pain disability: the U.S. and Sweden compared with Japan. IASP abstracts, *8th World Congress on Pain* [Abstract]. Seattle: IASP Press, 1996, p 68.

Von Korff M, Dworkin SF, LeResche L, Kruger A. An epidemiologic comparison of pain complaints. *Pain* 1988; 32:173–183.

Von Korff M, Ormel J, Keefe FJ, Dworkin SF. Grading the severity of chronic pain. *Pain* 1992; 50:133–149.

Walsh K, Cruddas M, Coggon D. Low back pain in eight areas of Britain. *J Epidemiol Community Health* 1992; 46: 227–230.

Waluyo L, Ekberg K, Eklund J. Assembly work in Indonesia and in Sweden—ergonomics, health and satisfaction. *Ergonomics* 1996; 39:199–212.

Wang XS, Mendoza TR, Gao SZ, Cleeland CS. The Chinese version of the Brief Pain Inventory (BPI-C): its development and use in a study of cancer pain. *Pain* 1996; 67:407–416.

Weisenberg M, Caspi Z. Cultural and educational influences on pain of childbirth. *J Pain Symptom Manage* 1989; 4:13–19.

Weisenberg M, Kreindler ML, Schachat R, Werboff J. Pain: anxiety and attitudes in black, white and Puerto Rican patients. *Psychosom Med* 1975; 37:123–135.

Weller SC, Romney AK. *Systematic Data Collection.* Newbury Park, CA: Sage, 1988.

Wolff BB, Langley S. Cultural factors and the response to pain: a review. *Am Anthropologist* 1968; 70:494–501.

Wynder EL. The American Health Foundation's Nocebo Conference. *Prev Med* 1997; 26:605–606.

Zatzick DF, Dimsdale JE. Cultural variations in response to painful stimuli. *Psychosom Med* 1990; 52:544–557.

Zborowski M. *People in Pain.* San Francisco: Jossey-Bass, 1969.

Zenz M. Barriers to effective care. In: *Refresher Course Syllabus.* Seattle: IASP Publications, 1993, pp 197–200.

Ziegler DK. Headache. Public health problem. *Neurol Clin* 1990; 8:781–791.

Zola JK. Culture and symptoms: An analysis of patients presenting complaints. *Am Soc Rev* 1966; 31:615–630.

Correspondence to: Rod Moore, DDS, PhD, Royal Dental College, Aarhus University, Vennelyst Boulevard, 8000 Aarhus C, Denmark. Tel: +45-89-424078; Fax: +45-86-136550; email: rmoore@odont.aau.dk.

Epidemiology of Pain, edited by
I.K. Crombie, IASP Press, Seattle, © 1999.

7

Chronic Pain in Children

Patricia A. McGrath

*Department of Paediatrics, The University of Western Ontario,
and Paediatric Pain Program, Child Health Research Institute, London, Ontario, Canada*

During the last decade, unprecedented attention has focused on the special pain problems of infants, children, and adolescents. As a result of much research, we have gained better insights into how children perceive pain, how to assess their pain, and how to use various pharmacological therapies more effectively to alleviate their pain and distress (for review see McGrath and Unruh 1987; Ross and Ross 1988; Pichard-Leandri and Gauvain-Piquard 1989; McGrath 1990, 1994; Tyler and Krane 1990; Schechter et al. 1993; Barr 1994; Houck et al. 1994; McGrath and Hillier 1996). However, while we know much more about the treatment of specific types of acute, recurrent, and chronic pain in children, we know little about the prevalence of these pain problems (McGrath 1990; Goodman and McGrath 1991). In addition, we know very little about the individual costs (to children and families), the economic costs, and the factors that may predispose certain children to develop debilitating pain problems.

This chapter reviews the epidemiological research on chronic pain in children to document the prevalence of different types of pain related to disease and trauma, nonspecific pain, and pain associated with emotional distress. Although chronic pain is often defined as any pain that persists (almost continuously) for a period of 3 months, many children experience intermittent episodes of pain over a long period. Thus, for this review, chronic pain is defined as any prolonged pain that lasts a minimum of 3 months or any pain that recurs throughout a minimum period of 3 months. Review of the existing epidemiological data on chronic pain in children began with a search of MEDLINE and Psych INFO databases for the period 1984–1998 (April). The main textbooks on pain in children were searched manually, as were reference lists of all relevant papers to identify studies published prior to 1984.

To provide a comprehensive review of all types of chronic pain, the literature search included the general topic of pain in children and 20 specific pain problems (i.e., headache, abdominal pain, limb pain, chest pain, knee pain, back pain, head injury, psychosomatic pain, somatization disorder, cancer, neuropathic pain, reflex sympathetic dystrophy, complex regional pain syndrome, phantom limb pain, musculoskeletal pain, fibromyalgia, arthritis, sickle cell anemia, orofacial pain, and dysmenorrhea) cross-referenced to children and cross-referenced separately to three terms—epidemiology, prevalence, and survey. All searches revealed a similar pattern: many citations related to prevalence, survey, or epidemiology; relatively few citations for the specific type of pain in children; and very few citations linking the pain problem in children and prevalence. In addition to specific pain problems, the review included major epidemiological studies of the childhood diseases usually associated with chronic pain, such as arthritis, so as to capture all potential data on the prevalence of chronic pain related to disease.

All studies were reviewed and graded as major if they satisfied the following criteria: well-defined purpose, adequate definition of pain, appropriate study design, adequate sample size, appropriate statistical analysis, and valid interpretation of findings. The study design was judged appropriate only when the methods of data collection and case identification were adequately described and the response rate from the study sample was sufficiently high (>75%) so that investigators could achieve their stated study objective.

Although most studies did not satisfy criteria for inclusion as major studies in the tables, several provided valuable documentation that children experience many types of chronic pain. These studies are described briefly in the text and are listed in the references. Epidemiological data are presented for five general categories of chronic pain: disease-related, trauma-related, nonspecific, recurrent pain syndrome, and mental health-related. Information on prevalence, natural history, and effect of pain is presented for each type of chronic pain, when such information is available.

PAIN RELATED TO CHRONIC DISEASE

The review of articles on pain related to chronic disease (e.g., arthritis, cancer, hemophilia, sickle cell disease, and fibromyalgia) did not yield any studies that satisfied fully the criteria of a major study exclusively focused on chronic pain in children. However, three epidemiological studies on juvenile arthritis satisfied many criteria, included some reference to pain, and provided prevalence estimates for a childhood disease usually associated with chronic pain (Gare et al. 1987; Gare and Fasth 1992; Manners and Diepeveen 1996). A population study provided estimates for juvenile arthritis and sickle cell disease (Newacheck and Taylor 1992). A study on psychiatric symptoms of pre-

adolescents with musculoskeletal pain provided prevalence data on fibromyalgia in children (Mikkelsson 1997).

Other studies of chronic diseases in children either provided epidemiological data on only disease prevalence or incidence, without explicitly including pain as part of the criteria for disease definition, or described the characteristics of a clinical sample—patient demographics and disease characteristics, perhaps including some information about the quality, location, intensity, and duration of pain. Although these latter studies did not present sufficient data to enable readers to extrapolate meaningful information about the prevalence of chronic pain in children, a few are presented in order to demonstrate the magnitude of chronic disease in childhood (Table I). Because these diseases often cause chronic pain, the available prevalence data constitute the only estimates for the prevalence of pain in children related to chronic disease.

JUVENILE RHEUMATOID/CHRONIC ARTHRITIS

Disease definition

Juvenile rheumatoid arthritis (JRA) or juvenile chronic arthritis (JCA) is a disease or group of diseases characterized by chronic synovitis and associated with extra-articular inflammatory manifestations (Schaller 1992). Diagnostic criteria include: age of onset less than 16 years; arthritis in one or more joints defined as swelling or effusion or two or more of the

Table I
Prevalence of chronic pain related to disease in children

Pain	Study Type	Disease Definition	Source of Sample	Sample Size	Prevalence Estimate	Age (years)	Prevalence per 100,000	Reference
Juvenile chronic arthritis	CS	EULAR	Sweden, clinic	400600	Period	0–16	56	Gare et al. 1987
Juvenile chronic arthritis	CS, longitudinal	EULAR	Sweden, clinic	386817	Period	0–15	64.1–86.3	Gare and Fasth 1992
Juvenile chronic arthritis	CS	EULAR	Australia, community	2241	Point	12	400	Manners and Diepeveen 1996
Juvenile arthritis	CS	Self-report	USA, population	17110	Point	0–8	460	Newacheck and Taylor 1992
Sickle cell disease	CS	Self-report	USA, population	17110	Point	0–8	120	Newacheck and Taylor 1992
Fibromyalgia	CS	ACR	Finland, school	1756	Point	9–12	57*	Mikkelsson et al. 1997

Abbreviations: ACR = American College of Rheumatology; CS = cross-sectional; EULAR = European League Against Rheumatism.
*Prevalence rate calculated from data presented in article.

following signs—limitation of the range of motion, tenderness or pain on motion, increased heat; minimum duration of 6 weeks (for JRA) or 3 months (for JCA); disease type during the first 4 or 6 months classified as polyarthritis (five joints or more), oligoarthritis (four joints or fewer), systemic disease (intermittent fever, rheumatoid rash, arthritis, visceral disease, lymphadenopathy); and exclusion of other rheumatic diseases (Brewer et al. 1972). The diagnosis of JRA requires a minimum 6-week duration and excludes juvenile ankylosing spondylitis (JAS) and juvenile psoriatic arthritis (JPA). In contrast, the diagnosis of JCA requires a minimum 3-month duration in the absence of trauma or other rheumatologic conditions, not excluding JAS and JPA.

As noted in this definition, pain is not a required criterion for a diagnosis of JRA or JCA. Yet, children with arthritis may develop chronic pain from inflammation of the joints, chronic changes in articular tissues, complications of the arthritis, systemic illness, medication side effects, and affective changes (Hart 1974). Clinical studies indicate that continuous or intermittent episodes of pain are common among the children treated (Thompson et al. 1987; Lovell and Walco 1989).

Prevalence data

The epidemiological data on juvenile arthritis yield conflicting prevalence rates of 3 to 460 cases per 100,000 children (Sury 1952; Laaksonen 1966; Bywaters 1968; Sullivan et al. 1975; Baum 1977; Bonham 1978; Gewanter et al. 1983; Towner et al. 1983; Manners and Diepeveen 1996; Hill 1977).

As shown in Table I, two large surveys were conducted in Sweden, using the European League Against Rheumatism (EULAR) criteria, diagnostic criteria described previously with a minimum disease duration of 3 months (Gare et al. 1987; Gare and Fasth 1992). Although the authors described these studies as population-based surveys, they identified arthritis cases from clinical records in pediatric rheumatology clinics and from local pediatricians. Both studies obtained high prevalence rates, 56 and 64 to 86 per 100,000, respectively (the latter estimate depending on whether children in remission were included). Girls predominated over boys in a ratio of 3:2.

However, results from three community studies suggest that the number of undiagnosed children with JCA significantly exceeds the number of known cases and that the true prevalence rate is higher than that reported in previous clinical studies. Mielants and colleagues (1993) conducted a community survey to determine the prevalence of inflammatory rheumatic diseases in 2990 adolescents, 12–18 years of age, in Belgium. After students completed a questionnaire about their history of joint pain, rheumatologists examined 524 students with a history of inflammatory joints or pain. Although the authors did not explicitly describe diagnostic criteria (this study thus does not satisfy the criteria for a major study), they obtained prevalence rates of 167 and 301 cases per 100,000 individuals for definite JCA and presumptive JCA, respectively.

In another cross-sectional community study, Manners and Diepeveen (1996) determined the point prevalence of inflammatory joint disease and other rheumatic disorders in 2241 12-year-old children in Australia. A pediatric rheumatologist examined all students. The prevalence rate for JCA was 4 cases per 1000 individuals. The authors conclude that this very high rate was due to their method of case ascertainment based on clinical examination by a rheumatologist of children within a community, which identified undiagnosed cases. A large population survey of childhood chronic illness obtained a similar high rate (4.6 cases per 1000) by using the 1988 National Health Interview Survey on 17,110 children from the United States under 18 years of age (Newacheck and Taylor 1992). The results of the community studies in three countries indicate a much higher than expected prevalence of JCA, a disease that probably causes some persistent pain in all affected children. However, we do not know the proportion of children who have different levels of pain (mild, moderate, severe) nor the proportion who experience almost continual pain.

Natural history and impact of pain

Although the pain of juvenile arthritis is related to the severity of the disease, there is usually no predictable course for children. Mild arthritis can cause little pain and disability, while severe arthritis may cause joint destruction, permanent deformity, and chronic pain. However, exacerbations and remissions may occur, or symptoms may persist for years (Schaller 1992). Interestingly, some clinical studies indicate that children with JRA may have less pain than do adults with arthritis (Laaksonen and Laine 1961; Scott et al.

1977) and that younger children (6–11 years old) have less pain than do older children (12–17 years old) (Beales et al. 1983). However, no study has yet followed the same cohort of children to evaluate developmental differences in the course of their pain.

Several studies have evaluated the roles of stress, personality, and familial factors in the cause or exacerbation of arthritis (Blom and Nicholls 1954; Heisel 1972; Varni and Jay 1984; Anderson et al. 1985; Ungerer et al. 1988) and the relationships among disease severity, pain, and psychological adjustment for children (McAnarney 1974; Ivey et al. 1981; Litt et al. 1982; Billings et al. 1987; Thompson et al. 1987; Timko et al. 1992). The results of studies are often contradictory because of the relatively small numbers of children drawn from clinic populations and differences in age groups, assessment procedures, and outcome measures. Thus, it is premature to make any firm conclusions about the specific impact of these factors on children's pain.

CANCER PAIN

Disease definition

Cancer pains are classified according to the primary source of noxious stimulation as disease-related, procedure-related, therapy-related, and incidental (Foley 1979). All children with cancer experience some acute pain during the disease course or treatment. Some children will experience chronic pain when the disease invades bone, compresses central or peripheral nerves, infiltrates blood vessels, and injures healthy tissue. Therapy-related chronic pain may develop as a result of surgery, neuropathy secondary to irradiation of a nerve plexus, chemotherapy administration (particularly vincristine), phantom limb pain, dermatitis/skin necrosis, corticosteroid-induced bone changes, and gastritis from protracted vomiting or drug-induced mucosal damage (Miser 1993).

Prevalence data

Cancer is a relatively rare disease in children, with an approximate incidence of 2 per 1000 in Western industrialized nations (Altman and Schwartz 1983; Diamond and Matthay 1988). Studies have indicated that approximately 60–70% of reported pain in adults is directly related to malignancy (Daut and Cleeland 1982), while procedure- and therapy-related pain are more common in children (Schechter 1985; Jay et al. 1986; Miser et al. 1987). It is presumed that children with cancer generally do not experience the same chronic debilitating pain as do adults with cancer because they are afflicted with different forms of the disease. Leukemia is the primary type of cancer that afflicts children, in contrast to the lung, breast, gastrointestinal, and skin cancers common in adults. In addition, most pediatric malignancies are highly responsive to the initial aggressive therapy regimens, so that complete remission occurs in most pediatric cancers, and many children in developed countries experience prolonged disease-free survival (Miser 1993).

However, we lack epidemiological data to determine whether children rarely have chronic cancer pain or whether we have simply failed to recognize this problem. Investigators have begun to specifically document the prevalence of childhood cancer pain within their own treatment centers, but no population-based prevalence estimates are available. Cornaglia and colleagues (1984) reported that 57% of 910 children treated over 10 years had experienced moderate to severe pain, but they did not specify the proportion of children who experienced chronic pain.

Two studies clearly demonstrate that some children with cancer suffer from chronic intractable pain. Miser and colleagues (1987a) surveyed the nature and prevalence of pain in all patients (139 children and young adults, 7–25 years of age; median 16 years) who were treated by the pediatric branch of the National Cancer Institute (United States) during a 6-month period. Seven patients had chronic pain for longer than 1 year after the eradication of all known tumors from the site of pain. In a second study, Miser (1987b) surveyed pain in 92 children and young adults (6 months to 24 years of age; median 16 years) with newly diagnosed malignancy. At the time of assessment, 72 patients had been experiencing pain for a median period of 74 days. Despite therapy, four patients experienced persistent pain for more than 9 months and another patient died 5 months later without obtaining adequate pain relief. The National Cancer Institute selects patients whose malignancies generally have a poor prognosis if treated by standard therapy, so the results may not be generalizable to all children with cancer. Thus, Elliott and colleagues (1991) surveyed the prevalence of pain in a more representative group of children whose cancer was managed in both community-based and tertiary care centers. They reported that 28 of 160 patients were in pain and that most pain was therapy-related, not disease-related. However, they did not distinguish between acute and chronic pain. At present, there is no accurate estimate of the prevalence of chronic cancer pain in children.

Natural history and impact of pain

The lack of prospective community studies on the prevalence of chronic cancer pain is paralleled by the lack of longitudinal, case-control, and cohort studies that could provide objective information to determine the usual course of chronic pain, identify relevant prognostic factors, and document the psychological, physical, social, and economic impact of children's pain. Although there is an extensive body of research on the impact of childhood cancer and acute procedural pain (Katz et al. 1980; Kellerman 1980), almost no research has been conducted on chronic cancer pain in children.

SICKLE CELL PAIN

Disease definition and prevalence

Sickle cell disease is an inherited painful blood disorder in which red blood cells are distorted into elongated sickle shapes that obstruct oxygen flow into capillaries. Although these cell distortions occur continuously, painful sickling crises occur when the rate of sickling increases so that many more cells are temporarily or irreversibly sickled. There is no known cure. Painful episodes are the most common problem affecting children, adolescents, and adults (Shapiro 1989).

The estimated prevalence of sickle cell disease in the population aged 0–20 in the United States ranges from 0.28 per 1000 (Perrin 1992, adapted from Gortmaker and Sappenfield 1984) to 1.2 per 1000 (Newacheck and Taylor 1992). It is presumed that all afflicted children will experience some pain, but there are no epidemiological data on the prevalence and severity of painful sickling crises in children, nor on the extent to which they may experience other types of chronic pain related to the disease.

Natural history and impact of pain

The hallmark of sickle cell pain is its extreme variability and unpredictability in timing, location, and intensity (Shapiro 1993). There is little information on the specific distribution of painful sites, probable precipitating factors, and possible age differences in pain patterns or pain experiences. Painful episodes can occur as early as 6 months of age, but some patients may not experience pain until adolescence or young adulthood (Serjeant 1985). In general, when pain occurs frequently during childhood, it continues at the same or increased frequency and intensity during adolescence and young adulthood (Baum 1987). Extremity pain is reported to be more common in children and abdominal pain in adolescents (Brozovic and Anionwu 1984; Serjeant 1985), but pain can occur in almost any site at any age. Several physical and psychological factors can precipitate painful episodes (For review, see Serjeant 1985; Platt and Nathan 1987; Thomas and Holbrook 1987; Shapiro 1993.)

Sergeant and colleagues (1994) described the clinical features of painful crises in 118 patients, 51 of whom were 3.5–19 years old. Within a 17-month study period, these 118 patients (of a total clinic population of 2490) experienced 183 painful episodes of sufficient severity to warrant opioid analgesia. Few children (~3%) under the age of 14 years had painful crises. Multiple pain sites were common (most frequently two or three sites), but pain occurred most often in the lumbar spine, femur, and abdomen. The pattern of distribution did not differ by age, gender, or reported precipitating factors.

The effect of painful sickling crises has not been well documented for children. The adverse effect may be progressive as children continue to experience repeated and perhaps uncontrolled episodes of pain. Two studies have shown that children with sickle cell disease did not differ psychologically from comparison groups matched for race and socioeconomic level (Kumar et al. 1976; Lemanek et al. 1986). Lemanek and colleagues noted that the psychosocial dysfunction observed in adults with sickle cell disease may first appear in adolescence. Shapiro (1989) questioned the specific impact of painful sickling crises on psychosocial function, noting that "the difference in degree of psychosocial dysfunction between children and adults with sickle cell disease is a concern. The potential role of cumulative pain argues for preventive intervention ..." (p 1033). Gil and colleagues conducted a series of studies to evaluate children's sickling pain, coping ability, and adjustment. They demonstrated that children's coping strategies affect their pain level and psychosocial adjustment, even after they controlled for frequency of painful episodes and disease severity (Gil et al. 1989, 1991, 1992, 1997). At present, though, we lack comprehensive information about prognostic factors, risk factors, and prevention strategies for children with sickle cell disease.

FIBROMYALGIA

Disease definition and prevalence

Fibromyalgia syndrome is a chronic rheumatologic syndrome characterized by diffuse musculoskeletal aching and tender points at multiple characteristic sites (Walco and Oberlander 1993). Diagnostic criteria for adults include a history of widespread pain and pain in at least 11 of 18 tender point sites on digital palpation, according to guidelines developed by the American College of Rheumatology (ACR) (Wolfe et al. 1990). The syndrome is discussed fully in Chapter 9.

Only one study provides prevalence data on fibromyalgia in children. Mikkelsson and colleagues (1997) interviewed 1756 Finnish schoolchildren, 9–12 years of age, about their pain history in the previous 3 months. Twenty-two children were classified with fibromyalgia in a blinded procedure based on palpation by a physiatrist of tender points according to the ACR criteria.

Natural history and impact of pain

There are almost no pediatric studies from which to determine the natural history of fibromyalgia, including the temporal course of pain and pain severity. In a clinical study of 33 children, 5–17 years of age, Yunus and Masi (1985) reported that disease onset was most frequent between the ages of 13 and 15. They report that children complained about back pain less frequently than reported in studies of adults, and had significantly fewer tender points in the lumbar spine/paraspinal area.

Similarly, there are almost no pediatric studies from which to determine the impact of the disease. Mikkelsson and colleagues (1997) evaluated the association of musculoskeletal pain with emotional and behavioral problems in Finnish preadolescents. Children with widespread pain had more emotional and behavioral problems, more depressive symptoms, and more sleep problems than did controls. Children with fibromyalgia had significantly more depressive symptoms than did other children with widespread pain.

TRAUMA-RELATED PAIN

Chronic pain related to trauma may be nociceptive, resulting from active peripheral stimulation due to severe tissue damage that requires many months for healing, or it may be neuropathic, resulting from altered excitability of the peripheral and central nervous systems due to injuries to nerves. Children may experience neuropathic pain related to amputation, plexus injuries, and central nervous system syndromes related to traumatic spinal cord injury or congenital paraplegia.

REFLEX SYMPATHETIC DYSTROPHY

Disease definition and prevalence

Reflex sympathetic dystrophy (RSD) in adults is characterized by intense pain, vasomotor dysfunction, delayed functional recovery, and associated trophic changes. According to the International Association for the Study of Pain (IASP), RSD pain follows trauma (usually mild) not associated with significant nerve injury; the pain is described as burning, continuous, exacerbated by movement, cutaneous stimulation, or stress (IASP 1986). Recently, the IASP taxonomy broadened the term RSD to complex regional pain syndrome, type I.

Clinical manifestations of RSD vary widely, particularly in children. At present, the appropriateness of the IASP classification for childhood RSD has not been demonstrated and there is no consensus as to a specific disease definition for RSD in children.

RSD has been recognized with increasing frequency in children (Bernstein et al. 1978; Silber and Majd 1988; Olsson et al. 1990; Wilder 1992), but no epidemiological studies or community prevalence studies have been conducted. Clinical referrals suggest that that the prevalence is highest for preadolescents (11–13 years old) and that there is a higher female to male ratio of 6:1 (Wilder et al. 1992; Olsson and Berde 1993).

Natural history and impact of pain

Almost no objective data are available on the natural history of RSD in children. Clinical follow-up studies show contradictory results as to the course of pain. Some studies report significant recovery in most patients (Bernstein et al. 1978; Ruggeri et al. 1982;

Kesler et al. 1988) while other studies report prolonged pain for most affected children (Greipp 1988) or for a substantial subset (Wilder et al. 1992). Similarly, we have almost no data on the impact of RSD.

Stress and competitive sports have been identified as associated factors (Wilder et al. 1992), which suggests that highly stressed adolescent girls involved in competitive sports are more likely to develop RSD, but the literature contains no case-control or cohort studies that could provide conclusive information on risk factors and prognostic factors.

PHANTOM LIMB PAIN

Disease definition and prevalence data

Phantom limb pain refers to painful sensations experienced in the absent portion of an extremity after amputation (see Chapter 11). There are no prospective studies on the prevalence of phantom limb pain in children. Clinical studies and retrospective surveys suggest that the prevalence is high among children and adolescents who require amputations (Browder and Gallagher 1948; Simmel 1962). Krane et al. (1991) reported that 85% of children and adolescents sur-

veyed in their clinical practice had phantom pain after amputation, and that pain persisted for months to years for half of the respondents.

Natural history and impact of pain

Data are almost entirely lacking on the natural history of phantom limb pain in children. While many children may experience some phantom sensations, no clear prognostic factors indicate which children will experience some phantom pain or prolonged pain.

CHRONIC NONSPECIFIC PAIN AND CHRONIC DYSMENORRHEA

While many pediatric studies address the lifetime prevalence of at least one occurrence of pain in different body sites, very few studies focus on chronic nonspecific pain. The literature review on chronic nonspecific pain yielded only four major studies on knee pain and back pain as summarized in Table II. These studies are cross-sectional, school-based surveys conducted in Finland that used questionnaires administered to children or their parents to identify

Table II
Prevalence estimates for chronic nonspecific pain in children and for dysmenorrhea

Pain	Study Type	Disease Definition	Source of Sample	Sample Size	Prevalence Estimate	Age (years)	Prevalence (%)			Reference
							Female	Male	All	
Chronic knee pain	CS	Pain >3 mo and several times weekly	Finland, school	856	Point	All 9–10 14–15	12.6 3.1 19.8	11.3 4.8 16.8	12.0 3.9 18.5	Vähäsarja 1995
Back and/or neck pain	CS	Self-report, continual or recurrent	Finland, school	370	Lifetime	11,13, 15,17			7.6	Salminen 1984
Low back pain	CS	Self-report, location and duration	Finland, school	1377	Period (1 y)	14			7.8	Salminen et al. 1992
Low back pain	Cohort, CS	Self-report, location of back pain	Finland, school	1171	Period (1 y)	7,10, 14,16	3.1*	2.8*		Taimela et al. 1997
Dysmenorrhea	CS	Self-report	USA, population	2699	Lifetime	12–17 12 17	39 72		59.7	Klein and Litt 1981
Dysmenorrhea	CS	Self-report	Finland, population	3370	Point	12.6–18.6 12 14 16 18	48 61 77 79			Teperi and Rimpela 1989

Abbreviation: CS = cross-sectional.

*Prevalence rate calculated from data presented in article.

children with pain. Only two major studies on dysmenorrhea reported the frequency or level of menstrual pain in adolescent girls.

CHRONIC KNEE PAIN

Disease definition and prevalence

Chronic knee pain (discussed more fully in Chapter 19) generally refers to persistent knee pain without a specific etiology. In some studies, frequent or persistent pain in the knee, usually triggered or intensified by prolonged sitting or by physical activity, is described as patellofemoral pain or chondromalacia patellae. An appropriate definition for studies on the epidemiology of chronic pain in children is that used by Vähäsarja (1995)—knee pain that has lasted longer than 3 months and that occurs several times weekly. At present, there are no generally accepted diagnostic criteria for chronic knee pain in children.

The prevalence of chronic knee pain in children increases significantly with age from 3.9% in 9–10-year-old children to 18.5% in 14–15-year-olds, with an almost equal prevalence among girls and boys, as shown in Table II (Vähäsarja 1995).

Natural history and impact of pain

Little information exists on the natural history and impact of chronic knee pain. Fairbank and colleagues (1984) evaluated the mechanical factors associated with the incidence of knee pain in 446 students, 13–17 years of age. They did not find any associations between knee pain and joint mobility or other mechanical factors, and authors concluded that chronic overloading, rather than faulty mechanics, was the dominant factor in anterior knee pain in adolescents. In this study, 46% of children reported that their pain was worse with exercise, consistent with Vähäsarja's (1995) finding that 56% of children experienced knee pain from athletic activities. Vähäsarja reported the extent to which children were disabled by knee pain: 4% had no disability, 51% had mild disability, 32% had moderate disability, 11% had a lot of disability, and 2% had severe disability. No other information is available on the usual course of pain, prognostic factors, or the psychological, physical, and economic consequences.

BACK PAIN

Disease definition and prevalence

Chronic back pain generally refers to persistent pain in the lower back without a specific etiology (see Chapter 18). This pain has been considered rare for children in that their complaints of back pain usually indicate a serious condition such as infection, neoplastic disease, developmental abnormalities, mechanical derangement, and inflammatory disorders (Winter and Lipscomb 1978; Bunnell 1982; Balague and Nordin 1992; Thompson 1993). At present, we lack generally accepted diagnostic criteria for nonspecific back pain in children. Most studies assess lifetime prevalence based on child or parent self-report, usually without specifying a minimum duration in the disease definition (Balague et al. 1988, 1994).

Five studies have provided lifetime prevalence estimates for at least one episode of back pain in children that vary from 7.6% to 34% (Salminen 1984; Balague et al. 1988; Salminen, et al. 1992; Balague et al. 1994; Taimela et al. 1997). Lifetime prevalence increases with age (e.g., from 1.1% for 7-year-olds to 18.4% for 15-year-olds; Taimela et al.1997). While these studies provide valuable information about factors associated with any lifetime back pain or with present pain, they do not provide detailed information on the prevalence of chronic back pain. Two studies by Balague and colleagues provide some general estimates. In a survey of 1715 Swiss schoolchildren aged 7–17, Balague and colleagues (1988) reported that 5% of children had frequent or continual back pain (but they did not report the duration). In another survey of 1716 schoolchildren aged 8–16, Balague and colleagues (1994) reported that 0.5% had constant disability due to back pain.

Only three studies specifically evaluated chronic pain. Salminen (1984) determined that 7.6% of children's neck and/or back (pain) symptoms had been continual or recurrent and had interfered with children's school work or leisure time. In this study, 19.7% of children reported present neck and/or back fatigue or pain, while 6.2% reported more chronic symptoms (previous and present back pain).

In a subsequent study, Salminen and colleagues (1992) reported that 7.8% of 14-year-old schoolchildren had recurrent or continual low back pain. Recently,

Taimela and colleagues (1997) investigated past and current back pain and classified low back pain based on timing, duration, and location. The prevalence of back pain was low among the 7-year-old (1%) and 10-year-old (6%) schoolchildren, but increased to 18% for 14- and 16-year-old adolescents. Among the children with low back pain, 26% of the boys and 33% of the girls had recurrent or chronic pain. The proportion of recurrent and chronic pain increased with age.

Natural history and impact of pain

Numerous studies have demonstrated a high lifetime prevalence of back pain, particularly low back pain, in children. Moreover, prevalence increases with age. Many associated factors and possible determinants of low back pain have been evaluated in children. These include physical findings related to structure and posture, physical activity, time spent watching television, smoking, competitive sports, grade point average, urban or rural residence, and parental history of back pain (Salminen 1984; Balague et al. 1988, 1994; Troussier et al. 1994). Among the possible risk factors evaluated, physical activities, positive family history of back pain, and gender are positively correlated with lifetime or period prevalence, while physical structure (posture and radiographic examination) are not. Studies evaluating most risk factors have yielded equivocal results, but no study has focused specifically on the risk factors for chronic low back pain in children. Thus, while we may speculate that certain factors are equally important for the onset or persistence of chronic back pain in children, we do not know their true predictive validity.

However, a history of low back pain in adolescence may have some predictive value for adult low back pain. Harreby and colleagues (1995) conducted a 25-year prospective cohort study of 640 14-year-old schoolchildren in Denmark to evaluate risk factors for adult low back pain. At ages 14 and 16 years, children were interviewed and had radiologic examinations of the thoracic and lumbar spine. At age 38, 90% (578) of the initial cohort completed a self-administered questionnaire about the history of back pain. Although radiologic changes in the spine showed no correlation to low back pain in adolescence or adulthood, low back pain in adolescence, particularly combined with familial occurrence of back disease, was associated with continuing pain in adulthood.

DYSMENORRHEA

Disease definition and prevalence

Dysmenorrhea is a syndrome characterized by recurrent, cramping, lower abdominal pain, often accompanied by nausea, vomiting, increased frequency of defecation, headaches, and muscular cramps occurring during menses (Klein and Litt 1981). Primary dysmenorrhea implies the absence of any pelvic abnormalities.

In studies on menstrual pain in adolescent girls, prevalence rates ranged widely from about 7% to 79% (Goldwasser 1938; Gallagher 1955; Golubet al. 1958; Widholm and Kantero 1971; Widholm 1979; Klein and Litt 1981; Teperi and Rimpela 1989). Teperi and Rimpela reported that while almost half of adolescents experience at least mild menstrual pain, the proportion of girls reporting severe pain increased from 5% for 12-year-olds to 23% for 16- and 18-year-olds. Klein and Litt (1981) analyzed data from the National Health Examination survey to determine prevalence and possible correlates of dysmenorrhea in adolescents. They reported a striking overall prevalence of nearly 60%, with 51% of girls who report pain describing the pain as moderate to severe. Dysmenorrhea increased with chronological age and with sexual maturity. However, no study has explicitly defined dysmenorrhea with respect to a level of pain (i.e., moderate to severe) or a minimum frequency (i.e., minimum number of episodes per year).

Natural history and impact of pain

Longitudinal studies of dysmenorrhea that would provide information on the natural history of pain from adolescence through adult life are lacking. However, the prevalence of dysmenorrhea in 12–18-year-olds positively correlates with all biological variables such as chronological age, sexual maturity, and gynecological age. Klein and Litt (1981) found no association between pain and whether girls reported they had been prepared for menarche, and noted a small positive association for socioeconomic status but not for race. Studies have shown significant morbidity from dysmenorrhea related to excessive school absence (Golub et al. 1958; Klein and Litt 1981; Teperi and Rimpela 1989). Teperi and Rimpela reported that both the use of medication and absenteeism due to menstrual pain were correlated with the severity of pain. Their results indicated that gynecological age and indicators of self-reported poor physical condition (e.g., several colds in the previous 6 months, or seldom or never feeling active in the morning) and unhealthy practices (e.g., smoking daily, alcohol consumption) were associated with menstrual pain in 16-year-old girls.

RECURRENT PAIN SYNDROMES

Many otherwise healthy children and adolescents suffer from frequent debilitating episodes of migraine or tension headache, abdominal pain, or limb pain. These recurrent pains are not symptoms of an underlying physical disorder. Instead, the pain syndrome is the disorder, and the situational factors responsible

Table III
Prevalence estimates for migraine headache in children

Study Type	Disease Definition	Source of Sample	Sample Size	Prevalence Estimate	Age (years)	Prevalence (%)			Reference
						Female	Male	All	
CS	Vahlquist 1955	Sweden, community	2609	Lifetime	10–12 16–19			4.5 7.4	Vahlquist 1955
CS	Vahlquist 1955	Sweden, school	8993	Lifetime	All 7 8 9 10 11 12 13 14 15	4.4 1.7 2.7 2.9 3.3 5.7 6.9 5.9 4.8 8.2	3.3 1.1 2.7 3.5 4.0 3.7 3.5 4.0 5.4 1.5	3.9 1.4 2.7 3.2 3.6 4.7 5.2 5.0 5.1 5.3	Bille 1962
CS	Ad Hoc Committee 1962	Denmark, school	2027	Point	7–9 9–11 11–13 13–15 15–17	2.8 4.3 6.0 7.7 9.5	3.1 4.5 6.0 7.3 8.4	2.9 4.4 6.0 7.5 9.0	Dalsgaard-Nielsen et al. 1970
CS	Vahlquist 1955	Finland, school	4235	Point	7			3.2	Sillanpää 1976
CS	Vahlquist 1955	South Wales, community	600	Lifetime	10–20	6.2–22.1	3.3–15.5		Deubner 1977
CS	Modified from Vahlquist 1955	Great Britain, school	15785	Point	10–18	2.5	3.4		Sparks 1978
CS	Modified from Vahlquist 1955	Israel, community	4899	Point	15–65+ 15–24	~10*	~5*		Abramson et al. 1980
CS	Vahlquist 1955	Finland, school	3784	Period (1 y)	13	14.5	8.1	11.3	Sillanpää 1983a
CS, longi- tudinal, cohort	Vahlquist 1995	Finland, school	2921	Period (1 y)	7 14	2.5 14.8	2.9 6.4	2.7 10.6	Sillanpää 1983b
CS	Modified IHS 1988	USA, population	10169 3161	Point	12–29 12–17	7.4 6.6	3.0 3.8		Linet et al. 1989
CS	HIS 1988	Scotland, school	1754	Period (1 y)	All 5 6 7 8 9 10 11 12 13 14 15	11.5 3.0 8.1 4.1 5.9 5.9 11.6 11.4 18.0 23.7 27.0 13.6	9.7 3.7 6.8 2.8 8.5 6.6 11.4 15.3 20.2 14.8 4.0 14.0	10.6 3.4 7.4 3.5 7.3 6.3 11.5 13.2 19.1 19.0 16.2 13.8	Abu-Arefeh and Russell 1994

Abbreviations: CS = cross-sectional; IHS = Headache Classification Committee of the International Headache Society.
*Prevalence estimate for age group interpreted from data presented in histogram.

for triggering painful episodes must be managed. Recurrent pain syndromes constitute a chronic pain condition, and this chapter reviews the epidemiological studies on headache, abdominal pain, and limb pain. Nineteen studies satisfied the criteria for designation as major studies and are summarized in Tables III and IV; most studies have focused on migraine headache. Six studies provide supplemental data on the prevalence of frequent nonmigraine headaches in children 7–19 years of age. These rates vary from 6.3% to 29% (Vahlquist 1955; Bille 1962; Sillanpää 1976, 1983a,b; Egermark-Eriksson 1982).

MIGRAINE HEADACHE

Disease definition

The definition of migraine is based almost entirely on clinical experience, given the lack of standardized and universally accepted diagnostic criteria (Linet and Stewart 1984). Investigators in early pediatric studies generally defined migraine based on criteria proposed by Vahlquist (1955), Bille (1962), or the 1962 Ad Hoc Committee on the Classification of Headache. Children must experience paroxysmal headaches separated by symptom-free intervals and accompanied by two to four of the following symptoms: unilateral pain, nausea or vomiting, visual aura in connection with headache, and family history of migraine.

In 1988, the Headache Classification Committee of the International Headache Society (IHS) proposed a new set of criteria for migraine headaches based on expert consensus. Pediatric migraine was defined as at least five headache attacks, lasting 2–48 hours, with at least two of the following features: unilateral location, pulsating quality, moderate to severe intensity, or aggravation by routine physical activity; and at least one of the following features: nausea or vomiting, photophobia, or phonophobia.

Maytal and colleagues (1997) used clinical diag-

Table IV
Prevalence estimates for recurrent abdominal pain and recurrent limb pain in children

Pain	Study Type	Disease Definition	Source of Sample	Sample Size	Prevalence Estimate	Age (years)	Prevalence (%) Female	Male	All	Reference
Recurrent abdominal pain	CS, case-control	Apley	Great Britain, school	1000	Period (1 y)		12.3	9.5	10.8	Apley and Naish 1958
Recurrent abdominal pain	CS	Apley	Great Britain, school	439	Point	5–6			24.5–26.9	Faull and Nicol 1986
Stomachache	CS	Maternal report, past and present	Great Britain, clinic	308	Point	3			9	Zuckerman et al. 1987
Recurrent abdominal pain	CS	Chronicity and impairment	Great Britain, school	250	Point	8–12			10	Sharrer and Ryan-Wenger 1991
Recurrent abdominal pain	CS	Apley	Great Britain, clinic	1083	Period (1 y)	3–11	9	8		Mortimer et al. 1993
Abdominal migraine	CS	Strict diagnostic criteria	Great Britain, clinic	1083	Period (1 y)	3–11			2.4	Mortimer et al. 1993
Abdominal migraine	CS	Modified from Symon and Russell (1986)	Aberdeen, school	1754	Period (1 y)	5–15			4.1	Abu-Arefeh and Russell 1995
Recurrent limb pain	CS	Strict diagnostic criteria	Aberdeen, school	1754		5–15	2.9	2.3	2.6	Abu-Arefeh and Russell 1996

Abbreviation: CS = cross-sectional.

nosis by pediatric neurologists to evaluate the validity of the IHS criteria for diagnosing migraine without aura in 253 children and adolescents. The IHS criteria had poor sensitivity (27.3%), high specificity (92.4%), and high positive predictive value (80%). The authors applied alternative case definitions to determine if they could increase sensitivity without sacrificing specificity, but were unable to develop criteria that accurately replicated clinical diagnosis. They concluded that the IHS criteria should be less restrictive for children (e.g., fewer number of attacks, only one rather than two specified features), but that further work is required in order to delineate developmental differences in headache characteristics. Abu-Arefeh and Russell (1994) concluded that the IHS criteria were generally adequate for their study on 5–15-year-old children and adolescents, but that the minimum acceptable duration of headache should be reduced from 1 to 2 hours because in their study 5% of children with severe headache fulfilled all the criteria for migraine diagnosis except that their headaches lasted less than 2 hours.

Prevalence data

Many studies have estimated the prevalence of migraine. As shown in Table III, community-based surveys in Sweden, Denmark, Finland, the United States, Israel, and Great Britain have yielded widely varying prevalence rates (1.4–27%). Although migraine is regarded as a chronic pain condition, studies have distinguished between the prevalence of "occasional" versus chronic migraines. As expected, prevalence rates for childhood migraine vary depending on the type of estimate, age and gender of the study population, and the criteria for diagnosis. However, most studies have found that migraine prevalence increases with age and after age 10–12, prevalence is higher for girls.

In most school-based studies of childhood migraine, children or the parents of younger children complete an initial screening questionnaire as to whether the child has had a headache. If children respond yes, they then complete another series of questions about their experiences to enable the investigators to ascertain whether their reported headache features satisfy the study criteria for migraine (Vahlquist 1955; Bille 1962; Sparks 1978; Sillanpää 1983a,b). In some studies, these children or a subset also receive a medical examination (Dalsgaard-Nielsen et al. 1970;

Sillanpää 1976; Deubner 1977; Abramson et al. 1980; Abu-Arefeh and Russell 1994). In one study, higher prevalence rates were obtained from cases identified through questionnaire responses than from cases identified through the clinical interview and exam (Deubner 1977). One study (Sparks 1978) had markedly different methods in that students were recruited from a posted notice inviting self-selected migraine sufferers to participate in a survey.

Natural history

Many studies have reported data on the age of onset, associated symptoms, possible headache triggers, and risk factors. Migraine without aura is more common then migraine with aura in children. Migraine onset is reported at 7–12 years of age (Vahlquist 1955), 6.9 years (Michael and Williams 1952), 7.3 years (Burke and Peters 1956), and younger than 9 years (Krupp and Friedman 1953). The prevalence increases with age (Bille 1962; Russell 1994). Although most studies report a higher prevalence rate for girls (Vahlquist 1955; Bille 1962; Dalsgaard-Nielsen et al. 1970; Deubner 1977; Linet et al. 1989), some studies have found higher rates in boys (Michael and Williams 1952; Burke and Peters 1956) or no gender differences (Sillanpää 1976). Reported gender differences in prevalence probably reflect age by gender interactions. Linet and colleagues (1989) reported that migraine prevalence decreased with age among males compared with an age-related increase among females. Similarly, Abu-Arefeh and Russell (1994) found that migraine was more common in boys by a ratio of 1.14:1 for children aged 12 years or younger, but for children over 12 years old, migraine was more common in girls with a ratio of 2:1. In addition, they found that significantly more girls than boys had migraine with aura.

The usual course of migraine in children has not been established. Frequency, intensity, and length of headache attacks vary widely. Pains are triggered by a variety of external and internal factors, particularly events that provoke stress. No prospective studies trace the natural history of migraine headaches from childhood into adult life. The proportion of children who continue to experience recurrent headaches has been estimated at 40–60% (Apley et al. 1978; Jay and Tomasi 1981; Larsson and Melin 1986). Bille (1962) conducted a 6-year follow-up study on 205 children with headaches and a comparison group of 73 children aged 13–21. The study showed that 35–50% of the children with migraine had become symptom-free. In a 7-year follow-up of 2291 7-year-old schoolchildren, Sillanpää (1983) obtained different remission rates depending on a child's age at onset. Migraine had remitted fully in 20% of the children with onset at 8–14 years of age, but in only 5% of the children with onset at 0–7 years of age. As Linet and Stewart (1987, p 462) concluded: "It is commonly held that the incidence of new cases of migraine and the frequency of attacks in existing cases begins to decrease with age beginning in the fourth decade. However, data are not available to clarify whether in fact attacks decrease or remit, whether the characteristics of migraine actually undergo marked change, or whether the incidence rapidly declines in older age groups (Dalsgaard-Nielsen [et al.] 1970; Clarke and Waters 1974; Waters 1974)."

Risk factors and triggers

Family and twin studies of adult migraine provide evidence that supports the role of familial and genetic factors (Burke and Peters 1956; Bille 1962), although environmental factors common to both twins or family members may play a role (Linet and Stewart 1984). Although many physiological constitutional factors have been evaluated in studies of adult migraine, studies of risk factors in children have focused primarily on precipitants or triggers for migraine attacks, such as mental stress, physical stress, food allergies, and menses. Studies have not found an association with scholastic achievement, ambition, or intellectual ability, but have found some association with reported levels of anxiety and migraine (Bille 1962). Other factors that are not consistently associated with migraine include socioeconomic level and travel sickness. Abu-Arefeh and Russell (1994) compared children with migraine with asymptomatic controls matched for age and sex, and found no significant differences in social background (defined by parents' occupations), parents' marital status, and parent-described personalities of children.

The Linet et al. (1989) population study differs from the other community-based studies listed in Table III because the investigators attempted to evaluate a subject's most recent headache (in contrast to their report of usual headache characteristics or lifetime occurrence of specific headache symptoms). Subjects provided socioeconomic data, information about headaches occurring in the previous 4 weeks, age of onset

of 14 symptoms that commonly accompany migraine and muscle contraction headaches, headache-related physician visits, exposure to common headache precipitators, and a history of other related symptoms linked to childhood migraine. They also described pain intensity, pain duration, and associated disability for their most recent headache. The report, stratified by age (13–17, 18–23, 24–29) and gender, provides data on pain characteristics, accompanying symptoms, risk factors, and the economic impact of migraine. In each age group, a higher proportion of females than males reported headaches. Females also reported a higher frequency of headaches than males. The proportion of males and females with frequent headaches (four or more in the previous 4 weeks) increased substantially between the youngest and the two oldest age groups.

Bille (1962) reported high absence rates from school for both children with migraine (mean 43.5 hours per term) and those with nonmigraine headache (mean 38.1 hours per term). Girls had significantly more absences than did boys; they missed a mean 49.7 hours versus a mean 27.6 hours for boys. Linet and colleagues (1989) reported substantial disability (school and work absences) due to recent headaches, with 10.1% of boys and 8.6% of girls aged 13–17 indicating absence for part of a day and 2.4% and 2.7%, respectively, for an entire day. Abu-Arefeh and Russell (1994) reported that children with migraine lost more school days due to any illness including headache than did controls. For children with migraine and controls, the mean number of days lost to migraine was 2.8 and 0, respectively, and the mean number of days lost to other illness was 5.0 and 3.7, respectively.

ABDOMINAL PAIN

Disease definition and prevalence

Recurrent abdominal pain is defined as at least three episodes of incapacitating pain, usually diffusely localized in the epigastric or periumbilical areas over not less than 3 months, in the absence of physical findings (Apley 1975). Abdominal migraine has been regarded as a migraine equivalent without the headache (Barlow 1984). Although it is not included in the IHS criteria, an adaptation of Symon and Russell's (1986) diagnostic criteria was used in the only community study on the prevalence of abdominal migraine (Abu-Arefeh and Russell 1995). Diagnostic criteria include pain severe enough to interfere with normal activities, dull or colicky pain, periumbilical or poorly localized pain, an attack that lasts for at least 1 hour, associated with two of the following features: anorexia, nausea, vomiting, pallor, and complete resolution of symptoms between attacks (Table IV).

The reported prevalence rates for recurrent abdominal pain have varied between 6% and 15% in children (Apley and Naish 1958; Pringle et al. 1966; Oster 1972). The prevalence is usually equal for boys and girls, peaking between 5 and 7 years of age. Abu-Arefeh and Russell (1995) reported that 32% of 1754 children aged 5–15 had at least one episode of severe abdominal pain in the previous year, while nearly 8% had at least two episodes. The estimated prevalence rate for abdominal migraine was about 4%.

Natural history

The frequency, intensity, and length of painful episodes vary widely and the prognosis is unclear; children may continue to suffer from gastrointestinal pains as adults (Christensen and Mortensen 1975; Stickler and Murphy 1979). Clinical studies indicate that stress, learning, modeling, emotional factors, familial behaviors, genetic predisposition, autonomic instability, and gut motility are associated with recurrent abdominal pain (Green 1967; Rubin et al. 1967; Apley et al. 1971; Bain 1975; Barr et al. 1979, 1981; Levine 1984; Hodges et al. 1985; and for reviews, see Levine and Rappaport 1984; McGrath and Feldman 1986; Zeltzer 1986; Barr 1989).

Several studies have shown an association between childhood abdominal pain and migraine (Mortimer et al. 1993). In fact, children with abdominal migraine, compared with children with migraine defined by IHS criteria, have similar demographic features, associated recurrent conditions, precipitating trigger factors, associated symptoms during attacks, and relieving factors (Abu-Arefeh and Russell 1995). The peak prevalence for abdominal migraine is 5–7 years of age.

LIMB PAIN

Disease definition

Recurrent limb pain occurs late in the day or awakens the child at night and is not specifically related to joints. Criteria include a pain history of at least 3 months; intermittent pain with symptom-free intervals of days, weeks, or months; and pain of sufficient severity to interrupt normal activities, including sleep. Physical examination results, laboratory data, and radiographic studies are normal (Naish and Apley 1951). "Growing pain" is a common term used to describe recurrent limb pain in children, although there is no evidence that the pain derives from maturation and growth.

Prevalence data

Prevalence estimates for recurrent limb pain vary widely from 4.2% to 33.6% (Hawksley 1938; Naish and Apley 1951; Brenning 1960; Oster and Nielsen 1972; Oberklaid et al. 1997). Boys and girls are almost equally affected. However, prevalence has been obtained in most studies by children's affirmative response to a question such as, "Do you have pain in your arms and legs—growing pains?" and not by a more precise classification of their pain as a recurrent or chronic condition. For example, Oster and Nielsen (1972) report an overall affirmative rate of 15.5% in their study of 2178 Danish schoolchildren aged 6–19, but they did not describe the proportion of children who had more chronic complaints or more frequent episodes.

Recently, Abu-Arefeh and Russell (1996) reported a prevalence rate of 33% for children who had at least one episode of limb pain over the past year, a 7.2% rate for children who had had at least two episodes, and a 2.6% rate for children with severe recurrent limb pain of unknown etiology (diagnosed with strict criteria after medical examination). Episodes of limb pain occurred on an average of 12 times per year and lasted for an average of 10 hours. The prevalence rate varied little according to the age of children (5–15 years), ranging from 1.2% to 4.5% with no specific trends.

Natural history and impact of pain

Recurrent limb pains are considered a relatively benign condition, but some children have considerable disability and pain. Symptoms may begin as early as 2 years of age, but one study reports a mean onset of 7.8 years (Abu-Arefeh and Russell 1996). Frequency and duration of pain episodes vary widely.

Oberklaid and colleagues (1997) found several differences between children with growing pains and a comparison group. Children with growing pains were significantly more likely to have headaches and abdominal pain, a negative mood, behavioral problems, and to be aggressive, anxious, and hyperactive. However, the group of children with growing pains was not carefully defined so that children with any pains in the previous year were included, as were children who had more chronic conditions.

PAIN RELATED TO MENTAL HEALTH

Chronic pain has unique psychological consequences. And, for many individuals with pain related to chronic disease or trauma, psychological factors are secondary contributing factors that can intensify pain and increase disability. However, for some persons, psychological factors are the primary cause of chronic pain. In somatoform disorders a person complains of physical symptoms that suggest a medical condition but are not fully explained by clinical findings, by the direct effects of a substance, or by another mental disorder (American Psychiatric Association 1994). The symptoms must cause clinically significant distress or impairment in social, occupational, or other areas of functioning. Pain, usually chronic pain, is a primary presenting symptom in two somatoform disorders—pain disorder and somatization disorder. The diagnostic criteria for the somatoform disorders were established for adults and are applied to children for lack of a child-specific research base and a developmentally appropriate alternative system (Fritz et al. 1997).

PAIN DISORDER

Disease definition

Pain disorder is a new classification in the *Diagnostic and Statistical Manual of Mental Disorders* (DSM-IV). The diagnostic criteria for pain disorder include: pain occurs in one or more anatomical sites as the predominant focus of clinical attention, and of sufficient severity to warrant clinical attention; pain causes clinically significant distress or impairment in social, occupational, or other important areas of functioning; pain is not intentionally produced or feigned; and the pain is not better accounted for by another mental disorder (American Psychiatric Association 1994).

Prevalence data and natural history

Pain disorder may occur at any age, but no prevalence data are available for the disorder in children and adolescents. Faravelli et al. (1997) surveyed the prevalence of somatoform disorders in 673 subjects, 15–65+ years of age, in Florence, Italy. Adolescents 15–19 years of age constituted 4% of their sample. They obtained 1-year prevalence rates of 0.6% and 0.7% for somatoform pain disorder and somatization disorder, respectively. However, they did not delineate rates by age groups. There is no information on the natural history of pain disorders in children.

SOMATIZATION DISORDER

Disease definition

The essential feature of somatization disorder is a pattern of recurring, multiple, clinically significant somatic complaints. Diagnostic criteria include: a history of many physical complaints before age 30 that occur over several years and result in treatment being sought or significant impairment; a history of pain related to at least four different body sites; a history of at least two gastrointestinal symptoms (other than pain); one sexual symptom; and one pseudoneurological symptom. The diagnosis of somatization disorder is rare, perhaps because of the inappropriateness of some diagnostic symptoms for prepubertal children. Several studies have been conducted in which children complete checklists of various somatic

Table V
Prevalence estimates for chronic pain related to mental health in children

Pain	Study Type	Disease Definition	Source of Sample	Sample Size	Prevalence Estimate	Age (years)	Prevalence (%)			Reference
							Female	Male	All	
Somatization	CS	DSM III	Canada, community	3294	Period (6 mo)	4–11 12–16	10.7	4.5		Offord et al. 1987
Somatization symptoms	CS	Study-defined	USA, school	540	Point	8–17			1.1	Garber et al. 1991

Abbreviation: CS = cross-sectional.

complaints (Aro et al. 1987; Larson 1991), but only a few studies have applied DSM-III (and none DSM-IV) criteria for diagnosing specific disorders.

Prevalence data, natural history, and impact of pain

Offord and colleagues (1987) found recurrent distressing somatic symptoms in 10.7% of girls and 4.5% of boys aged 12–16 years (Table V). In a small sample, Garber and colleagues (1991) reported that about 1% of children had sufficient somatization symptoms to qualify for somatization disorder.

The natural history is unknown. Bass and Murphy (1995) have proposed that somatization disorder is closely related to personality disorder as it has a persistent course, long duration, and early age of onset, and occurs more often in conjunction with personality disorders than other DSM-IV clinical disorders.

SUMMARY

Four common themes emerge from a review of the diverse articles on children's chronic pain. First, the literature includes relatively few major epidemiological studies of chronic pain in children. Second, the available studies yield widely varying results due to differences in pain definitions, methods for identifying children, age and gender of study populations, country of origin, and presentation and analysis of data. Third, specific disease/pain definitions are lacking for most types of chronic pain in children, so we have few uniform, consistent, and standard diagnostic criteria. In addition, the disease definition and diagnostic criteria for many types of chronic pain in children are based on the clinical signs and symptoms in adults, even though clinicians and investigators report that the presentation is different in children. Fourth, longitudinal, case-control, and cohort studies have not been conducted for most types of chronic pain in children, so we know almost nothing about the natural history of their pain, the personal and economic impact for children and families, prognostic factors, and specific risk factors for children and adolescents.

Table VI lists prevalence estimates for different types of chronic pain in children. The prevalence of many types of chronic pain either is unknown (i.e., cancer, reflex sympathetic dystrophy, phantom limb pain, and pain disorder) or is based on a single study (i.e., fibromyalgia, knee pain, or somatization disorder). As noted, there are few estimates of the prevalence of chronic disease-related pain. Most of the available estimates derive from epidemiological studies of disease prevalence; some information on pain prevalence can be extrapolated on the basis that the disease usually or always causes some persistent pain. No study has explicitly defined a chronic pain problem as a target condition. No study has yet provided explicit information about the proportion of children who experience mild, moderate, and severe pain and the proportion of children who experience pain on a seldom, occasional, frequent, or continual basis. Data on pain severity and pain persistency is essential to obtain an accurate estimate of the prevalence of chronic debilitating pain in children.

At present, without specific epidemiological data on the proportion of children with a chronic disease who experience severe persistent pain, the prevalence estimates in Table VI represent the best available data. The community studies on juvenile arthritis indicate a higher prevalence than had been originally estimated in several clinical studies. The method of case ascertainment by rheumatological examination provides the most accurate estimates because the examinations identify undiagnosed cases within the community.

Table VI
Prevalence estimates for chronic pain in children
and basis for estimate

Pain	Prevalence	Basis
Related to Disease		
Arthritis	3–460/100,000	Disease/pain
Cancer	Unknown	
Sickle cell disease	28–120/100,000	Disease
Fibromyalgia	57/100,000	Mikkelsson et al. 1997
Related to Trauma		
Reflex sympathetic dystrophy	Unknown	
Phantom limb	Unknown	
Nonspecific Pain		
Knee	3.9–18.5%	Vähäsarja 1995
Back	2.8–7.8%	Pain
Dysmenorrhea	7.2–7.9%	Pain
Recurrent Pain		
Migraine	1.4–37%	Pain
Nonmigraine headache	6.3–29%	Pain
Abdominal	6.0–15%	Pain
Limb	4.2–33.6%	Pain
Related to Mental Health		
Pain disorder	Unknown	
Somatization disorder	4.5–10.7%	Offord et al. 1987

Note: Based on epidemiological studies of disease/pain or a single study.

Thus, the upper limits for the estimates on chronic pain related to disease pain are those that more accurately represent its prevalence in children.

Most epidemiological studies on chronic pain in children have focused on nonspecific pain and on recurrent pain syndromes. Most studies show that the lifetime prevalence of nonspecific pain increases with age. The few studies that reported on the proportion of children with more chronic nonspecific pain (defined by frequency, intensity, or disability) also reported that these more chronic problems increased with age. In Table VI, the higher prevalence rates for knee and back pain generally reflect the proportion of children who had nonspecific pain for some defined time period, while the lower rates reflect the proportion of children who reported constant or continual pain. Thus, at present, these lower rates may be the more appropriate prevalence estimates for chronic knee and low back pain.

The prevalence of migraine increases with age, with the ratio of male to female reversing with age. After approximately 12 years of age, the prevalence of migraine is higher in females. In contrast, the prevalence of recurrent abdominal pain and of recurrent limb pain decreases with age, and most studies report an equal prevalence among females and males. However, recurrent abdominal pain and recurrent limb pain have not been studied as extensively as childhood migraine. Moreover, most studies have not defined the disease or the diagnostic criteria for these types of pain, so that additional prevalence information is required to clarify age- and gender-related difference.

Almost no epidemiological data document the prevalence of chronic pain due to emotional distress. Several studies have shown a high prevalence of recurrent somatic complaints in children, but the current diagnostic criteria for somatization disorder are not developmentally appropriate, so the true prevalence of this disorder may be significantly underestimated in children and adolescents.

CHALLENGES FOR THE FUTURE

Extensive epidemiological research is required for all types of chronic pain in children. For diseases or conditions (such as migraine) in which childhood prevalence has been established, research should focus on determining the prevalence of severe chronic pain and the consequences for children and families.

For all other pain conditions, accurate estimates of prevalence by age and gender should be obtained.

COMMUNITY STUDIES

Clinical investigations provide valuable information on childhood chronic pain, but clinical study samples may not wholly represent the population at large due to referral biases. Children referred for treatment may differ from those not referred in important characteristics (such as age, gender, pain severity, pain duration, disability behaviors, concurrent health or psychosocial problems, and family history), so that information obtained about associated factors, probable risk factors, and prognostic factors is distorted. Instead, prospective cross-sectional population studies are required to provide accurate estimates of prevalence by age and gender, to provide detailed information about the pain characteristics in children so as to facilitate developmentally appropriate definitions and diagnostic criteria, and to provide descriptive data on associated child, family, and environmental factors.

These studies must include an objective definition of the pain as a chronic problem according to its duration, intensity, and frequency, and explicit diagnostic criteria for case ascertainment. The most efficient study design is probably two-staged; probable cases could be identified in a preliminary screening procedure and then children could be interviewed in-depth or examined to determine who satisfies the diagnostic criteria. In addition, data on potentially relevant associated factors and on the personal and economic impact of the pain should be obtained for children who fulfill the criteria and for an age- and gender-matched cohort of children without the pain problem.

DEVELOPMENTALLY APPROPRIATE DISEASE DEFINITIONS

The definitions of many types of chronic pain are based on the disease characteristics described in adults, even though clinical and community studies indicate that the presentation of the pain is different or may be different in children. Moreover, there may be age-related differences in the presentation of chronic pain problems as well as in the prevalence. Thus, the results of initial community studies on chronic pain in children must be used to establish developmentally appropriate pain definitions. These definitions are essential to enable us to understand the continuity of some types of chronic pain from childhood into adult life and to perhaps understand the antecedents of some types of adult chronic pain.

LONGITUDINAL STUDIES

Longitudinal case-control and cohort studies are needed to document the natural history of chronic pain in children, to determine prognostic factors, to identify risk factors, and to identify any high-risk groups that require special intervention to reduce the likelihood that disabling pain will continue into adult life. These studies enable us to test causal hypotheses and determine whether the presumed effects of certain risk factors preceded children's exposure to those factors.

Many studies demonstrate that a substantial proportion of children experience various types of chronic pain. However, we do not have specific prevalence rates for most types of chronic pain related to disease, trauma, and emotional factors. Similarly, we lack data on the extent to which children experience severe pain and the extent to which their pain is constant and debilitating. Yet it is exceedingly important to obtain this information. Many types of acute pain were undertreated in children until relatively recently because their problems were under-reported. After the magnitude of acute pain in infants and children was documented, major changes occurred in the clinical management of acute pain. Similarly, unrecognized chronic pain is untreated chronic pain. The extent to which children may suffer from inadequately managed chronic pain is unknown. Our current assumption that children's chronic pain is adequately controlled must be confirmed with epidemiological data. Thus, a major challenge for the future is to develop a balanced, coordinated, cohesive, and comprehensive plan for conducting the necessary epidemiological research. This research is essential, but it is expensive and lengthy, so investigators from different centers (and preferably countries) should work together to develop a feasible plan of action and timetable to maximize the collection of needed data in comparable studies with appropriate methods, while minimizing any unnecessary duplication.

REFERENCES

Ad Hoc Committee on Classification of Headache. Classification of headache. *JAMA* 1962; 179(9):127–128.

Altman AJ, Schwartz AD. *Malignant Diseases of Infancy, Childhood and Adolescence*. Philadelphia: W.B. Saunders, 1983.

American Psychiatric Association. *Diagnostic and Statistical Manual of Mental Disorders: DSM-IV*. Washington, DC: American Psychiatric Association, 1994.

Anderson KO, Bradley LA, Young LD, McDaniel LK, Wise CM. Rheumatoid arthritis: review of psychological factors related to etiology, effects, and treatment. *Psychol Bull* 1985; 98:358–387.

Apley J. *The Child with Abdominal Pains*. Oxford: Blackwell Scientific, 1975.

Apley J, Haslam DR, Tulloh CG. Pupillary reaction in children with recurrent abdominal pain. *Arch Dis Child* 1971; 46:337–340.

Apley J, MacKeith R, Meadow R. *The Child and His Symptoms: A Comprehensive Approach*. Oxford: Blackwell Scientific, 1978.

Aro H, Paronen O, Aro S. Psychosomatic symptoms among 14–16 year old Finnish adolescents. *Soc Psychiatry* 1987; 22:171–176.

Bain HW. Abdominal pain in children. *Prim Care* 1975; 2:121–133.

Balague F, Nordin M. Back pain in children and teenagers. *Bailliere's Clinical Rheumatology* 1992; 6:575–593.

Balague F, Dutoit G, Waldburger M. Low back pain in schoolchildren: an epidemiological study. *Scand J Rehab Med* 1988; 20:175–179.

Balague F, Nordin M, Skovron ML. et al. Non-specific low-back pain among schoolchildren: a field survey with analysis of some associated factors. *J Spinal Disord* 1994; 7:374–379.

Barlow CF. *Clinics in Developmental Medicine: Vol. 91. Headaches and Migraine in Childhood*. Philadelphia: J.B. Lippincott, 1984.

Barr RG. Pain in children. In: Wall PD, Melzack R (Eds). *Textbook of Pain*, Vol. 2. Edinburgh: Churchill Livingstone, 1989, pp 568–588.

Barr RG. Pain experience in children: developmental and clinical characteristics. In: Wall PD, Melzack R (Eds). *Textbook of Pain*, Vol. 3. London: Churchill Livingstone, 1994, pp 739–765.

Barr RG, Levine MD, Wilkinson RH, Mulvihill D. Chronic and occult stool retention. *Clin Pediatr* 1979; 18:674–686.

Barr RG, Watkins JB, Perman JA. Mucosal function and breath hydrogen excretion: comparative studies in the clinical evaluation of children with nonspecific abdominal complaints. *Pediatrics* 1981; 68:526–533.

Bass C, Murphy M. Somatoform and personality disorders: syndromal comorbidity and overlapping developmental pathways. *J Psychosom Res* 1995; 39:403–427.

Baum J. Epidemiology of juvenile rheumatoid arthritis (JRA). *Arthritis Rheum* 1977; 20:158–160.

Baum KF, Dunn DT, Maude GH, Serjeant GR. The painful crisis of homozygous sickle cell disease. *Arch Intern Med* 1987; 147:1231–1234.

Beales JG, Keen JH, Holt PJL. The child's perception of the disease and the experience of pain in juvenile chronic arthritis. *J Rheumatol* 1983; 10:61–65.

Bernstein BH, Singsen BH, Kent JT, et al. Reflex neurovascular dystrophy in childhood. *J Pediatr* 1978; 93:211–215.

Billings AG, Moos RH, Miller JJ, Gottlieb JE. Psychosocial adaptation in juvenile rheumatic disease: a controlled evaluation. *Health Psychol* 1987; 6:343–359.

Blom GE, Nicholls G. Emotional factors in children with rheumatoid arthritis. *Am J Orthopsychiatry* 1954; 24:588–601.

Bonham GS. Prevalence of chronic skin and musculoskeletal conditions. United States 1976. In: Anonymous. *National Health Interview Survey*, Series 10. Udshew, 1978.

Brenning R. Growing pains. *Acta Societatis Medicorum Upsaliensis* 1960; 65:185–201.

Brewer EJ Jr, Bass JC, Cassidy JT. Criteria for the classification of juvenile rheumatoid arthritis. *Bull Rheum Dis* 1972; 23:712–719.

Browder J, Gallagher JP. Dorsal cordotomy for painful phantom limb. *Ann Surg* 1948; 128(3):456–469.

Brozovic M, Anionwu E. Sickle cell disease in Britain. *J Clin Pathol* 1984; 37:1321–1326.

Bunnell WP. Back pain in children. *Orthoped Clin N Am* 1982; 13:587–604.

Burke EC, Peters GA. Migraine in childhood. *AMA J Dis Child* 1956; 92:330–336.

Bywaters EGL. Diagnostic criteria for Still's disease (juvenile RA). In: Benett PH, Wood PH (Eds). *Population Studies of Rheumatic Diseases, Excerpta Medica.* New York, 1968, pp 235–240.

Christensen MF, Mortensen O. Long-term prognosis in children with recurrent abdominal pain. *Arch Dis Child* 1975; 50:110–114.

Clarke GJR, Waters WE. Headache and migraine in a London general practice. In: Waters WE (Ed). *The Epidemiology of Migraine,* Bracknell, Berks: Boehringer Ingelheim, 1974.

Cornaglia C, Massimo L, Haupt R, et al. Incidence of pain in children with neoplastic diseases. *Pain* 1984; (Suppl 2):28

Daut RL, Cleeland CS. The prevalence and severity of pain in cancer. *Cancer* 1982; 50(9):1913–1918.

Diamond CA, Matthay KK. Childhood acute lymphoblastic leukemia. *Pediatr Ann* 1988; 17:156–170.

Egermark-Eriksson I. Prevalence of headache in Swedish schoolchildren. *Acta Paediatr Scand* 1982; 71:135–140.

Elliott SC, Miser AW, Dose AM, et al. Epidemiologic features of pain in pediatric cancer patients: a co-operative community-based study. *Clin J Pain* 1991; 7:263–268.

Fairbank JCT, Pynsent PB, van Poortvliet JA, Phillips H. Mechanical factors in the incidence of knee pain in adolescents and young adults. *J Bone Joint Surg Br* 1984; 66-B:685–693.

Faravelli C, Salvatori S, Galassi F et al. Epidemiology of somatoform disorders: a community survey in Florence. *Society for Psychiatric Epidemiology* 1997; 32:24–29.

Foley K. Pain syndromes in patients with cancer. In: Bonica JJ, Ventafridda V (Eds). *Advances in Pain Research and Therapy,* New York: Raven Press, 1979, pp 59–75.

Fritz GK, Fritsch S, Hagino O. Somatoform disorders in children and adolescents: a review of the past 10 years. *J Am Acad Child Adolesc Psychiatr* 1997; 36:1329–1338.

Gallagher JR. Dysmenorrhea and menorrhagia in adolescence. *Conn Med* 1955; 19:469–471.

Gewanter HL, Roghmann KJ, Baum J. The prevalence of juvenile arthritis. *Arthritis Rheum* 1983; 26 599–603.

Gil KM, Abrams MR, Phillips G, Keefe FJ. Sickle cell disease pain: relation of coping strategies to adjustment. *J Consult Clin Psychol* 1989; 57(6):725–731.

Gil KM, Williams DA, Thompson RJ Jr, Kinney TR. Sickle cell disease in children and adolescents: the relation of child and parent pain coping strategies to adjustment. *J Pediatr Psychol* 1991; 16:643–663.

Gil KM, Abrams MR, Phillips G, Williams DA. Sickle cell disease pain. II: Predicting health care use and activity level at nine-month follow-up. *J Consult Clin Psychol* 1992; 60:267–273.

Gil KM, Edens JL, Wilson JJ, et al. Coping strategies and laboratory pain in children with sickle cell disease. *Ann Behav Med* 1997; 19:22–29.

Goldwasser M. Primary dysmenorrhea: a local manifestation of a constitutional disease and its treatment. *California and West Med* 1938; 48:418–421.

Golub LJ, Lang WR, Menduke H. The incidence of dysmenorrhea in high school girls. *Postgrad Med* 1958; 23:38–40.

Goodman JE, McGrath PJ. The epidemiology of pain in children and adolescents: a review. *Pain* 1991; 46:247–264.

Green M. Diagnosis and treatment: psychogenic, recurrent, abdominal pain. *Pediatrics* 1967; 40:84–89.

Greipp ME. Children and young adults with reflex sympathetic dystrophy syndrome. *Clin J Pain* 1988; 4:217–221.

Harreby M, Neergaard K, Hasselsoe G, Kjer J. Are radiologic changes in the thoracic and lumbar spine of adolescents risk factors for low back pain in adults? A 25-year prospective cohort study of 640 school children. *Spine* 1995; 20:2298–2302.

Hart FA. Pain in osteoarthrosis. In: *Anonymous Practitioner,* 1974, pp 244–250.

Hawksley JC. The incidence and significance of "growing pains" in children and adolescents. *J Royal Inst Public Health Hyg* 1938; 1:798–805.

Headache Classification Committee of the International Headache Society. Classification and diagnostic criteria for headache disorders, cranial neuralgias and facial pain. *Cephalalgia Supplement* 1988; 8:44–45.

Heisel JS. Life changes as etiologic factors in juvenile rheumatoid arthritis. *J Psychosom Res* 1972; 16:411–420.

Hill R. Juvenile arthritis in various racial groups in British Columbia. *Arthritis Rheum* 1977; 20:162

Hodges K, Kline JJ, Barbero G. Anxiety in children with recurrent abdominal pain and their parents. *Psychosomatics* 1985; 26:859–866.

Houck CS, Troshynski T, Berde CB. Treatment of pain in children. In: Wall PD, Melzack R (Eds). *Textbook of Pain,* Vol. 3. London: Churchill Livingstone, 1994, pp 1419–1434.

Ivey J, Brewer EJ, Giannini EH. Psychosocial functioning in children with juvenile rheumatoid arthritis. *Arthritis Rheum* 1981; S100.

Jay GW, Tomasi LG. Pediatric headaches: a one year retrospective analysis. *Headache* 1981; 2:15–9.

Jay SM, Elliott C, Varni JW. Acute and chronic pain in adults and children with cancer. *J Consult Clin Psychol* 1986; 54(5):601–607.

Katz ER, Kellerman J, Siegel SE. Behavioral distress in children with cancer undergoing medical procedures: Developmental considerations. *J Consult Clin Psychol* 1980; 48(3):356–365.

Kellerman J. *Psychological Aspects of Childhood Cancer.* Springfield: Charles C. Thomas, 1980.

Kesler RW, Saulsbury FT, Miller LT, Rowlinson JC. Reflex sympathetic dystrophy in children: treatment with transcutaneous electric nerve stimulation. *Pediatrics* 1988; 82(5):728–732.

Krane EJ, Heller LB, Pomietto ML. Incidence of phantom sensation and pain in pediatric amputees. *Anesthesiology* 1991; 75A69

Krupp GR, Friedman AP. Migraine in children. *AMA J Dis Child* 1953; 85:146–150.

Kumar S, Powars D, Allen J, Bellvue R, Dosik H. Anxiety, self-concept, and personal and social adjustments in children with sickle cell anemia. *J Pediatr* 1976; 8:859–863.

Laaksonen A.-L. A prognostic study of juvenile rheumatoid arthritis. *Acta Paediatr* 1966; 166.

Laaksonen A-L, Laine V. A comparative study of joint pain in adults and juvenile rheumatoid arthritis. *Ann Rheum Dis* 1961; 20 386–387.

Larson BS. Somatic complaints and their relationship to depressive symptoms in Swedish adolescents. *J Child Psychol Psychiat* 1991; 32:821–832.

Larsson B, Melin L. Chronic headaches in adolescents: Treatment in a school setting with relaxation training as compared with information-contact and self-registration. *Pain* 1986; 25:325–336.

Lemanek LK, Moure SL, Gresham FM, Williamson DA, Kelly ML. Psychological adjustment of children with sickle cell anemia. *J Pediatr Psychol* 1986; 11:397–409.

Levine MD, Rappaport LA. Recurrent abdominal pain in school children: the loneliness of the long-distance physician. *Pediatr Clinics N Am* 1984; 31:969–992.

Linet MS, Stewart WF. Migraine headache: epidemiologic perspectives. *Epidemiol Rev* 1984; 6:107–139.

Linet MS, Stewart WF. The epidemiology of migraine headache. In: Blau JN (Ed). *Migraine: Clinical and Research Aspects*, Baltimore: Johns Hopkins University Press, 1987, pp 451–477.

Litt IF, Cuskey WR, Rosenberg A. Role of self-esteem and autonomy in determining medication compliance among adolescents with juvenile rheumatoid arthritis. *Pediatrics* 1982; 15–17.

Lovell DJ, Walco GA. Pain associated with juvenile rheumatoid arthritis. *Pediatr Clinics N Am* 1989; 36(4) 1015–1028.

Maytal J, Young M, Shechter A, Lipton RB. Pediatric migraine and the International Headache Society (IHS) criteria. *Neurology* 1997; 48:607.

McAnarney ER, Pless IB, Satterwhite B, Friedman SB. Psychological problems of children with chronic juvenile arthritis. *Pediatrics* 1974; 53:523–528.

McGrath PA. *Pain in Children: Nature, Assessment and Treatment.* New York: Guilford Press, 1990.

McGrath PA. Alleviating children's pain: a cognitive-behavioural approach. In: Wall PD, Melzack R (Eds). *Textbook of Pain, Vol. 3.* London: Churchill Livingstone, 1994, pp 1403–1418.

McGrath PA, Hillier LM. Controlling children's pain. In: Gatchel RD, Turk D (Eds). *Psychological Treatment for Pain: A Practitioner's Handbook.* New York: Guilford Press, 1996, pp 331–370.

McGrath PJ, Feldman W. Clinical approach to recurrent abdominal pain in children. *Dev Beh Pediatr* 1986; 7:56–63.

McGrath PJ, Unruh A. *Pain in Children and Adolescents.* Amsterdam: Elsevier, 1987.

Michael MI, Williams JM. Migraine in children. *J Pediatr* 1952; 41:18–24.

Mielants H, Veys EM, Goemaere S, et al. Prevalence of inflammatory rheumatic diseases in an adolescent urban student population, age 12 to 18, in Belgium. *Clin Exp Rheumatol* 1993; 563–567.

Miser AW. Management of pain associated with childhood cancer. In: Schechter NL, Berde CB, Yaster M. (Eds). *Pain in Infants, Children, and Adolescents.* Baltimore: Williams and Wilkins, 1993, pp 411–423.

Miser AW, Dothage JA, Wesley RA, Miser JS. The prevalence of pain in pediatric and young adult cancer populations. *Pain* 1987a; 29:73–83.

Miser AW, McCalla J, Dothage JA, Wesley M, Miser JS. Pain as a presenting symptom in children and young adults with newly diagnosed malignancy. *Pain* 1987b; 29:85–90.

Naish JM, Apley J. "Growing pains": a clinical study of non-arthritic limb pains in children. *Arch Dis Child* 1951; 26:134–140.

Oberklaid F, Amos D, Liu C. "Growing pains": clinical and behavioral correlates in a community sample. *Dev Beh Pediatr* 1997; 18:102–106.

Olsson G, Berde C. Neuropathic pain in children and adolescents. In: Schechter NL, Berde CB, Yaster Y (Eds). *Pain in Infants, Children and Adolescents.* Baltimore: Williams and Wilkins, 1993, pp 473–493.

Olsson GL, Arner S, Hirsch G. Reflex sympathetic dystrophy in children. In: Tyler DC, Krane EJ (Eds). *Advances in Pain Research and Therapy*, Vol. 15. New York: Raven Press, 1990, pp 323–331.

Oster J. Recurrent abdominal pain, headache and limb pains in children and adolescents. *Pediatrics* 1972; 50:429–436.

Oster J, Nielsen A. Growing pains: a clinical investigation of a school population. *Acta Paediatr Scand* 1972; 61:329–334.

Perrin JM. Chronic illness in childhood. In: Behrman RE (Ed). *Textbook of Pediatrics.* Philadelphia: W.B. Saunders, 1992, pp 91–94.

Pichard-Leandri E, Gauvain-Piquard A. *La douleur chez l'enfant.* Paris: Medsi/McGraw-Hill, 1989.

Platt OS, Nathan DG. Sickle cell disease. In: Nathan DG, Oski FA (Eds). *Hematology of Infancy and Childhood*, Vol. 2. Philadelphia: W.B. Saunders, 1987, pp 655–698.

Pringle ML, Butler NR, Davie R. 11,000 seven-year-olds: *First report of the National Child Development Study.* London: Longmans, Green, 1966.

Ross DM, Ross SA. *Childhood Pain: Current Issues, Research, and Management.* Baltimore: Urban and Schwarzenberg, 1988.

Rubin LS, Barbero GJ, Sibinga MS. Pupillary reactivity in children with recurrent abdominal pain. *Psychosom Med* 1967; 29:111–120.

Ruggeri SB, Athreya BH, Doughty R, Gregg JR, Das, MM. Reflex sympathetic dystrophy in children. *Clin Orthop* 1982; 163:225–230.

Schaller JG. Juvenile rheumatoid arthritis. In: Behrman RE (Ed). *Textbook of Pediatrics*, Philadelphia: W.B. Saunders, 1992, pp 612–638.

Schechter NL. Pain and pain control in children. *Curr Prob Pediatr* 1985; 15:1–67.

Schechter NL, Berde CB, Yaster M (Eds). *Pain in Infants, Children and Adolescents.* Baltimore: Williams and Wilkins, 1993.

Scott PJ, Ansell BM, Huskisson EC. Measurement of pain in juvenile chronic polyarthritis. *Ann Rheum Dis* 1977; 36:186–187.

Serjeant GR. *Sickle Cell Disease.* Oxford: Oxford University Press, 1985.

Sergeant GR, Ceulaer CDE, Lethbridge R, et al. The painful crisis of homozygous sickle cell disease: clinical features. *Br J Haematol* 1994; 87:586–591.

Shapiro BS. The management of pain in sickle cell disease. *Pediatr Clinics N Am* 1989; 36:1029–1045.

Shapiro BS. Management of painful episodes in sickle cell disease. In: Schechter NL, Berde CB, Yaster M (Eds). *Pain in Infants, Children and Adolescents.* Baltimore: Williams and Wilkins, 1993, pp 385–410.

Silber TJ, Majd M. Reflex sympathetic dystrophy syndrome in children and adolescents. *Am J Dis Child* 1988; 142:1325–1330.

Simmel ML. Phantom experiences following amputation in childhood. *J Neurol Neurosurg Psychiatr* 1962; 25:69–78.

Stickler GB, Murphy DB. Recurrent abdominal pain. *Am J Dis Child* 1979; 133:486–489.

Sullivan DB, Cassidy JT, Petty RE. Pathogenic implications of age of onset in juvenile rheumatoid arthritis. *Arthritis Rheum* 1975; 18:251–255.

Sury B. *Rheumatoid Arthritis in Children. A Clinical Study.* Copenhagen: Munksgaard, 1952

Symon DNK, Russell G. Abdominal migraine: a syndrome defined. *Cephalalgia* 1986; 6:223–228.

Thomas R, Holbrook T. Sickle cell disease: ways to reduce morbidity and mortality. *Postgrad Med* 1987; 81:265–280.

Thompson GH. Back pain in children. *J Bone Joint Surg* 1993; 75-A:928–938.

Thompson KL, Varni JW, Hanson V. Comprehensive assessment of pain in juvenile rheumatoid arthritis: an empirical model. *J Pediatr Psychol* 1987; 12:241–255.

Timko C, Stovel KW, Moos RH, Miller JJ. Adaptation to juvenile rheumatic disease: a controlled evaluation of functional disability with a one-year follow-up. *Health Psychol* 1992; 11:67–76.

Towner SR, Michet CJ Jr, O'Fallon WM, et al. The epidemiology of juvenile arthritis in Rochester, Minnesota 1960–1979. *Arthritis Rheum* 1983; 26:1208–1208.

Troussier B, Davoine P. de-Gaudemaris R, Fauconnier J, Philip X. Back pain in schoolchildren. A study among 1178 pupils. *Scand J Rehabil Med* 1994; 26:143–146.

Tyler DC, Krane EJ (Eds). *Advances in Pain Research and Therapy.* New York: Raven Press, 1990.

Ungerer JA, Horgan B, Chaitow J, Champion GD. Psychosocial

functioning in children and young adults with juvenile arthritis. *Pediatrics* 1988; 81:195–202.

Varni JW, Jay SM. Biobehavioral factors in juvenile rheumatoid arthritis: implications for research and practice. *Clin Psychol Review* 1984; 4:543–560.

Varni JW, Thompson KL, Hanson V. The Varni/Thompson Pediatric Pain Questionnaire: I. Chronic musculoskeletal pain in juvenile rheumatoid arthritis. *Pain* 1987; 28:27–38.

Walco GA, Oberlander TF. Musculoskeletal pain syndromes in children. In: Schechter NL, Berde CB, Yaster M (Eds). *Pain in Infants, Children and Adolescents*. Baltimore: Williams and Wilkins, 1993, pp 459–471.

Waters WE. The Pontypridd headache survey. *Headache* 1974; 14:81–90.

Widholm O. Dysmenorrhea during adolescence. *Acta Obstet Gynecol Scand Suppl* 1979; 87:61–66.

Widholm O, Kantero RL. Menstrual patterns of adolescent girls according to chronological and gynecological ages. *Acta Obstet Gynecol Scand Suppl* 1971; 14.

Wilder RT, Berde CB, Wolohan M, et al. Reflex sympathetic dystrophy in children. *J Bone Joint Surg* 1992;74-A(6):910–919.

Winter RB, Lipscomb PR Jr. Back pain in children. *Minn Med* 1978; 61:141–147.

Wolfe F, Smythe HA, Yunus MB. The American College of Rheumatology 1990 criteria for the classification of fibromyalgia. Report of the multicenter criteria committee. *Arthritis Rheum* 1990; 63:160–172.

Yunus MB, Masi AT. Juvenile primary fibromyositis syndrome. A clinical study of thirty-three patients and matched normal controls. *Arthritis Rheum* 1985; 28:138

Zeltzer L. Commentary on "Clinical approach to recurrent abdominal pain in children." *J Devel Behav Pediatr* 1986; 7:62–63.

REFERENCES FOR MAJOR STUDIES

Abramson JH, Hopp C, Epstein LM. Migraine and non-migrainous headaches: a community survey in Jerusalem. *J Epidemiol Community Health* 1980; 34:188–193.

Abu-Arefeh I, Russell G. Prevalence of headache and migraine in schoolchildren. *BMJ* 1994; 309:765–769.

Abu-Arefeh I, Russell G. Prevalence and clinical features of abdominal migraine compared with those of migraine headaches. *Arch Dis Child* 1995; 72:413–417.

Abu-Arefeh I, Russell G. Recurrent limb pain in schoolchildren. *Arch Dis Child* 1996; 74:336–339.

Apley J, Naish N. Recurrent abdominal pains: a field survey of 1,000 school children. *Arch Dis Child* 1958; 33:165–170.

Bille B. Migraine in school children. *Acta Paediatr Scand* 1962; 51(Suppl 136):1–151.

Dalsgaard-Nielsen T, Engberg-Pedersen H, Holm HE. Clinical and statistical investigations of the epidemiology of migraine: an investigation of the onset age and its relation to sex, adrenarche, menarche and the menstrual cycle in migraine patients, and of the menarche age, sex distribution and frequency of migraine. *Dan Med Bull* 1970; 17:138–148.

Deubner DC. An epidemiologic study of migraine and headache in 10–20 year olds. *Headache* 1977; 17:173–180.

Faull C, Nicol AR. Abdominal pain in six–year-olds: an epidemiological study in a new town. *J Child Psychol Psychiat* 1986; 27:251–260.

Garber J, Walker LS, Zeman J. Somatization symptoms in a community sample of children and adolescents: further validation of the Children's Somatization Inventory, Psychological Assessment. *J Consult Clin Psychol* 1991; 3:588–595.

Gare AB, Fasth A. Epidemiology of juvenile chronic arthritis in southwestern Sweden: a 5-year prospective population study. *Pediatrics* 1992; 950–958.

Gare AB, Fasth A, Anderson J, et al. Incidence and prevalence of juvenile chronic arthritis: a population survey. *Ann Rheum Dis* 1987; 277–281.

Gortmaker SL, Sappenfield W. Chronic childhood disorders: prevalence and impact. *Pediatr Clinics N Am* 1984; 31:3–18.

Klein JR, Litt IF. Epidemiology of adolescent dysmenorrhea. *Pediatrics* 1981; 68:661–664.

Linet MS, Stewart WF, Celentano DD, Ziegler D, Sprecher M. An epidemiologic study of headache among adolescents and young adults. *JAMA* 1989; 261:2211–2216.

Manners PJ, Diepeveen DA. Prevalence of juvenile chronic arthritis in a population of a 12-year-old children in urban Australia. *Pediatrics* 1996; 98:84–90.

Mikkelsson M, Sourander A, Piha J, Salminen JJ. Psychiatric symptoms in preadolescents with musculoskeletal pain and fibromyalgia. *Pediatrics* 1997; 100:220–227.

Mortimer MJ, Kay J, Jaron A. Clinical epidemiology of childhood abdominal migraine in an urban general practice. *Develop Med Child Neurol* 1993; 35:243–248.

Newacheck PW, Taylor WR. Childhood chronic illness: prevalence, severity and impact. *Am J Public Health* 1992; 82:364–371.

Offord DR, Boyle MH, Szatmari P, et al. Ontario Child Health Study II. Six-month prevalence of disorder and rates of service utilization. *Arch Gen Psychiatry* 1987; 44:832–836.

Salminen JJ. The adolescent back: a field survey of 370 Finnish schoolchildren. *Acta Paediatr Scand* 1984; (Suppl) 315:1–122.

Salminen JJ, Pentti J, Terho P. Low back pain and disability in 14-year-old schoolchildren. *Acta Paediatr* 1992; 81:1035–1039.

Sharrer VW, Ryan-Wenger NM. Measurements of stress and coping among school-aged children with and without recurrent abdominal pain. *J School Health* 1991; 61:86–91.

Sillanpää M. Prevalence of migraine and other headache in Finnish children starting school. *Headache* 1976; 16:288–290.

Sillanpää M. Prevalence of headache in prepuberty. *Headache* 1983a; 23:10–14.

Sillanpää M. Changes in the prevalence of migraine and other headaches during the first seven school years. *Headache* 1983b; 23:15–19.

Sparks JP. The incidence of migraine in schoolchildren: a survey by the Medical Officers of Schools Association. *Practitioner* 1978; 221:407–411.

Taimela S, Kujala UM, Salminen JJ, Viljanen T. The prevalence of low back pain among children and adolescents. *Spine* 1997; 22:1132–1136.

Teperi J, Rimpela M. Menstrual pain, health and behavior in girls. *Soc Sci Med* 1989; 29:163–169.

Vähäsarja V. Prevalence of chronic knee pain in children and adolescents in northern Finland. *Acta Paediatr* 1995; 84:803–805.

Vahlquist B. Migraine in children. *Int Arch Allergy* 1955; 7:348–355.

Zuckerman B, Stevenson J, Bailey V. Stomachaches and headaches in a community sample of preschool children. *Pediatrics* 1987; 79:677–682.

Correspondence to: Patricia A. McGrath, Ph.D. Paediatric Pain Program, Child Health Research Institute, 800 Commissioners Road East, London, Ontario, Canada N6C 2V5, Tel: 519-685-8107; Fax: 519-685-8186; email: pamcgrat@julian.uwo.ca.

Epidemiology of Pain, edited by
I.K. Crombie, IASP Press, Seattle, © 1999.

8

Pain in Older People

Robert D. Helme and Stephen J. Gibson

National Ageing Research Institute, Parkville, Victoria, Australia

According to self-report measures, acute pain probably occurs at much the same rate across all age groups. Chronic pain is experienced more by older people, but this increase does not continue beyond the seventh decade. The elderly often experience chronic pain in the joints, back, legs, and feet; they appear to suffer less visceral pain and headache than younger people. The plateau in overall chronic pain prevalence with age may reflect a balance between age-related impairment of the nociceptive function of the nervous system and an increase in the pathological load that accompanies old age. The contribution of other dimensions of the pain experience to this equation can only be discovered through longitudinal studies that focus primarily on pain rather than addressing pain as an ancillary to other aspects of aging.

PREVALENCE OF PAIN IN OLDER PEOPLE

The population prevalence and characteristics of pain are difficult to ascertain, and comparisons across studies are complex. Moreover, many common pain problems (e.g., the suffering associated with fractures or cancer) may seriously afflict the person involved, but are short-lived because of rapid resolution or mortality and so are not reflected in cross-sectional prevalence studies. Even chronic conditions well known to increase with age, such as central post-stroke pain (Leijon et al. 1989) and postherpetic neuralgia (Portenoy et al. 1986), rarely feature because of their low incidence compared to the overwhelming frequency and chronicity of degenerative joint disease. Most prevalence studies are also unable to incorporate the large number of questions needed to adequately describe the pain experience: where is the site of pain; is it continuous or intermittent; what has been its duration; what is its quality and severity at different times; how is it aggravated and relieved; and how has it been treated? We might also address the effect of pain on quality of life and mood, how pain relates to comorbidity, and its effect on caregivers, and then shift our focus of attention to another pain complaint (Ferrell et al. 1990; Mobily et al. 1994) and repeat this entire battery of questions.

This complexity is compounded by the fact that most epidemiological studies of pain in older people were not designed with the primary object of examining the problem of pain. Pain is either an afterthought or a minor aspect of the study in hand, or the results on pain prevalence were derived later from more general data by a second group of researchers. Presumably the difficulty is the cost of such studies, particularly if a longitudinal element is incorporated into the study design.

Yet the epidemiological study of pain is important as it assists us to define the extent of the problem, which in turn helps determine resource allocation and generates important questions relevant to the pathophysiology, psychopathology, and pathogenesis of pain itself. Such factors are usually hidden in the morass of details that must be interpreted for the typical clinic patient with chronic pain. We must consider several factors in reviewing epidemiological studies of pain prevalence in the elderly. These include the selection of the study population, which may comprise random samples of individuals from the community or convenience samples from pain clinics, general practice groups, or institutions. The method of contact, response rates, age distribution of the sample, and questions asked are also important considerations.

FIELD STUDIES

One of the most quoted studies is that by Crook et al. (1984), who randomly sampled the patients of a group of general practitioners located near Toronto, Canada. Their telephone survey had a gratifying 95% response rate, but there were few participants over the age of 80, a problem common to most community studies that explore issues relevant to the elderly. Questions regarding the temporal nature of pain did not follow the usual pattern of description for acute and chronic pain, and this study's classification of pain as temporary or persistent is not easily compared with classifications used in other studies. Nevertheless, it was one of the first studies to clearly demonstrate increased pain prevalence with increasing age, and it highlighted pain as a frequent problem for a large number of older people. Its finding that temporary pain had the same prevalence at all ages is intriguing, and it remains the only study to have reported age-related prevalence for acute pain of any type.

However, other studies were not necessarily able to replicate Crook's results on persistent or chronic pain. Table I summarizes recent studies that report pain prevalence among older people. Fig. 1 contains prevalence data from 11 studies that contain sufficient detail to allow comparison of overall pain rates across a wide age range. Gibson and Helme (1995) recently reviewed these studies, which collectively suggest a peak or plateau in the prevalence of pain by age 65 (Brattberg et al. 1989, 1996; Andersson et al. 1993) and a decline in reported pain in the old old (75–84 years) and oldest old (85+) (Roy and Thomas 1987; Mobily et al. 1994; Brattberg et al. 1996).

We recently completed a study of a community sample from Melbourne, Australia (Health Status Of Older People [HSOP]; Kendig et al. 1996). A sample of 1000 English-speaking persons aged 65 years and over was randomly selected from electoral rolls (voting is compulsory for all Australian citizens between the ages of 18 and 70, and the names of all adults are maintained on the rolls, regardless of age). Only 12% of residents over age 70 were not Australian citizens, and most of this group were of non-English-speaking background and were beyond the scope of the study. The response rate among participants was 70%, which is common for this type of study. Trained researchers interviewed subjects and obtained answers to a wide

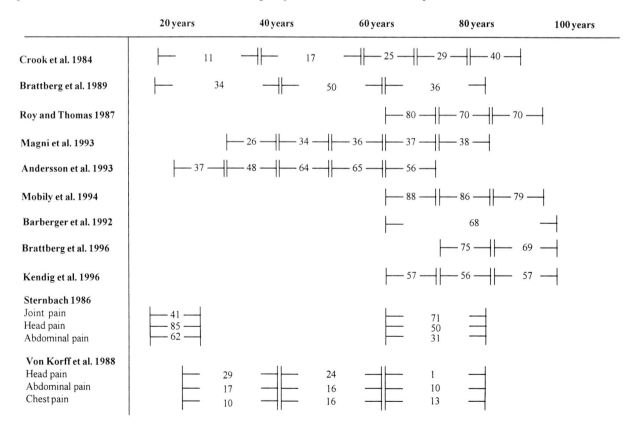

Fig. 1. Pain prevalence (%) across the adult lifespan.

Table I
Studies of pain prevalence that include older persons

Reference	Type of Study	Type of Pain	Source of Sample	Sample Size (>65 y)	Pain Severity	Duration of Symptoms	Type of Prevalence Estimate
Crook et al. 1984	Telephone survey	All types	GP practice	827 (107*)	Often troubled by pain	Previous 2 wk	Period
Sternbach 1986	Telephone survey	Headache, backache, muscle, joint, stomach, premenstrual, dental	Random population sample	1254 (179)	Any pain	Previous 12 mo	Period
Roy and Thomas 1987	Telephone survey	All types	Convenience sample	205 (205)	Not stated	Not stated	Point
Von Korff et al. 1988	Postal survey	Back, head, abdomen, face, chest	Stratified random population sample	1016 (77)	Mild to severe of >1 d duration	Previous 6 mo	Period
Brattberg 1989	Postal survey	All types	Random population sample	1009 (183)	Affected to severe degree	<1 mo to >6 mo	Period
Magni et al. 1993†	Interview	Musculo-skeletal	Stratified random population sample	3023 (333)	Not asked	Previous 12 mo	Period
Andersson et al. 1993	Postal survey	All types	Random population sample	1806 (285)	Weak to intense	>3 mo	Period
Mobily et al. 1994‡	Interview	Legs, joints, back, chest	Random rural population sample	3097 (3097)	Been troubled, persistent, bothersome	Previous 12 mo	Period
Barberger et al. 1996	Interview	Joint pain	Random population sample	2792 (2792)	Not stated	Not stated	Period
Brattberg et al. 1996	Telephone interview	All types	Stratified random population sample	537 (537)	Mild to severe	Previous 12 mo	Period
Kendig et al. 1997	Interview	All types	Random population sample	1000 (1000*)	Weak to severe	Previous 12 mo	Period

* Persons >60 years old.
† See also Magni et al. 1990, 1992.
‡ See also Herr et al. 1991, Lavsky-Shulan et al. 1985.

range of demographic and social questions as well as details about active disease states, functional ability, and attitudes to health. A brief physical examination completed the interview. The interview included a brief series of questions on pain, its expectation, frequency, site, severity, presumed cause, and treatment. Representative data are shown in Table II (adapted from Helme and Gibson 1997). The prevalence of pain considered to be "persistent, or bothersome, or limiting activities" over the preceding 12 months was essentially the same at all ages above 65. The stability of pain prevalence with increasing age is best shown for the group who did not report pain at all over this time interval; 44% of subjects within each of the three age cohorts had no pain. These figures are in general agreement with the studies shown in Fig. 1, and include a reasonable sample of persons over the age of 85. The sociodemographic factors that were associated with increased pain report were low educational status (odds ratio [OR] = 1.6) and a history of unpaid em-

Table II
Health status of older people

	Young Old	Old Old	Oldest Old
Pain Prevalence	*n* = 638	*n* = 310	*n* = 42
Frequent	32	36	34
Occasional	25	20	23
Never	43	44	43
Pain Duration			
Acute	6	7	6
Chronic	51	48	55
No Pain	51	45	43
Pain Site	*n* = 364	*n* = 172	*n* = 24
Joints	49	50	50
Back	45	40	42
Legs/feet	38	37	50
Abdomen	7	9	0
Chest	8	10	0
Head	5	3	8
Other	7	4	0

Source: Adapted from Helme and Gibson (1997).
Note: "Young old" represents persons aged 65–74 years, "old old" 75–84 years, and "oldest old" 85+ years. Pain prevalence figures are percentage of positive responses in three categories (frequent = once or twice a week to daily, occasional = a few times a year to once or twice a month, never) to the question: "In the past 12 months how often have you felt pain that is persistent or bothersome or limits your activities?" Pain duration figures are percentage of responses in three categories (acute = less than 3 months, chronic = more than 3 months, or no pain) to the question: "About how long ago did you start having (your most severe) pain?" Pain site figures are percentage of positive responses to the question: "In the past 12 months, where is your pain?" (respondents were restricted to a maximum of three sites).

ployment, such as household duties (OR = 1.5). The prevalence of acute pain in the HSOP sample, defined as pain with onset within the previous 3 months, was stable at 6% across the entire age range. This finding adds support to the notion that the prevalence of temporary pain is remarkably constant across the age spectrum (Crook et al. 1984).

METHODOLOGICAL CONSIDERATIONS

The question remains as to why the studies in Fig. 1 demonstrate such widely disparate prevalence figures for chronic pain. Many reasons can be put forward, most notably methodological variations such as whether the means of data acquisition is by personal or proxy interview, telephone interview, or postal survey (postal surveys have a selection bias toward healthier older persons; Von Korff et al. 1990). Other considerations include the number of subjects in each age group

and response rates, especially for the oldest old. The unreliability of memory of previous pain may be particularly important in older samples, where the effects of age-associated memory impairment and incipient dementia are frequent enough to seriously affect data acquisition in large-scale prevalence surveys. However, the most likely reason for the variation in absolute prevalence figures is the nature of the questions. Questions may involve the pain "window" (the time period over which pain is sampled), the time in pain within this window, the severity of pain, or the level of its interference with daily life (often recorded as whether the pain is "troubling" or "bothersome"), and the effect of cueing.

Most epidemiological studies differ on several of these points, making direct comparison difficult. For example, Roy and Thomas conducted their 1987 study on a convenience sample using telephone survey methods; the numbers of oldest old were small, and the measure of pain poorly specified. In contrast, Mobily et al. (1994) examined a randomly selected rural sample using direct interview techniques and limited questions regarding pain to the back, chest, legs, and joints. Given such fundamental differences, it is not surprising that absolute prevalence figures vary.

As might be expected, studies with a longer time frame tend to report higher pain prevalence (compare Crook et al. 1984 with Andersson et al. 1993). However, more subtle influences on the way the pain is defined are also important. Brattberg et al. (1989) examined the prevalence of pain in response to different questions in the same population. Positive answers to the question "any" pain were reported by 66% of respondents, pain "to a high degree" by 51%, "obvious" pain over one month by 44%, "obvious" pain over 6 months by 40%, and "continuous or nearly continuous" pain by 23%. The HSOP study (Kendig 1996) reported a slight increase in pain with age in females of 4.6% per decade if it occurred daily, but a decrease if the pain occurred from once or twice a month to a few times a year. Thus, it appears that both an age-related increase and a decrease in pain prevalence can be supported from the same database, depending on the stringency of the criteria used for describing pain as "bothersome."

Cueing is more difficult to recognize because the nature and sequencing of the questions asked are rarely reported with the data. Nonetheless, the prevalence of pain in studies that ask for "any" pain before asking where that pain is located (Crook et al. 1984; Roy and

Thomas 1987; Andersson et al. 1993) is often strikingly different to that reported in studies that ask about pain in each anatomical location and then request specific details (Sternbach 1986; Von Korff et al. 1988; Brattberg et al. 1989, 1996; Mobily et al. 1994). For example, Mobily et al. asked respondents if they had experienced any pain in their legs at night or while walking, and then asked similar questions about joint pain, back pain, and chest pain prior to asking about any other pain condition. This type of rich contextual information is likely to provide a more salient prompt to the recollection of pain symptoms than studies like that of Crook et al. (1984) that simply ask whether the subject is often troubled by pain.

SITE OF PAIN

The site of reported pain is a major source of variation in prevalence figures between different studies. Several studies have examined pain at particular body sites, and while the absolute prevalence figures vary according to the temporal definition of pain, some consistent trends have emerged. The prevalence of articular joint pain more than doubles in adults over 65 years old compared to young adults (Sternbach 1986; Von Korff et al. 1990; Barberger-Gateau et al. 1992; Andersson et al. 1993; Harkins et al. 1994). The frequency of foot and leg pain also increases markedly with advancing age (Herr et al. 1991; Mobily et al. 1994; Benvenuti et al. 1995; Helme and Gibson 1997). Conversely, the prevalence of headache shows a progressive decrease with increasing age after a peak prevalence at 45–50 years of age (Sternbach 1986; D'Allesandro et al. 1988; Kay et al. 1992; Andersson et al. 1993; Harkins et al. 1994). The frequency of facial/dental pain and abdominal/stomach pain also appears to decline during old age (Kay et al. 1992). Chest pain probably is most prevalent during late middle age at the peak of ischemic heart disease, but declines thereafter despite the continuing high mortality from this disease (Sternbach 1986; Korff et al. 1988; Tibblin et al. 1990; Andersson et al. 1993). The findings are more equivocal with respect to back pain. Harkins et al. (1994) and Von Korff et al. (1988) report a small but significant increase in back pain with advancing age, whereas other studies have shown the reverse (Sternbach 1986; Tibblin et al. 1990; Andersson et al. 1993). A summary view would be that head, abdominal, and chest pain frequency are reduced in older

people and that joint pain is increased. Age-related back pain prevalence varies among studies, so no definite opinion can be provided on how age affects that condition (Gibson and Helme 1995).

GENDER AND PAIN

Almost 60% of persons more than 65 years old are women, and by the year 2020, 73% of those aged 85 and above will be women (Ruda 1993). Given this disproportionate representation within older segments of the population, any gender differences in pain complaint could greatly affect age-specific pain prevalence estimates. Most epidemiological studies have indicated that women have a significantly higher prevalence of pain when compared to men of similar age (Crook et al. 1984; Lavsky-Shulan et al. 1985; Sternbach 1986; Von Korff et al. 1988; Magni et al. 1990, 1993), although there have been some exceptions (Brattberg et al. 1989; Anderssen et al. 1993). The magnitude of gender differences in pain prevalence may depend upon the type of disease. Rheumatoid arthritis, osteoarthritis, headache, and fibromyalgia are more common in women, whereas gout, ankylosing spondylitis, and coronary heart disease are more common in men (Berkeley 1993). Biological factors probably contribute to some of these differences, and there are documented changes in pain report during pregnancy and during the different stages of the menstrual cycle (Ryan and Maier 1988; Polleri 1992). Socialization and lifestyle factors in self-report of pain must also be considered, and at least some of these influences are unlikely to change across the adult lifespan. Biological factors may be less important in persons of advanced age, but unfortunately little systematic research has focused on gender differences beyond the reproductive years. The prevalence of headache is 15% higher in middle-aged women than middle-aged men, but this apparent gender difference disappears in persons over the age of 70 years (D'Allesandro et al. 1988; Von Korff et al. 1988). Abdominal and visceral pain complaints are more common in women aged 18–40 years than in men of the same age, but are approximately equal in older men and women (Von Korff et al. 1988; Tibblin et al. 1990; Brattberg et al. 1996). Conversely, gender differences in backache, joint and leg pain, and multiple pain complaints may be preserved with advancing age (Lavsky-Shulan et al. 1985; Tibblin et al. 1990; Mobily et al. 1994). Gender differences in pain report may diminish during the later years of life, at least for certain types of pain, but further research is needed in order to fully clarify this issue.

REASONS FOR AGE-RELATED CHANGES IN PAIN PREVALENCE

Gerontologists would most likely agree that pathological load is the overriding factor contributing to increased pain complaint with advancing age. Most illnesses increase in prevalence with advancing age, and the interplay of multiple diseases in an individual case is the hallmark of geriatric medicine. The HSOP study (Helme and Gibson 1997) detected a modest association between age and number of self-reported diseases, despite the truncated age range of subjects ($r = 0.12$, $P = 0.0001$). One of the burdens of disease is an increased risk of pain, although not all diseases are painful. Older patients with occasional or regular pain are likely to suffer from a circumscribed list of complaints including osteoarthritis in its numerous clinical manifestations, osteoporosis with crush fractures, other fractures of the spine or limbs, headache, and postherpetic neuralgia (Farrell et al. 1996).

Leaving aside the increase in pain-associated diseases in older people, it is easier to postulate reasons for decline in pain report than for any increase. First, there are issues related to selection bias. For instance, older persons with painful disease may be sequestered into institutional care, thereby reducing pain prevalence estimates among older persons in the community. The response rates among the very old in community surveys may be poor, especially for those who are disabled by disease and hence more likely to suffer from pain. The very oldest (85+) also represent a select sample of survivors, and these individuals may experience less pain-causing disease. Second, there may be an age-specific response bias. The elderly may de-emphasize pain due to other significant life events such as death of a spouse, loss of independence, and high levels of morbidity and disability. There is a general perception that older persons are more stoic (Foley 1994) and more likely to misattribute pain symptoms to the aging process. Furthermore, pain may not be present at the time of questioning, especially if it is arthritic in nature (subjects are normally seated during an interview, and arthritic pain "right now" is often relieved in this posture). Lastly, age-related

changes in the function of nociceptive pathways could lead to reduced pain sensitivity during senescence.

ISSUES RELATED TO SELECTION BIAS

The sequestration of elderly pain sufferers into nursing home care appears an unlikely explanation of reduced pain prevalence in older persons in the community. Studies of pain prevalence in institutional settings have largely been conducted in North American nursing homes and independent but supervised living accommodations for the frail elderly (Roy and Thomas 1986; Ferrell et al. 1990; Parmelee et al. 1991, 1993; Sengstaken and King 1993). Although the methods of pain measurement are not always clear and vary among studies, all such studies showed pain prevalence to be high, ranging between 70% and 83%, with severity ranging from mild to severe. Most reported pain was in the back and joints. Ferrell et al. (1990) used a measure of present pain intensity from the McGill Pain Questionnaire (MPQ) and found that 66% of subjects had no pain at the time of interview. These prevalence figures are approximately commensurate with those from community samples (Roy and Thomas 1986; Mobily et al. 1994). Depression, a common problem among institutionalized patients, is also likely to influence the prevalence of pain (Parmelee et al. 1991; Casten et al. 1995). Magni et al. (1985) found that 96% of the depressed and 80% of others reported pain in a geriatric hospital setting. Thus, institutionalized persons appear to be a cohort of the very old with high rates of pain, although they seem to have the same disorders at the same prevalence rates as people of similar age who reside in the community. No large-scale study has compared the same measures of pain in community and institutionalized samples, although a small study by Roy and Thomas (1986) directly supports the view that pain is equally prevalent in elderly persons in the community and in institutions. Given the relatively similar pain prevalence figures between institutionalized and community-dwelling persons over the age of 80, even high rates of institutionalization approaching 30% would be expected to have little overall effect on community prevalence rates. Moreover, most of the reported decrease in pain occurs at an age when institutionalization rates are less than 1%.

The high response rates in most large-scale epidemiological surveys suggests that the prospect of an age-specific drop-out of older persons with pain should not be viewed as a major concern. However, response rates may depend upon the method of data acquisition, as personal interview appears to result in a higher yield of older persons when compared to postal surveys, and response rates vary across different age groups when postal survey methods are used (Von Korff et al. 1990). Recent epidemiological investigations in which the study population was restricted to persons aged 65 and older have generally noted a higher overall prevalence of pain than has been found in cross-sectional studies that cover the entire age range of the adult population (Lavsky-Shulan et al. 1985; Barberger-Gateau et al. 1992; Mobily et al. 1994). These restricted sample studies have used methods tailored specifically to recruit older individuals, and they usually contain a much larger sample of adults in the seventh, eighth, and ninth decades of life. The findings of higher pain prevalence in restricted elderly samples are of concern; however, the difference between these and cross-sectional population studies is not large, and both types of investigation support a decline in pain prevalence from younger elderly adults (aged 65–75 years) to those of more advanced age (85+ years).

Finally, the issue of survivorship as an explanation for decreased pain report among the very oldest also appears unlikely. In general, studies that report prevalence rates of asymptomatic pathology, such as that of the spine (Wiesel et al. 1984; Jensen et al. 1994), show a progressive increase with increasing age. Rates of disability also increase into the very extremes of old age. A retrospective investigation showed pain report to be even more frequent during the last years of life (Moss et al. 1991).

AGE-SPECIFIC RESPONSE BIAS AND MISATTRIBUTION

The context in which painful symptoms are processed and the meaning attributed to them are recognized as important factors in shaping the pain experience (Melzack 1973). Older adults may attribute pain symptoms to the normal aging process rather than perceiving them as a warning sign of injury or disease (Stoller et al. 1993). Several studies have demonstrated that mild pain symptoms do not affect self-rated perceptions of health in older adults as they do in the young (Tornstam 1975; Ebrahim et al. 1991). Mis-attribution of mild aches and pains to the normal aging process greatly reduces the importance attached to this

symptom and may even alter the fundamental meaning of pain. Pain may also be judged as a relatively minor problem when compared to other concurrent life circumstances such as the loss of a lifetime partner or increasing levels of morbidity and disability that threaten loss of functional independence. One important consequence of such life events and the misattribution of pain symptoms is that older adults will be less likely to endorse questions pertaining to the presence of "bothersome pain" or "being often troubled by pain." However, severe pain symptoms are always interpreted as signs of serious illness, irrespective of age (Leventhal et al. 1993), and the elderly are more likely to seek medical attention than are younger persons when faced with severe pain (Stoller et al. 1993).

Another form of age-specific response bias that could affect pain report relates to stoicism, or alternatively, a decreased willingness to label a sensation as painful. There is a commonly held view that older adults are more stoic in reporting clinical pain sensations (Portenoy and Farkash 1988; Hofland 1992; Foley 1994), although empirical studies have yet to substantiate this view. In an extensive series of studies, Botwinick (1984) has shown an age-related increase in the tendency toward cautious response patterns for most tasks involving sensory threshold processing. Psychophysical studies of pain perception are consistent with this view and suggest that elderly persons adopt a more stringent response criterion for the threshold report of pain when faced with low-intensity noxious stimulation (Clark and Mehl 1971; Harkins and Chapman 1976, 1977). It is difficult to estimate the extent to which stoicism, misattribution, or cautiousness might influence pain prevalence figures in older persons. The effect of response bias (either stoicism or cautiousness) and misattribution appears to be most pervasive at lower intensities of noxious sensation. This could result in the under-reporting of mild or weak pain symptoms by older persons, but would be unlikely to affect reports of moderate to severe pain.

AGE-RELATED CHANGES IN NOCICEPTIVE FUNCTION

One of the reasons for a decline in pain complaint after the age of 65 years despite increasing morbidity from pain-associated disease may be reduced function in nociceptive pathways. The results from psychophysical studies using experimentally controlled levels of noxious stimulation are somewhat equivocal with regard to age differences in pain perception. Many studies have shown a progressive decrease in pain sensitivity with advancing age, but there have also been numerous reports of no age difference, particularly when using electrical stimulation (for review see Gibson and Helme 1995; Harkins et al. 1996). A recent study using differential nerve fiber blockade has shown that older persons rely on C-fiber activation before reporting the presence of pain, whereas younger adults utilize the additional information from A-delta nociceptive fibers (Chakour et al. 1996). Moreover, when A-delta-fiber input was blocked in young adults, the observed age differences in pain threshold and subjective ratings of pain intensity disappeared. Age differences in the temporal summation of nociceptive input also varies as a function of nociceptive fiber type (Harkins et al. 1996), and such differential age effects on A-delta and C-fiber function may help explain some of the disparity in psychophysical findings.

Studies of clinical pain states have also indicated that older persons exhibit a relative absence of pain in the presentation of certain visceral disease states such as ischemic heart pain and abdominal pain associated with acute infection (Albano et al. 1975; MacDonald et al. 1983; Norman and Yoshikawa 1983; Clinch et al. 1984; Solomon et al. 1989; Muller et al. 1990). Unfortunately, most of the clinical studies are difficult to interpret because the severity of pathology is seldom reported. Nonetheless, controlled investigations of myocardial pain during exercise-induced ischemia provide support for the view of a clinically significant decrease in ischemic pain perception with advancing age (Miller et al. 1990; Ambepitiya et al. 1993, 1994).

There is limited evidence of age-related changes in the physiological functioning of peripheral and central nervous system (CNS) nociceptive pathways. For instance, a marked decrease in the density of myelinated and unmyelinated nerve fibers has been noted in older adults (Ochoa and Mair 1969), and nerve conduction studies indicate prolonged latencies in peripheral sensory nerves in apparently healthy older persons (Desmedt and Cheron 1980). Stimulation of cutaneous nociceptors on some finely myelinated A-delta and unmyelinated C-fibers produces impulses that travel both to the CNS to signal pain and along axon collaterals to initiate a neurogenic vasodilatation or flare around the site of stimulation. Older persons

show a significant reduction in the neurogenic flare size, which provides further indirect evidence of altered primary afferent nociceptive function (Helme and McKernan 1985; Parkhouse and Le Quesne 1988; Ardron et al. 1991). Under certain conditions, the size of axon flare is highly correlated with the perception of pain (Helme and McKernan 1985; Gibson et al. 1994), and these responses are thought to play an important role in primary hyperalgesia and wound healing.

With regard to CNS processing, the Cerebral Event Related Potential (CERP) in response to noxious thermal CO_2 laser stimulation is also altered with advancing age (Gibson et al. 1990, 1994). This electroencephalographic response to a noxious stimulus shows a strong relationship between peak amplitude and subjective ratings of pain in response to increasing strength of stimulation. The CERP is a sensitive measure of analgesic efficiency and is affected by levels of arousal and attention. It is therefore thought to represent integrated CNS processing of afferent noxious input. A recent study has shown an age-related increase in the latency of CERP components and a reduction in peak amplitude in older people (Gibson et al. 1990). These findings suggest an age-related slowing in the cognitive processing of noxious information and a reduced cortical activation in response to noxious input.

In summary, limited evidence from physiological studies and psychophysical investigations suggest age-related alterations in the function of peripheral and CNS nociceptive pathways. These changes are likely to influence sensitivity to painful sensation and would be expected to contribute to a decline in pain report in persons of advanced age. However, most of the evidence of age differences in nociceptive function is indirect, and the clinical relevance of reduced pain sensitivity to experimental pain stimuli is still the subject of considerable debate (see Harkins et al. 1994). It seems likely that pain report does decline as a consequence of age-related changes in nociceptive function, but more definitive studies on physiological changes in nociceptive pathways are needed in order to fully resolve this issue.

CONCLUSIONS

Most cross-sectional epidemiological studies have shown that the overall prevalence of pain increases with advancing age. Absolute prevalence rates vary considerably among different investigations, which probably reflects the nature of questions asked, including the time window for pain assessment, the time in pain within this window, and the severity and site of pain included within the prevalence estimate. The well-documented increase in pathological load, particularly degenerative joint and spine disease and leg and foot disorders, may help explain the increased frequency of pain report in surveys of older persons. However, it is also apparent that the age-related increase in overall pain prevalence does not continue beyond the seventh decade of life. The reasons for maintaining a steady frequency of pain report beyond that time remain largely unknown. Issues relating to selection bias, response bias, or misattribution of pain symptoms and possible age-related changes in the function of nociceptive pathways may play some role in explaining this trend. Future studies will need to focus on the development of pain over the life-span of the individual and on the influence on pain report of losses in independence brought about by diminished functional capacity, death of spouse, and altered socioeconomic status as well as the effects of dementia and depression. There remains the more difficult task of accurately determining the effects of pain from uncommon or short-lived disease states such as cancer, fractures, and infections on health outcomes and costs.

REFERENCES

Albano W, Zielinski CM, Organ CH. Is appendicitis in the aged really different? *Geriatrics* 1975; 30:81–88.

Ambepitiya GB, Iyengar EN, Roberts ME. Review: Silent exertional myocardial ischaemia and perception of angina in elderly people. *Age Ageing* 1993; 22:302–307.

Ambepitiya G, Roberts M, Ranjadayalan K, Tallis R. Silent exertional myocardial ischemia in the elderly: a quantitative analysis of anginal perceptual threshold and the influence of autonomic function. *J Am Geriatr Soc* 1994; 42:732–737.

Andersson HI, Ejlertsson G, Leden I, Rosenberg C. Chronic pain in a geographically defined general population: studies of differences in age, gender, social class, and pain localization. *Clin J Pain* 1993; 9:174–182.

Ardron ME, Helme RD, Gibson SJ. Microvascular skin responses in elderly people with varicose leg ulcers. *Age Ageing* 1991; 20:124–128.

Barberger-Gateau P, Chaslerie A, Dartigues J, Commenges D, Gagnon M, et al. Health measures correlates in a French elderly community population: the PAQUID study. *J Gerontol* 1992; 472:S88–95.

Benvenuti F, Ferrucci L, Guralnik JM, Gangemi S, Baroni A. Foot pain and disability in older persons: an epidemiologic survey. *J Am Geriatr Soc* 1995; 43:479–484.

Berkeley KJ. Sex and chronobiology: opportunities for focus on the positive. *Newsletter of the International Association for the Study of Pain*, January 1993.

Botwinick J. *Aging and Behavior*. New York: Springer, 1984.

Brattberg G, Thorslund M, Wikman A. The prevalence of pain in the general community: the results of a postal survey in a county of Sweden. *Pain* 1989; 37:215–222.

Brattberg G, Parker MG, Thorslund M. The prevalence of pain amongst the oldest old in Sweden. *Pain* 1996; 67:29–34.

Casten RJ, Parmelee PA, Kleban MH, Powell-Lawton M, Katz IR. The relationship among anxiety, depression, and pain in a geriatric institutionalised sample. *Pain* 1995; 61:271–276.

Chakour MC, Gibson SJ, Bradbeer M, Helme RD. The effect of age on A-delta and C-fibre thermal pain perception. *Pain* 1996; 64:143–152.

Clark WC, Mehl L. Thermal pain: a sensory decision theory analysis of the effect of age and sex on d', various response criteria, and 50% pain threshold. *J Abnorm Psychol* 1971; 78:202–212.

Clinch D, Banjeree AK, Ostick G. Absence of abdominal pain in elderly patients with peptic ulcer. *Age Ageing* 1984; 13:120–123.

Crook J, Rideout E, Browne G. The prevalence of pain complaints in a general population. *Pain* 1984; 18:299–314.

D'Alessandro R, Benassi G, Lenzi PL, et al. Epidemiology of headache in the republic of San Marino. *J Neurol Neurosurg Psychiatry* 1988; 51:21–27.

Desmedt JE, Cheron G. Somatosensory evoked potentials to finger stimulation in healthy octogenarians and in young adults: waveforms, scalp topography and transit times of parietal and frontal components. *EEG Clin Neurophysiol* 1980; 50:404–425.

Ebrahim S, Brittis S, Wu A. The valuation of states of ill health: the impact of age and disability. *Age Ageing* 1991; 20:37–40.

Farrell MJ, Gibson SJ, Helme RD. Chronic nonmalignant pain in older people. In: Ferrell BR, Ferrell BA (Eds). *Pain in the Elderly*. Seattle: IASP Press, 1996, pp 81–89.

Ferrell BA, Ferrell BR, Osterweil D. Pain in the nursing home. *J Am Geriatr Soc* 1990; 38:409–414.

Foley KM. Pain management in the elderly. In: Hazzard WR, Bierman EL, Blass JP, Ettinger WH, Halter JB (Eds). *Principles of Geriatric Medicine and Gerontology*. 3rd ed. New York: McGraw Hill, 1994: 317–331.

Gibson SJ, Helme RD. Age differences in pain perception and report: a review of physiological, psychological, laboratory and clinical studies. *Pain Reviews* 1995; 2:111–137.

Gibson SJ, Gorman MM, Helme RD. Assessment of pain in the elderly using event-related cerebral potentials. In: Bond MR, Charlton JE, Woolf CJ (Eds) *Proceedings of the VIth World Congress on Pain*. Amsterdam: Elsevier Science, 1990, pp 523–529.

Gibson SJ, Helme RD, Gorman MM. Age related changes in the scalp topography of cerebral event related potentials following noxious CO_2 laser stimulation. In: Gebhart GF, Hammond DL, Jensen TS. (Eds) *Proceedings of the 7th World Congress on Pain*. Seattle: IASP Press, 1994, p 159.

Harkins SW, Chapman CR. Detection and decision factors in pain perception in young and elderly men. *Pain* 1976; 2:253–264.

Harkins SW, Chapman CR. The perception of induced dental pain in young and elderly women. *J Gerontol* 1977; 32:428–435.

Harkins SW, Price DD, Bush FM, Small RE. Geriatric pain. In: Wall PD, Melzack M (Eds). *Textbook of Pain*, 3rd ed. New York: Churchill Livingstone, 1994, pp 769–784.

Harkins SW, Davis MD, Bush FM, Kasberger J. Suppression of first pain and slow temporal summation of second pain in relation to age. *J Gerontol* 1996; 51A:M260–M265.

Helme RD, McKernan S. Neurogenic flare responses following topical application of capsaicin in humans. *Ann Neurol* 1985; 18:505–509.

Helme RD, Gibson SJ. Pain in the elderly. In: Jensen TS, Turner JA, Wiesenfeld-Hallin Z (Eds). *Proceedings of the 8th World Congress on Pain*. Seattle: IASP Press, 1997, pp 919–944.

Herr KA, Mobily PR, Wallace RB, Chung Y. Leg pain in the rural Iowa 65+ population: prevalence, related factors, and association with functional status. *Clin J Pain* 1991; 7:114–121.

Hofland SL. Elder beliefs: blocks to pain management. *J Geriatr Nurs* 1992; 18:19–24.

Jensen MC, Brant-Zawadzki MN, Obuchowski N, et al. Magnetic resonance imaging of the lumbar spine in people without back pain. *N Engl J Med* 1994; 331:69–73.

Kay L, Jorgensen T, Schultz-Larsen K. Abdominal pain in a 70-year old Danish population. *J Clin Epidemiol* 1992; 45:1377–1382.

Kendig H, Helme RD, Teshuva K, et al. *Health Status of Older People Project: Data from a Survey of the Health and Lifestyles of Older Australians.* Melbourne: Victorian Health Promotion Foundation, 1996.

Lavsky-Shulan M, Wallace RB, Kohout FJ, Lemke JH, Morris MC. Prevalence and functional correlates of low back pain in the elderly: the Iowa 65+ rural health study. *J Am Geriatr Soc* 1985; 33:23–28.

Leijon G, Boivie J, Johansson I. Central post-stroke pain: neurological symptoms and pain characteristics. *Pain* 1989; 36:13–25.

Leventhal EA, Leventhal H, Schaefer P, Easterling D. Conservation of energy, uncertainty reduction, and swift utilization of medical care among the elderly. *J Gerontol* 1993; 48:P78–86.

MacDonald JB, Ballie J, Williams BO, Ballantyne D. Coronary care in the elderly. *Age Ageing* 1983; 12:17–20.

Magni G, Schifano F, De Leo D. Pain as a symptom in elderly depressed patients. *Eur Arch Psychiatr Neurol Sci* 1985; 235:143–145.

Magni G, Caldieron C, Rigatti-Luchini S, Merskey H. Chronic musculoskeletal pain and depressive symptoms in a general population. An analysis of the 1st National Health and Nutrition Examination survey data. *Pain* 1990; 43:299–307.

Magni G, Rossi MR, Rigatti-Luchini S, Merskey H. Chronic abdominal pain and depression. Epidemiological findings in the United States. Hispanic health and nutrition survey. *Pain* 1992; 49:77–85.

Magni G, Marchetti M, Moreschi C, Mersky H, Luchini SR. Chronic musculoskeletal pain and depressive symptoms in the National Health and Nutrition Examination. *Pain* 1993; 53:163–168.

Melzack R. *The Puzzle of Pain.* New York: Basic Books, 1973.

Miller PF, Sheps DS, Bragdon EE, et al. Ageing and pain perception in ischemic heart disease. *Am Heart J* 1990; 120:22–30.

Mobily PR, Herr KA, Clark MK, Wallace RB. An epidemiologic analysis of pain in the elderly: the Iowa 65+ Rural Health Study. *J Aging and Health* 1994; 6:139–154.

Moss MS, Powell-Lawton, Glicksman A. The role of pain in the last year of life of older persons. *J Gerontol* 1991; 46:P15–P57.

Muller RT, Gould LA, Betzu R, Vacek T, Pradeep V. Painless myocardial infarction in the elderly. *Am Heart J* 1990; 119:202–205.

Norman DC, Yoshikawa TT. Intraabdominal infections in the elderly. *J Am Geriatr Soc* 1983; 31:677–684.

Ochoa J, Mair WGP. The normal sural nerve in man. II. Changes in the axon and Schwann cells due to ageing. *Acta Neuropathol (Berlin)* 1969; 13:217–239.

Parkhouse N, Le Quesne PM. Quantitative objective assessment of peripheral nociceptive C fibre function. *J Neurol Neurosurg Psychiatry* 1988; 51:28–34.

Parmelee PA, Katz IR, Powell Lawton M. The relation of pain to depression among institutionalized aged. *J Gerontol* 1991; 46:P15–P21.

Parmelee PA, Smith B, Katz IR. Pain complaints and cognitive status among elderly institution residents. *J Am Geriatr Soc* 1993; 41:517–522.

Polleri A. Pain and sex steriods. *Adv Pain Res Ther* 1992; 20:253–259.

Portenoy RK, Farkash A. Practical management of non-malignant pain in the elderly. *Geriatrics* 1988; 43:29–47.

Portenoy RK, Duma C, Foley KM. Acute herpetic and postherpetic neuralgia: clinical review and current management. *Ann Neurol* 1986; 20:651–664.

Roy R, Thomas M. A survey of chronic pain in an elderly population. *Can Fam Physician* 1986; 32:513–516.

Roy R, Thomas M. Elderly persons with and without pain: a comparative study. *Clin J Pain* 1987; 3:102–106.

Ruda MA. Gender and pain. *Pain* 1993; 53:1–2.

Ryan SM, Maier SF. The estrous cycle and estrogen modulate stress-induced analgesia. *Behav Neurosci* 1988; 102:371–380.

Sengstaken EA, King SA. The problems of pain and its detection among geriatric nursing home residents. *J Am Geriatr Soc* 1993; 41:541–544.

Solomon CG, Lee TH, Cook EF, et al. Comparison of clinical presentation of acute myocardial infarction in patients older than 65 years of age to younger patients: the multicenter chest pain study experience. *Am J Cardiol* 1989; 63:772–776.

Sternbach RA. Survey of pain in the United States: the Nuprin pain report. *Clin J Pain* 1986; 2:49–53.

Stoller EP, Forster LE, Portugal S. Self care responses to symptoms by older people. *Med Care* 1993; 31:24–42.

Tibblin G, Bengtsson C, Furness B, Lapidus L. Symptoms by age and sex. *Scand J Prim Health Care* 1990; 8:9–17.

Tornstam L. Health and self-perception. A systems theoretical approach. *Gerontologist* 1975; 27:264–270.

Von Korff M, Dworkin SF, Le Resche L, Kruger A. An epidemiologic comparison of pain complaints. *Pain* 1988; 32:173–183.

Von Korff M, Dworkin SF, Le Resche L. Graded chronic pain status: an epidemiologic evaluation. *Pain* 1990; 40:279–291.

Wiesel SW, Tsourmas N, Feffer HL, Citrin CM, Patronas N. A study of computer-assisted tomography. 1. The incidence of positive CAT scans in an asymptomatic group of patients. *Spine* 1984; 9:549–551.

Correspondence to: Robert D. Helme, MBBS, PhD, FRACP, National Ageing Research Institute, PO Box 31, Parkville, Victoria 3052, Australia. Fax: 61-3-389-7148; email: r.helme@medicine.unimelb.edu.au

Epidemiology of Pain, edited by
I.K. Crombie, IASP Press, Seattle, © 1999.

9

Fibromyalgia and Chronic Widespread Pain

Gary J. Macfarlane

Arthritis Research Campaign Epidemiology Unit, School of Epidemiology and Health Services,
University of Manchester, Manchester, United Kingdom

Epidemiological research on chronic widespread pain is a relatively recent phenomenon. In a seminal paper of 1977, Smythe and Moldofsky described the cardinal symptoms and associated features and offered hypotheses about how they may be related. Since that time descriptive and analytical research in this area has grown exponentially. While there is little evidence that chronic widespread pain has become more common, there is no doubt that today it is an important source of disability among clinic patients and in the general population.

DEFINITION AND DIAGNOSTIC CRITERIA

CLASSIFICATION OF CHRONIC WIDESPREAD PAIN

Early studies on chronic widespread pain (called fibromyalgia or fibrositis when associated with additional features) were difficult to interpret and compare because different criteria were used to define this syndrome. Smythe and Moldofsky (1977) described the nature and location of tenderness in patients with the "fibrositis" syndrome, and noted that pain symptoms and generalized tenderness were often accompanied by a cycle of disturbed sleep, fatigue, and emotional distress.

Wolfe and colleagues (1985) examined three groups of patients: (1) those previously diagnosed with fibrositis, (2) those diagnosed with other rheumatic diseases, and (3) a group of normal controls. They found that while a lack of pain symptoms easily distinguished the group of normal controls, patients with fibrositis and other rheumatic conditions were best distinguished by a high level of tenderness on examination, and that no other information significantly improved the ability to differentiate between them. Subsequent criteria proposed by Yunus et al. (1989) were similarly derived by comparing a group of clinical patients diagnosed with "primary fibromyalgia syndrome" to both normal controls and subjects with other types of pain (mild rheumatoid arthritis and local fibromyalgia secondary to trauma). To satisfy the criteria, subjects were required to have had pain or stiffness at four or more anatomic sites for 3 months or longer (with bilateral involvement counting as one site), and the existence of an underlying condition must have been excluded. In addition, subjects were required to have either (1) at least two of six "historical" variables and pain on palpation at four or more specific anatomical sites (so-called "tender points") or (2) at least three of six "historical" variables and two or more "tender points." The "historical" variables were general fatigue, poor sleep, anxiety/tension, irritable bowel syndrome, and pain in seven or more areas. These criteria (with some minor modifications) were subsequently used in several population surveys, while studies based in clinics used a wide array of similar, but not identical sets of criteria.

In 1990, the American College of Rheumatology (ACR) published classification criteria for fibromyalgia (Wolfe et al. 1990) developed in a comparison study of clinic patients seen by individual rheumatologists with an interest in fibromyalgia. Each identified a group of their clinic patients diagnosed with fibromyalgia (by whatever criteria they considered appropriate), and also a comparison group of age- and sex-

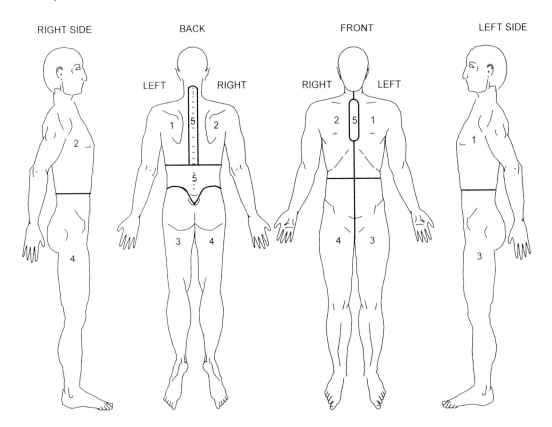

Fig. 1. Body areas used in the American College of Rheumatology definition of chronic widespread pain, as part of the classification criteria for fibromyalgia (from Wolfe et al. 1990; reprinted with permission).

matched clinic patients with other painful conditions. The subjects selected included both those with primary fibromyalgia (occurring in the absence of another rheumatic disorder) and those with secondary fibromyalgia (occurring as part of an underlying disease process such as osteoarthritis or rheumatoid arthritis) Discrimination between fibromyalgia and nonfibromyalgia patients was best achieved using two factors: the presence of chronic widespread pain and multiple "tender points." Widespread pain was considered present if a subject reported axial skeleton pain, pain in the left and right sides of the body, and pain above and below the waist. Subjects were to indicate pain on a body manikin with areas defined as in Fig. 1. To be classified with widespread pain, subjects must shade at least some parts of areas 1, 4, and 5 or areas 2, 3, and 5. Pain of at least 3 months' duration was considered chronic. The criterion for multiple "tender points" was satisfied if subjects reported pain at 11 or more of 18 specified anatomical locations when a pressure of 4 kg was applied (Fig. 2, Table I). However, despite the fact that such points are referred to as "tender points," a subject must report *pain* (not tenderness) or must flinch or withdraw when pressure is applied be-

fore the result can be recorded as positive. Overall, the proposed criteria correctly classified 85% of patients in the fibromyalgia and nonfibromyalgia groups and discriminated as least as well as any previous set of criteria. The criteria proposed by the ACR were applicable to both clinical and epidemiological studies since the required information on chronic widespread pain could be collected simply and quickly through a self-completed questionnaire and brief examination. In addition, the ACR suggested that it was not necessary to distinguish between primary and secondary fibromyalgia patients because their symptoms and physical examination findings did not differ.

The ACR criteria have been widely used in recent studies and have greatly facilitated the standardization of studies and the comparison of results from studies conducted in clinics, in the general population, and in diverse geographical locations. However, further studies have shown that these criteria do not define a distinct disease entity of fibromyalgia. Although generalized tenderness is associated with widespread pain, most people with generalized tenderness have either no pain or regional pain. Moreover, associations between generalized tenderness and some features asso-

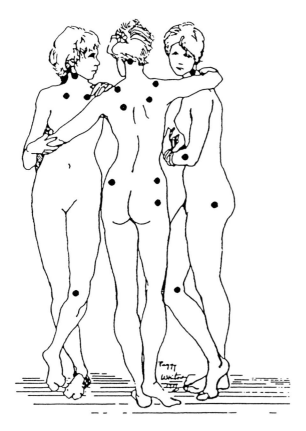

Fig. 2. Tender point locations for the American College of Rheumatology classification criteria for fibromyalgia (from Wolfe et al. 1990; reprinted with permission).

ciated with fibromyalgia such as psychological distress, fatigue, and sleep disturbance are observed independently of the extent of concomitant pain symptoms. Consequently, Macfarlane et al. (1996a) suggested a refinement of the criteria for chronic widespread pain because they believed that the individual components of fibromyalgia lacked validity when considered alone. It is possible to satisfy the ACR criteria for chronic widespread pain with, for example, pain in the lower back, right thumb, and left ankle—a combination that clearly does not represent widespread pain in the true sense. The revised "Manchester" criteria still require the presence of axial pain and contralateral limb pain. However, each limb is divided into four anatomical areas, and pain must be present in at least two areas before a limb is considered to be "painful." The modified criteria require that pain be more genuinely diffuse and have been found to be more strongly related to associated features such as tenderness, fatigue, and psychological distress. In contrast, subjects who satisfy ACR criteria for chronic widespread pain but not the modified Manchester criteria are more similar to subjects with regional pain.

EVALUATION OF TENDERNESS

Tenderness is usually assessed either by manual palpation or using a dolorimeter. The ACR criteria for fibromyalgia specify that specific anatomical locations (Fig. 2) should be examined by manual palpation with a pressure of 4 kg. This approach had greater power to discriminate between subjects with fibromyalgia and those with other rheumatic pain than did attempts to determine pain threshold levels by dolorimeter. However, there is still considerable scope for variation in conducting the examination—such as in the precise determination of examination sites, the position of the subject, and the rate of force applied—and in the recording of results. Okifugi and colleagues (1997) recently proposed a standard for the recording of pain, although it is more appropriate for clinical settings than for population studies that may involve examination in the subjects' homes. Based on their analysis of results in groups of patients with fibromyalgia and chronic headache, the authors propose that rather than recording each examination site as painful or not painful, researchers should score pain on a continuous scale. This may be particularly useful when considering the natural history of symptoms or response to treatment, where the level of tenderness may improve but not completely resolve. Examination of tender points according to a specified protocol has moderate to high levels of both test/retest stability and interobserver agreement (Jacobs et al. 1995; Tunks et al. 1995).

Instead of the manual palpation techniques, some studies evaluate tenderness by using a dolorimeter to measure the amount of force at which subjects report pain. This technique also lacks a standard of assessment, and at least two variables, the dolorimeter surface area and rate of force application, can substantially influence results (Smythe et al. 1992a,b; White et al. 1993).

PREVALENCE

Although most research in the broad area of widespread pain has focused on fibromyalgia, there is little evidence that this combination of symptoms and signs comprises a distinct entity (Croft et al. 1994). Tender points appear to be a general measure of distress, with fibromyalgia at one extreme of a continuous spectrum of distress and pain (Croft et al. 1996; Wolfe 1997).

Table I
Studies estimating the prevalence of chronic widespread pain/fibromyalgia

Study type	Disease Definition	Source of Sample	Sample Size	Duration of Symptoms	Prevalence (%)	Reference
Clinical						
Cross-sectional	Primary fibromyalgia (not precisely specified)	Rheumatology clinic	285	—	20	Yunus et al. 1981
Cross-sectional	7 tender points and diffuse musculoskeletal aching in 3 areas	Rheumatology clinic (private)	1473	≥3 mo§	primary 3.7 secondary 11 overall 15	Wolfe and Cathey 1983
Cross-sectional	Questionnaire and physical exam	Medical clinics	596	1.5–24 y mean 7.6 y	5.7	Campbell et al. 1983
Prospective	Multiple tender points, diffuse musculoskeletal aching and skin fold tenderness	Rheumatology clinic	280	Mean 13 y	13.6	Wolfe et al. 1984
Cross-sectional	Unexplained chronic diffuse muscular aching	Family practice clinic	692	≥3 mo	2.1	Hartz and Kirchdoefer 1987
Cross-sectional	Spontaneous pain, multiple tender points, psychological changes	Hospital	11500	—	7.5	Muller 1987
Cross-sectional	7 tender points, diffuse musculoskeletal aching	Rheumatology clinic	2781	≥3 mo§	4.6	Greenfield et al. 1992
Cross-sectional	ACR	SLE clinic (public)	102	≥3 mo§	22.0	Middleton et al. 1994
Prospective	Score of 6 on 10-point pain scale and 11 of 18 tender points	Spine clinic	125	—	primary 4.8 secondary 7.2 overall 12.0	Borenstein 1995
Population						
Cross-sectional	Yunus	Population	876	≥6 wk§	1.0	Jacobsson et al. 1989
Cross-sectional	Yunus	Population	7217	≥3 mo§	0.75	Mäkelä and Heliövaara 1991
Cross-sectional	ACR	School	338	≥3 mo§	6.2	Buskila et al. 1993‡
Cross-sectional	ACR	Population	2038	≥3 mo§	10.5	Forseth and Gran 1992†
Cross-sectional	ACR	Population	1219	≥3 mo§	0.66	Prescott et al. 1993
Cross-sectional	ACR	Population	1340	≥3 mo§	11.2	Croft et al. 1993*
Cross-sectional	ACR	Population	3006	≥3 mo§	10.6*/2.0	Wolfe et al. 1995
Cross-sectional	Chronic pain with multiple localization	Population	1609	≥3 mo§	10.7	Andersson et al. 1996*

Abbreviations: ACR = American College of Rheumatology; SLE = systemic lupus erythematosus.
* Chronic widespread pain. † Women only. ‡ Children only. § Defined duration of chronic widespread pain.

This chapter will review the descriptive epidemiology of chronic widespread pain, where such information is available, and then discuss the epidemiology of fibromyalgia.

The variety of definitions used to study widespread pain and tenderness hampers the direct comparison of measures of occurrence between studies. Studies that have estimated the prevalence of such symptoms are listed in Table I (general population studies) and Table II (general, rheumatology, or other specialist clinic studies) with details of the disease definitions used.

CHRONIC WIDESPREAD PAIN

Two large studies have examined the descriptive epidemiology of chronic widespread pain in the general population. The first, in the United States, involved a random sample of 3006 adult subjects in the community (a participation rate of approximately 75%) who completed a mailed questionnaire (Wolfe et al. 1995).

Overall, the prevalence of chronic widespread pain according to the ACR criteria was 10.6% (95% CI = 9.5–11.7%). Prevalence was higher in women than men at all ages. The pattern of age-specific prevalence rates in adults was broadly similar in both sexes, however, increasing with age and reaching a peak between 60 and 69 years in 23% of men and 13% of women, and thereafter declining (see Fig. 7b in Chapter 5). Croft et al. (1993) conducted a similar mailed questionnaire survey in the United Kingdom involving 1340 subjects (75% participation rate) registered with two general practices. The crude prevalence of chronic widespread pain in this population was 13%, with higher rates in women (16%) than men (9%). Applying age- and sex-specific rates derived from the study population to the adult population of England and Wales produced an estimated national prevalence of 11%. In women, the prevalence of chronic widespread pain was around 10% below the age of 45, while at older ages the prevalence was slightly higher than 20%. In men the prevalence was between 5% and 10% up to age 55 and between 65 and 74 years, with a higher prevalence (15–20%) noted between the ages of 55–64 and over 74 years. The findings that around 1 of 10 subjects from these populations have chronic widespread pain is broadly in line with other population studies. For example, Crook and colleagues (1984) reported a prevalence of 11% for persistent pain (defined as "often troubled by pain") in Canada, and the first American National Health and Nutrition Examination Survey in the United States reported a prevalence of 14% for chronic pain in the back, hip, knee, or other joints (Magni et al. 1990).

In summary, these studies clearly show that chronic widespread pain occurs more commonly among women, and that it is generally more prevalent at older ages, although the precise relationship of age to the prevalence of chronic widespread pain has not been consistently defined.

FIBROMYALGIA

Several population studies have been conducted using the ACR criteria for fibromyalgia. In the study by Wolfe et al. (1995) discussed in the previous section, subjects were classified as to whether they had chronic widespread pain according to responses on the mailed questionnaire, and were then examined for tenderness. The overall prevalence of fibromyalgia was 2% (95% CI = 1.4–2.7%). In women, rates rose from

1% in those aged 18–29 years to 7% at age 70–79 years, with a small decrease in the oldest age group. In men, rates increased very slightly with age, reaching a peak of only 1% among 70–79-year-olds (see Fig. 7c in Chapter 5). Divorced subjects were significantly more likely to have fibromyalgia than were married persons (odds ratio [OR] = 4.3 (95% CI = 1.03–18), and the risk increased as levels of education and income declined. The risk of fibromyalgia was similar among Caucasians and non-Caucasians. Buskila and colleagues (1993) conducted a survey involving 338 healthy schoolchildren aged 9–15 years in Israel, and found a high prevalence of fibromyalgia (6.2%) in this age group, with the prevalence in girls (8.8%) more than double that in boys (3.9%). Mäkelä and Heliövaara (1991), in an early study from Finland, used the criteria of Yunus et al. (1989), which requires widespread pain in addition to specific combinations of characteristic symptoms and tender points, to determine the prevalence and determinants of fibromyalgia in a community study of more than 7000 adults aged over 30 years. The overall prevalence was 0.8% (females 1%; males 0.5%). Prevalence increased from 0.1% at age 30–44 years to a peak prevalence of 1.4% at 55–64 years. Those who did not complete elementary-level education had a considerably higher prevalence (2.8%) in comparison to those with elementary (0.7%) or secondary education (0.2%).

Prevalence estimates of fibromyalgia derived from clinic populations are more difficult to interpret. By definition, they are concerned with persons who have sought consultation for these or related symptoms, and will be highly influenced by the type of clinic population considered and the definition of fibromyalgia used. For example, published prevalence estimates in clinical studies range from 5.7% in a U.S. study based within medical clinics (excluding rheumatology) that defined "fibrositis" based on answers to a 15-item questionnaire (Campbell et al. 1983), to 22% among patients attending a systemic lupus erythematosus (SLE) clinic who were diagnosed according to ACR criteria (Middleton et al. 1994). Within a private general rheumatology clinic, Wolfe and Cathey (1995) reported the prevalence of "fibrositis" (seven or more tender points and diffuse aching in at least three areas for 3 months) at 4% in patients with no other clinically discernible significant disease; rates were more than three times higher among patients diagnosed as having rheumatoid arthritis, osteoarthritis, or symptoms of neck or back pain. Within a population of pa-

Table II
Factors associated with chronic widespread pain/fibromyalgia

Study Type	Risk Factor	Strength and Type of Association	Reference
Cross-sectional	Smoking	—	Vaeroy et al. 1988
Cross-sectional and mixed longitudinal	Psychological stress	Predictive	Leino 1989
Cross-sectional	Sex Age Occupation Education level Physical stress level	F > M (1.0% vs. 0.5%) Peak prevalence at ages 55–64 y Highest prevalence in "never employed" Inverse association Direct association	Mäkelä and Heliövaara 1991
Cross-sectional	Physical trauma, surgery, or medical illness	Present in 23% of fibromyalgia patients	Greenfield et al. 1992
Cross-sectional	Sex Age Difficulty coping with problems Poor sleep Depression Somatic symptoms	F > M (16% vs. 9%) Direct association OR = 2.9 (CI = 2.0–4.4) OR = 2.1 (CI = 1.4–3.1) OR = 1.9 (CI = 1.3–2.8) OR = 2–5 for specific somatic symptoms	Croft et al. 1993*
Cross-sectional	Sex Age Education Somatization Depression, past or present Depression, family history	F > M (2–6-fold depending on age) Direct association. Inverse association OR = 10 (CI = 2.6–4.1) OR = 4.2 (CI = 1.9–9.5) OR = 2.2 (CI = 1.1–4.6)	Wolfe et al. 1995
Cross-sectional	Sexual abuse	History of sexual abuse in 65% of fibromyalgia patients and 52% of controls	Taylor et al. 1995
Cross-sectional	Sexual and physical abuse	No significant difference in history of abuse between fibromyalgia and other rheumatic disease patients	Boisset-Pioro et al. 1995
Cross-sectional	No. lifetime psychiatric disorders	Direct association only in consulting subjects	Aaron et al. 1996
Prospective	Negative major life events	Associated with increased pain and disturbed sleep at 4.5 y follow-up	Wigers 1996

* Studies of chronic widespread pain.

tients with rheumatoid arthritis (RA), those with fibromyalgia (according to the previous criteria plus skinfold tenderness) were more likely to be women and married, but there was no difference according to level of income, education employment status, or RA-specific measures (Wolfe et al. 1984).

Little information exists to describe the epidemiology of tenderness (specifically a high tender point count) in the general population. Wolfe and Cathey (1985) examined 1520 consecutive patients with a variety of rheumatic diseases for tenderness at 14 anatomical locations previously described by Smythe (1985). Tender points were present in 40% of patients: 23% had 4 or more, 14% had 7 or more, and 4% had at least 12 tender points. Women had more tender points than did men, as did Caucasians in comparison to blacks and persons of Hispanic origin. The number of tender points generally increased with age, and was also correlated with neck or low back pain, anxiety levels, disability, fatigue, and disturbed sleep. However, the sites of tenderness in patients with rheumatic disease did not generally correspond to the site of joint pathology.

In summary, despite differing criteria and different designs and population settings, the studies discussed above do provide some consistent information about the descriptive epidemiology of fibromyalgia in the community. Prevalence increases with age until about the sixth decade, and thereafter decreases slightly. Fibromyalgia is considerably more common in women than men and tends to be more prevalent in persons of low education. Clinic studies have shown that it is particularly common among certain clinic populations and generally shows an even greater female/male ratio than that observed in the general population.

CONSEQUENCES OF CHRONIC WIDESPREAD PAIN

COSTS FOR HEALTH CARE SYSTEMS

Although chronic widespread pain and fibromyalgia are common, there is little information on the associated health care costs. In a community survey in the United Kingdom, 75% of subjects satisfying ACR criteria for chronic widespread pain had previously consulted their general practitioner with symptoms, which suggests a potentially large burden to the health care system (Macfarlane et al. 1999). In the United States, Cathey et al. (1986) compared health care utilization in a group of 81 patients with (primary) fibromyalgia and a group of age- and sex-matched community controls. Fibromyalgia patients recorded a higher average number of physician visits (3.5) in comparison to controls (2.2), and more visits to other health care professionals (fibromyalgia patients, 5.6; controls, 0.4). Medication usage was slightly higher (mean number of medications: fibromyalgia patients, 4.7; controls, 3.8), with 98% of fibromyalgia patients using some form of medication. Nonsteroidal anti-inflammatory drugs (NSAIDs), analgesics, and muscle relaxants were the most common medications taken. While very high hospitalization rates were noted among fibromyalgia patients, they were confined to the year prior to diagnosis and fell sharply thereafter. Simms et al. (1995) estimated the cost of treating a patient with fibromyalgia for 1 year at 1991 prices. Most of the costs related to medication (~$700), with lower costs for consultation visits (~$200), imaging, and laboratory investigations (both <$100). Total costs were only slightly lower than those for patients with osteoarthritis and rheumatoid arthritis.

COSTS TO THE PATIENT

The cost of fibromyalgia involves not only direct health care costs, but also indirect costs to the patient in terms of disability (including inability to work or carry out daily tasks). Wolfe et al. (1995), using the Health Assessment Questionnaire (HAQ) Disability Index (on a scale of 0–3), reported mean scores of 1.0 and 1.3 in community and clinic fibromyalgia subjects, respectively, and a mean score in clinic patients of 1.1 over a 12-month period (Hawley et al. 1988); these scores are consistent with a mild functional loss. Fibromyalgia patients were much more likely than normal controls to consider their health to be "poor" and to be "very dissatisfied" with their state of health. A further study by the same authors of 81 patients with fibromyalgia suggested, however, that the syndrome's impact on work was relatively modest. Subjects reported a higher number of working hours (40 hours) than the United States average (35 hours); more than half had not reported any lost working days, and the mean number of days lost in the previous working year (9 days) was heavily skewed by a few patients with work loss of greater than 30 days (Cathey et al. 1986)

A specific instrument to measure the effect of fibromyalgia on patients' lives—the Fibromyalgia Impact Questionnaire (FIQ)—was developed by Buckhardt et al. (1991). This instrument includes items on physical, psychological, social, and global well-being. The section on physical activities requires subjects to record whether they were able to carry out each of a list of activities "Always," "Most times," "Occasionally," or "Never," and the physical activities listed include "Walk several blocks," "Make beds," "Vacuum a rug," and "Do Shopping." The questionnaire includes items on the impact of symptoms on the ability to work and an assessment of the number of work days lost because of symptoms. Among the initial 89 clinic patients used to validate the FIQ, scores on a scale of 0–10 for interference with work (4.1), for impeding physical functioning (3.2), and for loss of work days (0.8) implied that symptoms did have a significant effect on everyday life., A recent study from Brazil, using the FIQ, suggested that in the clinic setting, FIQ scores were higher for fibromyalgia patients than for those with rheumatoid arthritis (Martinez et al. 1995).

NATURAL HISTORY

Although population studies have shown that chronic widespread pain is common, relatively little information is available on the natural history of symptoms. Studies of clinic patients have generally suggested that it is a difficult condition to treat and that symptoms rarely resolve. For example, in a study from the United Kingdom of 84 patients diagnosed with (primary) fibromyalgia, 72 patients were followed up for a mean of 4 years. Seventy patients (97%) still had symptoms consistent with fibromyalgia, while 61 (85%) continued to satisfy the criteria used for diagnosis (Ledingham et al. 1993). In the United States, Hawley and colleagues (1988) found that the severity of symptoms and level of pain were remarkably stable in 75 patients with fibromyalgia over 1 year, while Felson and Goldenberg (1986) found that 60% of patients had moderate or severe symptoms throughout a 2-year follow-up period. Clinic studies, often conducted within specialist referral centers, inevitably include patients with more severe and persistent symptoms and therefore may not accurately reflect the natural history of symptoms among all subjects.

The only reported prospective study of chronic widespread pain in the community found a rather more favorable outcome than was suggested by clinic studies. A group of 141 subjects who completed a mailed questionnaire and were examined for tenderness by a research nurse were reevaluated approximately 2 years later. Only 35% of the original group still satisfied the criteria for chronic widespread pain. Those with additional symptoms and signs such as a high number of tender points, a high score on the General Health Questionnaire (a measure of psychological distress; Goldberg and Williams 1988), high levels of fatigue, or sleep problems were least likely to have symptom improvement (Macfarlane et al. 1996b). This high rate of improvement may indicate that chronic widespread pain in the community has a better prognosis in comparison to that of clinic patients, whose symptoms were usually more severe. Alternatively, subjects may have experienced intermittent symptoms and simply failed to meet the criteria around the time of the follow-up survey, or perhaps the ACR criteria for widespread pain used in the study were too loose to define a group of patients with truly widespread pain. Further community studies are needed to provide more information on the natural history of symptoms.

RISK FACTORS AND HIGH-RISK GROUPS

Etiological factors relative to chronic widespread pain or fibromyalgia have been evaluated primarily through cross-sectional studies involving clinic patients or the general population. These studies consider factors that are *associated* with chronic widespread pain symptoms, rather than, necessarily, etiological

factors. Subjects with chronic widespread pain commonly report a variety of other symptoms such as high levels of fatigue, sleep disturbance, psychological distress (in particular anxiety and depression), and somatic symptoms such as numbness, paraesthesia, and disorders of bowel function (Mäkelä and Heliövaara 1991; Croft et al. 1993; Wolfe et al. 1995). However, the temporal relationship between such potential "exposures" and symptom onset cannot normally be determined. For example, it could be hypothesized either that adverse psychological factors, through a process of somatization, result in the subsequent onset of pain symptoms, or alternatively, that adverse psychological factors such as depression are a consequence of the chronic pain experience.

The relationship between depression and chronic pain has been examined in one major prospective study, the National Health and Nutrition Examination Survey (NHANES I) in the United States (Magni et al. 1994). Chronic pain was defined as pain occurring for most days in at least one of the past 12 months. There was no requirement for the pain to be widespread. Among those who were pain free at the initial survey, depressive symptoms (assessed using the Centre for Epidemiologic Studies Depression Scale; Radloff 1977) predicted chronic musculoskeletal pain at follow-up approximately 8 years later (OR = 2.1). Conversely however, among subjects without depression at baseline, chronic pain was the most powerful predictor of its onset (OR = 2.9). This study provides evidence not only that depression may be an etiological factor in the onset of chronic pain, but also that the reverse relationship holds (Magni et al. 1994).

Retrospective studies have also investigated the relationship between psychological disturbance and chronic widespread pain. In their assessment of lifetime rates of psychiatric diagnoses, Hudson et al. (1992) found higher rates in clinic patients with fibromyalgia compared to those with rheumatoid arthritis (64% vs. 22% for major mood disorders), and noted that in most cases psychiatric symptoms predated the onset of pain. Similarly, Aaron et al. (1996) found higher rates of lifetime psychiatric diagnoses when comparing subjects with fibromyalgia (both clinic patients and community volunteers) in comparison to healthy community volunteers. However, this study reported that higher rates of lifetime psychiatric disorders were confined to subjects with fibromyalgia who had sought treatment for symptoms, and the authors suggested that the association of fibromyalgia with psychological factors may in part be due to the influences associated with seeking treatment.

Finally, recent studies have investigated the relationship between a history of abuse and the onset of fibromyalgia symptoms. In general, physical and sexual abuse has been reported to be more common in subjects with fibromyalgia in comparison to control groups (Boisset-Pioro et al. 1995; Taylor et al. 1995). However, the differences observed have been small in magnitude and the studies have involved relatively few subjects, with unsatisfactory control groups or low participation rates. Given the inherent difficulties in collecting this sort of information retrospectively from symptomatic and nonsymptomatic subjects, the results to date could only be considered as "hypothesis-generating" rather than indicative of any link between abuse and later symptoms.

Smythe and Moldofsky (1977) discussed the association of sleep disturbance in relation to "fibrositis" in an early paper and provided preliminary evidence from experimental studies that disturbance of sleep itself increased the likelihood of subsequently reporting pain symptoms. Seven university students were studied first during a period of undisturbed sleep and later during a period when sleep was interrupted. The experience of disturbance in non–rapid eye movement (REM) sleep deprivation was followed by a significant increase in tenderness as assessed by dolorimeter, and in fatigue and sluggishness. The symptoms disappeared with subsequent uninterrupted sleep, and did not recur with further deprivation of REM sleep.

Overall, the ability to define risk factors for chronic widespread pain is limited, based on current information. However, the data suggest that female sex, older age (particularly above 50 years), and lower educational level predispose to widespread pain symptoms, while psychological distress and sleep disturbance may also increase the likelihood of future symptoms.

SCOPE FOR PREVENTION

Epidemiological studies have concentrated principally on measuring the prevalence of chronic widespread pain and on determining features associated with the symptoms. These studies have shown that in the population, approximately 13% of adults report chronic widespread pain during any given month. This figure remains relatively constant when subjects are followed over time, although there may be two subgroups, one whose symptoms persist and are chronic, and the other whose symptoms are intermittent. In the former group, pain is associated with other psychological and physical symptoms. It is still unclear whether adverse psychological factors are simply a consequence of chronic pain symptoms or are important etiological factors. This important question must be resolved if we are to understand why some persons experience these chronic, disabling symptoms, which in turn may help us to alleviate their symptoms.

To determine the etiology of symptoms, studies must collect information on potential etiological factors among pain-free subjects from unselected populations and then follow them to determine the future occurrence of widespread pain. Such prospective studies are necessarily long-term and require considerable effort to ensure high participation rates during follow-up. Such studies are already under way, and the results of initially short-term follow-up are eagerly awaited. Even prospective, population studies conducted on adults may have difficulty determining true etiological factors for pain if the relevant factors were present in childhood and if most subjects have previously experienced (or are experiencing) chronic pain episodes. In addition, determining the relationship between chronic pain and other somatic symptoms will be important since the available evidence indicates that their occurrences may have much in common.

Only when such information on the etiology of chronic pain is available will we have a strong scientific basis on which to propose and evaluate intervention studies, with the ultimate aim of reducing the burden of chronic pain for both new episodes and persistent symptoms.

ACKNOWLEDGMENTS

The author thanks colleagues Alan Silman, Ann Papageorgiou, and Isabelle Hunt from the Arthritis Research Campaign Epidemiology Unit at the University of Manchester and Peter Croft at the University of Keele, with whom he has collaborated on studies of widespread pain. Particular thanks are due to John McBeth from the ARC Epidemiology Unit, who provided assistance with tables and references, and to Lesley Jordan for her help with the preparation of the manuscript.

REFERENCES

Aaron LA, Bradley LA, Alarcon GS, et al. Psychiatric diagnoses in patients with fibromyalgia are related to health care-seeking behaviour rather than to illness. *Arthritis Rheum* 1996; 39(3):436–445.

Andersson HI, Ejlertsson E, Leden I, Rosenberg C. Characteristics of subjects with chronic pain, in relation to local and widespread pain report. Scand J Rheumatol 1996; 25:146–154.

Boisset-Pioro MH, Esdaile JM, Fitzcharles M-A. Sexual and physical abuse in women with fibromyalgia syndrome. *Arthritis Rheum* 1995; 38(2):235–241.

Borenstein D. Prevalence and treatment outcome of primary and secondary fibromyalgia in patients with spinal pain. *Spine* 1995; 20:796–800.

Buckhardt CS, Clark SR, Bennett RM. The fibromyalgia impact questionnaire: development and validation. *J Rheumatol* 1991; 18:728–733.

Buskila D, Press J, Gedalia A, et al. Assessment of non articular tenderness and prevalence of fibromyalgia in children. *J Rheumatol* 1993; 20:368–370.

Campbell SM, Clark S, Tindall EA, Forehand ME, Bennett RM. Clinical characteristics of fibrositis. I: A "blinded" controlled study of symptoms and tender points. *Arthritis Rheum* 1983; 26:817–824.

Cathey MA, Wolfe F, Kleinheksel SM, Hawley DJ. Socioeconomic impact of fibrositis: a study of 81 patients with primary fibrositis. *Am J Med* 1986; 81:78–84.

Croft PR, Rigby AS, Boswell R, Schollum J, Silman AJ. Prevalence of chronic widespread pain in the general population. *J Rheumatol* 1993; 20:710–713.

Croft PR, Schollum J, Silman AJ. Population study of tender point counts and pain as evidence of fibromyalgia. *BMJ* 1994; 309:696–699.

Croft PR, Burt J, Schollum J, et al. More pain, more tender points: is fibromyalgia just one end of a continuous spectrum? *Ann Rheum Dis* 1996; 55:482–485.

Crook J, Rideout E, Browne G. The prevalence of pain complaints in a general population. *Pain* 1984; 18:299–314.

Felson D, Goldenberg DL. The natural history of fibromyalgia. *Arthritis Rheum* 1986; 29:1522–1526.

Forseth KO, Gran JT. The prevalence of fibromyalgia among women aged 20–49 years in Arendal, Norway. *Scand J Rheumatol* 1992; 21:74–78.

Goldberg D, Williams P. *A User's Guide to the General Health Questionnaire.* Windsor: FEFR-Nelso, 1988.

Greenfield S, Fitzcharles M-A, Esdaile JM. Reactive fibromyalgia syndrome. *Arthritis Rheum* 1992; 35:678–681.

Hartz A, Kirchdoefer E. Undetected fibrositis in primary care practice. *J Fam Pract* 1987; 25:365–369.

Hawley DJ, Wolfe F, Cathey MA. Pain, functional disability, and psychological status: a 12-month study of severity in fibromyalgia. *J Rheumatol* 1988; 15:1551–1556.

Hudson JI, Goldenberg DL, Pope HG, Keck PE, Schlesinger L. Comorbidity of fibromyalgia with medical and psychiatric disorders. *Am J Med* 1992; 92:363–367.

Jacobs JWG, Greenan R, Van Der Heide A, Rasker JJ, Bijlsma JWJ. Are tender point scores assessed by manual palpation in fibromyalgia reliable. *Scand J Rheumatol* 1995; 24:243–247.

Jacobsson L, Lindegarde F, Manthorpe R. The commonest rheumatic complaints of over six weeks' duration in a twelve month period in a defined Swedish population. *Scand J Rheumatol* 1989; 18:353–360.

Ledingham J, Doherty S, Doherty M. Primary fibromyalgia syndrome: an outcome study. *Br J Rheumatol* 1993; 32:139–142.

Leino P. Symptoms of stress predict musculoskeletal disorders. *J Epidemiol Community Health* 1989; 43:293–300.

Macfarlane GJ, Croft PR, Schollum J, Silman AJ. Widespread pain: is an improved classification possible? *J Rheumatol* 1996a; 23:1628–1632.

Macfarlane GJ, Thomas E, Papageorgiou AC, et al. Natural history of chronic pain in the community: a better prognosis than in the clinic? *J Rheumatol* 1996b; 23:1617–1620.

Macfarlane GJ, Hunt IM, McBeth J, Papageorgiou AC, Silman AJ. Chronic widespread pain in the community: influences on healthcare seeking behaviour. *J Rheumatol* 1999; 26:413–419.

Magni G, Caldieron C, Rigatti-Luchini S, Merskey H. Chronic musculoskeletal pain and depressive symptoms in the general population. An analysis of the 1st National Health and Nutrition Examination Survey Data. *Pain* 1990; 43:299–307.

Magni G, Moreschi C, Rigatti-Luchini S, Merskey H. Prospective study on the relationship between depressive symptoms and chronic musculoskeletal pain. *Pain* 1994; 56:289–297.

Mäkelä M, Heliövaara M. Prevalence of primary fibromyalgia in the Finnish population. *BMJ* 1991; 303:216–219.

Martinez JE, Ferraz MB, Sato EI, Atra E. Fibromyalgia versus rheumatoid arthritis: a longitudinal comparison of the quality of life. *J Rheumatol* 1995; 22:270–274.

Middleton GD, McFarlin JE, Lipsky PE. The prevalence and clinical impact of fibromyalgia in systemic lupus erythematosus. *Arthritis Rheum* 1994; 8:1181–1188.

Muller W. The fibrositis syndrome: diagnosis, differential diagnosis and pathogenesis. *Scand J Rheumatol Suppl* 1987; 65:40–53.

Okifugi A, Turk DC, Sinclair JD, Starz TW, Marcus DA. A standardised manual tender point survey. I. Development and determination of a threshold point for the identification of positive tender points in fibromyalgia syndrome. *J Rheumatol* 1997; 24:377–383.

Prescott E, Kjoller M, Jacobson S, et al. Fibromyalgia in the adult Danish population: I. Prevalence study. *Scand J Rheumatol* 1993; 22:233–237.

Radloff L. The CES-D scale: a self-report depression scale for research in the general population. *J Appl Psychol Meas* 1977; 1:385–401.

Simms RW, Cahill L, Prashker M, Meenan RF. The direct costs of fibromyalgia treatment: comparison with rheumatoid arthritis and osteoarthritis. *J Musculoskeletal Pain* 1995; 3:127–132.

Smythe HA. Fibrositis and other diffuse musculoskeletal syndromes. In: Kelley WN, Harris ED Jr, Russy S, et al. (Eds). *Textbook of Rheumatology.* Philadelphia: WB Saunders, 1985, pp 481–489.

Smythe HA, Moldofsky H. Two contributions to understanding of the "fibrositis" syndrome. *Bull Rheum Dis* 1977; 28:928–931.

Smythe HA, Gladman A, Dagenais P, Kraishi M, Blake R. Relation between fibrositic and control site tenderness; effects of dolorimeter scale length and footplate size. *J Rheumatol* 1992a; 19:284–289.

Smythe HA, Buskila D, Urowitz S, Langevitz P. Control and "fibrositic" tenderness: comparison of two dolorimeters. *J Rheumatol* 1992b; 19:768–771.

Taylor ML, Trotter DR, Csuka ME. The prevalence of sexual abuse in women with fibromyalgia. *Arthritis Rheum* 1995; 2:229–234.

Tunks E, McCain GA, Hart LE, et al. The reliability of examination for tenderness in patients with myofascial pain, chronic fibromyalgia and controls. *J Rheumatol* 1995; 22:944–952.

Vaeroy H, Helle R, Forre O, Kass E, Terenius L. Elevated CSF levels of substance P and high incidence of Raynaud phenomenon in patients with fibromyalgia: new features for diagnosis. *Pain* 1988; 32:21–26.

White KP, McCain GA, Tunks E. The effects of changing the painful stimulus upon dolorimetry scores in patients with fibromyalgia. *J Musculoskeletal Pain* 1993; 1:43–58.

Wigers SH. Fibromyalgia outcome: the predictive values of symptom duration, physical activity, disability pension, and critical life events: a 4.5 year prospective study. *J Psychosom Res* 1996; 41:235–243.

Wolfe F. The relation between tender points and fibromyalgia symptom variables: evidence that fibromyalgia is not a discrete disorder in the clinic. *Ann Rheum Dis* 1997; 56:268–271.

Wolfe F, Cathey MA. Prevalence of primary and secondary fibrositis. *J Rheumatol* 1983; 10:965–968.

Wolfe F, Cathey MA. The epidemiology of tender points: a prospective study of 1520 patients. *J Rheumatol* 1985; 12:1164–1168.

Wolfe F, Cathey MA, Kelinheksel SM. Fibrositis (fibromyalgia) in rheumatoid arthritis. *J Rheumatol* 1984; 11:814–818.

Wolfe F, Hawley DJ, Cathey MA, Caro X, Russell IJ. Fibrositis: symptom frequency and criteria for diagnosis. *J Rheumatol* 1985; 12:1159–1163.

Wolfe F, Smythe HA, Yunus MB, et al. The American College of Rheumatology 1990 criteria for the classification of fibromyalgia: report of the multicenter criteria committee. *Arthritis Rheum* 1990; 33:160–172.

Wolfe F, Ross K, Anderson J, Russell IJ, Hebert L. The prevalence and characteristics of fibromyalgia in the general population. *Arthritis Rheum* 1995; 38:19–28.

Yunus MB, Masi AT, Calabro JJ, Miller KA, Feigenbaum SL. Primary fibromyalgia fibrositis: Clinical study of 50 patients with matched normal controls. *Semin Arthritis Rheum* 1981; 11:151–171.

Yunus MB, Masi AT, Aldag JC. Preliminary criteria for primary fibromyalgia syndrome (PFS): multivariate analysis of a consecutive series of PFS, other pain patients and normal subjects. *Clin Exp Rheumatol* 1989; 7:63–69.

Correspondence to: Gary J. Macfarlane, PhD, Arthritis Research Campaign, Epidemiology Unit, School of Epidemiology and Health Services, University of Manchester, Stopford Building, Oxford Road, Manchester M13 9PT, United Kingdom. Fax: 44-161-275-5043.

Epidemiology of Pain, edited by
I.K. Crombie, IASP Press, Seattle, © 1999.

10

Chronic Postsurgical Pain

William Andrew Macrae[a] and Huw Talfryn Oakley Davies[b]

[a]Department of Anaesthesia, University of Dundee, Ninewells Hospital and Medical School, Dundee, United Kingdom; and [b]Department of Management, University of St Andrews, St Katharine's West, The Scores, St Andrews, Fife, United Kingdom

In some patients, postsurgical pain persists long after natural healing processes should have been completed. Some operations, such as thoracotomy, breast surgery, hernia repair, and amputation, are well known to cause chronic pain problems, and several research studies have been published in each of these areas. However, chronic postsurgical pain (CPSP) in general is neglected as an area of study; for many relatively common surgical procedures the literature is sparse, and for many others the problem appears to have been ignored altogether.

One reason for the neglect of CPSP may be the wide variety of surgical procedures that can cause long-term problems. A further difficulty lies in the range and diversity of pain syndromes that can follow surgery. Patients complain of differing symptoms, sometimes using specific descriptors that may lead the clinician to infer a cause. For example, descriptors such as burning, tingling, or shooting usually imply that nerve injury is the cause. The finding of specific sensory changes such as anesthesia, allodynia (pain from a stimulus that is not normally painful, e.g., cotton wool), or hyperalgesia (more pain than you would expect from a painful stimulus, e.g., a pinprick) would tend to confirm the diagnosis. In other cases, the symptoms and signs that the patient brings to the doctor are vague and ill defined, and the pathophysiology remains obscure.

The diversity of surgical procedures that can lead to pain and the multitude of pain syndromes reported have led in turn to a disparate, scattered, and incoherent literature on CPSP. This chapter seeks to further our understanding of CPSP by reviewing studies that have attempted to document the size and scope of the problem. Our objectives are three-fold: (1) to assess the extent and severity of CPSP after a range of common surgical operations; (2) to highlight the organizational and attitudinal changes needed to foster a better recognition of the problem and its prevention and management; and (3) to identify the key research issues that will help us to better understand this complex phenomenon and open up new avenues in prevention and treatment. This chapter is not concerned with investigating the underlying pathophysiological mechanisms of the different CPSP syndromes; much work remains to be done in that area.

DEFINING THE PROBLEM

CHRONICITY

The first obstacle to be overcome in defining CPSP is the need to distinguish a chronic pain problem from the "normal" acute pain associated with the surgical insult. It is hard to give fixed times for when acute postoperative pain ends and chronic postsurgical pain starts. Postsurgical pain comes in many guises: sometimes it is transient and at other times it is enduring or even permanent; sometimes its onset is immediate and at other times it develops slowly or after some delay. Nascent CPSP may be present when the patient recovers from the anesthetic (perhaps masked by the expected acute pain), or it may take some time to become apparent. For example, immediately after the operation, the patient may have both postoperative pain and nerve injury pain, but the "normal" postoperative pain will usually resolve over the first 2–10 days, leaving persistent nerve injury pain.

Researchers have never agreed how long patients must suffer from postsurgical pain before it can be termed "chronic." In general, chronic pain has been described variously, and somewhat loosely, as pain lasting over 3 (or sometimes 6) months, as pain that is unlikely to resolve, or as pain lasting longer than the usual healing time (Sternbach 1984; Merskey and Bogduk 1994; Working Group of the National Medical Advisory Committee 1994). However, as understanding of the pathophysiology of pain has advanced, a sharp distinction between acute and chronic pain has become less helpful; a cascade of changes can be initiated by injury or surgery, some short-term and self-limiting, and others long-term and seemingly irreversible (Wall 1987; Woolf and Walters 1991; Coderre et al. 1993).

While CPSP clearly has no defined point of onset, some common definition of duration is helpful to describe the epidemiology of CPSP. Many studies of pain following specific surgical procedures have suggested a time frame of 2 or 3 months. It would seem reasonable to use 2 months in a common definition, as this is well past the point when acute postoperative pain would be expected to have resolved, and pain that is present at 2 months seldom resolves over the next month.

PRE-EXISTING PAIN

A further problem in defining postsurgical pain is that many operations are performed to treat pre-existing painful conditions. If pain persists after surgery, was the operation ineffective, or has it caused a new problem? An example might be cholecystectomy. This is usually performed because the patient has gallstones or suffers bouts of acute cholecystitis, an extremely painful condition. If gallstones remain in the common bile duct, the patient may continue to experience the same kind of pain that was present prior to the operation. However, in some patients pain in the right upper quadrant of the abdomen may persist despite the absence of stones (Stiff et al. 1994). In other patients the incision may damage nerves, giving rise to a neurogenic (nerve injury) type of pain syndrome. Another example would be a patient who has had coronary artery bypass surgery for angina. Chest pain after the operation could be continuing angina or CPSP. Often careful history taking, listening closely to the patient's description, and thorough physical examination are sufficient to differentiate the two. Sometimes more so-

phisticated tests may be needed (e.g., nerve conduction studies). Clearly, careful research with rigorously applied criteria is needed to disentangle the epidemiology of CPSP from that of pre-existing painful conditions.

WORKING DEFINITION

A single universal definition of CPSP may not be possible or even desirable. Different definitions may be needed for different purposes. For example, a definition that is useful in assessing patients and directing their pain management may lack utility in unraveling basic pathophysiological mechanisms. We developed a working definition to describe and collate the epidemiological findings on CPSP from diverse studies. In order to qualify as CPSP the following criteria must be met: (1) the pain developed after a surgical procedure; (2) the pain is of at least 2 months duration; (3) other causes for the pain have been excluded, for example, continuing malignancy (following surgery for cancer) or chronic infection; (4) the possibility that the pain is continuing from a pre-existing problem should be explored and exclusion attempted. (There is an obvious gray area here in that surgery may simply exacerbate a pre-existing condition, but it is clearly not possible to attribute escalating pain to the surgery as natural deterioration cannot be ruled out.) Needless to say, most of the existing published studies are less explicit about how CPSP is defined and assessed. Such ambiguity limits (but does not preclude) interpretation of these studies.

LITERATURE REVIEW

SEARCH PROCEDURE

The literature review began with a search of MEDLINE using the search terms "Pain-Postoperative" with all subheadings. Other terms used to narrow the search were "long-term"(and variations on this), "perioperative," and "chronic." Subsequently, we searched for specific surgical procedures using key words such as "mastectomy," "thoracotomy," and "cholecystectomy." We performed additional searches using surgical specialty names such as "orthopedics" and "gynecology." We reviewed the reference lists of all papers retrieved in search of further relevant papers. More detailed searching of other electronic sources, or hand searching of journals, was not considered warranted: the quality of papers retrieved even from major journals abstracted in MEDLINE was often poor, and further accumulation of dubious studies seemed unlikely to substantially alter the conclusions. We need more thorough primary research, not further aggregation of inadequate studies.

QUALITY OF STUDIES

Most of the studies retrieved were poorly designed, executed, analyzed, and interpreted. The major problems are reviewed here to prevent repetition later. Studies that were especially well conducted are noted in the text. Most papers that primarily reported on operative techniques or that merely recorded personal case series have been excluded from this review.

The patients in many of the studies were convenience samples or, at best, time-delimited samples drawn from a given service. Frequently the source of the study sample was unclear, with all the problems this entails for interpretation (Crombie and Davies 1998). Study design was usually some sort of cross-sectional survey (albeit with historical analysis) or else a retrospective cohort study that left considerable doubt as to the origins and composition of the original cohort. Details on duration of follow-up, exclusions, and losses to follow-up were usually poorly documented. Prospective studies were rare.

In most studies, patient descriptions and categorizations were nonstandardized, and pain characteristics and severity were recorded using simple, crude, and idiosyncratic measures. No studies attempted to replicate findings from earlier work using the same standard definitions. The poor quality of reporting often made it difficult to identify the extent of patient problems that could be truly attributed to the surgery (rather than pre-existing problems or concomitant independent pain problems). Nonetheless, when assessing the findings from individual studies, the key question was not whether flaws and biases are present, but whether these defects vitiate the findings. In our judgment, despite the presence of many deficiencies in the primary studies, clear messages about CPSP have emerged from our review of existing empirical work.

PRESENTATION OF FINDINGS

This review of literature on CPSP is structured around the different major operations on which there is a substantial body of research, with a focus on procedures that can lead to pain (breast surgery, thoracotomy, cholecystectomy, orthopedic surgery, and dental surgery). For many other surgical procedures little systematic research has been done, but sporadic studies provide some insight. Pain after amputation is excluded from this chapter as this frequent and debilitating affliction is addressed elsewhere (Chapter 11).

The tables in this chapter are constructed around a common template and report the following information: (1) The design of the research study: survey, retrospective cohort study, prospective cohort study, or (rarely) prospective trial. In some cases, due to poor reporting, the design itself is not clear. (2) The definition or description of the pain (or other) problems examined. (3) The source of patients described in the study (when reported) and the size of the sample. (4) The pain measures used (if described). These may include verbal rating scales (VRS), visual analogue scales (VAS), and the McGill Pain Questionnaire (MPQ). (5) The duration of follow-up post operation (if reported). (6) The estimated prevalence of pain at given time periods following surgery (if discernible from the reported data). (6) The reference to the published report.

Because of the huge diversity (and general poor quality) of the reported studies, we made no attempt to aggregate data from the different studies into a single estimate of the prevalence of CPSP. Even for specific surgical procedures, such aggregation would be unreliable and probably meaningless. Instead, we have provided a narrative review of the long-term pain sequelae for each type of surgery to identify areas of clinical concern and allow more focused future research.

FINDINGS ON CPSP

CHRONIC PAIN AFTER BREAST SURGERY

Many studies have investigated chronic pain after breast surgery, which vary in both design and quality. Most of the existing studies focus on pain after mastectomy for breast cancer, although one paper looked at chronic pain after breast reconstruction, which included patients with and without cancer (Wallace et al. 1996). Studies that enabled some assessment of the size and scope of chronic pain after breast surgery are summarized in Table I; additional studies that shed some light on the nature and implications of the prob-

Table I
Chronic pain after breast surgery

Study Type	Outcomes Studied	Source of Subjects	Sample Size	Pain Measure	Duration of Follow-up	Estimated Prevalence	Reference
Survey	Various	Patient support group volunteers	314 in sample; 251 responses, of which 223 usable	Descriptive, VRS	16 mo–32 y (mean 8 y)	Phantom breast 36%; numbness 39–78%; paresthesia 19–35%; sensitivity 23–34%; pain 22–32%	Polinsky 1994
Prospective cohort	Phantom breast pain; scar pain	Oncology and radiotherapy depts.	120 patients; 110 at 1 y	Descriptive	1 y	Phantom breast pain at: 3 wk 13%, 1 y 13%; scar pain at: 3 wk 35%, 1 y 23%	Kroner et al. 1989
Prospective cohort	Phantom breast pain; scar pain	Oncology and radiotherapy depts.	120 patients; 110 at 1 y; 69 at 6 y	Descriptive	6 y	Phantom breast pain at 6 y 17%; scar pain at 6 y 1%	Kroner et al. 1992
Retrospective cohort	Pain, strange sensations, and paresthesia	Breast cancer patients from surgery dept.	569 contacted; 467 analyzed	VAS, VRS, MPQ, drug use	9–58 mo	Pain 49%; paresthesia 54%; "strange sensations" 50%	Tasmuth et al. 1995
Retrospective cohort	Pain	Breast cancer patients from medical center	479 contacted; 282 responses	VAS, MPQ	2–6 y	Pain at 1 y after: mastectomy 31%; mastectomy /reconstruction 49%; breast augmentation 38%; breast reduction 22%	Wallace et al. 1996
Survey	Pain	Oncology out-patients (grab sample)	95 patients	MPQ, CPQ	Not stated	Post-mastectomy pain 20%	Stevens et al. 1995
Survey	Morbidity after axillary dissection	Patients attending breast clinic	126 patients	Not stated	6 mo–4 y	1 y 45%; 1–2 y 37%; 2–4 y 28%; >4 y 20%	Ivens et al. 1992

Abbreviations: CPQ = Cancer Pain Questionnaire; MPQ = McGill Pain Questionnaire; VAS = visual analogue scale; VRS = verbal rating scale.

lem are discussed below.

Overall, seven studies revealed considerable long-term morbidity associated with breast surgery: typically a quarter (or more) of women are still reporting pain over a year after the operation (Table I). However, pain after mastectomy is not a simple syndrome. Several different types of pain have been described: phantom breast pain, pain around the operative site, chest wall pain, and pain in the ipsilateral arm. In a careful study of 38 patients with pain in the ipsilateral arm following mastectomy, Vecht et al. (1989) found nine different categories of problems. In only eight of these patients was the pain definitely caused by the surgery, with clear evidence of nerve injury. Other causes for arm pain after mastectomy included bra-

chial plexus neuropathy, due to infiltration by the cancer or radiotherapy; cervical radiculopathy; carpal tunnel syndrome; and pericapsulitis of the shoulder joint. The authors point out that postsurgical pain develops soon after the operation (sometimes directly after, with a mean interval of 6 weeks but sometimes with a delay of up to 26 weeks). However, pain from cancer infiltration or radiotherapy develops after a median delay of around 5 years. In none of the patients could severe pain be sufficiently relieved, so that prevention was of the utmost importance.

Phantom breast syndrome has been studied by Kroner et al. (1989, 1992). Many patients have phantom breast sensations after surgery, and these may be painful or painless. The incidence of phantom pains varied from 13% at 3 weeks to 17% at 6 years, although the numbers in the study had fallen from 120 to 69 over that period. Pain in the scar over the same time intervals was recorded in around one third of patients and showed little diminution over time.

Wallace et al. (1996) investigated the effect of type of surgery on long-term pain in a study of 282 women, some of whom had cancer. They looked at pain after several different breast operations: mastectomy, mastectomy with reconstruction, cosmetic augmentation, and breast reduction. The results showed that the incidence of breast pain varied and was related to the procedure carried out: 49% of those having mastectomy with reconstruction had pain at 1 year, compared to 31% of those having mastectomy alone and 22% of those having breast reduction. Further, women who had implants had a higher incidence of pain (53%) than those who did not (30%). Some research has also shown that chronic pain is more common if the patient receives chemotherapy and/or radiotherapy in addition to surgery (Tasmuth et al. 1995), but this finding is not universal (Kroner et al. 1992).

Existing studies that indicate that the type of surgery performed may influence the development of long-term pain are observational and nonrandomized. Hence, we must be cautious about asserting a causal relationship between type of surgery and deleterious long-term outcomes. However, further investigation of the effects of different surgical approaches may be fruitful in providing accurate information for patients and may provide clues on the scope for safer surgery.

Many patients with chronic pain after breast surgery may be misdiagnosed. Watson et al. (1989) found that only 2 of 18 patients in their study of post mastectomy pain syndrome were referred with the correct diagnosis. They comment that most were thought by the referring physician to have "emotionally derived pain." The authors were unable, however, to support the concept that the pain was related to moderate to severe depression; using the Beck Depression Inventory (BDI), only six of the patients scored in the mildly depressed range. The authors stressed the need for careful evaluation, paying attention to the history (particularly the timing of onset), the character of the pain, and the findings from sensory examination.

Pain is the most obvious unpleasant symptom experienced by women after breast surgery, but many other symptoms can develop. In a large study of breast cancer survivors from five American Cancer Society units, Polinsky (1994) found that considerable morbidity was related to treatment, including chemotherapy and radiotherapy as well as surgery. Pain was only one of many problems that interfered considerably with patients' lives. Ivens et al. (1992) studied the morbidity of 126 women who had axillary dissection as part of their surgical treatment, but who had neither radiotherapy nor chemotherapy. They found that 70% of cases complained of numbness, 33% of pain, 25% of weakness, 24% of arm swelling, and 15% of stiffness. Objective tests confirmed that these symptoms affected the daily lives of 39% of the patients. Tasmuth et al. (1995) studied 569 women who had undergone modified radical mastectomies with axillary evacuation or breast resection with axillary evacuation. They also found a high incidence of morbidity from a range of symptoms, with about a third to half the patients suffering from pain, paresthesia, edema, strange sensations, or muscle weakness. These symptoms had a marked effect on the daily lives of about 25% of patients.

In summary, many women suffer long-term problems after breast surgery, at least some of which are related to the surgery itself. Pain is just the most obvious of a whole range of unpleasant sensations that contribute to long-term morbidity. It appears that the more careful the search for evidence of long-term problems, the greater was the extent of the problem uncovered. However, the pain syndromes reported are disparate, and their diverse underlying mechanisms are poorly differentiated and understood. There is some evidence of under-recognition of the problem, misattribution of the pain, and undermanagement of the patients.

CHRONIC PAIN AFTER THORACOTOMY

The postero-lateral thoracotomy produces one of the worst types of suffering that it is possible to inflict on patients. Failure to anticipate and manage it adequately is not only inhumane but the consequences of unrelieved severe post-operative pain are diverse and profound. To the long list of these consequences must be added post-thoracotomy neuralgia, for in some unfortunate individuals chest wall pain persists in a very severe and chronic form (Richardson et al. 1994).

Although pain after thoracotomy had been recognized for many years, it was not until 1991 that its incidence or prevalence were studied systematically (Dajczman et al. 1991). Until that time, many researchers had reported on pain in the immediate postoperative period, and some anecdotal studies mentioned longer term pain. However, most of these reports suggest an incidence of less than 5% (Conacher 1992). Subsequently, studies specifically designed to estimate the incidence or prevalence of chronic post-thoracotomy pain have found a much higher rate of between 10% and 50% (Table II), but many of these studies have some or all of the methodological problems outlined earlier.

Pain after thoracotomy varies widely in severity. Dajczman et al. (1991) carried out a retrospective case-note review, following up 56 post-thoracotomy patients. Just over half of these (54%) had pain at the thoracotomy site at the time of interview, but pain severity was generally low, with 80% of patients choosing a visual analogue score (VAS) of 4 or less on a 10-point scale. Nonetheless, a third of patients with pain described it as "constant," and 44% complained that the pain interfered with their lives. Only five patients (9%) were receiving ongoing treatment for their pain, and the authors considered that the prevalence was often underestimated because some studies report only on patients presenting for treatment.

Similar findings were reported in a careful series of studies by Richardson and colleagues from Bradford, United Kingdom (1994). In a retrospective review of 1000 consecutive thoracotomies (883 suitable for analysis), they found a point prevalence of post-thoracotomy neuralgia of 22% at 2 months and 14% at 12 months. These figures are likely to underestimate the true extent of the problem, since to be included in the study, the continuation of the wound pain had to be severe enough to warrant recording in the surgical follow-up notes. This study confirms that post-thoracotomy pain can be a severe problem, as 15% of all patients had pain that was sufficiently troublesome to require a pain clinic referral.

Chronic post-thoracotomy pain is usually continuous, dating from the immediate postoperative period. Where pain appears after a pain-free period, doubts should be raised as to its pathology. In their retrospective review of 238 patients, Keller et al. (1994) found that worsening pain following an interval of adequate pain control occurred in 20 patients, all of whom were found to have tumor recurrence.

Some studies offer intriguing glimpses that the quality of postoperative pain relief may have some influence over the subsequent development of CPSP. In a retrospective study of 90 patients, Matsunaga et al.

(1990) asked about chronic pain 6–18 months after thoracotomy (response rate 86%). Fifty-two patients (67%) complained of continuing post-thoracotomy pain. The proportion reporting *chronic* pain varied according to their need for pain relief in the *acute* postoperative phase: 32 patients needed analgesics every day during the first 14 days after surgery, and of this group 91% had pain at 6 months. However, of the 45 patients who did not need analgesics every day after surgery, only 44% had pain at 6 months. In another retrospective cohort study, Kalso et al. (1992) reviewed the charts of all 150 surviving patients who had undergone thoracotomies over a 2-year period. The response rate was 89%, and 44% of subjects reported pain lasting more than 6 months. Compared to patients without chronic pain, those with ongoing pain were significantly more likely to report that their acute postoperative pain had been "excruciating" and that the acute pain relief provided to them was "poor." In a further small (but prospective) study, Katz et al. (1996) reported similar findings. They found that early postoperative pain was the only factor that significantly predicted long-term pain.

Preoperative pain may also play a role in the development of CPSP (Keller et al. 1994). Of the 238 thoracotomy patients in this study, 23 were taking narcotics (opioids) prior to the operation, and 12 of these (52%) subsequently developed chronic post-thoracotomy pain. This compares to just 13 of the 215 patients who were not taking narcotics preoperatively (6%). It is not clear whether the chronic pain reported was a continuation or exacerbation of pre-existing pain (perhaps related to malignancy) or the development of new pain as a result of surgery.

Type of surgery may also have an effect on long-term outcomes. However, existing studies have failed to clarify the situation. In Keller and colleagues' retrospective review (1994), pain occurred in 10 of 20 patients (50%) who had chest wall resections, 5 of 25 (20%) who underwent pleurectomy, and 10 of 193 (5%) who received thoracotomies. However, these numbers are too small to draw definitive conclusions, and in any case the type of surgery is confounded with the nature of any pre-existing conditions. Richardson and colleagues (1994) found a significant association between the development of post-thoracotomy neuralgia and transthoracic surgery for benign esophageal disease, and reported that the lowest incidence of CPSP occurred with operations for malignant lung disease. Rib resection was also associated with a lower inci-

Table II
Chronic pain after thoracotomy

Study Type	Outcomes Studied	Source of Subjects	Sample Size	Pain Measure	Duration of Follow-up	Estimated Prevalence	Reference
Survey of records	Post-thoracotomy neuralgia	Hospital records, 10-y period	3109 records	Not stated	≥3 mo	5%	Conacher 1992
Retrospective cohort	Post-thoracotomy neuralgia	1000 consecutive thoracotomy patients	1000 records; 883 analyzed	Not stated	≥2 mo	Pain at 2 mo 22%; at 12 mo 14%; severe enough for referral in 15% of patients	Richardson et al. 1994
Retrospective cohort	Post-thoracotomy pain	Hospital records: patients after thoracotomy and video-assisted thoracic surgery	391 contacted; 343 responses	VAS, VRS	>3 mo	Pain after lateral thoracotomy at: <1 y 44%, >1 y 29%; after video-assisted surgery at: <1 y 30%, >1 y 22%	Landreneau et al. 1994
Retrospective cohort	Post-thoracotomy pain	Hospital records	56 patients	VAS	≥2 mo	54%	Dajczman et al. 1991
Retrospective cohort	Chest pain	Hospital records: 50 consecutive patients	50 patients	VAS, MPQ, and analgesic requirement	≤6 mo	Pain at 6 mo: non-serratus sparing antero-axillary thoractomy 8%; posterolateral thoracotomy 12%	Nomori et al. 1997
Prospective randomized and blind trial of cryoanalgesia	Post-thoracotomy pain	60 consecutive thoracotomy patients	53 patients	VAS, analgesic use	6 wk and 6 mo	Pain in cryoanalgesia group 23%, vs. 7% in control group	Roxburgh et al. 1987
Retrospective cohort	Post-thoracotomy pain	Additional phone follow-up of post-thoracotomy patients	30 patients; only 23 contacted	VAS, MPQ	About 1.5 y after thora-cotomy	52%	Katz et al. 1996
Retrospective cohort	Post-thoracotomy pain	Medical records of post-thoracotomy patients	214 records; 150 survivors; 134 replies	Analgesic use	≥6 mo	44%	Kalso et al. 1992
Retrospective cohort	Post-thoracotomy pain	238 consecutive patients	238 patients	Pain assessment card; pain impact statement	≥3 mo	11%	Keller et al. 1994
Retrospective cohort	Post-thoracotomy pain	Surgical records	90 contacted; 77 responses	Not stated	6–18 mo	67%; 20% required medication	Matsunaga et al. 1990

dence of pain, while chest drains and postoperative radiotherapy were associated with an increased incidence. These authors speculated that effective perioperative analgesia and gentle surgery can reduce the incidence of post-thoracotomy neuralgia.

Other prospective studies have attempted to evaluate the role of different surgical procedures in the development of chronic post-thoracotomy pain. In a randomized and blinded study that compared standard posterolateral thoracotomy with muscle-sparing thoracotomy, significantly less *acute* postoperative pain affected the muscle-sparing group, but there was no difference in longer term pain (Hazelrigg et al. 1991). In a second prospective, randomized study to investigate the effect of cryoanalgesia in the control of pain after thoracotomy, Roxburgh at al. (1987) found that direct cryotherapy to the intercostal nerves did not improve postoperative pain control. Of more concern is that their results suggest an *increase* in long-term pain in the cryotherapy group (although no proper statistical analysis was performed). Both of these studies were small (about 50 patients) and so would be unlikely to detect even large differences in long-term outcome.

In summary, recognition has grown over the past decade that chronic post-thoracotomy pain is serious and widespread. The high prevalence of both severe and relatively mild (though not inconsequential) pain requires attention. Some studies suggest that operative approach, perioperative care, and level of immediate postoperative pain may all have a bearing on the subsequent development of a chronic pain problem. If this is true, then these discoveries hold out great hope for prevention. However, the quality of the existing studies is inadequate to support the inferential demands made of them. New high-quality studies (preferably prospective and randomized studies, but also well-conducted, properly adjusted cohort analyses) are needed to test existing hypotheses and develop preventative strategies.

CHRONIC PAIN AFTER CHOLECYSTECTOMY

An anonymous editorial in the *Lancet* (1988) stated: "Almost half the patients who undergo elective cholecystectomy will be dissatisfied with the outcome. Can this be true of such a safe and 'popular' operation? Probably, because most surgeons do not bother with long term follow-up."

Cholecystectomy is one of the most problematic

operations to study for evidence of CPSP. Almost all patients who have a cholecystectomy were subject to pre-existing pain (that is usually the reason they have the operation), which is often severe: "of the symptoms experienced by patients with gallstones, pain is the most dramatic, being severe, protracted, and persistent" (Gunn and Keddie 1972). Patients frequently have pain in the right upper abdomen, together with dyspepsia (indigestion) and heartburn. Hence it can be difficult to separate a continuation of this pre-existing condition from the development of a new (and pathologically distinct) pain problem.

One of the first researchers to study long-term problems after cholecystectomy was Bodvall. In a seminal 1964 monograph, he assessed the extent of postoperative "biliary distress," which he defined as biliary colic or dyspepsia, similar to the symptoms prior to the cholecystectomy. The period of follow-up varied between 2 and 9 years. In a review of the literature up to 1964, 34 studies showed an incidence of severe biliary distress between 2.3% and 32%. The number of patients free of symptoms after cholecystectomy varied from 78% to as few as 53%. In Bodvall's study, the total frequency of postoperative biliary distress was 40%, of which 2.4% was classified as severe pain. He found the incidence of the syndrome to be increased in women, those with a long preoperative history, and those with a functioning gallbladder. It decreased with advancing age, varied according to the stage of the cholecystitis, and decreased among those whose gallstones had been removed. The type of gallbladder disease influenced the incidence, but the size and number of stones did not. Radiographic studies showed that, for those with mild symptoms, a decreased width of the common bile duct was associated with an increased incidence of pain, but those with severe symptoms showed dilatation of the duct. Surprisingly, Bodvall makes no mention of pain related to the incision or scar.

Subsequently, several retrospective cohort studies have examined pain after cholecystectomy, and these are summarized in Table III. Pain prevalence estimates vary from less than 5% to more than 20%, with the prevalence of severe pain problems at the lower end of this range. However, in general, the studies did not make careful assessment of the impact of pre-existing pain problems, and therefore their findings are hard to interpret.

Patients who undergo cholecystectomy hope to be cured of biliary pain and to avoid further attacks of

Table III
Chronic pain after cholecystectomy

Study Type	Outcomes Studied	Source of Subjects	Sample Size	Pain Measure	Duration of Follow-up	Estimated Prevalence	Reference
Retrospective cohort	Upper abdominal pain	Hospital patients after open and laparoscopic cholecystectomy	450 contacted; 360 responses	Not stated	Mean for: laparoscopic 15 mo; open 32 mo	Pain after: laparoscopic 3.4%; open procedure 10%	Stiff et al. 1994
Survey	Stomach pain	Hospital patients after open and laparoscopic cholecystectomy	315 contacted; 267 responses	Not stated	At least 12 mo; mean 14 mo	Pain after: laparoscopic 7%; open procedure 7%	Wilson and Macintyre 1993
Retrospective cohort	Symptoms after cholecystectomy	Hospital patients after open cholecystectomy	1930	Dyspepsia or abdominal pain similar to preoperative symptoms	2–9 y	Prevalence of all symptoms 40%; dyspepsia 11%; mild pain 24%; severe pain 6%	Bodvall 1964
Prospective cohort	Pain and other symptoms after cholecystectomy	Elective patients scheduled for cholecystectomy	130	Not stated	2 y	Dull upper abdominal pain 21%	Ros and Zambon 1987
Retrospective cohort	Symptoms after cholecystectomy	Hospital patients after open cholecystectomy	1716 patients initially; 862 contacted; 800 analyzed	Not stated	4 y	Prevalence of all symptoms 31%; severe pain 4%	Stefanini et al. 1974
Prospective cohort	Pain after cholecystectomy	Consecutive patients after cholecystectomy	115 patients	Not stated	12 mo	Persistent abdominal pain 27%	Bates et al. 1984

acute cholecystitis, pancreatitis, or jaundice (Ros and Zambon 1987). Most also assume that their dyspepsia will be relieved. These expectations are conveyed to patients by their physicians. Unfortunately, such expectations are frequently unmet. In a prospective study of 130 patients in Barcelona (75% available for follow-up), Ros and Zambon (1987) reported that just 53% of patients were satisfied with the operation and that 21% were still suffering upper abdominal pain at their 2-year follow-up visit. They state that the pain "was usually referred as due to the scar." In a second prospective study, Bates and colleagues (1984) found that 43% of patients rated their operation as less than completely successful 12 months after surgery. About half (46%) still complained of indigestion, and 27% complained of abdominal pain, most often in or deep to the scar.

LAPAROSCOPIC CHOLECYSTECTOMY

Laparoscopic cholecystectomy has been widely practiced over the past 10 years. In this procedure, the instruments are introduced through small punctures, so that there is no large incision. It may therefore be expected to produce a reduced incidence of CPSP because the chance of nerve injury should be greatly reduced.

Several review articles have investigated the safety, efficacy, and complications of laparoscopic cholecystectomy since 1990, some of them examining very large cohorts of patients. Although operative technique is often described in some detail in these papers, pain and other long-term complications are rarely mentioned and even then are covered only briefly (Cuschieri et al. 1991; Peters et al. 1991; Southern Surgeons Club 1991; Deziel et al. 1993).

In a study of long-term right upper quadrant pain after open or laparoscopic cholecystectomy, Stiff and colleagues (1994) found that 9.7% of patients complained of chronic pain after open cholecystectomy compared to 3.4% after laparoscopic cholecystectomy. The incidence of mild gastrointestinal symptoms such as heartburn and indigestion was the same in both groups, suggesting that the different incidence of pain was due to the operative technique rather than the success or failure of the procedure. In the open cholecystectomy group, 10.3% of patients felt the same or worse after the operation, and in the laparoscopy group 4.9% felt worse. However, these results are far from conclusive. In an earlier study that looked at several symptoms after open and laparoscopic procedures Wilson and Macintyre (1993) found an incidence of abdominal pain of around 6% in both groups. Regrettably, neither of these studies was a prospective randomized study with appropriate blinding.

In summary, patients are frequently dissatisfied with the results of their cholecystectomy (whether open or laparoscopic); their dissatisfaction mostly revolves around continuing symptoms, especially pain. Despite several large studies, the relative contributions to long-term pain of the pre-existing condition and the operation itself remain unclear. Differing levels of long-term problems between patients who underwent open versus laparoscopic surgery suggest that the operation may indeed contribute to subsequent pain problems. It is to be hoped that in future, well-designed and rigorously conducted studies will address the important issue of long-term pain and other distressing symptoms after undergoing different techniques of cholecystectomy.

CHRONIC PAIN AFTER ORTHOPEDIC SURGERY

Orthopedics has two main components: trauma (patients with injuries, usually involving broken bones), and elective work, such as joint replacement and spinal surgery. In both these groups, many patients have pain prior to their operations, making this (again) a difficult area to study. After trauma, the injury that the patient suffers will often have caused widespread damage, and the operation is usually centered on the area of damage. A good example is an ankle injury. Five main nerves pass from the leg to the foot around the ankle. If the injury causes a major deformity of the ankle joint (for example a dislocation, with or without bone fracture), it is likely that one or more of the nerves have been injured and that the soft tissues have been severely damaged. It is thus impossible to distinguish the relative contribution of these factors and the surgery itself. It is clear that many patients suffer long-term pain after trauma and that surgery may play at least some part in the etiology. It must be stressed, however, that the surgery is usually essential if the patient is to regain function after the injury. Perhaps because this is such a difficult and complex area, no good studies have examined chronic pain after surgery for trauma.

Turning to elective orthopedic surgery, few studies have specifically addressed long-term pain (Table IV). Swanson's study (1983) showed that nerve injury pain is common after open meniscectomy. However, the advent of arthroscopic surgery has made this type of operation rare. Nerve injury can still occur with minimally invasive surgery, but is less common. Many

Table IV
Chronic pain after orthopedic surgery

Study Type	Outcomes Studied	Source of Subjects	Sample Size	Pain Measure	Duration of Follow-up	Estimated Prevalence	Reference
Prospective cohort	Prepatellar neuropathy	Patients after open meniscectomy	87	Dysesthesia in area of operation	6 mo	44% at 6 mo	Swanson 1983
Prospective trial of two types of hip prostheses	Thigh pain after total hip replacement	Patients having two types of total hip replacement	215	Thigh pain	1 and 2 y	Pain at 1 y: 13% and 7% in each group; pain at 2 y: 23% and 3% in each group	Burkart et al. 1993
Retrospective cohort	Pain after total hip replacement	Hospital patients after total hip replacement	505	Not stated	Mean 102 mo (range 42–171 mo)	Pain when sitting 16%; pain when walking 35%	Johnsson and Thorngren 1989

Table V
Chronic pain after dental surgery

Study Type	Outcomes Studied	Source of Subjects	Sample Size	Pain Measure	Duration of Follow-up	Estimated Prevalence	Reference
Survey	Phantom tooth pain	Endodontic therapy patients	732 contacted, 463 usable replies	Not stated	Not stated	3%	Marbach et al. 1982
Survey	Pain	Surgical endodontic patients	206 contacted; 118 responses	Not stated	Not stated	5%	Campbell et al. 1990
Prospective cohort	Pain after endodontic treatment	Surgical endodontic patients	198 contacted; 165 responses	Not stated	1 y	13%	Lobb et al. 1996

publications have looked at the failure of joint replacements, but few of them have looked at the incidence of pain in a systematic way. Studies of pain after hip replacement have shown that different prostheses are associated with differing incidences of pain following surgery (Johnsson and Thorngren 1989; Burkart et al. 1993).

In a review of patient outcomes after lumbar spinal fusions, Turner and colleagues (1992) found 47 articles, although none of these were randomized trials (which makes it difficult to disentangle the natural history of back pain from surgically induced chronic pain). Presumably, most of these operations were performed because of pre-existing back or leg pain, although when reporting long-term outcomes only six of the studies gave details on continuing back pain and only two provided information on chronic leg pain. There was, however, a reported incidence of 9% of chronic pain at the bone graft donor site (Turner et al. 1992), which is almost certainly a complication arising from the surgery.

Orthopedic procedures, whether carried out as emergencies for trauma or used electively, are aimed at remedying obvious defects and improving long-term function. Given this, the lack of systematic attention paid to important long-term outcomes (especially pain) is both surprising and disappointing, particularly in the light of evidence that many patients who receive orthopedic surgery subsequently end up in chronic pain clinics (Crombie and Davies 1991; Crombie et al. 1998).

CHRONIC PAIN AFTER DENTAL SURGERY

While many studies address pain after dental surgery, few of them are concerned with chronic pain; the assumption seems to be that dental pain is largely short lived and self limiting. However, two distinct chronic clinical entities have been reported: post-traumatic dysesthesia and phantom tooth pain (Table V). Moreover, there is some confusion in the terminology, and another term, "atypical odontalgia," has also been used to describe long-term problems after dental surgery.

The term "phantom tooth pain" was first used by Marbach in 1978. However, in a subsequent paper (1993), Marbach does not confine phantom tooth pain to the absent tooth, but includes within the definition pain in the area around the removed tooth. He also states that phantom tooth pain can occur as a consequence of routine dental and surgical procedures, as well as resulting from physical trauma to the face. Given our current understanding of the pathophysiology of pain after traumatic insults, it seems plausible that chronic pain may result from any injury to the tissues in the mouth and face (especially nerve injury). Thus, phantom tooth pain is a specific entity that arises when the original pain is in the area of an extracted tooth.

The reported incidence of pain after endodontic therapy varies from 3% to 13% (Marbach et al. 1982; Campbell et al. 1990; Lobb et al. 1996). Lobb and colleagues reported that most of the patients who experienced pain after their treatment did not revisit the endodontist. There are many possible explanations for this, but endontists are undoubtedly underestimating the morbidity of the procedures they carry out. The shortage of good studies leaves much to be uncovered about the epidemiology of chronic pain after dental surgery.

OTHER CPSP SYNDROMES

This section comments on various other surgical procedures for which there is at least some published literature (Table VI), although the paucity and poor quality of the available information severely limit the scope of any conclusions drawn.

Table VI
Chronic pain after other surgical procedures

Study Type	Outcomes Studied	Source of Subjects	Sample Size	Pain Measure	Duration of Follow-up	Estimated Prevalence	Reference
Hernia							
Prospective randomized trial of three surgical techniques	Pain	Trial patients having hernia repair	315 patients	VAS	6, 12, and 24 mo	Pain at 12 mo 63%, with 12% moderate or severe; pain at 2 y 54%, with 11% moderate or severe.	Cunningham et al. 1996
Prospective study of trans-peritoneal laparoscopic herniorrhaphy	Pain	Trial patients having hernia repair	60 patients	Not stated	Average 9 mo	15%	Cornell and Kerlakian 1994
Sympathectomy							
Unclear	Neuralgia after phenol sympathectomy	Patient records	1028 patients; 1666 operations	Not stated	Not stated	Pain after 9% of operations in 15% of patients	Reid et al. 1970
Survey	Post-sympathectomy neuralgia	Patients having open sympathectomy	100 patients; 142 operations	Not stated	Not stated	13%	Postle-thwaite 1973
Prospective cohort	Post-sympathectomy neuralgia	Patients having open sympathectomy	56 patients; 96 operations	Not stated	6 mo	35%	Raskin et al. 1974
Prospective cohort	Neuralgia after sympathectomy with phenol or alcohol	Patients having sympathectomy	386 patients	Pain description "mild" to "severe"	6 mo	Pain after use of: alcohol 40%; phenol 20%	Cousins et al. 1979
Cardiac Surgery							
Retrospective cohort	Chest wall pain	Patients after coronary artery bypass grafting	178 patients	Pain affecting daily life or return to work	Minimum 1 y, maximum 22 mo	5–70%, depending on site of harvested bypass conduit	Eng and Wells 1991
Rectal Amputation							
Survey	Perineal pain	Patients after abdomino-perineal resection for rectal cancer	286 contacted; 177 replies	Presence of perineal pain	5 y plus	12%	Boas et al. 1993
Retrospective cohort	Phantom pain	Patients after rectal amputation	22 (21 with cancer)	Phantom sensations and pain	Mean 44 mo (range 14–90)	68% with phantom sensations; 18% with pain	Ovesen et al. 1991

(continued)

Table VI
Continued

Study Type	Outcomes Studied	Source of Subjects	Sample Size	Pain Measure	Duration of Follow-up	Estimated Prevalence	Reference
Vasectomy							
Retrospective cohort	Testicular pain	Hospital records	172 men	Not stated	4 y	33% had chronic discomfort; 15% regarded it as "troublesome" and 5% sought further medical help	McMahon et al. 1992
Retrospective cohort	Testicular pain	Hospital records	396 men	Not stated	Mean 19 mo (range 8–39)	5% had chronic testicular pain and 10% reported pain on intercourse	Ahmed et al. 1997
Randomized control trial	Testicular discomfort	Men having vasectomy, enrolled in trial	70 men	VAS	1 y	37% of control group had pain for 2–24 wk; no pain reported in active group (use of anesthetic injections)	Paxton et al. 1995

Chronic pain after hernia repair

Despite the fact that hernia repair is a common procedure, and that chronic pain is a recognized complication, no study has succeeded in shedding much light on the epidemiology of this problem. Many studies have examined outcome after hernia surgery, but most of them do not even mention long-term pain. In most published work, the study design, research methods, and data analysis either are not described in detail or are so poor that the studies cannot be included in any meaningful analysis. In contrast to the lack of methodological detail, the surgical technique used is usually explained in full, with diagrams.

Only one study evaluates the incidence of pain in a randomized prospective clinical trial known as the Cooperative Hernia Study (Cunningham et al. 1996). The authors identified three distinct chronic pains, of which the most common and severe was a somatic pain, the second a neuropathic pain (caused by nerve injury), and the third a visceral, ejaculatory pain. Moderate to severe pain was persistent, with the incidence at 2 years (11%) being only slightly less than that at 1 year (12%). This is in contrast to the comments made in many surgical textbooks and reports that the pain is usually transient. Pain was not the only long-term problem reported; numbness was also present in about a quarter of the patients at 2 years.

Chronic pain after lumbar sympathectomy

Lumbar sympathectomy was originally carried out as an open operation involving a large incision. Now it is usually done percutaneously, using needles, under X-ray control. After the procedure patients may develop pain in the thigh (post-sympathectomy neuralgia). The incidence after open sympathectomy is quoted in many studies and varies between 12% and 35% (Postlethwaite 1973; Raskin et al. 1974). The incidence is similar following percutaneous phenol sympathectomy (Reid et al. 1970; Cousins et al. 1979). This suggests that the sympathectomy itself, not the generalized damage caused by the operation, causes the problem.

Chronic pain after cardiac surgery

Cardiac surgery involves a thoracotomy, so some of the pain syndromes are similar to post-thoracotomy pain (described in detail above). Most cardiac operations involve splitting the sternum, which can produce a separate chronic pain problem. Operations to revascularize the heart using either arteries or veins produce their own syndromes, and use of the internal mammary artery has been reported as carrying a higher incidence of chronic pain than procedures using veins (Eng and Wells 1991).

Chronic pain after rectal amputation

Ovesen et al. (1991), in a small study, found phantom phenomena to be common after rectal amputation (68% of patients), while phantom pain was less common but still significant (18%). The incidence was not affected by age, sex, stage of the tumor, or healing of the wound, and it was no more common in patients with preoperative pain (although small numbers mean that few conclusions can be drawn). None of the patients had been informed that phantom phenomena could appear postoperatively, and only one had received medical help. Boas et al. (1993) looked at all types of chronic pain after rectal surgery and found a significant number of patients with chronic pain at 5 years (11%). The patients fell into two groups, those who developed pain within a few weeks of the operation, and those with late-onset pain. The late-onset group had an 80% chance of dying from tumor recurrence, while those in the early-onset group had a 26% chance of tumor recurrence. Thus, once again the temporal pattern of chronic pain can be an important indicator of the underlying pathology.

Chronic pain after gynecological surgery

We found no high-quality studies that specifically examined chronic pain after gynecological surgery. However, the incidence of pain after endometrial resection has been reported to be 13% at 1 year (Jacobs and Blumenthal 1994). It is unclear from this study whether this represents continuation of preoperative pain or development of a new pain. Thirteen percent of patients had pelvic pain prior to surgery, but the paper did not clarify whether these were the same women as those experiencing pain at 1 year.

In a systematic review of choice of suture materials and techniques for repair of perineal trauma, Grant (1989) located a number of studies reporting long-term pain. Estimates of the proportion of women suffering long-term pain were mostly in the range of 7–12%, but one study reported a prevalence of 38%.

Chronic pain after urological surgery

In a study of long-term results of colposuspension, Wheelan (1990) states that 27% of patients had pain persisting for 2 months or longer, but that this discomfort had disappeared within 4 months. Pain after prostatectomy was evaluated by Niesel et al. (1996) in a review of 200 cases (response rate 89%). After a mean duration of 20 weeks, 33% of patients were still reporting pain either around the incision or at the site of the drain. Pain intensities recorded were usually low, however, with a mean of 1.3 and a maximum of 6 on a numeric intensity scale of 0–10.

Chronic pain after vasectomy

Vasectomy is the second most common operation performed on men (circumcision is the most common). Chronic testicular pain after vasectomy is a recognized complication, occurring in between 5% (Ahmed et al. 1997) and 33% (McMahon et al. 1992) of patients. It may occur spontaneously or at the time of intercourse (McMahon et al. 1992; Ahmed et al. 1997). Paxton et al. (1995) reported that injecting a local anesthetic into the vas deferens at the time of surgery prevented the development of chronic pain after vasectomy; however, chronic pain can also occur after vasectomy performed under local anesthesia (although the local anesthetic could have been incomplete in these cases).

Given that almost all men who opt for a vasectomy are pain free beforehand, and that the operation is being performed for social rather than medical reasons, there is a double imperative to ensure that no long-term harm results. Therefore, it is essential to identify predisposing factors (of the patient and the procedure) and clearly describe the risks if men are to make sensible and informed decisions. Regrettably, the epidemiology is not yet clear even for this common surgical procedure.

DISCUSSION

EXTENT OF THE PROBLEM

Chronic pain is a common sequel to surgery; up to 20% of patients seen in chronic pain clinics have surgery as the main or a contributory cause of their pain (Davies et al. 1992; Crombie et al. 1998). The extent of CPSP is difficult to assess because few really well-conducted studies have been carried out. With rare exceptions, the studies reported here were retrospective cohort studies documenting the experiences of disparate patient groups (often convenience samples). They largely used idiosyncratic measures of pain, and most paid scant attention to methodological issues such as the representativeness of samples and the completeness of follow-up. Many other papers that purported to be about long-term surgical outcomes were actually articles about surgical technique. That so little should be known about the long-term deleterious outcomes of such common procedures is as remarkable as it is lamentable.

Even from the mixed bag of studies uncovered in this review, certain messages are clear. First, well-designed studies that focus on the problem of CPSP find a higher prevalence than follow-up studies that merely mention pain as an incidental finding. In some of these better studies, a third or more of patients complain of ongoing problems. Second, pain is just one of a range of unpleasant chronic symptoms arising from sensory disturbance that cause long-term discomfort; phantom sensations, numbness, allodynia, and hyperalgesia also contribute to patients' distress. The presence of these symptoms is related to pain as they may arise from the same or similar pathological processes. Third, patients who have had operations for cancer and who subsequently develop pain after a prolonged pain-free period should be closely investigated for tumor recurrence (Vecht et al. 1989; Keller et al. 1994).

Surgical procedures are often undertaken to relieve symptoms, reduce long-term morbidity (and mortality), and improve function. Yet studies that have expressly examined the issue show a large gap between patients' expectations of their operation's ability to relieve pre-existing symptoms and their experiences postoperatively in terms of unresolved morbidity and new problems. It is ironic, therefore, that the beneficial impact of technically successful surgical procedures is blunted by unwanted long-term discomfort.

Finally, many people suffer symptoms at a relatively low level and do not seek further professional help. These people may be missing out on relief from modern pain management approaches (Davies et al. 1994, 1995). Patients who have severe problems may be referred for specialist care outside the surgical service (for example, in pain clinics). Some may even have further surgery in an attempt to ameliorate their (surgery-induced) problems.

RISK FACTORS FOR CPSP

Several studies conclude that CPSP is long lasting or permanent, and that it is hard to treat successfully. This makes prevention an important topic. Why some patients should develop CPSP, while others who have the same operation do not, remains a mystery. We found no studies that looked at genetic predisposition or examined whether other patient characteristics or concurrent illness could influence the incidence of chronic pain. There is some evidence that the type of surgical operation and differences in technique can influence the incidence, but existing studies are inadequate to shed light on the issue. It is to be hoped that modern innovations such as laparoscopic surgery will reduce the incidence of CPSP, but this hypothesis has yet to be exposed to serious scrutiny. More studies are needed that specifically focus on this question.

PROSPECTS FOR PREVENTION

Several studies suggest that effective treatment of acute pain after surgery can reduce the incidence of CPSP, and our emerging understanding of the pathophysiology of pain suggests that this is plausible. It seems that the actual method of pain relief is not as important as the degree of relief obtained, and that by using combinations of treatments it is possible to virtually eliminate postoperative pain. It is laudable to try and prevent postoperative pain as an end in itself, but given that it is also possibly a factor in the incidence of CPSP, there is an added impetus to concentrate efforts in this area. Although evidence exists in some areas (such as thoracotomy; Matsunaga et al. 1990; Kalso et al. 1992, 1996), prospective randomized studies are needed in all types of surgery to ascertain the best approach to postoperative analgesia and determine how different approaches can influence the incidence of CPSP. This evidence must be used to minimize both postoperative pain and CPSP.

IMPLICATIONS FOR PRACTICE

These findings have profound implications for preoperative counseling of patients and the obtaining of informed consent. Patients have a right to expect clear, accurate, and detailed information on the likely range of possible outcomes (including those that are deleterious) and on their relative frequencies. The lack of clear information in this area means that balanced assessment of risks against benefits is difficult for professionals, let alone patients.

The large variations in the reported levels of chronic problems after surgery may arise simply from the methodological variability of the studies examined. Alternatively, they may suggest that there is much to uncover about the influence of patient characteristics, surgical approach, and peri-operative care on the subsequent development of CPSP. As better studies provide a clearer picture, the knowledge gained must be incorporated into clinical decision making. In this way, patients and doctors together can assess the potential benefits of elective surgery against the risks of acquiring long-term morbidity, and can do so based on a realistic assessment of individual risk. For example, some urologists already advise against performing vasectomy on men with pre-existing testicular pain or discomfort.

The importance of meticulous attention to perioperative care has already been highlighted, but patients undergoing surgery need longer term follow-up to identify and deal with any emerging long-term sequelae. Because the prevalence of CPSP is largely underestimated, patients may have their pain misdiagnosed (for example, as psychogenic) or even denied. As a result, many patients' difficulties are compounded by their physicians' failure to address continuing problems.

IMPLICATIONS FOR RESEARCH

Further progress in unraveling the epidemiology of CPSP will only be made with proper attention to important design issues (Crombie et al. 1994; see Chapters 2 and 3 in this volume). A major advance would be to use explicit prior hypotheses testing them in prospective studies and using clearly defined groups of patients and psychometrically sound measurement tools (for both initial characteristics and final outcomes). At the design stage, researchers must recognize that many surgical procedures are carried out on patients with pre-existing pain. These methodological criteria are well understood (at least by epidemiologists), but adhering to them in practice is not so easy. The hope is that the epidemiology of CPSP can move beyond being merely a collection of disparate studies (although some may offer tantalizing glimpses of insight) and can become a mature research field that will build a substantial and robust body of knowledge with wide practical application.

CONCLUDING REMARKS

For many years acute postoperative pain was a neglected part of clinical practice. Patients had technically successful operations, but suffered greatly for days or weeks. Despite accumulating evidence over many decades, prevention and treatment were accorded low priority. Since the 1980s, however, a revolution in acute postoperative care has swept the developed world. New approaches to therapy and systematic application of existing knowledge have greatly improved patient comfort in the immediate postoperative period. Many of these changes were underpinned by a clear understanding of the nature, etiology, and pathophysiology of acute pain. Unfortunately, the advances made have not extended into the post-discharge period. The findings from this review highlight the scale of chronic suffering and hint at the complexity of the web of causation. If chronic postsurgical pain is to be diminished, a shift in attitudes is needed in both research and practice similar to that which revolutionized acute postoperative care.

REFERENCES

Ahmed I, Rasheed S, White C, Shaikh NA. The incidence of post-vasectomy chronic testicular pain and the role of nerve stripping (denervation) of the spermatic cord in its management. *Br J Urol* 1997; 79:269–270.

Anonymous. Cholecystectomy: the dissatisfied customer [editorial]. *Lancet* 1988; 339.

Bates T, Mercer JC, Harrison M. Symptomatic gall stone disease: before and after cholecystectomy. *Gut* 1984; 24:579–50.

Boas RA, Schug SA, Acland RH. Perineal pain after rectal amputation: a 5-year follow-up. *Pain* 1993; 52:67–70.

Bodvall B. Late results following cholecystectomy in 1930 cases and special studies on postoperative biliary distress. *Acta Chir Scand* 1964; (Suppl):329.

Burkart BC, Bourne RB, Rorabeck CH, Kirk PG. Thigh pain in cementless total hip arthroplasty. A comparison of two systems at 2 years follow-up. *Orthop Clin North Am* 1993; 24:645–663.

Campbell RL, Parks KW, Dodds RN. Chronic facial pain associated with endodontic therapy. *Oral Surg Oral Med Oral Pathol* 1990; 69:287–290.

Coderre TJ, Katz J, Vaccarino AL, Melzack R. Contribution of central neuroplasticity to pathological pain: review of clinical and experimental evidence. *Pain* 1993; 52:259–285.

Conacher ID. Therapists and therapies for post-thoracotomy neuralgia. *Pain* 1992; 48:409–412.

Cornell RB, Kerlakian GM. Early complications and outcomes of the current technique of transperitoneal laparoscopic herniorraphy and a comparison to the traditional open approach. *Am J Surg* 1994; 168:275–279.

Cousins MJ, Reeve TS, Glynn CJ, Walsh JA, Cherry DA. Neurolytic lumbar sympathetic blockade: duration of denervation and relief of rest pain. *Anaesth Intensive Care* 1979; 7:121–135.

Crombie IK, Davies HTO. Audit of outpatients: entering the loop. *BMJ* 1991; 302:1437–1439.

Crombie IK, Davies HTO. Selection bias in pain research, [editorial] *Pain* 1998; 74:1–3.

Crombie IK, Davies HTO, Macrae WA. The epidemiology of chronic pain: time for new directions [editorial]. *Pain* 1994; 57:1–3.

Crombie IK, Davies HTO, Macrae WA. Cut and thrust: antecedent surgery and trauma among patients attending a pain clinic. *Pain* 1998;76:167–671.

Cunningham J, Temple WJ, Mitchell P, et al. Cooperative Hernia Study. Pain in the post-repair patient. *Ann Surg* 1996; 224:598–602.

Cuschieri A, Dubois F, Mouiel J, et al. The European experience with laparoscopic cholecystectomy. *Am J Surg* 1991; 161:385–387.

Dajczman E, Gordon A, Kreisman H, Wolkove N. Long-term post-thoracotomy pain. *Chest* 1991; 99:270–274.

Davies HTO, Crombie IK, Macrae WA, Rogers KM. Pain Clinic patients in northern Britain. *Pain Clinic* 1992; 5:129–135.

Davies HTO, Crombie IK, Macrae WA. Why use a pain clinic? Management of neurogenic pain before and after referral. *J R Soc Med* 1994; 87:382–385.

Davies HTO, Crombie IK, Macrae WA. Back pain in the pain clinic: nature and management. *Pain Clinic* 1995; 8:191–199.

Deziel DJ, Millikan KW, Economou SG, et al. Complications of laparoscopic cholecystectomy: a national survey of 4,292 hospitals and an analysis of 77,604 cases. *Am J Surg* 1993; 165:9–13.

Eng J, Wells FC. Morbidity following coronary artery revascularisation with the internal mammary artery. *Int J Cardiol* 1991; 30:55–59.

Grant A. The choice of suture materials and techniques for repair of perineal trauma: an overview of the evidence from controlled trials. *Br J Obstet Gynaecol* 1989; 96:1281–1289.

Gunn A, Keddie N. Some clinical observations on patients with gallstones. *Lancet* 1972; 239–241.

Hazelrigg SR, Landreneau RJ, Boley TM, et al. The effect of muscle-sparing versus standard posterolateral thoracotomy on pulmonary function, muscle strength and postoperative pain. *J Thorac Cardiovasc Surg* 1991; 101:394–401.

Ivens D, Hoe AL, Podd TJ, et al. Assesssment of morbidity from complete axillary dissection. *Br J Cancer* 1992; 66:136–138.

Jacobs SA, Blumenthal NJ. Endometrial resection follow-up: late onset of pain and the effect of depot medroxyprogesterone acetate. *Br J Obstet Gynaecol* 1994; 101:605–609.

Johnsson R, Thorngren KG. Function after total hip replacement for primary osteoarthritis. *Int Orthop* 1989; 13:221–225.

Kalso E, Perttunen K, Kaasinen S. Pain after thoracic surgery. *Acta Anaesthesiol Scand* 1992; 36:96–100.

Katz J, Jackson M, Kavanagh BP, Sandler AN. Acute pain after thoracic surgery predicts long-term post-thoracotomy pain. *Clin J Pain* 1996; 12:50–55.

Keller SM, Carp NZ, Levy MN, Rosen SM. Chronic post thoracotomy pain. *J Card Surg* 1994; 35:161–164.

Kroner K, Krebs B, Skov J, Jorgenson HS. Immediate and long-term phantom breast syndrome after mastectomy: incidence, clinical characteristics and relationship to pre-mastectomy breast pain. *Pain* 1989; 36:327–334.

Kroner K, Knudsen UB, Lundby L, Hvid H. Long term phantom breast syndrome after mastectomy. *Clin J Pain* 1992; 8:346–350.

Landreneau RJ, Mack MJ, Hazelrigg SR, et al. Prevalence of chronic pain after pulmonary resection by thoracotomy or video-assisted thoracic surgery. *J Thorac Cardiovasc Surg* 1994; 107:1079–1086.

Lobb WK, Zakariasen KL, McGrath PJ. Endodontic treatment outcomes: do patients perceive problems? *J Am Dent Assoc* 1996; 127:597–600.

Marbach JJ. Phantom tooth pain. *J Endod* 1978; 4:362–372.

Marbach JJ. Is phantom tooth pain a deafferentation (neuropathic) syndrome? *Oral Surg Oral Med Oral Pathol* 1993; 75:95–105.

Marbach JJ, Hulbrook J, Hohn C, Segal AG. Incidence of phantom tooth pain: an atypical facial neuralgia. *Oral Surg Oral Med Oral Pathol* 1982; 53:190–193.

Matsunaga M, Dan K, Manabe FY, et al. Residual pain of thoractomy patients with malignancy and non-malignancy. *Pain* 1990; (Suppl) 5:S148.

McMahon AJ, Buckley J, Taylor A, et al. Chronic testicular pain following vasectomy. *Br J Urol* 1992; 69:188–191.

Merskey H, Bogduk N (Eds). *Classification of Chronic Pain. Descriptions of Chronic Pain Syndromes and Definitions of Pain Terms.* Seattle: IASP Press, 1994.

Niesel T, Partin AW, Walsh PC. Anatomic approach for placement of surgical drains after radical prostatectomy: long-term effects on postoperative pain. *Urology* 1996; 48:91–94.

Nomori H, Horio H, Fuyuno G, Kobayashi R. Non-serratus-sparing antero-axillary thoracotomy with disconnection of anterior rib cartilage. *Chest* 1997; 111:572–576.

Ovesen P, Kroner K, Ornsholt J, Bach K. Phantom-related phenomena after rectal amputation: prevalence and clinical characteristics. *Pain* 1991; 44:289–291.

Paxton LD, Huss BK, Loughlin V, Mirakhur RK. Intra-vas deferens bupivacaine for prevention of acute pain and chronic discomfort after vasectomy. *Br J Anaesth* 1995; 74:612–613.

Peters JH, Ellison EC, Innes JT, et al. Safety and efficacy of laparoscopic cholecystectomy. *Ann Surg* 1991; 213:3–12.

Polinsky ML. Functional status of long-term breast cancer survivors. *Health Soc Work* 1994; 19:165–173.

Postlethwaite JC. Lumbar sympathectomy. *Br J Surg* 1973; 60:878–879.

Raskin NH, Levinson SA, Hoffman PM, Pickett JBE, Fields HL. Postsympathectomy neuralgia. *Am J Surg* 1974; 128:75–78.

Reid W, Kennedy Watt J, Gray TG. Phenol injection of the sympathetic chain. *Br J Surg* 1970; 57:45–50.

Richardson J, Sabanathan S, Mearns AJ, Sides C, Goulden CP. Post-thoracotomy neuralgia. *Pain Clinic* 1994; 7:87–97.

Ros E, Zambon D. Post-cholecystectomy symptoms. A prospective study of gall stone patients before and two years after surgery. *Gut* 1987; 28:1500–1504.

Roxburgh JC, Markland CG, Ross BA, Kerr WF. Role of cryoanalgesia in the control of pain after thoracotomy. *Thorax* 1987; 42:292–295.

Southern Surgeons Club. A prospective analysis of 1518 laparoscopic cholecystectomies. *N Engl J Med* 1991; 324:1073–1078.

Stefanini P, Carboni M, Patrassi N, et al. Factors influencing the long term results of cholecystectomy. *Surgery, Gynecology and Obstetrics* 1974; 139:734–738.

Sternbach RA. Acute versus chronic pain. In: Wall PD, Melzack R (Eds). *Textbook of Pain.* Edinburgh: Churchill Livingstone, 1984, pp 173–177.

Stevens PE, Dibble SL, Miaskowski C. Prevalence, characteristics, and impact of postmastectomy pain syndrome: an investigation of women's experiences. *Pain* 1995; 61:61–68.

Stiff G, Rhodes M, Kelly A, et al. Long-term pain: less common after laparoscopic than open cholecystectomy. *Br J Surg* 1994; 81:1368–1370.

Swanson AJG. The incidence of prepatellar neuropathy following medial meniscectomy. *Clin Orthop* 1983; 181:151–153.

Tasmuth T, von Smitten K, Hietanen P, Kataja M, Kalso E. Pain and other symptoms after different treatment modalities of breast cancer. *Ann Oncol* 1995; 6:453–459.

Turner JA, Ersek M, Herron L, et al. Patient outcomes after lumbar spinal fusions. *JAMA* 1992; 268:907–911.

Vecht CJ, Van der Brand HJ, Wajer OJM. Post-axillary dissection pain in breast cancer due to a lesion of the intercostobrachial nerve. *Pain* 1989; 38:171–176.

Wall PD. Recent advances in the knowledge of mechanisms of intractable pain. *International Disability Studies* 1987; 9:22–23.

Wallace MS, Wallace AM, Lee J, Dobke MK. Pain after breast surgery: a survey of 282 women. *Pain* 1996; 66:195–205.

Watson CPN, Evans RJ, Watt VR. The post-mastectomy pain syndrome and the effects of topical capsaicin. *Pain* 1989; 38:177–186.

Wheelan JB. Long-term results of colposuspension. *Br J Urol* 1990; 65:329–332.

Wilson RG, Macintyre IMC. Symptomatic outcome after laparoscopic cholecystectomy. *Br J Surg* 1993; 80:439–441.

Woolf CJ, Walters ET. Common patterns of plasticity contributing to nociceptive sensitization in mammals and Aplysia. *Trends Neurosci* 1991; 14:74–78.

Working Group of the National Medical Advisory Committee. *The Management of Patients with Chronic Pain*. HMSO, 1994.

Correspondence to: William Andrew Macrae, MB ChB, FRCA, Department of Anaesthesia, University of Dundee, Ninewells Hospital and Medical School, Dundee, DD1 9SY, United Kingdom. Email: w.a.macrae @dundee.ac.uk.

Epidemiology of Pain, edited by
I.K. Crombie, IASP Press, Seattle, © 1999.

11

Phantom Limb Pain

Donna A.K. Kalauokalani[a,b,d] and John D. Loeser[a,c,d]

Departments of [a]Anesthesiology, [b]Health Services, and [c]Neurological Surgery, and [d]Multidisciplinary Pain Center, University of Washington, Seattle, Washington, USA

Phantom limb pain is a well-recognized problem in the amputee population. Reports of prevalence range from 0% to 100% (De Gutierrez-Mahoney 1948; Cronholm 1951; Solonen 1962; Carlen et al. 1978; Sherman and Sherman 1983; Jensen and Rasmussen 1994). This chapter reviews information on the epidemiology of phantom limb pain and highlights what is known and not known about the incidence and prevalence of this perplexing problem. Such a review may offer insight into how our knowledge and understanding can be refined through further investigation and serve as foundation for allocation of resources for further research.

DEFINITION AND DIAGNOSTIC CRITERIA

It is essential to distinguish between phantom limb sensation, phantom limb pain, and stump pain because they are distinct in character and may represent different underlying mechanisms. In preparing this chapter we considered only studies that explicitly demonstrated some distinction between these entities.

Phantom limb sensations are a variety of sensory phenomena including the perception that the limb is present. Often the limb is perceived to be foreshortened, distorted in position, or movable with conscious thought. Variable over time, the phantom sensation may consist of kinesthetic, kinematic, or paresthetic sensations, may telescope into the stump, or fade away (Haber 1956). Reports indicate that patients' attitudes toward phantom sensations range from bothersome to inconsequential to helpful in ambulating.

Stump pain refers to pain perceived in the region of the amputation at the location of existing body parts. It may be associated with poor wound healing, ischemia, inadequate prosthesis fit, or palpable neuromata.

Phantom limb pain refers to pain perceived in the absent body part. As with phantom sensations, phantom pain may occur in varying frequency, duration, and intensity over time. Phantom limb pain was described as early as the middle of the 16th century by the great military surgeon Ambroise Paré (Price and Twombly 1972). The term "phantom limb pain" was introduced by S. Weir Mitchell (1872), based on his experiences and observations during the American Civil War. Since then, phantom phenomena have attracted the attention of researchers from several disciplines. Unfortunately, early investigators did not discriminate between phantom pain, phantom sensations, and stump pain, so ambiguity hinders interpretation of their results.

The phenomena of phantom sensations and phantom pain are not unique to the limbs. Simmel (1966) reports that the loss of a breast may result in phantom breast sensations in 95% of patients and suggests that the occurrence is nearly as predictable as phantom sensations following amputation of extremities. Several series of mastectomies report a 25% occurrence of phantom breast sensations, 50% of which are painful (Weinstein et al. 1970; Jamison et al. 1979; Staps et al. 1985; Kroner et al. 1989). What is not clear is whether these studies used the methods advocated by Simmel (1966) to achieve optimal conditions for data collection. The extent to which the conditions for data collection are responsible for the relative discrepancies between studies remains unclear. We are also

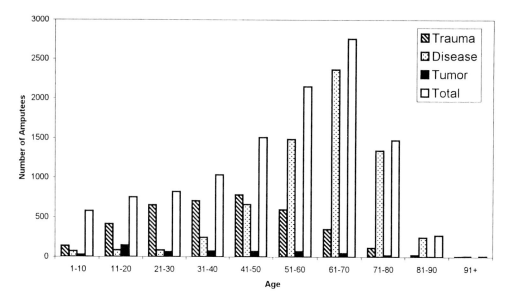

Fig. 1. Age and cause for amputation among 12,000 amputees receiving prosthetic fitting in the United States (adapted from Glattly 1964).

aware of case reports of phantom sensations following the removal of body parts such as eyeball, nose, teeth, tongue, penis, rectum, and others (Heusner 1950; Weinstein 1968; Hanowell and Kennedy 1979; Ovesen et al. 1991). Apart from case reports, no epidemiological data are available to describe pain syndromes specific to these situations. Other than to note that phantom pain can be found following the loss of many body parts, we will consider only phantom limb pain in this chapter; postsurgical pain is addressed in Chapter 10.

Meaningful assessment of the epidemiological data on phantom limb pain requires that we understand the prevalence of amputation in the population, as amputees define the population at risk for this condition. Furthermore, we must consider the frequency of amputation and the reasons for amputation when comparing the prevalence rates of phantom pain in different populations. Therefore, the first part of this chapter describes what is known of the incidence and reasons for amputation. The descriptive epidemiology of phantom limb pain that follows can then be put into the context of the relative burden of amputation on the general population.

AMPUTATION

In 1961–1963 Glattly (1964) surveyed 12,000 new amputees receiving prosthetic fitting in the United States and found a male to female ratio of 3.3:1. Most amputations were of the lower extremity (85.4%).

Causes of amputation were limited to four categories: trauma (amputations due to physical and thermal injuries), disease (amputations due to vascular disease and infections), tumor (all types of growths for which an amputation is performed), and congenital (those fitted with a prosthesis). Most amputations were attributed to disease (male, 54.7%; female, 69.9%), followed by trauma (male, 39.2%; female, 13.6%), tumor (male, 3.3%; female, 8.9%), then congenital (male, 2.8%; female, 7.6%). Fig. 1 shows the relative numbers of amputations by age and cause as reported in this survey.

The source sample for Glattly's survey was based on data collection at U.S. prosthetic service departments, and the results refer only to amputees who sought prosthetic fittings. The disparity between percentages of males and females and the percentage of amputees over age 65 must be interpreted in the context of Bureau of Vocational Rehabilitation policies of the early sixties. Some states accepted as beneficiaries only those who were employable and arbitrarily established age limits at 60 to 65; some states did not accept housewives as legitimate beneficiaries. Hence, the apparent proportion of amputations in older men may, at least in part, be due to these attendant biases.

In the attempt to detect significant differences in population trends over the ensuing decade, Kay and Newman (1974) repeated Glattly's survey. A series half the size of Glattly's (6000 amputees) showed only minor differences in distribution patterns with regard to gender and cause of amputation, including a slightly higher proportion of women (28% vs. 23%). The per-

Table I
Ethnic differences in crude population rates of lower extremity amputation

	Rate of Amputation*		
	American Indians	Caucasians	References
Diabetes mellitus	1280[a] (1972–1989)	376[b] (1978–1991)	a) Nelson et al. 1988; Moss et al. 1992; Farrell et al. 1993; Lee et al. 1993; Rith-Najarian et al. 1993; Valway et al. 1993
			b) Most and Sinnock 1983; Waugh 1988; Deerochanawong et al. 1992; Lawee and Csima 1992; Gujral et al. 1993; Siitonen et al. 1993
No diabetes mellitus	220[c]† (1972–1984)	23[d] (1978–1985)	c) Nelson et al. 1988
			d) Most and Sinnock 1983; Pohjolainen and Alaranta 1988; Kald et al. 1989; Jones 1990; Gujral et al. 1993; Siitonen et al. 1993

* Rates are reported as number of cases per 10^5 individuals per year. Rate estimates were obtained by averaging crude rates reported in cited references (denoted by superscript letters). Years in parentheses are cumulative time periods for all studies used to calculate given rates.
† Rate was reported for "general population" and may include persons with diabetes.

centage of amputations deriving from trauma was slightly lower, while the reverse was true for disease-related amputation (Kay and Newman 1975).

Many subsequent smaller surveys have looked at the distribution of subgroups of amputees in the United States and other countries. Amputees with diabetes mellitus have been a primary focus (Most and Sinnock 1983; Bild et al. 1989; Ebskov 1991; Moss et al. 1992; Siitonen et al. 1993). Interestingly, diabetic studies conducted around the world have elucidated ethnic differences in rates of lower extremity amputation that are not solely attributable to differences in disease incidences (Gujral et al. 1993). Table I summarizes the crude rates of amputation among diabetics and nondiabetics in different ethnic groups. The 17-fold difference in the relative rates of amputation in Caucasians emphasizes that diabetics face substantially increased risk for amputation. Even more compelling, though, is the comparison of amputation rates in diabetics across different racial groups. Indians with diabetes are 3.4 times more likely to have an amputation of a lower extremity than are whites with diabetes. This finding suggests that other factors influence amputation apart from the disease state. More information is necessary to allow adjustment for socioeconomic status and health service factors.

SEARCH STRATEGY

Literature review began with a computerized MEDLINE search using the terms phantom limb, prevalence, incidence, amputation, amputation-stumps, amputation-traumatic, amputees, limb, extremity, foot, leg, hand, and arm. The search included articles published between 1966 and 1996. We scanned reference lists of retrieved articles, reference textbooks (Bonica 1990; Wall and Melzack 1994), and personal reprint files for additional reports not identified in the MEDLINE search. We included studies published in English whose primary purpose was the assessment of prevalence and excluded case reports; letters to the editor; editorials; studies that lacked original data, an analysis of treatment strategy, or a method of distinguishing between phantom limb pain, phantom sensations, and stump pain; and studies that did not focus on limb amputees.

PREVALENCE OF PHANTOM LIMB PAIN

In the last two decades 10 studies have specifically described the prevalence of phantom limb pain among amputees. Studies that demonstrated some attempt to distinguish phantom limb pain from phantom sensations or stump pain are summarized in Table II.

Only three investigators included point estimates at different follow-up times in their studies to assess changes in prevalence rates of phantom limb pain over time. Retention of subjects was an issue in all these studies due to death or other unspecified causes. Pohjolainen (1991) studied 155 consecutive referrals to a prosthetic factory by physical exams and interviews at the time of prosthetic fitting and 1 year after

Table II
Summary of phantom limb pain point prevalence estimates

Sampling Method	Sample Source	Sample Size	Features Assessed	Observation Period (Time after Amputation)	Prevalence			Reference
					PLP	SP	PS	
Interview	Soldiers injured in October 1973 war	73 (18 UE, 55 LE)	N/A	Single interview at 1–6 mo (see Steinbach et al. 1982)	67%	43%	100%	Carlen et al. 1978
Interview	War veteran traumatic amputees	42 of 73 survivors	Frequency of PLP	5 y after amputation (follow-up from Carlen et al. 1978)	72.5% (constant 7.5%, occasional 45%, frequent 20%)		85.7%	Steinbach et al. 1982
Questionnaire	Members of National Amputation Foundation	764 of 1321 members	0–100 scale (mean 68.7 ± 29.99)	Single questionnaire at variable times; no follow-up	85%			Sherman et al. 1983
Questionnaire	5000 military amputees	2694	0–10 scale	Single questionnaire at variable times; no follow-up	78%	62%	99.9%	Sherman 1984
Exam and interview	Adult amputees at university affiliated hospitals during 2 y	58 (51 at 6 mo [7 deaths]; 34 at 2 y)	N/A; pain character descriptions given	Pre-amputation pain: 98% / 8 d after amputation / 6 mo after amputation / 2 y after amputation	72% / 67% / 59%	57% / 22% / 21%	84% / 90% / 71%	Jensen et al. 1983, 1985
Interview	624 adult amputees during 1970–1977	86 of 95 living in 1983 (9 excluded for dementia)	N/A	Median time since amputation: 7.2 y	52.3%	23.3%	76.7%	Krebs et al. 1985
Interview	Amputees using Canadian prosthetic facilities 1979–1980	716	N/A	No follow-up	62.4%		84.1%	Buchanan and Mandel 1986
Exam and interview	LE amputees (consecutive referrals to prosthetic factory)	155 (124 at 1 y)	Mild, moderate, or severe pain	16 wk after amputation / 1 y after amputation	59% Mild 73% Mod. 27% Sev. 0% / 53% Mild 70% Mod. 30% Sev. 0%	5% Mild 72% Mod. 14% Sev. 14% / 6% Mild 57% Mod. 43% Sev. 0%	41% Mild 84% Mod. 16% Sev. 0% / 18% Mild 86% Mod. 14% Sev. 0%	Pohjolainen 1991
Questionnaire	338 LE amputees at single center	176 of 212 replies	Pain scores by recall (0–10 scale) medians reported	Single questionnaire at variable times; no follow-up	78%		82%	Houghton et al. 1994
Questionnaire and Medical Record Review	54 children (age 5–19) amputees 1980–1990	24	Pain intensity since onset assessed by recall	Single questionnaire at variable times; no follow-up	83%		100%	Krane and Heller 1995

Abbreviations: LE = lower extremity; N/A = not assessed; PLP = phantom limb pain; PS = phantom sensations; SP = stump pain; UE = upper extremity.

amputation. Notably, 20% of the original sample was lost to follow-up at 1 year. This study uses exams and interviews to characterize the severity of pain (mild, moderate, severe) at 16 weeks and 1 year following amputation.

In contrast, Steinbach and colleagues (1982) characterize the duration of pain symptoms (constant, frequent, occasional, or never) as part of their interview process. At 5 years following amputation only 42 (58%) of the sample of war veterans, originally identified and reported by Carlen et al. (1978), were alive and available to interview. Phantom limb pain was present in 72.5% compared with 67% within 6 months following amputation (Carlen et al. 1978). Carlen et al. (1978) and Jensen et al. (1985) provide lists of terms used to describe phantom pain symptoms. In Jensen's series, nearly all patients having amputations within the same 2-year time period had pre-amputation pain (98%). The prevalence of phantom limb pain was 72% at 8 days, 65% at 6 months, and 59% at 2 years.

To summarize the estimates drawn from these studies that incorporated follow-up, it appears that the prevalence of phantom limb pain ranges between 53% and 72% and remains relatively constant for at least 5 years. It is worth noting the relatively small numbers of subjects from which these estimates are made. In addition, the prevalence rates given are group rates and do not reflect the potential variability among individuals. These studies do not present data for individuals, so the findings cannot be analyzed further. The degree to which an individual's pain varies over time has not been studied.

Other investigators made single observations without structured follow-up. The largest of the surveys were conducted by Sherman et al. in 1983 ($n = 764$) and by Sherman in 1984 ($n = 2694$), and reported prevalence rates for phantom limb pain to be 85% and 78%, respectively. These estimates are slightly higher than those reported in the prospective studies. Participants in both surveys varied widely in time since amputation. Potential bias was introduced into these surveys; respondents (58% in 1983 and 54% in 1984) to a survey about phantom symptoms were more likely to be those who were actually experiencing symptoms, and respondents to a survey based on a Veteran's Affairs Medical Center questionnaire may have perceived that eligibility for future services might be contingent on a positive response.

Similarly, Houghton and colleagues (1994) achieved a response rate of 52% to their questionnaire mailed to a group of lower extremity amputees all under the care at the same facility, and reported the prevalence of phantom limb pain to be 78%. Variation in the time since amputation ranged from 7 to 10 years. Subjects were asked to recall pain scores at specified times ranging from immediately post-surgery to 5 years after the amputation. Obviously, a study based on subjective recall, particularly over a 10-year period, is not optimal for studying the natural history of any disease. Moreover, little evidence supports the allegation that phantom limb pain usually improves with time.

Krane and Heller (1995) administered a similar questionnaire to a series of pediatric amputees. They also relied on subject recall for the time of onset since amputation and comparative intensities of phantom limb pain between the time of onset and the time of the interview. They received a response rate of 57% and reported the prevalence of phantom limb pain in this patient group to be 83%.

The remaining two studies were based on personal contact interviews. Buchanan and Mandel (1986) used a sample population similar to Glattly's (1964) in that he studied amputees using prosthetic service departments across Canada. He reports the prevalence of phantom limb pain among this patient population to be 62.4%. In 1983, Krebs (1985) interviewed all survivors of a cohort who had amputations during 1970–1977 (median age at the time of amputation was 60 years) and reported a 52.3% prevalence of phantom limb pain in the survivors (15% of the 624 amputees).

EXPLANATIONS FOR DISPARITY IN REPORTED PREVALENCE

Several explanations alone or in combination may account for the disparity in reported prevalence of phantom limb pain: disagreement in classification among investigators (Stannard 1993); misclassification by investigators when interpreting subjective reports; differences in methods of ascertaining the presence of pain (Sherman et al. 1980); and failure to recognize the temporal relationship of symptoms to the time of amputation (Jensen et al. 1985). Because the method of ascertaining symptoms can affect the results, we excluded studies that did not collect information about pain symptoms as the primary purpose of the study.

Furthermore, difficulties in eliciting information about phantom pain and sensations apart from those inherent in the processing of that information (i.e., interpretation and communication) make it important to consider studies that incorporate the collection of such data as a primary objective. For example, Persson and Liedberg (1983) reported that a consecutive series of 86 amputees revealed the occurrence of stump pain and phantom limb pain in 20%. This study, however, focused on stump measurement and classification and the use of a new standard data collection form developed for the International Society for Prosthetics and Orthotics. Information on stump and phantom pain were incidental to the process of systematic examinations to identify important qualities of major amputation stumps to increase the possibility for analyzing problems and correcting malfunction. In fact, the reported phantom limb pain incidence of 20% corresponds to that fraction of patients who sought treatment for pain, in contrast to a much higher proportion reporting pain symptoms in two separate series of interviewed amputees (Sherman and Sherman 1983; Sherman 1984). This finding underscores the importance of considering the methods of study design, data collection, and reporting in interpreting the results of such studies.

NATURE OF PHANTOM LIMB PAIN

Worz and Worz (1990) selected 100 amputees with phantom limb pain and determined that 68% experienced constant pain, whereas 32% described their pain as intermittent in nature. This is in contrast to Steinbach's smaller series where most patients reporting phantom limb pain described it as occasional, while a minority reported constant pain. It is unclear how these differences are related to sample size or time since amputation. Data collection techniques and differences in how classification schemes are defined for "constant," "intermittent," "frequent," or "occasional" also probably contributed to the discrepancy.

RISK FACTORS

Few data exist on risk factors for the development of phantom limb pain. Several hypotheses have been offered to explain the mechanism of phantom limb pain (Mitchell 1872; Riddoch 1941; Henderson and Smyth 1948; Cronholm 1951; Simmel 1956; Melzack 1974; Melzack and Loeser 1978). An extensive review of these theories is beyond the scope of this chapter. It is important, however, to note that the evolution of theories affected secular trends in how phantom pain was

perceived by both subjects and investigators and has, undoubtedly, affected the reporting and interpretation of symptoms. Ewalt (1947) reported phantom sensations occurring in 95% and phantom pain occurring in only 4% of a subgroup of 100 amputees (of 2284) who were considered "persons who were making a normal adjustment to their amputation." He concludes that phantom pain is merely the interpretation of a phantom sensation by certain individuals who show psychopathology. Henderson and Smyth (1948) also reported a similar prevalence of phantom pain at less than 5% among 300 prisoners of war in Germany between 1940 and 1945. The occurrence of this severe "unnatural attitude" of the phantom is considered to be psychogenically determined and distinct from the "natural phantom." We can only speculate to what degree such bias affected investigators' interpretations, and how the social stigma affected patient's reports. Given this apparent selection/investigator bias, we have focused our review on studies that have emerged in the past two decades since the theoretical advances of Melzack and Loeser (1978).

Without information on the true incidence of disease, which would require a large population-based prospective study, we cannot accurately discern attributable risks. Amputation is necessary by virtue of the definition of phantom limb; however, amputation alone is not sufficient to establish causality for phantom limb pain. Table III lists the factors considered to be associated with the development of phantom limb pain. Unfortunately, stratification of risk factors is limited by the size of the studies conducted to date. Moreover, varying styles of presenting data do not allow for even crude relative risk calculations. Based on the limited information on potential risk factors, there does not appear to be a relationship to age or gender. Preoperative pain may be a factor, but universal agreement across studies is lacking. Jensen et al. (1985) reported the association between preoperative pain with phantom limb pain at 8 days and at 6 months, but not at 2 years, which indicates that perhaps the association is also time dependent. Other factors pertinent to primary or secondary prevention may not have been systematically studied.

PRIMARY PREVENTION

Preventing the need for amputation would certainly decrease the absolute numbers of persons at risk

Table III
Phantom limb pain risk factors

Study Type and Size	Risk Factor	Association*	Reference
Cross-sectional $N = 764$	Cause for amputation	0	Sherman and Sherman 1983
	Pre-amputation interpersonal relations	0	
	Age	0	
	War served	0	
	Pre-amputation pain	0	
	Years since amputation	0	
	Prosthetic use	0	
	Site: above/below knee/elbow	0	
	Limb(s) amputated	0	
	Stump pain	$+ P < 0.05$	
Longitudinal, cross-sectional $N = 58$ at 8 d	Preoperative pain	$+ P < 0.01$	Jensen et al. 1983
Cross-sectional, correlational $N = 2694$	Age	0	Sherman 1984
	Preoperative familiarity with amputee	0	
	Cause of amputation	0	
	Pre-amputation pain	0	
	Years of pain prior to amputation	0	
	Years since amputation	0	
	Prosthesis use	0	
	Site: above/below knee/elbow	0	
	Site: upper vs. lower extremity	0	
	Stump pain	$+ P < 0.001$	
Longitudinal, cross-sectional $N = 51$ at 6 mo	Gender	0	Jensen et al. 1985
	Proximal amputation	0	
	Previous amputation	0	
	Diabetes mellitus	0	
	Pre-amputation pain <1 mo	$- P < 0.05$	
	Preoperative pain	$+ P < 0.01$	
	Stump pain	0	
	Side of amputation	0	
Longitudinal, cross-sectional $N = 34$ at 2 y	Gender	0	Jensen et al. 1985
	Proximal amputation	0	
	Previous amputation	0	
	Diabetes mellitus	0	
	Pre-amputation pain <1 mo	0	
	Preoperative pain	0	
	Stump pain	$+ P < 0.05$	
	Side of amputation	0	
Cross-sectional $N = 338$	Cause of amputation: vascular vs. trauma	0	Houghton et al. 1994
	Preoperative pain	$+ P < 0.005$	
Correlational $N = 92$	Ethnicity (Caucasian)	$+ P < 0.01$	Weiss and Lindell 1996
	Clot etiology	$+ P < 0.05$	
	Non-clot diabetic	0	
	Miscellaneous circulation problems	0	
	Gangrene with/without infection	$+ P < 0.001$	
	Number of medical conditions	0	

* Direction of association: positive (+), negative (−), or none found (0); strength of association with phantom pain is indicated by P value.

for developing phantom limb pain. Furthermore, it is readily apparent that the treatment of diabetes and vascular disease is of great importance in lowering the incidence of amputation. Preventive measures in this area should target early screening for populations at risk. Given that more than half of all lower extremity amputations are performed on diabetics, with the vast majority preceded by traumatic or vascular ulceration, much effort has been focused on prevention in this group. Several studies have suggested that a multidisciplinary and multifactorial program for preventive foot care can reduce the amputation rate by more than 50% (Larsson and Apelqvist 1995). In addition, behavior modifications focusing on tobacco use, nutrition, and exercise and on early treatment of vascular foot lesions potentially can reduce the number of amputees (Reiber 1996). It is yet unclear what role these factors play on the risk of developing phantom limb pain subsequent to amputation.

Kegel and colleagues (1977) emphasized the need for disseminating information and improved communication between hospital staff and patients prior to amputation based on his survey of lower-limb amputees. Specifically, patients felt they should have been warned of the likely or possible sequelae to the amputation (e.g., possible complications from surgery, persistence of peripheral vascular disease, physical and mental fatigue, societal reactions and the "handicapped" label, anticipated difficulties with restaurant seating, prosthesis fitting, and complications such as the loss of suction when doing twisting actions) and that phantom sensations are normal.

Continuing investigations are examining the role of preemptive measures in the anesthetic preparation of patients undergoing amputation so as to reduce risk of developing phantom limb pain. These investigations vary in the interventions employed and in the imputed etiology upon which the hypothesis for the intervention is based. In addition, the selected outcome measure may not be in the pathway of the intervention's effect or may be insensitive to its effect (Fleming and DeMets 1996). Such methodological concerns have made comparison across "preemptive" studies difficult.

SECONDARY PREVENTION

Abramson and Feibel (1981) presented compelling support for prevention of phantom limb pain by early counseling intervention and aggressive enhancement of function. They found that less than 2% of patients in a series of 2000 amputees over 10 years developed phantom limb pain. Steinbach et al.'s (1982) observation that the percentage of amputees complaining of pain was greater when the artificial limb was received more than 7 months post-surgery supports Abramson's active rehabilitative approach to reducing the risk of phantom limb pain. Though Abramson's study reports a prevalence that is suspiciously low, no

other study has rigorously evaluated the effects of psychosocial and rehabilitative interventions to affirm or refute such suspicion. Such a study would require care to separate investigators from providers to avoid reporting bias due to perceived threat to the provider-patient relationship.

Other behavioral factors such as use of tobacco, alcohol, and caffeine have not been studied as potential risk factors for developing phantom pain. Behavioral factors may influence the level of amputation (Stewart 1987). In addition, it is unclear how certain behaviors potentially augment or ameliorate the abnormal vascular response following amputation (Backman et al. 1991). Other physiologic or genetic factors have yet to be explored. Recent animal and human studies have evaluated the relationship between resting blood pressure and threshold to noxious stimuli (Stewart and France 1996). This line of investigation may also have implication for amputees, given the possible role of vascular responsiveness in the manifestation and maintenance of pain.

FUTURE CHALLENGES

Questions about the natural history of phantom limb pain, who gets it, when it occurs, and how it changes over time, need to be studied prospectively with periodic follow-up. Prevalence estimates from the literature ranging from 0 to 100% are not helpful to the physician advising a patient of the risk of developing phantom limb pain, nor do they clarify the burden of the problem to society so that appropriate resources for research and treatment can be made available.

If predisposing risk factors are to be elucidated, at least some of the data collection (particularly behavioral factors) needs to predate the amputation to avoid recall bias. What we know about potential risk factors is limited and poses a great challenge to future research. What is compelling about the collective table of risk factors we have synthesized is what is absent from the list. Risk factors that may potentially influence vascular pathology such as smoking, hypertension, cholesterol, and glycosylated hemoglobin have yet to be considered. Investigators reporting on potential risk factors should do so to allow independent analysis and comparisons by others.

A large sample size and multivariate analysis are necessary to detect differences among subgroups of amputees. Such a study would require multicenter participation much like the global effort proposed by the Lower Extremity Amputation Study Group (1995). Attention to specific study design issues to address the posed question(s) including adherence to standard definitions, procedural protocols, methods of data collection, and quality control is paramount. Furthermore, when comparing prevalence rates of phantom limb pain in different populations, the frequency of and reasons for amputation must be taken into account.

In addition to understanding the natural history of phantom limb pain, there are at least two related outstanding issues. First, there is the issue of testing for plausible cause(s) of phantom pain. The literature includes more than a century of observations of phantom limb pain among amputees. Several investigators attempt to analyze characteristics that distinguish affected from unaffected persons. The findings of such studies generally guide the formation of inferences as to which of these characteristics, or other unmeasured ones, play a role in causing phantom limb pain, i.e., the influence of certain risk factors. Unfortunately, the failure of authors to report data in a way that allows an independent observer to validate conclusions or to combine similar findings across studies has been an obstacle in the advancement of our knowledge. A second issue is treatment of phantom limb pain. Given a multitude of possible though unsubstantiated causes, clinical trials designed to evaluate the efficacy of interventions for phantom limb pain or its prevention do so with varying assumptions of the underlying causal mechanism. When these assumptions are not explicitly stated, results from such trials are often confusing or contradictory.

Ideally, assessing the occurrence of phantom limb pain among amputees would involve frequent monitoring for symptoms following amputation that continued indefinitely. The advantages of this approach would be a decrease in recall error and the opportunity to assess an individual's changes in the prevalence of phantom limb pain. Cross-sectional studies are subject to selection bias due to differential survival (or completeness of follow-up) and the reason for entry into the study (e.g., fitting for prosthesis).

Historically, investigators often attempted to answer multiple questions concurrently and, as a result, compromised the strength of their study designs to answer any question. Such an attempt is often accompanied by failure to minimize foreseeable biases. With careful attention to the design and implementation of clinical trials, meaningful information can be presented

and used along with other such studies to guide the progressive advancement of understanding this complex phenomenon. It is critical to recognize the importance of adequate sample size when assessing treatment outcomes (Weiss 1996).

Continued interdisciplinary contributions among the fields of physical medicine, internal medicine, neurosurgery, anesthesia, surgery, physical therapy, and prosthetic manufacture are necessary. Potential areas for further investigation include establishing a plausible role for vasoactivity (i.e., use of vasoactive agents during amputation), cortical reorganization associated with amputation and its implications for therapy, experiences of individuals with congenitally absent limbs, and randomized clinical trials of aggressive rehabilitation as described by Abramson and Feibel (1981). This list of suggestions is not intended to be exhaustive. There is yet much to learn about this perplexing and painful problem.

REFERENCES

Abramson AS, Feibel A. The phantom phenomenon: its use and disuse. *Bull N Y Acad Med* 1981; 57(2):99–112.

Backman C, Nystrom A. Cold-induced arterial spasm after digital amputation. *J Hand Surg Br* 1991; 16(4):378–381.

Bild DE, Selby JV, Sinnock P, et al. Lower-extremity amputation in people with diabetes. Epidemiology and prevention. *Diabetes Care* 1989; 12(1):24–31.

Bonica JJ. *The Management of Pain,* 2nd ed. Philadelphia: Lea and Febiger, 1990.

Buchanan DC, Mandel AR. The prevalence of phantom limb experience in amputees. *Rehabilitation Psychology* 1986; 31(3):183–188.

Carlen PL, Wall PD, Nadvorna H, Steinbach T. Phantom limbs and related phenomena in recent traumatic amputations. *Neurology* 1978; 28:211–217.

Cronholm B. Phantom limbs in amputees. *Acta Psychiatr Scand* (Suppl) 1951; 72:1–310.

Deerochanawong C, Home PD, Alberti KG. A survey of lower limb amputation in diabetic patients. *Diab Med* 1992; 9:942–946.

De Gutierrez-Mahoney CG. The treatment of painful phantom limb. *Surg Clin North Am* 1948; 28:481–483.

Ebskov LB. Epidemiology of lower limb amputations in diabetics in Denmark (1980 to 1989). *Int Orthop* 1991; 15(4):285–288.

Ewalt JR. The phantom limb. *Psychosom Med* 1947; 9:118–123.

Farrell MA, Quiggins PA, Eller JD, et al. Prevalence of diabetes and its complications in the eastern band of Cherokee Indians. *Diabetes Care* 1993; 16(1):253–256.

Fleming TR, DeMets DL. Surrogate end points in clinical trials: are we being misled? *Ann Intern Med* 1996; 125(7):605–613.

Glattly HW. A statistical study of 12,000 new amputees. *South Med J* 1964; 57:1373–1378.

Gujral JS, McNally PG, O'Malley BP, Burden AC. Ethnic differences in the incidence of lower extremity amputation secondary to diabetes mellitus. *Diabet Med* 1993; 10(3):271–274.

Haber WB. Observations on phantom limb phenomena. *Arch*

Neurol Psychiatry 1956; 75:624–636.

Hanowell ST, Kennedy SF. Phantom tongue pain and causalgia: case presentation and treatment. *Anesth Analg* 1979; 58(5):436–438.

Henderson WR, Smyth GE. Phantom limbs. *J Neurol Neurosurg Psychiatry* 1948; 11:88–112.

Heusner AP. Phantom genitalia. *Trans Am Neurol Assoc* 1950; 75:128–134.

Houghton AD, Nicholls G, Houghton AL, Saadah E, McColl L. Phantom pain: natural history and association with rehabilitation. *Ann R Coll Surg Engl 1994*; 76(1):22–25.

Jamison K, Wellisch DK, Katz RL, Pasnau RO. Phantom breast syndrome. *Arch Surg* 1979; 114(1):93–95.

Jensen TS, Rasmussen P. Phantom pain and other phenomena after amputation. In: Wall PD, Melzack R (Eds). *Textbook of Pain.* New York: Churchill Livingstone, 1994, pp 651–665.

Jensen TS, Krebs B, Nielsen J, Rasmussen P. Phantom limb, phantom pain and stump pain in amputees during the first 6 months following limb amputation. *Pain* 1983; 17(3):243–256.

Jensen TS, Krebs B, Nielsen J, Rasmussen P. Immediate and long-term phantom limb pain in amputees: incidence, clinical characteristics and relationship to pre-amputation limb pain. *Pain* 1985; 21(3):267–278.

Jones LE. Lower limb amputation in three Australian states. *Int Disabil Stud* 1990; 12(1):37–40.

Kald A, Carlsson R, Nilsson E. Major amputation in a defined population: incidence, mortality and results of treatment. *Br J Surg* 1989; 76(3):308–310.

Kay HW, Newman JD. Amputee survey, 1973–74: preliminary findings and comparisons. *Orthotics and Prosthetics* 1974; 28(2):27–32.

Kay HW, Newman JD. Relative incidences of new amputations. *Orthotics and Prosthetics* 1975; 29(2):3–16.

Kegel B, Carpenter ML, Burgess EM. A survey of lower-limb amputees: prostheses, phantom sensations, and psychological aspects. *Bull Prosthetics Research* 1977; 10(27):43–60.

Krane EJ, Heller LB. The prevalence of phantom sensation and pain in pediatric amputees. *J Pain Symptom Manage* 1995; 10(1):21–29.

Krebs B, Jensen TS, Kroner K, Nielsen J, Jorgensen HS. Phantom limb phenomena in amputees 7 years after limb amputation. In: Fields HL, Dubner R, Cervero F (Eds). *Advances in Pain Research and Therapy.* Vol. 9. New York: Raven Press, 1985, pp 425–429.

Kroner K, Krebs B, Skov J, Jorgensen HS. Immediate and long-term phantom breast syndrome after mastectomy: incidence, clinical characteristics and relationship to pre-mastectomy breast pain. *Pain* 1989; 36(3):327–334.

Larsson J, Apelqvist J. Towards less amputations in diabetic patients. Incidence, causes, cost, treatment, and prevention—a review. *Acta Orthop Scand* 1995; 66(2):181–192.

Lawee D, Csima A. Diabetes-related lower extremity amputations in Ontario: 1987–88 experience. *Can J Public Health* 1992; 83(4):298–302.

Lee JS, Lu M, Lee VS, et al. Lower-extremity amputation. Incidence, risk factors, and mortality in the Oklahoma Indian Diabetes Study. *Diabetes* 1993; 42(6):876–882.

Lower Extremity Amputation Study Group. Comparing the incidence of lower extremity amputations across the world: the global lower extremity amputation study. *Diabet Med* 1995; 12:14–18.

Melzack R. Central neural mechanisms in phantom limb pain. *Adv Neurol* 1974; 4:319–326.

Melzack R, Loeser JD. Phantom body pain in paraplegics: evidence for a central pattern generating mechanism for pain.

Pain 1978; 4(3):195–210.

Mitchell SW. *Injuries of Nerves and Their Consequences.* Philadelphia: J.B. Lippincott, 1872.

Moss SE, Klein R, Klein BE. The prevalence and incidence of lower extremity amputation in a diabetic population. *Arch Intern Med* 1992; 152(3):610–616.

Most RS, Sinnock P. The epidemiology of lower extremity amputations in diabetic individuals. *Diabetes Care* 1983; 6(1):87–91.

Nelson RG, Gohdes DM, Everhart JE, et al. Lower-extremity amputations in NIDDM. 12-yr follow-up study in Pima Indians. *Diabetes Care* 1988; 11(1):8–16.

Ovesen P, Kroner K, Ornsholt J, Bach K. Phantom-related phenomena after rectal amputation: prevalence and clinical characteristics. *Pain* 1991; 44(3):289–291.

Persson BM, Liedberg E. A clinical standard of stump measurement and classification in lower limb amputees. *Prosthet Orthot Int* 1983; 7(1):17–24.

Pohjolainen T. A clinical evaluation of stumps in lower limb amputees. *Prosthet Orthot Int* 1991; 15(3):178–184.

Pohjolainen T, Alaranta H. Lower limb amputations in southern Finland 1984–1985. *Prosthet Orthot Int* 1988; 12(1):9–18.

Price DD, Twombly SJ. *The Phantom Limb: An 18th Century Latin Dissertation* [text and translation with a medical-historical and linguistic commentary]. Washington, DC: Georgetown University Press, 1972.

Reiber GE. The epidemiology of diabetic foot problems. *Diabet Med* 1996; 1:S6–11.

Riddoch G. Phantom limbs and body shape. *Brain* 1941; 64(4):197–222.

Rith-Najarian SJ, Valway SE, Gohdes DM. Diabetes in a Northern Minnesota Chippewa Tribe. Prevalence and incidence of diabetes and incidence of major complications, 1986–1988. *Diabetes Care* 1993; 16(1):266–270.

Sherman RA. Chronic phantom and stump pain among American veterans: results of a survey. *Pain* 1984; 18:83–95.

Sherman RA, Sherman CJ. Prevalence and characteristics of chronic phantom limb pain among American veterans. Results of a trial survey. *Am J Phys Med Rehab* 1983; 62(5):227–238.

Sherman RA, Sherman CJ, Gall NG. A survey of current phantom limb pain treatment in the United States. *Pain* 1980; 8(1):85–99.

Siitonen OI, Niskanen LK, Laakso M, Siitonen JT, Pyorala K. Lower-extremity amputations in diabetic and nondiabetic patients. A population-based study in eastern Finland. *Diabetes Care* 1993; 16(1):16–20.

Simmel ML. On phantom limbs. *Arch Neurol Psychiatry* 1956; 75:637–647.

Simmel ML. A study of phantoms after amputation of the breast. *Neuropsychologia* 1966; 4:331–350.

Solonen KA. The phantom phenomenon in amputated Finnish war veterans. *Acta Orthop Scand* 1962; (Suppl) 54:7–37.

Stannard CF. Phantom limb pain [see comments]. *Br J Hosp Med* 1993; 50(10):583–584.

Staps T, Hoogenhout J, Wobbes T. Phantom breast sensations following mastectomy. *Cancer* 1985; 56(12):2898–2901.

Steinbach TV, Nadvorna H, Arazi D. A five year follow-up study of phantom limb pain in post traumatic amputees. *Scand J Rehabil Med* 1982; 14(4):203–207.

Stewart CP. The influence of smoking on the level of lower limb amputation. *Prosthet Orthot Int* 1987; 11(3):113–116.

Stewart KM, France CR. Resting systolic blood pressure, parental history of hypertension, and sensitivity to noxious stimuli. *Pain* 1996; 68(2,3):369–374.

Valway SE, Linkins RW, Gohdes DM. Epidemiology of lower-extremity amputations in the Indian Health Service, 1982–1987. *Diabetes Care* 1993; 16(1):349–353.

Wall PD, Melzack R. (Eds). *Textbook of Pain*, 3rd ed. New York: Churchill Livingstone, 1994.

Waugh NR. Amputations in diabetic patients—a review of rates, relative risks and resource use. *Community Med* 1988; 10(4):279–288.

Weinstein S. Phantoms following orchiectomy. *Neuropsychologia* 1968; 6:61–63.

Weinstein S, Vetter RJ, Sersen EA. Phantoms following breast amputation. *Neuropsychologia* 1970; 8(2):185–197.

Weiss NS. *Clinical Epidemiology: the Study of the Outcome of Illness.* New York: Oxford University Press, 1996.

Weiss SA, Lindell B. Phantom limb pain and etiology of amputation in unilateral lower extremity amputees. *J Pain Symptom Manage* 1996; 11(1):3–17.

Worz R, Worz E. Pain syndromes following amputation. Analysis of 100 affected patients with chronic stump and phantom pain. (In German.) *Fortschr Med* 1990; 108(4):53–65.

Correspondence to: John D. Loeser, MD, Multidisciplinary Pain Center, 4245 Roosevelt Way NE, Seattle, WA 98105, USA. Tel: 206-548-4429; Fax: 206-548-8776; email: jdloeser@u.washington.edu.

Epidemiology of Pain, edited by
I.K. Crombie, IASP Press, Seattle, © 1999.

12

Central Post-Stroke Pain

Karsten Vestergaard,[a] Grethe Andersen,[b] and Troels S. Jensen[b]

[a]*Department of Neurology, Aalborg Hospital, Aalborg, Denmark; and*
[b]*Department of Neurology, Aarhus University Hospital, Aarhus, Denmark*

Central pain following a stroke, previously termed thalamic pain syndrome, is a severe chronic pain condition that constitutes a major burden for those afflicted. While our knowledge of symptoms and signs has improved since the syndrome was first defined at the beginning of the 20th century, we know little about the incidence and prevalence of this and other central pain conditions because epidemiological studies are few or nonexistent. This chapter reviews all relevant studies on central post-stroke pain and highlights the need for further prospective epidemiological studies.

METHODS

We performed a literature search using MEDLINE 1963–1998. A search using the key words central post-stroke pain, post-stroke pain, and thalamic syndrome identified 67 papers. We performed a further search among the selected papers using the key words incidence, prevalence, survey, cohort, prospective, retrospective, case-control, etiology, and aetiology and found 14 papers suitable for review.

DEFINITION

In the classic description by Dejerine and Roussy (1906), "thalamic syndrome" was caused by thalamic lesions and included slight hemiplegia, sensory abnormalities, hemiataxia, hemiastereognosis, choreoathetoid movements, and severe pain. Since then it has become clear that lesions at other sites of the somatosensory pathway can give rise to similar pain symptoms (Leijon et al. 1989; Lewis-Jones et al. 1990;

Vestergaard et al. 1995). Other names have been given to this condition, such as thalamic pain, central pain, and dysesthetic pain, but the most commonly accepted term for this condition is central post-stroke pain (CPSP).

Precise definition is a prerequisite for the epidemiological study of CPSP. The International Association for the Study of Pain (IASP) defined CPSP in 1986 as pain following an unequivocal stroke episode, where a psychogenic, nociceptive, or peripheral neurogenic cause is considered highly unlikely; the pain can be constant or intermittent (Merskey et al. 1986). Leijon et al. (1989) further proposed that somatosensory abnormalities should be included in the diagnostic criteria, but noted that in a few cases sensory abnormalities could not be demonstrated.

The IASP definition has been used in the most recently published studies. The definition contains no positive criteria, and in a clinical situation it might be difficult to judge whether the pain (e.g., shoulder pain) is of central or peripheral origin or both. So far, no studies have dealt with the interobserver variability of the diagnosis.

CLINICAL SIGNS

CPSP is associated with partial sensory loss. In clinical tests, sensitivity to cold, warmth, and touch (a pinprick) is abnormal in 81–94% of patients (Andersen et al. 1995; Bowsher 1996). However, quantitative sensory testing has revealed that all CPSP patients had raised detection thresholds to cold or warm stimuli, whereas few patients had altered sensory thresholds for touch (von Frey hairs) or pinprick (using argon laser tests) (Vestergaard et al. 1995). Bowsher (1996) found that all but one of 92 patients with CPSP had abnormally low responses to thermal and/or pinprick stimuli. The almost invariable loss of thermal sensation suggests that spinothalamic function is always impaired in CPSP. However, a similar loss of thermal sensation is seen in more than half of stroke patients who experience somatosensory loss without pain. The essential feature of CPSP may be evoked dysesthesia or allodynia to cutaneous stimuli, as this is present in more than 75% of CPSP patients, compared to almost no patients with sensory loss but no pain (Leijon et al. 1989; Andersen et al. 1995; Bowsher 1996). Cold stimuli evoke the dysesthetic response most frequently, so clinical testing for CPSP should include thermal response tests. Bowsher (1996) was the first to describe allodynia to movement (isotonic or isometric muscle contraction) as a unique feature of CPSP, present in 22% of patients. Further prospective studies must confirm this finding.

The severity and quality of pain vary over time in the individual patient, and can be provoked or exacerbated by factors such as cold and warmth, stress, fatigue, or exercise (Bowsher 1996). A minor injury to the skin or muscles of affected limbs may result in long-lasting and sometimes excruciating pain. One patient with CPSP was admitted to hospital with a minor crural injury that mimicked a deep venous thrombosis (Vestergaard et al., personal observation). Most CPSP patients describe a constant pain sensation, but pain episodes may be intermittent, possibly due in part to autonomic instability (Bowsher 1996). This is supported by the observation that pain is often less severe when patients are sleeping, while it is aggravated by emotional stress (Bowsher 1996). Pain is most commonly described as burning, aching, or lacerating (Leijon et al. 1989; Andersen et al. 1995; Bowsher 1996); similar descriptors are used for other central or peripheral neurogenic pain syndromes. Standards such as the McGill Pain Questionnaire (MPQ) that rely on patients' descriptions of pain may be in-

adequate to distinguish different neurogenic pain syndromes. Bowsher mentions, however, that the words "cold" or "freezing" in the MPQ are commonly used to describe CPSP (Andersen et al. 1995), but are rarely used by patients with other types of pain (Bowsher 1996).

The area of pain distribution varies from hemipain to pain in discrete parts of the body, e.g., half the face or a finger; pain intensity may vary within the total area of pain. The sensory deficit to thermal stimuli seems to be most marked in areas where the pain is most intense (Bowsher 1996). The pain is located in areas of sensory abnormality that often extend beyond the site of pain (Vestergaard et al. 1995; Bowsher 1996), which suggests that loss of sensory input is a prerequisite for CPSP. Brain stem lesions, often in the lateral medulla, may give rise to crossed pain symptoms (pain in half the face and in the contralateral body half) (Vestergaard et al. 1995; Bowsher 1996). Eye pain has also been proposed as a manifestation of CPSP (Andersen et al. 1995).

INCIDENCE AND PREVALENCE

Only one prospective epidemiological study of CPSP has been reported (Andersen et al. 1995) (Table I). The study population included 207 patients, aged 25–80 years, who survived more than 6 months after having a stroke and were followed for 1 year. The follow-up rates were 98% at 1 month, 95% at 6 months, and 97% at 12 months. By the IASP definition, the 1-year incidence of central pain was 8% (95% CI = 5–13%), of which 5% had moderate to severe pain, while 3% characterized their pain as mild and did not take any analgesic medication. The lifetime risk for developing CPSP thus seems to be more frequent than previous estimations of 0.5–2% of surviving stroke victims. It is not clear how these incidence rates were estimated, since the literature search revealed only one recent retrospective study, where the

Table I
Epidemiological studies of central post-stroke pain

Study Design	Pain Def.	Sample Size	Pain Severity	Pain Duration	Prevalence Rate	Incidence	Reference
Prospective community	IASP	207	1/3 light, 2/3 moderate or severe	> 6 mo	40/100,000	8% (5–13%)	Andersen et al. 1995; Vestergaard et al. 1995
Retrospective		400				2%	Bowsher 1993

lifetime risk was estimated to be 2% (Bowsher 1993) (Table I). Prospective studies may detect mild cases of CPSP that may otherwise be overlooked. In addition, hospital neurologists may overlook pain symptoms in severely handicapped elderly persons who do not attend rehabilitation clinics, causing an underestimation of CPSP in retrospective studies.

In the West the prevalence of stroke is 2.5 times its incidence. If we assume that CPSP is a chronic stable condition, then per 100,000 population the incidence and prevalence of stroke is 200 and 500, respectively, and the incidence of CPSP is 16 and the corresponding prevalence rate is 40.

DEMOGRAPHIC FACTORS IN PREVALENCE

The median age of the patients with central pain in the epidemiological study was 72 years, which did not differ significantly from patients without pain (Andersen et al. 1995). The median age of CSPS patients reported in other studies has been considerably younger than in unselected stroke populations (Leijon et al. 1989; Bowsher 1996). Thus, in the series reported by Bowsher the median age was 57, while in the 27 CPSP cases reported by Leijon et al. it was 67. The reason for this can be selection bias in retrospective studies and in stroke populations from rehabilitation clinics.

Incidence of CPSP does not vary by gender or by social or educational group (Andersen et al. 1995; Bowsher 1996). Differences in pain characteristics by gender have not been studied in detail, but one interesting difference has been found using the MPQ. Although no difference in pain severity was found, the number of words chosen was considerably higher in women than in men, reaching statistical significance in only 11 patients (Vestergaard et al., personal observation). This may, however, reflect a difference in the way women and men experience pain, and may not necessarily be a specific feature of CPSP.

NATURAL HISTORY

Onset of pain after stroke varies. In some patients pain occurs immediately after a stroke, and abrupt onset of left-sided pain may be mistaken for angina pectoris (Gorson et al. 1996). In most cases, however, the pain gradually increases in the first months after stroke. Median pain onset was 1 month (Leijon et al. 1989;

Andersen et al. 1995), whereas Bowsher (1996) found a median onset of 3 months using retrospective data. Leijon et al. (1989) reported pain onset as late as 2–3 years after a stroke. No studies have prospectively evaluated the duration of the pain or the variability of pain severity or pain characteristics over time.

CONSEQUENCES

Pain following a stroke is often incapacitating for the patient, and pain complaints are often more distressing than other stroke sequelae. Treatment of CPSP is still a challenge for the physician, and it is well known that this syndrome responds poorly or not at all to standard analgesics. This is not surprising, as much evidence shows that peripheral nociceptors and medullary pathways are relatively unaffected in CPSP.

RISK FACTORS

The etiology of CPSP is still unknown, but the spontaneous and evoked pain may be due to hyperexcitability of thalamic or cortical neurons that have lost part of their normal afferent input (Jensen and Lenz 1995). A prerequisite for CPSP is a spino-thalamo-cortical lesion with associated somatosensory dysfunction. The literature cannot predict which stroke patients with somatosensory dysfunction will develop CPSP. Computerized tomography (CT) scans of 16 unselected CPSP patients compared to 82 patients with somatosensory dysfunction but without pain revealed no difference in lesion type or location (Andersen et al. 1995). Magnetic resonance imaging (MRI) scans of CPSP patients have shown that at most half of the patients have lesions in the thalamus (Vestergaard et al. 1995; Bowsher 1996), and that both cortical and subcortical lesions may produce CPSP. MRI scans have detected a high number of brain stem lesions (Lewis-Jones et al. 1990; Vestergaard et al. 1995; Bowsher 1996), and in a retrospective study, MacGowan et al. (1996) found that one-third of 52 patients with lateral medullary infarction detected by MRI developed CPSP.

The distribution of right- or left-sided pain was found to be equal in the epidemiological study (Andersen et al. 1995) and in Bowsher's (1996) study. However, in patients with one acute lesion on CT scan, which includes patients with cerebral infarction and excludes patients with brain-stem infarction, nine patients had a right-sided lesion compared to two patients with a left-sided lesion (Andersen et al. 1995). This finding agrees with previous retrospective studies that have proposed an overrepresentation of lesions in the nondominant hemisphere (Leijon et al. 1989; Kameyama 1976–77).

Antidepressive drugs relieve CPSP (Leijon and Boivie 1989), which may in part be explained by their antidepressive effect. In the prospective study by Andersen et al. (1995), however, CPSP did not correlate with depression, although CPSP patients did score significantly higher on the Hamilton Depression Rating Scale. Further, in a preliminary report, treatment of post-stroke depression did not alleviate the concomitant pain of CPSP (Vestergaard et al. 1996). Post-stroke depression and CPSP thus seems to be separate entities that may follow stroke. However, the fact that both conditions are relieved by antidepressants suggests that ascending monoaminergic systems may be a common factor in both.

CHALLENGES FOR THE FUTURE

Further prospective studies are needed to clarify the magnitude of the CPSP problem, as only one prospective study has been conducted. Emphasis should be placed on the long-term prognosis of CPSP, which is unknown. Controlled pharmacological studies with receptor-selective drugs may help to elucidate the mechanisms of CPSP. Researchers have focused on the monoaminergic system, but manipulation of the excitatory amino acid and GABA-ergic system may be also be worthy of future research. Investigations using new imaging techniques such as positron emission tomography (PET) combined with treatment studies may be a valuable way to study the mechanisms of CPSP and may lead to a specific pharmacological treatment for this syndrome.

REFERENCES

Andersen G, Vestergaard K, Ingeman-Nielsen M, Jensen TS. Incidence of central post-stroke pain. *Pain* 1995; 61:187–193.

Bowsher D. Sensory consequences of stroke. *Lancet* 1993; 341:156.

Bowsher D. Central pain: clinical and physiological characteristics. *Neur Neurosurg Psych* 1996; 61:62–69.

Dejerine J, Roussy G. Le syndrome thalamique. *Rev Neurol* 1906; 14:521–532.

Gorson et al. Stroke with sensory symptoms mimicking myocardial ischemia. *Neurology* 1996; 46:548–551.

Jensen TS, Lenz FA. Central post-stroke pain. A challenge for the scientist and the clinician. *Pain* 1995; 61:161–164.

Kameyama M. Vascular lesions of the thalamus on the dominant and the non-dominant side. *Appl Neurophysiol* 1976–77; 39:171–177.

Leijon G, Boivie J. Central post-stroke pain—a controlled trial of amitriptyline and carbamazepine. *Pain* 1989; 36:27–36.

Leijon G, Boivie J, Johansson L. Central post-stroke pain—neurological symptoms and pain characteristics. *Pain* 1989; 36:13–25.

Lewis-Jones H, et al. Magnetic resonance imaging in 36 cases of central post stroke pain. *Pain* 1990 (Suppl 5):s278.

MacGowan DJL, et al. Central pain of the Dejerine-Roussy type is a frequent complication of lateral medullary infarction: a clinical and MRI study of 52 patients. [Abstract] *Neurology* 1996; 46:A302.

Merskey H, Lindblom U, Mumford JM, et al. Pain terms. A current list with definitions and notes on usage. *Pain* 1986 (Suppl)3:216–221.

Vestergaard K, Nielsen J, Andersen G, Arendt-Nielsen L, Jensen TS. Sensory abnormalities in consecutive unselected patients with central post stroke pain. *Pain* 1995; 61:177–186.

Vestergaard K, Andersen G, Jensen TS. Treatment of central post-stroke pain with a selective serotonin reuptake inhibitor. [Abstract] *Eur J Neurol* 1996; 3(Suppl 5):169.

Correspondence to: Karsten Vestergaard, MD, Department of Neurology, Aalborg Hospital, 9000 Aalborg, Denmark. Tel: +45 99 32 11 11; email: vest@dadlnet.dk.

Epidemiology of Pain, edited by
I.K. Crombie, IASP Press, Seattle, © 1999.

13

Migraine and Headache: A Meta-Analytic Approach

Ann I. Scher,[a] Walter F. Stewart,[b] and Richard B. Lipton[c]

[a]*Department of Epidemiology, The Johns Hopkins University, Baltimore, Maryland, USA; and Neuroepidemiology Branch, National Institute for Neurological Disorders and Stroke, National Institutes of Health, Bethesda, Maryland, USA;* [b]*Department of Epidemiology, The Johns Hopkins University, Baltimore, Maryland, USA; and Innovative Medical Research, Towson, Maryland, USA; and* [c]*Departments of Neurology, Epidemiology, and Social Medicine, Albert Einstein College of Medicine and Headache Unit, Montefiore Medical Center, Bronx, New York, USA; and Innovative Medical Research, Stamford, Connecticut, USA*

Prevalence estimates for headache and, in particular, for migraine have varied in many population studies worldwide. Understanding factors that explain variation in prevalence will help clarify the sociodemographic and geographic factors that determine the distribution of disease and will provide a more complete and realistic depiction of the scope and distribution of the public health problem posed by headache. Identifying the methodological factors that account for differences among studies will guide interpretation of these studies and inform future research.

In a previous meta-analysis (Stewart et al. 1995) of population studies of migraine headache published from 1962 to 1994, we found that approximately 70% of the variation in estimates among studies was explained by differences in migraine case definitions and differences in the age and gender composition of the study populations. In particular, differences in case definitions explained 36% of the overall variation in the estimates among 24 studies. It is noteworthy that little variation was observed among the studies that employed International Headache Society (IHS) standardized diagnostic criteria for migraine (Headache Classification Committee of the International Headache Society 1988). However, in that meta-analysis, only five population studies had used the IHS criteria. Since that publication, 16 additional epidemiological studies have used the IHS criteria. These new studies provide an important opportunity to use a consistent case definition to assess the influence of other factors.

In this chapter we present a summary of the population studies of headache and migraine prevalence. We review the surveys reported to date, describe the variation in reported prevalence, and estimate the proportion of this variation that is explained by age, geographic area, and study methods (e.g., sampling method, response method, response rate, recall period). While the previous analysis included all studies, we were primarily interested in understanding variation among studies explained by factors other than the case definition. For this reason, the meta-analysis of migraine prevalence was limited to those studies that have used the IHS criteria for migraine. In addition, we summarize findings on the overall prevalence of headache (including both migrainous and nonmigrainous headache). The two sets of studies are hereafter referred to as the "migraine" studies and the "headache" studies.

METHODS

LITERATURE SEARCH

We conducted a broad search of the literature to

Table I

Profile of epidemiological studies of migraine prevalence published between 1962 and 1997 that met minimal inclusion criteria

Reference, Country	Selected for Meta-Analysis	Population	No. Females	No. Males	Age Range	Method	Migraine Definition	Time Frame	Prevalence (%) Female	Prevalence (%) Male
Abu-Arefeh and Russell 1994, UK	✓	School	866	888	5–15	Clin. Exam	HIS	1 y	11.5	9.7
Alders et al. 1996, Malaysia	✓	Comm.	248	135	5+	In-person SAQ	HIS	1 y	11.3	6.7
Arregui et al. 1991, Peru	✓	Comm.	1091	1166	All	Clin. Exam	HIS	—	12.2	4.5
Barea et al. 1996, Brazil	✓	School	266	274	10–18	Clin. Exam	HIS	Lifetime	10.3	9.6
Bille 1962, Sweden		School	4553	4440	7–15	Mailed SAQ	FH	Lifetime	4.4	3.3
Breslau et al. 1991, USA	✓	HMO	621	386	21–30	Face-to-face	HIS	1 y	12.9	3.4
Clarke and Waters 1974, UK		Comm.	774	745	15–64	Mailed SAQ	Waters	1 y	40.4	26.0
Cruz et al. 1995, Ecuador	✓	Comm.	1260	1463	All	Clin. Exam	HIS	—	7.9	5.6
D'Alessandro et al. 1988, San Marino		Comm.	562	582	7–70	Face-to-face	FH	1 y	18.0	9.3
Deubner 1977, UK		Comm.	303	297	10–20	Face-to-face	2 of U/N/VA	1 y	22.1	15.5
Ekbom et al. 1978, Sweden		Military	—	9803	18	In-person SAQ	FH	Lifetime	—	1.7
Franceschi et al. 1997, Italy	✓	Comm.	148	164	65–84	Clin. Exam	HIS	1 y	2.0	0
Göbel et al. 1994, Germany	✓	Comm.	2123	1936	18+	Face-to-face	HIS	1 y	15.0	7.0
Henry et al. 1992, France		Comm.	2216	1988	5–65	Face-to-face	HIS	Lifetime	17.6	6.1
Honkasalo et al. 1995, Finland		Twin study	11783	11026	24+	Mailed SAQ	U+1 of NV/VA	1 y	10.1	2.5
Jaillard et al. 1997, Peru		Comm.	1752	1494	15+	Clin. exam	HIS	1 y	7.8	2.3
Linet et al. 1989, USA	✓	Comm.	5296	4836	12–29	Telephone	HIS	1 y	14.0	5.3
Michel et al. 1996, France		Comm.	4988	4423	18+	Mailed SAQ	HIS	3 mo	18.0	8.0
Mills et al. 1974, UK		Comm.	508	459	15–65	Mailed SAQ	Waters	1 y	32.2	17.0
Moss and Waters 1974, UK		School	536	—	11–16	In-person SAQ	Waters	1 y	48.3	—
Newland et al. 1978, UK	✓	Comm.	1126	939	18–65	Face-to-face	Waters	1 y	44.7	28.5
O'Brien et al. 1994, Canada	✓	Comm.	1572	1347	18+	Telephone	HIS	1 y	21.9	7.4
Osuntokun et al. 1982, Nigeria		Comm.	472	431	1–70	Face-to-face	3 of U/T/NV	Lifetime	8.9	4.6
Osuntokun et al. 1992, Nigeria		Comm.	9513	9441	All	Face-to-face	U+1 of N/VA/WK	—	5.6	5.0
Paulin et al. 1985, New Zealand		Comm.	590	549	10–80	Face-to-face	2 of U/N/VA	1 y	21	4
Raieli et al. 1995, Italy	✓	School	707	738	11–14		HIS	1 y	3.3	2.7
Rasmussen et al. 1991, Denmark	✓	Comm.	353	387	25–64	Clin. exam	HIS	1 y	15.3	5.9
Sakai and Igarashi 1997, Japan	✓	Comm.	684	340	15+	Mailed SAQ	HIS	1 y	13.0	3.6
Sillanpää 1983a, Finland		School	1873	1911	13	In-person SAQ	FH	Lifetime	14.5	8.1
Sillanpää 1983b, Finland		School	1448	1473	14	In-person SAQ	FH	1 y	14.8	6.4
Sillanpää and Anttila 1996, Finland		School	684	749	7	Clin. exam	FH	6 mo	5.0	6.3
Small and Waters 1974, UK		School	410	367	10–16	In-person SAQ	Waters	1 y	57.1	46.3
Stewart et al. 1992, USA	✓	Comm.	10808	9660	12–80	Mailed SAQ	IHS	1 y	17.6	5.7
Stewart et al. 1996, USA	✓	Comm.	7409	4919	18–65	Telephone	IHS	1 y	19.0	8.2
Tekle-Haimanot et al. 1995, Ethiopia	✓	Comm.	8000	7000	20–89	Clin. exam	IHS	1 y	4.2	1.7
Thomson et al. 1993, New Zealand	✓	Comm.	494	425	17+	Telephone	IHS	Lifetime	14.1	10.1
Waters 1970a, UK		Comm.	430	400	15–75	Face-to-face	Waters	1 y	27.7	11.8
Waters and O'Connor 1971, UK		Comm.	2933	—	20–64	Mailed SAQ	Waters	1 y	23.6	—
Wong et al. 1995, Hong Kong	✓	Comm.	3585	3771	15+	Telephone	IHS	1 y	1.5	0.6

Abbreviations: Comm. = community; FH = family history; HMO = health maintenance organization; IHS = International Headache Society; N = nausea; NV = nausea or vomiting; SAQ = self-administered questionnaire; T = throbbing/pulsating pain; U = unilateral; VA = visual aura; Waters = two of warning/unilateral/nausea; WK = weakness.

identify population studies of migraine and other headache. Search methods included MEDLINE, review articles, a review of specific journals in which such studies are most often reported, and a review of reference lists of published prevalence studies identified from the above sources. The MEDLINE search used the key words headache, migraine, and epidemiology for the years 1966 to 1997 and was limited to English language publications. Published manuscripts were reviewed if the abstract referenced a population study on headache. Studies based on nonrepresentative populations (e.g., employees, physicians, volunteers) were excluded.

We identified 90 such population studies. Of these, 39 studies of migraine prevalence and 44 studies of headache prevalence met the following initial minimal inclusion criteria: (1) gender-specific estimates of migraine or headache prevalence were reported; (2) the study population was selected to be representative of a defined community (e.g., local area, school, or managed care population); and (3) for migraine studies, the case definition was provided. These studies are summarized in Tables I and II for migraine and headache, respectively. Twenty-nine countries are represented, with publication dates ranging from 1962 to 1997. Half of the studies were published since 1992 (migraine) or 1991 (headache). More than half ($n = 21$) of the migraine studies used IHS diagnostic criteria.

Both age- and gender-specific prevalence estimates were needed for the meta-analysis. For studies that did not report prevalence by both age and gender, we attempted to obtain these data directly from the author. Authors of four studies (Linet et al. 1989; Henry et al. 1992; Stewart et al. 1992, 1996) provided information not reported in their publications. For migraine, 18 of 39 studies used IHS diagnostic criteria for migraine (or a close approximation)[1] and provided age-specific prevalence estimates. We selected these studies for the meta-analysis (check-marked in Table I); the remaining 21 studies used a variety of diagnostic criteria, including three that used IHS criteria but did not provide age- and gender-specific estimates, six that used criteria that included family history, seven studies by Waters and collaborators whose migraine definition required two of warning/nausea/unilateral pain, and five that used other diagnostic criteria as shown in Table I.

Of the 44 headache studies, 29 provided age- and gender-specific prevalence estimates and were used in the meta-analysis. No restrictions were placed on the case definition used to define overall headache prevalence.

DATA ABSTRACTING

We developed a standardized form and procedure to abstract study design information and prevalence data from the articles that met the initial criteria. Information on study design factors included the source of the population (community, school, other), method of selecting the sample (complete ascertainment, random or systematic, and other), response method (in-person interview, in-person self-administered questionnaire [SAQ], mailed SAQ, telephone), response rate, whether case status was clinically confirmed, and the time frame (1 year, lifetime) used to derive prevalence estimates. We also abstracted data on age- and gender-specific prevalence estimates and sample sizes. When we calculated prevalence using more than one case definition, we used the most inclusive criteria. For example, for the migraine studies, when estimates were reported for all cases with migraine and for both migraine with aura and migraine without aura, we used the prevalence estimate for all migraine cases. For the headache studies, estimates of overall headache prevalence included headache sufferers with and without migraine.

The 29 headache studies used a variety of case definitions that were categorized into five groups: (1) those requiring some measure of severity, e.g., "Do you suffer from bad headaches?"; (2) those requiring some measure of disability, e.g., "Do you suffer from headaches which limit your activities?"; (3) those requiring both severity and disability; (4) those with unrestricted case definitions, e.g., "Have you ever had a headache?" or "Have you had a headache in the last year?"; and (5) those with nonspecified or other criteria.

The time frame for period prevalence differed within and among studies. Where different time frames were used in the same study, we selected the estimates of 1-year period prevalence. Lifetime prevalence, which should reflect cumulative lifetime risk, is a less reliable measure because cumulative prevalence declines with advancing age (Rasmussen and Olesen

---

[1] One study (Linet et al. 1989) used a close approximation of the IHS criteria. Estimates were provided directly by the author. In this study, cases were defined as having any two of nausea/vomiting, unilateral pain, or visual aura. In addition, these cases had to be reliable and report the same criteria symptoms in two interviews spaced 6–8 weeks apart.

Table II

Profile of epidemiological studies of headache prevalence published between 1962 and 1997 that met minimal inclusion criteria

Reference, Country	Selected for Meta-Analysis	Population	No. Females	No. Males	Age Range	Method	Headache Definition	Time Frame	Prevalence (%) Female	Prevalence (%) Male
Abramson et al. 1980, Israel		Comm.	2651	2248	15+	Clin. exam	Unk	–	80.7	70.8
al Rajeh et al. 1993, Saudi Arabia		Comm.	3210	3148	0–6	Clin. exam	D	Lifetime	0.8	0.5
al Rajeh et al. 1993, Saudi Arabia		Comm.	8239	8122	7+	Clin. exam	D	Lifetime	20.2	12.5
Alders et al. 1996, Malaysia	✓	Comm.	248	135	5+	In-person SAQ	U	1 y	68.7	60.5
Arregui et al. 1991, Peru	✓	Comm.	1091	1166	All	Clin. exam	IHS (TTH+MHA)	–	24.7	11.8
Barea et al. 1996, Brazil	✓	School	266	274	10–18	Clin. exam	IHS (TTH+MHA)	Lifetime	87.9	77.9
Bille 1962, Sweden	✓	School	4553	4440	7–15	Mailed SAQ	S	Lifetime	59.3	58.0
Carlsson 1996, Sweden	✓	School	556	588	7–15	Mailed SAQ	U	1 mo	28.1	23.0
Cheng et al. 1986, China	✓	Comm.	1374	1354	15+	Face-to-face	S/D	Lifetime	5.8	2.7
Clarke et al. 1974, UK		Comm.	774	745	15–64	Mailed SAQ	Unk	1 y	90.4	83.6
D'Alessandro et al. 1988, San Marino	✓	Comm.	562	582	7–70	Face-to-face	S	1 y	46.2	35.3
Deubner 1977, UK	✓	Comm.	303	297	10–20	Face-to-face	U	1 y	81.5	74.4
Duckro et al. 1989, USA		Comm.	249	251	21+	Telephone	SD	Lifetime	20.4	11.2
Egermark-Eriksson 1982, Sweden	✓	School	194	208	7,11,15	In-person SAQ	U	Lifetime	57.2	54.3
Ekbom et al. 1978, Sweden	✓	Military		9803	18	In-person SAQ	U	Lifetime		4.4
Franceschi et al. 1997, Italy	✓	Comm.	148	164	65–84	Clin. exam	SD	1 y	9.5	3.1
Garcia-Pedroza et al. 1991, Mexico	✓	Comm.	444	289	10+	Clin. exam	U	Lifetime	10.6	8.9
Henry et al. 1992, France		Comm.	2216	1988	5–65	Face-to-face	U	Lifetime	39.2	21.6
Honkasalo et al. 1993, Finland	✓	Twin study	11783	11026	24+	Mailed SAQ	U	1 y	67.0	29.2
Jaillard et al. 1997, Peru		Comm.	1752	1494		Clin. exam	S	1 y	46.0	19.8
Kristjánsdóttir and Wahlberg 1993, Iceland	✓	School	1045	1084	11–16	Mailed SAQ	U	1 mo	57.3	45.8
Lavados and Tenham 1997, Chile	✓	Comm.	648	737	15+	Face-to-face	IHS TTH	1 y	35.2	18.1
Levy 1983, Zimbabwe		Comm.	1385	3643		Face-to-face	U		27.0	17.6
Michel et al. 1996, France		Comm.	4988	4423	18+	Mailed SAQ	U	3 mo	58.0	39.0
Mills and Waters 1974, UK		Comm.	508	459	15–65	Mailed SAQ	Unk	1 y	86.0	70.8
Mitsikostas et al. 1996, Greece		Comm.	1764	1737	15–75	Face-to-face	S	1 y	40.0	19.0
Moss and Waters 1974, UK	✓	Comm.	536	–	11–16	In-person SAQ	U	1 y	93.1	73.1
Newland et al. 1978, UK		Comm.	1126	939	18–65	Face-to-face	U	1 y	81.4	73.1
Nikiforow and Hokkanent 1978, Finland		Comm.	1623	1444	15–65	Mailed SAQ	Unk	1 y	73.1	57.6
O'Brien et al. 1994, Canada		Comm.	1572	1347	18+	Telephone	Unk	1 y	90.6	83.9
Oster 1972, Denmark		Comm.	1116	1062	6–19	Clin. exam	U	–	22.8	18.3
Osuntokun et al. 1992, Nigeria	✓	Comm.	9513	9441	All	Face-to-face	Unk	Lifetime	52.0	50.0
Passchier and Orlebeke 1985, Netherlands	✓	School	1049	1132	10–17	Face-to-face	Unk	1 y	91.2	84.5
Paulin et al 1985, New Zealand		Comm.	590	549	16+	Face-to-face	U	1 y	60.0	39.0
Raieli et al. 1995, Italy	✓	School	707	738	11–14	Face-to-face	U	1 y	28.0	19.9
Rasmussen et al. 1991, Denmark		Comm.	353	387	25–64	Clin. exam	U	1 y	99.0	93.0
Sachs et al. 1985, Ecuador	✓	Comm.	569	544	All	Clin. exam	Unk	–	2.6	10.9
Sillanpää 1983a, Finland	✓	School	1873	1911	13	In-person SAQ	D	1 y	84.2	79.4
Small and Waters 1974, UK	✓	School	410	367	10–16	In-person SAQ	Unk	1 y	92.9	84.5
Stewart et al. 1992, US	✓	Comm.	10808	9660	12–80	Mailed SAQ	S	1 y	27.3	13.9
Stewart 1996, USA	✓	Comm.	7409	4919	18–65	Telephone	U	1 y	74.2	59.9
Thomson et al. 1993, New Zealand	✓	Comm.	494	425	17+	Telephone	S	Lifetime	45.5	34.6
Waters 1970, UK	✓	Comm.	221	194	15–75	Face-to-face	U	1 y	78.7	64.9
Waters and O'Connor 1971, UK	✓	Comm.	2933	–	20–64	Mailed SAQ	Unk	1 y	78.7	
Wong et al. 1995, Hong Kong	✓	Comm.	3585	3771	15+	Telephone	U	1 y	5.9	2.7

Abbreviations: D = disability; (headache resulting in disruption of activity); IHS = International Headache Society; MHA = migraine headache; S = severity ("severe," "bad," "troublesome," or "moderate"); SD = self-administered questionnaire; TTH = tension-type headache; U = unrestricted ("headache," "headache more than rarely," or "recurrent headache").

Table III
Summary profile of migraine and headache prevalence studies which met final inclusion criteria

Study Factor	Category	Migraine Studies ($N = 18$)	Headache Studies ($N = 29$)
Method of selection	Random/systematic	13	15
	Complete population	14	12
	Other/unknown	1	2
Source of sample	Community	14	15
	School	3	11
	Other	1	2
Response method	Face-to-face	2	6
	Telephone	5	3
	Mailed SAQ	2	7
	In-person SAQ	1	6
	Clinical exam	7	6
Case status clinically confirmed	Yes	6	8
	No	6	11
	No, clinically validated	6	10
Time period for prevalence estimate	1 mo	0	2
	1 y	12	17
	Lifetime	4	7
	Unknown	2	3
Headache definition (overall)	Unrestricted	—	12
	Severe	—	4
	Disabling	—	1
	Severe and disabling	—	2
	Unknown/other	—	10
Area	Africa	1	1
	Asia	3	3
	Central/S. America	3	5
	Europe	5	9
	N. America	5	1

1992), which suggests that poor recall is associated with advancing age. When shorter time periods are used (e.g., 1 year) to recall headache history, underreporting is less likely.

Studies were assigned to the following regional categories: Asia (China, Japan, Hong Kong, Malaysia), Africa (Ethiopia, Nigeria, Zimbabwe), Middle East (Israel, Saudi Arabia), Europe (Denmark, Finland, France, Germany, Greece, Iceland, Italy, Netherlands, San Marino, Sweden, United Kingdom), South/Central America (Chile, Brazil, Ecuador, Mexico, Peru), and North America (Canada, United States). Abstracting errors were identified by comparing computerized data to the original reports.

DATA ANALYSIS

Linear regression was used to determine the proportion of variance in age- and gender-specific preva-

lence estimates explained by each sociodemographic and study design variable. Gender- and age-specific estimates from the same study are likely to be correlated. To control for this lack of independence, we defined each study as a cluster and relaxed the requirement for independence of observations for those prevalence estimates produced by the same study.

For the analysis, age was defined by the midpoint of the published age range. Predictor variables in the linear regression model included: age (Age, Age^2, Age^3), case definition (Case), method of selecting the sample (Random), source of the sample (Pop), response method (Survey), response rate (Response), time period for estimating prevalence (Period), whether or not case status was clinically confirmed (Clindx), and the publication time frame (Pubyear).

Prevalence estimates were modeled separately by gender. Variables for age (Age, Age^2, and Age^3) and area were first added to the model because prior

Table IV
Gender- and age-specific migraine prevalence as reported in 18 population studies of migraine
that used International Headache Society (IHS) diagnostic criteria

Reference	Age Range	Prevalence (%) Female	Prevalence (%) Male	Reference	Age Range	Prevalence (%) Female	Prevalence (%) Male
Abu-Arefeh and Russell 1974	5–15	11.5	9.7	Raeli et al. 1991	11–11	1.1	4.2
Alders et al. 1996	5–15	4.4	2.6		12–12	4.8	4.7
	16–25	11.3	8.1		13–13	3.8	2.1
	26–35	11.5	6.7		14–14	5.2	1.5
	36–45	20.3	17.7	Rasmussen and Olesen 1992	25–34	18.0	5.0
	46–55	22.7	7.7		35–44	14.0	7.0
	56–65	6.7	0.0		45–54	12.0	6.0
	66–87	5.3	0.0		55–64	19.0	7.0
Arregui et al. 1991	0–9	0.0	0.8	Sakai and Igarashi 1997	15–19	11.5	2.0
	10–19	3.7	1.5		20–29	13.0	7.0
	20–29	8.8	0.0		30–39	20.0	6.0
	30–39	8.5	0.0		40–49	18.0	2.5
	40–49	18.0	2.3		50–59	11.0	3.0
	50–59	8.1	3.1		60–69	9.0	0.5
	60–69	4.0	0.0		70–79	3.0	0.0
	0–9	4.8	0.7	Stewart et al. 1996	18–25	22.7	10.0
	10–19	20.1	8.1		26–30	22.1	11.5
	20–29	16.8	5.0		31–35	19.0	8.2
	30–39	22.1	10.0		36–40	21.2	9.8
	40–49	21.5	16.1		41–45	21.0	9.1
	50–59	38.1	12.0		46–55	20.9	6.5
	60–69	15.4	0.0		56–65	9.8	3.2
Barea et al. 1996	10–18	10.2	9.5	Stewart et al. 1992	12–19	8.1	4.3
Breslau et al. 1991	21–30	12.9	3.4		20–29	19.8	7.1
Cruz et al. 1995	0–9	1.4	1.5		30–39	28.7	8.9
	10–19	8.2	8.4		40–49	24.4	7.4
	20–29	9.7	6.2		50–59	18.7	6.0
	30–39	10.1	5.8		60–69	10.5	3.4
	40–49	13.0	6.6		70–85	6.6	2.5
	50–59	10.3	7.1	Tekle-Haimanot et al. 1995	20–29	4.8	1.1
	60–69	3.1	6.5		30–39	5.6	4.3
Franceschi et al. 1997	65–84	2.0	0.0		40–49	3.8	1.4
Henry et al. 1992	15–24	6.0	2.0		50–59	3.4	1.6
	25–34	12.0	3.9		60–69	1.9	0.6
	35–49	12.0	2.4		70–79	0.6	0.6
	50–64	6.7	2.2		80–89	0.0	0.0
	65–75	2.8	0.9	Thomson et al. 1993	17–29	15.5	13.4
Linet et al. 1989	12–17	10.2	5.4		30–49	14.4	10.7
	18–23	13.1	5.2		50–70	12.1	5.3
	24–29	18.8	5.4	Wong et al. 1995	15–24	0.8	0.4
O'Brien et al. 1994	18–24	18.3	10.9		25–34	2.6	0.9
	25–34	23.0	9.1		35–44	2.7	1.0
	35–44	33.3	8.7		45–54	1.4	0.2
	45–54	32.3	5.9		55–64	0.6	0.4
	55–64	28.7	5.4		65–74	0.4	0.2
	65–74	11.7	1.5				

studies have shown that migraine prevalence varies significantly by these variables (Stewart et al. 1992). Subsequently, each study design variable was individually added to the model to estimate its additional contribution to explained variance. Regression analysis was weighted by the gender- and age-specific sample size.

RESULTS

MIGRAINE META-ANALYSIS

Eighteen studies used IHS criteria for migraine and contributed one or more gender- and age-specific estimate of migraine prevalence. Most studies ($n = 14$) were community based (Table III) and either used a clinical exam ($n = 6$) or a clinically validated inter-

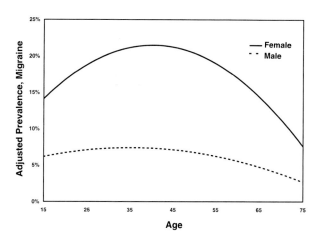

Fig. 1. Gender- and age-specific estimates of migraine prevalence (North America) based on 18 population studies that used International Headache Society (IHS) diagnostic criteria.

view ($n = 6$) to ascertain cases. With the exception of one study, either the total population or a random sample of the population was surveyed. Most studies ($n = 12$) estimated 1-year period prevalence; two studies estimated lifetime prevalence. A total of 182 gender- and age-specific migraine prevalence (Table IV) were obtained from these 18 studies completed on five continents. Five or more age-specific estimates were obtained from each of 11 studies.

Linear regression was used to examine factors that explained variation in age-specific estimates of migraine prevalence. Estimates were modeled separately for males and females. Each specific estimate was

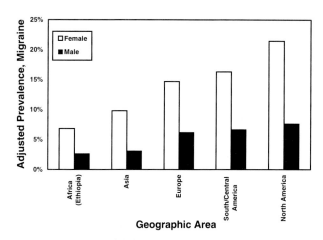

Fig. 2. Gender- and area-specific estimates of migraine prevalence (age 40) based on 18 population studies that used IHS diagnostic criteria.

Table V
Estimated proportion of variance (R^2) in age and gender-specific migraine prevalence estimates from 18 studies explained by sociodemographic and study design factors

Variable(s) in Weighted Model	R^2
Female	
Intercept	0.0000
Age	0.0114
Age + Age^2	0.1977
Age + Age^2 + Area	0.7112
Age + Age^2 + Area + Pop	0.7419
Age + Age^2 + Area + Survey	0.7599
Age + Age^2 + Area + Random	0.7161
Age + Age^2 + Area + Period	0.7277
Age + Age^2 + Area + Response	0.7690
Age + Age^2 + Area + Clindx	0.7280
Age + Age^2 + Area + Pubyear	0.7170
Male	
Intercept	0.0000
Age	0.0757
Age + Age^2	0.1392
Age + Age^2 + Area	0.5613
Age + Age^2 + Area + Pop	0.6544
Age + Age^2 + Area + Survey	0.6682
Age + Age^2 + Area + Random	0.5860
Age + Age^2 + Area + Period	0.6183
Age + Age^2 + Area + Response	0.6204
Age + Age^2 + Area + Clindx	0.6082
Age + Age^2 + Area + Pubyear	0.6392

Abbreviations: Area = geographic area; Clindx = clinical diagnosis; Period = prevalence period (e.g., 1 year, lifetime); Pop = source of sample; Pubyear = publication time frame; Random = selection method; Response = response rate; Survey = survey type (e.g., phone, in-person).

weighted by the age-specific sample size. Age, Age^2, and Age^3 terms were entered into the model first because estimates were age specific. Age and Age^2 accounted for 20% ($P < 0.005$) of the variation in females and 14% ($P < 0.005$) of the variation in males (Table V). Age^3 was not statistically significant. This finding is consistent with the well-established nonlinear relationship between migraine prevalence and age, where prevalence of active cases peaks between ages 35 and 45 and declines thereafter (Waters 1970).

The most important variable accounting for variation in age- and gender-specific estimates was geographic location (i.e., Area). The variable Area, which

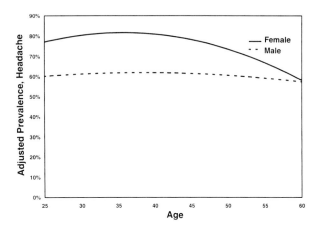

Fig. 3. Gender- and age-specific estimates of headache prevalence (North America) based on 29 population studies.

included five categories, substantially increased the explained variance (i.e., R^2) from 20% to 71% for females and from 14% to 56% for males ($P < 0.0001$).

The final linear regression model was used to derive predicted gender- and age-specific prevalence estimates of migraine by geographic area, using the explanatory variables Age, Age^2, and Area. As shown in Fig. 1, the predicted age-specific prevalence of migraine increases up to age 40 in both males and females and declines thereafter. This pattern reflects the Age and Age^2 terms in the model. Among females, the prevalence is higher and increases considerably faster when compared to males. After we adjusted for age, we found that migraine prevalence was lowest in Asia and Africa for females and males and increased as follows: Europe, Central/South America, and North America (Fig. 2).

HEADACHE META-ANALYSIS

Twenty-nine studies contributed one or more gender- and age-specific prevalence estimates (Table VI). Most studies were community ($n = 15$) or school based ($n = 11$) (Table III) and used either a clinical exam ($n = 8$) or clinically validated interview ($n = 10$) to ascertain cases. Most studies ($n = 17$) estimated 1-year period prevalence; seven studies estimated lifetime prevalence. In total, 271 gender- and age-specific prevalence estimates were included in the analysis (Table VI).

Linear regression was used to understand factors that explained variation in age specific estimates of headache prevalence. Headache prevalence varied with

age for females, accounting for 19% of the variation ($P < 0.005$). The age covariate did not significantly explain variation in headache prevalence in males (Table VII).

As in the migraine regression, geographic area accounted for significant variation in age-specific estimates. When Area (the area term for Africa was dropped from the model due to collinearity) was added to the model, the R^2 value for the combination of age and geographic area increased to 69% in females and 30% in males ($P < 0.0001$). The case definition also accounted for a significant amount of variation in the prevalence estimates. When Case was added to the model, the proportion of variation explained by the model increased to 78% in females and 68% in males ($P < 0.0001$).

The final linear regression model was used to derive predicted gender and age specific prevalence estimates of headache by geographic area and case definition, using the explanatory variables Age, Age^2, Area, and Casedef. The gender-specific variation by age is shown in Fig. 3 (using North America as an example). The prevalence of headache in females varies by age, although not as strongly as seen in migraine. The pattern in males is essentially linear. The pattern of variation by area was again lowest in Asia and highest in North America. However, the adjusted prevalence of headache was higher in Europe than in South/Central America (in contrast to the pattern of migraine prevalence in those areas) (Fig. 4).

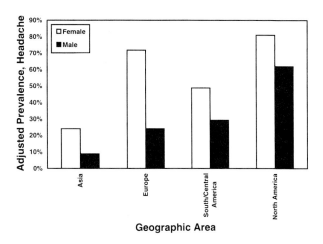

Fig. 4. Gender- and area-specific estimates of headache prevalence (age 40) based on 29 population studies.

Table VI
Gender- and age-specific headache prevalence as reported in 29 population studies of headache

Reference	Age Range	Prevalence (%) Female	Male	Reference	Age Range	Prevalence (%) Female	Male
Alders et al. 1996	5–15	42.4	50.7	Honkasalo et al. 1995	24–29	72.9	28.2
	16–25	87.1	64.9		30–39	78.6	31.5
	26–35	76.9	76.7		40–49	71.6	31.0
	36–45	72.5	73.5		50–64	51.2	28.8
	46–55	90.9	34.6		65–74	17.4	10.2
	56–65	56.7	50.0	Kristjánsdóttir and Wahlberg 1993	11–12	54.6	50.0
	66–87	36.8	44.4		15–16	59.8	42.1
Arregui et al. 1991	0–9	0.9	1.6	Lavados and Tenham 1997	15–29	32.1	17.3
	10–19	21.6	10.0		30–39	37.4	18.7
	20–29	27.5	6.2		40–49	40.3	21.0
	30–39	23.4	3.5		50–59	40.2	17.2
	40–49	40.0	9.3		60–69	29.5	16.8
	50–59	29.7	9.4	Moss and Waters 1974	11–12	88.9	
	60–69	20.0	3.7		13–15	94.5	
	0–9	10.6	2.0		16–18	94.5	
	10–19	31.0	17.7	Nikiforow and Hokkanen 1978	15–24	80.0	62.2
	20–29	27.4	14.3		15–24	77.8	47.8
	30–39	34.9	20.0		25–44	82.6	66.3
	40–49	36.9	37.6		25–44	83.7	65.6
	50–59	52.4	20.0		45–64	67.4	59.3
	60–69	38.5	0.0		45–64	69.3	58.1
Barea et al. 1996	10–18	88.0	77.4		65–74	49.3	38.5
Bille 1962	7–7	37.1	40.3		65–74	53.5	36.7
	8–8	47.7	49.2	Oster 1972	6–19	22.7	18.3
	9–9	53.5	54.0	Osuntokun et al. 1992	0–9	33.0	33.0
	10–10	59.4	59.7		10–19	61.0	59.0
	11–11	62.4	65.2		20–29	64.0	60.0
	12–12	66.8	66.8		30–39	63.0	63.0
	13–13	69.3	63.7		40–49	58.0	59.0
	14–14	72.4	67.7		50–59	54.0	58.0
	15–15	82.8	65.0		60–69	58.0	57.0
Carlsson 1996	7–7	12.3	19.4		70–79	52.0	57.0
	8–8	16.9	17.3		80–89	50.0	53.0
	9–9	29.0	17.9	Passchier and Orlebeke 1985	10–17	91.2	84.5
	10–10	19.4	20.6	Raieli et al. 1995	11–11	17.2	17.5
	11–11	26.5	26.0		12–12	27.8	27.4
	12–12	26.9	31.5		13–13	35.1	25.9
	13–13	45.5	19.0		14–14	55.8	18.1
	14–14	36.7	30.7	Sachs et al. 1985	6–9	0.7	0.0
	15–15	55.9	27.3		10–19	4.9	4.0
Cheng et al. 1986	15–24	0.8	1.5		20–29	12.3	0.0
	25–34	8.8	3.2		30–39	21.8	0.0
	35–44	11.4	3.5		40–49	27.5	4.4
	45–54	12.1	7.1		50–59	27.8	6.1
	55–64	5.4	3.9		60–69	12.9	6.1
	15–24	2.5	1.4	Sillanpää 1983	13–13	84.3	79.4
	25–34	4.8	1.8	Small and Waters 1974	10–16	92.9	84.5
	35–44	3.5	2.0	Stewart et al. 1996	18–25	79.9	63.6
	45–54	6.3	2.5		26–30	81.4	66.8
	55–64	2.2	0.0		31–35	78.3	66.1
D'Alessandro et al. 1988	7–15	50.0	41.3		36–40	81.2	66.1
	16–20	40.2	31.5		41–45	78.2	65.1
	21–30	41.3	39.1		46–55	74.5	54.9
	31–40	58.2	37.5		56–65	52.3	37.7
	41–50	63.6	41.3	Thomson et al 1993	17–29	50.3	43.3
	51–60	55.4	37.5		30–49	42.3	32.6
	61–70	22.3	20.7		50–70	44.7	27.2
	71–80	20.1	21.7	Waters and O'Connor 1970	20–34	82.9	
Deubner 1977	10–12	79.1	72.0		35–54	80.1	
	13–15	84.0	76.1		55–64	68.4	
	16–20	81.5	75.0	Waters 1970	21–34	98.0	80.3
Egermark-Eriksson 1982	7–7	41.9	33.9		35–54	84.9	65.4
	11–11	63.9	67.1		55–64	61.6	47.3
	15–15	69.5	59.2	Wong et al. 1995	15–24	4.43	2.5
Ekbom et al. 1978	18–18		4.5		25–34	7.93	3.7
Franceschi et al. 1997	65–84	9.5	3.1		35–44	10.9	4.2
Garcia-Pedroza et al. 1991	0–14	3.1	3.9		45–54	5.4	1.9
	15–34	5.2	5.7		55–64	3.8	2.2
	35–54	18.3	13.2		65–74	1.5	0.2
	55–64	19.1	14.6				

Table VII
Estimated proportion of variance (R^2) in age- and
gender-specific headache prevalence estimates from
29 studies explained by sociodemographic and
study design factors

Variable(s) in Weighted Model	R^2
Female	
Intercept	0.0000
Age	0.0075
Age + Age^2	0.1890
Age + Age^2 + Area	0.6860
Age + Age^2 + Area + Case	0.7771
Age + Age^2 + Area + Case + Pop	0.7919
Age + Age^2 + Area + Case + Survey	0.8875
Age + Age^2 + Area + Case + Random	0.8487
Age + Age^2 + Area + Case + Period	0.8182
Age + Age^2 + Area + Case + Response	0.9025
Age + Age^2 + Area + Case + Clindx	0.8214
Age + Age^2 + Area + Case + Pubyear	0.8424
Male	
Intercept	0.0000
Age	0.0110
Age + Age^2	0.0119
Age + Age^2 + Area	0.3037
Age + Age^2 + Area + Case	0.6780
Age + Age^2 + Area + Case + Pop	0.8558
Age + Age^2 + Area + Case + Survey	0.8510
Age + Age^2 + Area + Case + Random	0.8364
Age + Age^2 + Area + Case + Period	0.8099
Age + Age^2 + Area + Case + Response	0.8565
Age + Age^2 + Area + Case + Clindx	0.7318
Age + Age^2 + Area + Case + Pubyear	0.8851

Abbreviations: As for Table V.

DISCUSSION

Despite the marked variation in migraine prevalence among the 18 population studies, 71% of the gender-specific variation for females and 56% of the gender-specific variation for males was accounted for by age (Age and Age^2) and geographic area. The prior meta-analysis, which explained 70% of the variation in migraine prevalence, did not analyze prevalence separately by gender. Thus, this meta-analysis explained relatively more of the variance.

Migraine was more prevalent in females than males, and varied strikingly with age, peaking between 35 and 45 years in both gender groups. This finding is consistent with those from our prior meta-analysis. Approximately half the variation in migraine preva-

lence was accounted for by the geographic area, with the lowest prevalence in the Asian and African surveys. This present result is consistent with an earlier report on racial differences in migraine prevalence (Stewart et al. 1996). That study of a U.S. population reported that migraine prevalence was lowest in Asian Americans, followed by African Americans and Caucasians. Accordingly, we suggest that the apparent geographic differences we identify may represent an effect of race. Unmeasured environmental factors, such as degree of urbanization, economic status, and living habits may also explain part of this marked regional variation in migraine prevalence. The fact that acculturized African Americans and Asians show these patterns suggests that individuals carry their reduced risk of migraine with them after migrating to the United States. This observation suggests the possibility of race-related differences in biological risk.

The model explained approximately 70% (78% female, 68% male) of the variation in the headache prevalence estimates. Most of the variation in females was explained by geographic area, while the largest explanatory variable for males was case definition. The influence of age on headache prevalence was statistically significant only for females, and was less marked than that seen for migraine.

The prevalence of headache was higher in females than males, but the gender ratio was less marked than that seen for migraine. As the headache studies included those with migraine, the prevalence ratio for headache partly reflects the influence of the migraine group, with its higher female to male prevalence ratio.

The results of this meta-analysis demonstrate a high degree of consistency between studies in which the case definition for migraine was based on IHS diagnostic criteria. In addition, while prevalence estimates for headache overall vary widely between studies, a high degree of this variability is explained by variation in sociodemographic attributes of the underlying populations, the geographic area in which the survey took place, and survey methodology.

REFERENCES

Abramson JH, Hopp C, Epstein LM. Migraine and non-migrainous headaches. A community survey in Jerusalem. *J Epidemiol Community Health* 1980; 34:188–193.

Abu-Arefeh I, Russell G. Prevalence of headache and migraine in schoolchildren. *BMJ* 1994; 309:765–769.

al Rajeh S, Bademosi O, Ismail H, et al. A community survey of neurological disorders in Saudi Arabia: the Thugbah study.

Neuroepidemiology 1993; 12:164–178.

Alders EE, Hentzen A, Tan CT. A community-based prevalence study on headache in Malaysia. *Headache* 1996; 36:379–384.

Arregui A, Cabrera J, Leon-Velarde F, et al. High prevalence of migraine in a high-altitude population. *Neurology* 1991; 41:1668–1669.

Attia RN, Ben HM, Mrabet A, et al. Prevalence study of neurologic disorders in Kelibia (Tunisia). *Neuroepidemiology* 1993; 12:285–299.

Barea LM, Tannhauser M, Rotta NT. An epidemiologic study of headache among children and adolescents of southern Brazil. *Cephalalgia* 1996; 16:545–954 [discussion].

Bille B. Migraine in schoolchildren. *Acta Paediatr Scand* (Suppl) 1962; 51:1–151.

Borge AI, Nordhagen R, Moe B, Botten G, Bakketeig LS. Prevalence and persistence of stomach ache and headache among children. Follow-up of a cohort of Norwegian children from 4 to 10 years of age. *Acta Paediatr* 1994; 83:433–437.

Brattberg G. The incidence of back pain and headache among Swedish school children. *Quality of Life Research* 1994; 3(Suppl 1):S27–S31

Breslau N, Davis GC, Andreski P. Migraine, psychiatric disorders, and suicide attempts: an epidemiologic study of young adults. *Psychiatry Res* 1991; 37:11–23.

Carlsson J. Prevalence of headache in schoolchildren: relation to family and school factors. *Acta Paediatr* 1996; 85:692–696.

Cheng XM, Ziegler DK, Li SC, et al. A prevalence survey of 'incapacitating headache' in the People's Republic of China. *Neurology* 1986; 36:831–834.

Clarke GJR, Waters WE. Headache and migraine in a London general practice. In: Waters WE (Ed). *The Epidemiology of Migraine.* Bracknell-Berkshire, UK: Boehringer Ingelheim, Ltd, 1974, pp 14–22.

Cook NR, Evans DA, Funkenstein HH, et al. Correlates of headache in a population-based cohort of elderly. *Arch Neurol* 1989; 46:1338–1344.

Crisp AH, Kalucy RS, McGuinness B, Ralph PC, Harris G. Some clinical, social and psychological characteristics of migraine subjects in the general population. *Postgrad Med J* 1977; 53:691–697.

Cruz G, Schoenberg BS, Portera-Sanchez A. Prevalence of neurological diseases in Madrid, Spain. *Neuroepidemiology* 1989; 8:43–47.

Cruz ME, Cruz I, Preux PM, Schantz P, Dumas M. Headache and cysticercosis in Ecuador, *South America Headache* 1995; 35:93–97.

D'Alessandro R, Benassi G, Lenzi PL, et al. Epidemiology of headache in the Republic of San Marino. *J Neurol Neurosurg Psychiatry* 1988; 51:21–27.

Dalsgaard-Nielsen T. Some aspects of the epidemiology of migraine in Denmark. *Headache* 1970; 10:14–23.

Deubner DC. An epidemiologic study of migraine and headache in 10–20 year olds. *Headache* 1977; 17:173–180.

Duckro PN, Tait RC, Margolis RB. Prevalence of very severe headache in a large US metropolitan area. *Cephalalgia* 1989; 9:199–205.

Egermark-Eriksson I. Prevalence of headache in Swedish schoolchildren. A questionnaire survey. *Acta Paediatr Scand* 1982; 71:135–140.

Ekbom K, Ahlborg B, Schele R. Prevalence of migraine and cluster headache in Swedish men of 18. *Headache* 1978; 18:9–19.

Fernandez E, Sheffield J. Descriptive features and causal attributions of headache in an Australian community. *Headache* 1996; 36:246–250.

Franceschi M, Colombo B, Rossi P, Canal N. Headache in a population-based elderly cohort. An ancillary study to the Italian Lon-

gitudinal Study of Aging (ILSA). *Headache* 1997; 37:79–82.

Garcia-Pedroza F, Chandra V, Ziegler DK, Schoenberg B. Prevalence survey of headache in a rural Mexican village. *Neuroepidemiology* 1991; 10:86–92.

Göbel H, Petersen-Braun M, Soyka D. The epidemiology of headache in Germany: a nationwide survey of a representative sample on the basis of the headache classification of the International Headache Society [see comments]. *Cephalalgia* 1994; 14:97–106.

Green JE. A survey of migraine in England 1975-1976. *Headache* 1977; 17:67–68.

Hall A, Leibrich J. Serious illness in 204 New Zealand families during a 16 year period. *N Z Med J* 1985; 98:135–138.

Hasvold T, Johnsen R, Forde OH. Non-migrainous headache, neck or shoulder pain, and migraine—differences in association with background factors in a city population. *Scand J Prim Health Care* 1996; 14:92–99.

Headache Classification Committee of the International Headache Society. Classification and diagnostic criteria for headache disorders, cranial neuralgias and facial pain. *Cephalalgia* 1988; 8(Suppl 7):1–96.

Henry P, Michel P, Brochet B, et al. A nationwide survey of migraine in France: prevalence and clinical features in adults. GRIM [see comments]. *Cephalalgia* 1992; 12:229–237.

Henryk-Gutt R, Rees WL. Psychological aspects of migraine. *J Psychosom Res* 1973; 17:141–153.

Honkasalo ML, Kaprio J, Winter T, Migraine and concomitant symptoms among 8167 adult twin pairs. *Headache* 1995; 35:70–78.

Jaillard AS, Mazetti P, Kala E. Prevalence of migraine and headache in a high-altitude town of Peru: a population-based study. *Headache* 1997; 37:95–101.

King NJ, Sharpley CF. Headache activity in children and adolescents. *J Paediatr Child Health* 1990; 26:50–54.

Kottke TE, Tuomilehto J, Puska P, Salonen JT. The relationship of symptoms and blood pressure in a population sample. *Int J Epidemiol* 1979; 8:355–359.

Kristjánsdóttir G, Wahlberg V. Sociodemographic differences in the prevalence of self-reported headache in Icelandic schoolchildren. *Headache* 1993; 33:376–380.

Kryst S, Scherl E. A population-based survey of the social and personal impact of headache. *Headache* 1994; 34:344–350.

Lavados PM, Tenham E. Epidemiology of tension type headache in Santiago, Chile: a prevalence study. *Cephalalgia* 1998; 18:553–558.

Lee LH, Olness KN. Clinical and demographic characteristics of migraine in urban children. *Headache* 1997; 37:269–276.

Levy LM. An epidemiological study of headache in an urban population in Zimbabwe. *Headache* 1983; 23:2–9.

Linet MS, Stewart WF, Celentano DD, Ziegler D, Sprecher M. An epidemiologic study of headache among adolescents and young adults. *JAMA* 1989; 261:2211–2216.

Liu HC, Wang SJ, Fuh JL, et al. The Kinmen Neurological Disorders Survey (KINDS): a study of a Chinese population. *Neuroepidemiology* 1997; 16:60–68.

Longe AC, Osuntokun BO. Prevalence of migraine in Udo, a rural community in southern Nigeria. *East African Medical Journal* 1988; 65:621–624.

Markush RE, Karp HR, Heyman A, O'Fallon WM. Epidemiologic study of migraine symptoms in young women. *Neurology* 1975; 25:430–435.

Merikangas KR, Angst J, Isler H. Migraine and psychopathology. Results of the Zurich cohort study of young adults. *Arch Gen Psychiatry* 1990; 47:849–853.

Michel P, Pariente P, Duru G, et al. MIG ACCESS: a population-based, nationwide, comparative survey of access to care in migraine in France [published erratum appears in Cephalalgia 1996 May; 16(3):213]. *Cephalalgia* 1996; 16:50–55 [discussion].

Mills C.H., Waters WE. Headache and migraine on the Isles of Scilly. In: Waters WE (Ed). *The Epidemiology of Migraine.* Bracknell-Berkshire, UK: Boehringer Ingelheim, Ltd, 1974, pp 23–34.

Mitsikostas DD, Tsaklakidou D, Athanasiadis N, Thomas A. The prevalence of headache in Greece: correlations to latitude and climatological factors. *Headache* 1996; 36:168–173.

Moss G, Waters WE. Headache and migraine in a girls' grammar school. In: Waters WE (Ed). *The Epidemiology of Migraine.* Bracknell-Berkshire,UK: Boehringer Ingelheim, Ltd, 1974, pp 49–58.

Munoz M, Dumas M, Boutros-Toni F, et al. Prevalence of headache in a representative sample of the population in a French department (Haute-Vienne-Limousin). *Headache* 1993; 33:521–523.

Nakashima K, Yokoyama Y, Shimoyama R, et al. Prevalence of neurological disorders in a Japanese town. *Neuroepidemiology* 1996; 15:208–213.

Newland CA, Illis LS, Robinson PK, Batchelor BG, Waters WE. A survey of headache in an English city. *Research and Clinical Studies in Headache* 1978; 5:1–20.

Nikiforow R, Hokkanen E. An epidemiological study of headache in an urban and a rural population in northern Finland. *Headache* 1978; 18:137–145.

O'Brien B, Goeree R, Streiner D. Prevalence of migraine headache in Canada: a population-based survey. *Int J Epidemiol* 1994; 23:1020–1026.

Oster J. Recurrent abdominal pain, headache and limb pains in children and adolescents. *Pediatrics* 1972; 50:429–436.

Osuntokun BO, Schoenberg B, Nottidge VA, et al. Migraine headache in a rural community in Nigeria: results of a pilot study. *Neuroepidemiology* 1982; 1:31–39.

Osuntokun BO, Adeuja AO, Nottidge VA, et al. Prevalence of headache and migrainous headache in Nigerian Africans: a community-based study. *East Afr Med J* 1992; 69:196–199.

Passchier J, Orlebeke JF. Headaches and stress in schoolchildren: an epidemiological study. *Cephalalgia* 1985; 5:167–176.

Paulin JM, Waal-Manning HJ, Simpson FO, Knight RG. The prevalence of headache in a small New Zealand town. *Headache* 1985; 25:147–151.

Phanthumchinda K, Sithi-Amorn C. Prevalence and clinical features of migraine: a community survey in Bangkok, Thailand. *Headache* 1989; 29:594–597.

Pryse-Phillips W, Findlay H, Tugwell P, et al. A Canadian population survey on the clinical, epidemiologic and societal impact of migraine and tension-type headache. *Can J Neurol Sci* 1992; 19:333–339.

Raieli V, Raimondo D, Cammalleri R, Camarda R. Migraine headaches in adolescents: a student population-based study in Monreale. *Cephalalgia* 1995; 15:5–12.

Rasmussen BK, Olesen J. Migraine with aura and migraine without aura: an epidemiological study. *Cephalalgia* 1992; 12:221–228.

Rasmussen BK, Jensen R, Schroll M, Olesen J. Epidemiology of headache in a general population: a prevalence study. *J Clin Epidemiol* 1991; 44:1147–1157.

Sachs H, Sevilla F, Barberis P, et al. Headache in the rural village of Quiroga, Ecuador. *Headache* 1985; 25:190–193.

Sakai F, Igarashi H. Prevalence of migraine in Japan: a nationwide survey. *Cephalalgia* 1997; 17:15–22.

Sillanpää M. Prevalence of migraine and other headache in Finnish children starting school. *Headache* 1976; 15:288–290.

Sillanpää M. Changes in the prevalence of migraine and other headaches during the first seven school years. *Headache* 1983a; 23:15–19.

Sillanpää M. Prevalence of headache in prepuberty. *Headache* 1983b; 23:10–14.

Sillanpää M, Anttila P. Increasing prevalence of headache in 7-year-old schoolchildren. *Headache* 1996; 36:466–470.

Sillanpää M, Piekkala P, Kero P. Prevalence of headache at pre-school age in an unselected child population. *Cephalalgia* 1991; 11:239–242.

Small P, Waters WE. Headache and migraine in a comprehensive school. In: Waters WE (Ed). *The Epidemiology of Migraine.* Bracknell-Berkshire, UK: Boehringer Ingelheim, Ltd, 1974, pp 59–67.

Sparks JP. The incidence of migraine in schoolchildren. A survey by the Medical Officers of Schools Association. *Practitioner* 1978; 221:407–411.

Stang PE, Osterhaus JT. Impact of migraine in the United States: data from the National Health Interview Survey. *Headache* 1993; 33:29–35.

Stewart WF, Lipton RB, Celentano DD, Reed ML. Prevalence of migraine headache in the United States. Relation to age, income, race, and other sociodemographic factors. *JAMA* 1992; 267:64–69.

Stewart WF, Simon D, Shechter A, Lipton RB. Population variation in migraine prevalence: a meta-analysis. *J Clin Epidemiol* 1995; 48:269–280.

Stewart WF, Lipton RB, Liberman J. Variation in migraine prevalence by race. *Neurology* 1996; 47:52–59.

Tekle-Haimanot R., Seraw B, Forsgren L, Ekbom K, Ekstedt J. Migraine, chronic tension-type headache, and cluster headache in an Ethiopian rural community [see comments]. *Cephalalgia* 1995; 15:482–488.

Thomson AN, White GE, West R. The prevalence of bad headaches including migraine in a multiethnic community. *N Z Med J* 1993; 106:477–480.

To T, Wu K. Health care utilization and disability of migraine: the Ontario Health Survey. *Can J Public Health* 1995; 86:195–199.

Ulfberg J, Carter N, Talback M, Edling C. Headache, snoring and sleep apnoea. *J Neurol* 1996; 243:621–625.

Vahlquist B. Migraine in children. *Int Arch Allergy* 1955; 7:348–355.

Waters WE. Community studies of the prevalence of headache. *Headache* 1970a; 9:178–186.

Waters WE. Headache and the eye. *Lancet* 1970b; 2:467–468.

Waters WE, O'Connor PJ. Epidemiology of headache and migraine in women. *J Neurol Neurosurg Psychiatry* 1971; 34:148–153.

Weiss NS. Relation of high blood pressure to headache, epistaxis, and selected other symptoms. The United States Health Examination Survey of Adults. *N Engl J Med* 1972; 287:631–633.

Wilkinson IA, Halliday JA, Henry RL, Hankin RG, Hensley MJ. Headache and asthma. *J Paediatr Child Health* 1994; 30:253–256.

Wong TW, Wong KS, Yu TS, Kay R. Prevalence of migraine and other headaches in Hong Kong. *Neuroepidemiology* 1995; 14:82–91.

Zhao F, Tsay JY, Cheng XM, et al. Epidemiology of migraine: a survey in 21 provinces of the People's Republic of China, 1985. *Headache* 1988; 28:558–565.

Ziegler DK, Hassanein RS, Couch JR. Characteristics of life headache histories in a nonclinic population. *Neurology* 1977; 27:265–269.

Correspondence to: Ann I. Scher, MS, Neuroepidemiology Branch, National Institute for Neurological Disorders and Stroke, National Institutes of Health, 7550 Wisconsin Avenue, Room 714, Bethesda, MD 20892, USA. Email: ScherA@ninds.nih.gov.

Epidemiology of Pain, edited by
I.K. Crombie, IASP Press, Seattle, © 1999.

14

Facial Pain

Joanna M. Zakrzewska[a] and Peter J. Hamlyn[b]

[a]Department of Oral Medicine, St. Bartholomew's and the Royal London School of Medicine and Dentistry, London, United Kingdom; and [b]Department of Neurological Surgery, St. Bartholomew's and the Royal London Hospital, London, United Kingdom

OVERVIEW

Most facial pain is due to dental causes and trauma and is acute rather than chronic pain. However, once these categories of pain are excluded, there remain more complex causes of chronic facial pain. Facial pain is defined as pain originating below the orbitomeatal line, above the neck, and anterior to the ears.

Diagnostic criteria for facial pain have been advocated both by the International Association for the Study of Pain (IASP) (Merskey and Bogduk 1994) and by the International Headache Society (IHS) (Headache Classification Committee 1988). The two classification systems differ significantly in structure, and it is not always easy to compare studies that used different systems. In the IASP handbook, *Classification of Chronic Pain* (Merskey and Bogduk 1994), trigeminal neuralgia, glossopharyngeal neuralgia, and pain from herpes zoster all fall under the same category. The IASP system recognizes "atypical odontalgia or tooth pain not associated with lesions" (code 034.X8b) but does not use the term atypical facial pain. Instead, it is suggested that these pains be classified under categories for other facial pains or as pain of psychological origin. The IHS classification uses the term "facial pain not fulfilling other criteria" for atypical facial pain and atypical odontalgia (12.8). The IASP classifies glossodynia or burning mouth under the section "the pains of the ear, nose and oral cavity" (code 051.X8), whereas the IHS system does not mention this condition. Both classifications deal with temporomandibular (TMD) pain separately.

Population studies using mailed questionnaires or interviewers who are not health care workers may not be sensitive enough to distinguish between the different types of orofacial pain. The broad categories of pain used in these settings are dental pain, jaw pain, and a burning sensation. Attempts to collect data on other forms of facial pain have specified only sharp, shooting, or dull aching pain. Therefore, apart from burning mouth syndrome, the current information on the epidemiology on facial pain allows only a general assessment rather than analysis of distinct conditions as classified above. This chapter will summarize these general studies before describing in more detail burning mouth syndrome, atypical facial pain, atypical odontalgia, trigeminal neuralgia, glossopharyngeal neuralgia, and maxillary sinusitis.

SURVEY OF OROFACIAL PAIN LITERATURE

We searched the literature using MEDLINE databases from 1966 to July 1997 and the Cochrane database, Issue 3. The following terms were used: "facial pain" from 1986 onward (MeSH heading) and "facial neuralgia" since 1966 (MeSH heading). This search yielded 2175 papers. To exclude TMD pain and trigeminal neuralgia, the search used the text words: temporomandibular, TMD, craniomandibular dysfunction, myofascial pain, and trigeminal neuralgia. The epidemiological search strategy was applied using the following words and phrases: epidemiological methods and factors, longitudinal studies (including fol-low-up studies and case controls), prevalence, cross-sectional studies, retrospective studies, prognosis, dis-ease progression, risk including case referent, risk factors, primary prevention, etiology, and aetiology. This search yielded 260 papers. The abstracts were read on screen and irrelevant papers were excluded.

We printed 65 abstracts and obtained paper cop-ies of the most relevant studies for close review. To identify additional references, we searched several major review articles, the author's collection of pa-pers, and the books *Textbook of Pain* (Wall and Melzack 1989) and *Oral Manifestations of Systemic Disease* (Mason and Jones 1990). The standards for inclusion were clear diagnostic criteria and a primary focus on epidemiological issues and risk factors. Due to the lack of randomized controlled trials, we included some studies that used observational data combined with clear diagnostic criteria. We rejected papers giv-ing prevalence data if they did not differentiate among different types of pain.

DEFINITION AND DIAGNOSTIC CRITERIA

The seven general studies on the epidemiology of facial and dental pain (Table I) are difficult to com-pare as they include acute and chronic pain, and five assessed pain in the previous month only. Of the six population studies, only one asked about pain experi-enced in the previous 6 months (Lipton et al. 1993). The one clinical study, by Speculand and colleagues (1979), assessed patients attending a facial pain clinic. Four studies collected data on "sharp, shooting pain across the face and cheeks," whereas the American study (Lipton et al. 1993) asked about "dull, aching pain across the face and cheek" and specifically ex-cluded sinus pain. The Malaysian population study (Jaafar et al. 1989) collected data on "other pains of the face." Speculand's retrospective data allowed clas-sification of facial pain but included data from patients who had intractable pain, and thus were not represen-tative of the population. These studies focused on de-termining the prevalence of dental and orofacial pain in general to assess their social impact and estimate the potential economic costs. They were not conducted to determine the prevalence of specific types of dental and orofacial pain. None of the studies specified the diagnosis they anticipated when asking patients whether they suffered from shooting or dull, aching pain across the cheek and face. The pain could, there-fore, have been trigeminal neuralgia, atypical facial pain, postherpetic neuralgia, maxillary sinusitis, or even dental in origin.

DEMOGRAPHIC FACTORS IN PREVALENCE

Prevalence data are presented in Table I. Although some studies have assessed age, sex, racial, educa-tional, and occupational groups, they report data col-lectively rather than for individual types of pain. The groups are so disparate that there is little value in at-tempting to evaluate the data for nondental pain, which includes a wide range of orofacial pains.

CONSEQUENCES

Only one study attempts to determine use of the health care system by patients with chronic facial pain; large numbers had TMD (Lundeen et al. 1991). It as-sessed 100 consecutive patients who had significant pain for at least 6 months and one prior treatment fail-ure. The patients completed the following question-naires: Patient Assessment Inventory, McGill Pain Questionnaire, Illness Behavior Questionnaire, a vi-sual analogue scale for pain intensity, and the Health Care Utilization Index. Clinicians then used a four-point scale to rate the patients regarding psychologi-cal factors, stress, and chronicity of pain. Results of the Health Care Utilization scale categorized patients as low utilizers (scores of 4 and below) or high utiliz-ers (scores of 5 or above). The high utilizers of ser-vices had greater concern for somatic symptoms and a stronger belief that they had physical symptoms. Clinicians, to the contrary, had assumed that high uti-lizers of services would be those with more psycho-logical features and stress. The authors suggest that behavioral methods (coping and living with pain) would provide more cost-effective treatment than would psychiatric care. Other studies have assessed consequences of facial pain, but they all include acute dental pain and a wide variety of chronic pain condi-tions such as TMD and so were excluded.

CAUSATION AND PREVENTION

Psychological disorders in facial pain patients

A number of studies have examined the psycho-logical profiles of patients with undifferentiated

Table I

Prevalence estimates of nondental orofacial pain excluding TMD pain

Study Type	Disease Definition	Source of Sample	Sample Size	Pain Severity	Duration of Symptoms	Type of Prevalence Estimate	Prevalence	Comments	Reference
CS population, mailed SCQ	Facial pain and discomfort	Randomized voters, City of Toronto	1014; R = 72%	10% severe, 40% moderate, 50% mild	Mean 6 d	Period, 1 mo	27% pain only, 13% pain and discomfort, 14% discomfort only, 4.9% sharp shooting pain across face	Difficult to assess which is dental, TMJ, or other type of facial pain; included acute and chronic	Locker and Grushka 1987, 1988
CS population, SCQ, interviewers	Orofacial pain: dull aching pain across face or cheek excluding sinus	NHIS, USA (1989)	45,711; R = 92%	NR	NR	Period, 6 mo	1.4% dull, aching facial pain	No diagnosis	Lipton et al. 1993
Industrial population, SCQ, interviewers	Orofacial pain, "other facial pain"	Two factories, Malaysia	355; R = NR	2% very severe, 7% severe, 44% moderate, 47% mild	NR	Period, 1 mo	3% nondental, non-TMJ facial pain	No diagnosis	Jaafar et al. 1989
CS population over 65 y, telephone and EX	Oral health status: "burning or shooting pains in the mouth"	Random sample non-business telephones, Ottawa-Carleton	791; R = 37% (telephone only); R = 38% (telephone and EX)	NR	NR	Period, 1 mo	38% facial pain incl. oral mucosal pain due to ulcers, excl. dental and TMJ pain	Only 65 y and older; overrepresented younger groups and females, especially on EX	Slade et al. 1990
Cohort retrospective, notes	Intractable facial pain, TMJ, AFP, neuralgias	Pain clinic, S. Australia	225 pain clinic patients, 29 with facial pain	NR	59% >2 y	Period, 3 y	8 per million	Based on population of 1.2 million; 50% had spine or limb pain, 13% facial pain	Speculand et al. 1979
CS general practice, SCQ	Oral ill health: "shooting pains in face"	General dental practice, Wales	997; R = NR	NR	NR	Period, 1 mo	3.1% sharp shooting pain across face	Emphasis on dental disease	Richards and Scourfield 1996
CS population over 50 y, Q and EX	Shooting pains in face/cheek	Independently living elderly, Ontario telephone lists	907; R = NR	25% moderately severe to severe	NR	Period, 1 mo	2.4% shooting pain	May be same groups as Slade et al. 1990	Locker 1992

Abbreviations: AFP = atypical facial pain; CS = cross-sectional; EX = examination; NHIS = National Health Interview Survey; NR = not reported; Q = questionnaire; R = response; SCQ = self-completed questionnaire.

"chronic facial pain," or have compared psychological factors among patients with various diagnoses. However, none of these studies are population based, and few used pain-free controls. Thus, they provide little information about psychological risk factors for facial pain.

Lascelles (1966) used his own questionnaire to conduct a psychiatric assessment of patients with facial pain. The diagnostic criteria were facial pain with no physical signs that could be interpreted as TMD pain, atypical facial pain, or atypical odontalgia. He diagnosed all patients as suffering from depression. A comparison with 50 general medical patients and 50 severely depressed patients revealed that obsessive personalities were most common in the facial pain group.

To assess the vulnerability to long-term consequences of pain, Lipton and Marbach (1983) studied the responses of 170 facial pain patients in four groups: myofascial pain (68), organic TMD pain (41), typical facial neuralgia (61), and mixed pain (41). They found that irrespective of diagnosis, increased perceived pain severity and increased level of psychological stress were the most important variables influencing response to pain, emotional expressiveness, and ability to function. These findings held even after controlling for personal background, sociocultural and sociomedical orientation, and pain history. The patient's psychological state, the authors suggest, will influence the reporting of pain and the degree of disability.

One study using the Illness Behaviour Questionnaire (IBQ) (Speculand et al. 1981) attempted to assess which patients may be at increased risk of developing facial pain. Three studies used the Minnesota Multiphasic Personality Inventory (MMPI) to assess vulnerability to chronic facial pain (Eversole et al. 1985; Harness and Peltier 1992; Mongini et al. 1992).

Speculand et al. (1981) applied the 52-item version of the IBQ to 24 patients with intractable facial pain and 24 age- and sex-matched controls seeking relief of toothache. No subjects in the control group had pain for more than 56 months, whereas 58% of patients in the intractable pain group had pain longer than 2 years. The intractable facial pain group had increased somatic preoccupation and were less likely to accept professional reassurance or a psychological reason for their pain. The authors suggest that patients with abnormal illness behavior patterns are more likely to develop chronic pain.

Mongini and colleagues (1992) used the diagnostic criteria of the IHS to identify 157 patients with chronic head and facial pain including temporomandibular disorders (53), trigeminal neuralgia (7), and atypical facial pain (AFP) (33). They administered the MMPI to two age- and sex-matched control groups; 27 had no pain problems, while 18 had constant or recurrent pain outside the head and neck region. Patients with AFP scored the highest and TMD the lowest on all but three of the MMPI scales. AFP patients showed a tendency toward neuroticism and psychosis, and personality disturbances were found in all pain patients but not in controls. Personality change was associated with the character of the pain rather than the chronicity; however, it is not clear whether personality change was a risk factor for the development of facial pain or occurred as a consequence of it.

Eversole and colleagues (1985) used the MMPI in three groups of patients attending a facial pain clinic: myogenic facial pain, i.e., pain in muscles of mastication with no disk changes (46); TMD internal derangement (51); and atypical facial pain, i.e., pain in jaws or teeth with no organic lesions (58). The study did not use controls, but compared results with other published results. In general, high scores on hypochondriasis with hysteria, depression with psychesthenia, and schizophrenia with psychesthenia were evident in all groups. However, myogenic facial pain and AFP patients scored higher on depression, hypochondriasis, and hysteria.

Harness and Peltier (1992) used the same questionnaire to compare three similar groups of facial pain patients: myogenic facial pain (25); TMD internal derangement (30), and AFP (39). The investigators also assessed bruxism and sleep patterns. The study did not use controls or provide details on age, sex, pain duration, or severity. Bruxism was not associated with psychiatric disturbance, whereas sleep disturbance was. The authors suggest that poor sleep is a more socially acceptable symptom than are emotional psychiatric symptoms, and that poor sleep thus could be used as a predictor of increased psychiatric disturbance.

Holzberg and colleagues (1996) assessed 70 facial pain patients with the Beck Depression Inventory, McGill Pain Questionnaire, and Sickness Impact Profile. Their only selection criteria were facial pain of longer than 6 months' duration and a minimum age of 19 years. Unfortunately, the study did not use controls, but the authors suggest that depression rather than subjective pain severity determines the ability to function. They accept the limitations of this study and urge further population studies to assess the causal relationship between pain and depression.

In a double-blind study of 30 patients with chronic facial pain, Seltzer and colleagues (1982) showed that a diet high in carbohydrate and low in fat and protein with the addition of 3 g of tryptophan per day resulted in decreased pain and greater tolerance of pain. The diet had no effect on anxiety or depression. Other studies have shown that patients with low levels of monoamines in brain cerebrospinal fluid have intractable facial pain. It is not known whether brain dopamine and serotonin systems first become dysfunctional and then result in facial pain or vice versa (Bouckoms et al. 1993).

CHALLENGES FOR THE FUTURE

Some researchers have suggested that more psychobehavioral assessment of patients with facial pain would enable clinicians to predict those who are more likely to develop intractable facial pain (Speculand et al. 1981; Lundeen et al. 1991; Holzberg et al. 1996). Such prediction could lead to earlier referral for psychological and behavioral management and possible prevention of chronicity. However, no studies have attempted to validate this hypothesis.

Data are scarce on the epidemiology of nondental, chronic facial pain other than TMD pain. Scientifically designed, large, multicenter population studies using tools sensitive to the many types of facial pain are needed to collect basic pain data. In addition to mailed questionnaires, data collection methods should also include trained interviewers and in some instances clinical investigations to make precise diagnoses. Nonresponders would need to be followed with a minimum of two mailings and the responders compared to the general population, because men are often underrepresented in such studies. The validity, reliability, and reproducibility of the questionnaires and examinations should be assessed and stated. The period of recall of symptoms should be at least 6 months.

Assessing the burden of disease to society requires analysis of the educational, ethnic, socioeconomic, and occupational characteristics of subjects and their use of health care services. As LeResche (1997) points out, objective measures are now available to measure pain perception, pain appraisal including coping strategies and psychological factors, pain behavior, and general pain-related disability. Studies using such measures may provide crucial data on the causes and risk fac-

tors of these various conditions and could lead to improved prevention strategies and treatment. Similar studies on patients treated in hospitals and other tertiary care settings for both facial pain and other chronic pain would provide further data on the risk factors and costs involved in the management of these more difficult patients with facial pain. These studies would highlight the differences between patients seeking health care and those not coming forward.

Keefe and Beckham (1990) stress the importance of evaluating behavioral factors, not only for assessment but also to monitor progress and treatment. Along the lines suggested by LeResche (1997) for TMD, an essential prerequisite for further studies on management of facial pain is an estimate of its prevalence and influence on the patients' quality of life. This knowledge will determine how many patients would be likely to participate in clinical trials and hence how applicable the trials would be to this population. Even if randomized controlled trials are not possible, well-designed prospective cohort studies using clear diagnostic criteria would help clarify many controversies in the literature. A systematic review of treatments used in chronic pain clinics reveals that cognitive behavior therapy is the most effective treatment for chronic pain and should be assessed in depth in this particular group of patients (McQuay et al. 1996).

BURNING MOUTH SYNDROME

Although the literature on burning mouth syndrome (BMS) is relatively extensive, few studies are of sound, scientific quality. Randomized controlled trials are lacking and the best evidence is from case-control studies. However, controversy remains as to whether burning mouth is a disease in its own right and hence a syndrome, or a symptom of other diseases.

We searched the literature using MEDLINE databases from 1966 to March 1997 and the Cochrane database of trials 1996, Issue 3. The term burning mouth syndrome (as a MeSH heading) yielded 228 listings. The text words dysaesthesia or dysesthesia, stomatodynia, glossopyrosis, sore tongue, glossodynia, and burning tongue yielded another 96 papers for a total of 324. The abstracts were read on screen and irrelevant papers excluded. We printed and read 75 abstracts and obtained paper copies of the most relevant for detailed review. Twenty articles were included

Table II
Studies of burning mouth syndrome (BMS) using patients with burning mouths
for which no medical or odontological causes were found

Source of Sample	Sample Size	No. Males	No. Females	Mean Age, Female (y)	Age Range, Female (y)	Mean Age, Male (y)	Age Range, Male (y)	Mean Age, Mixed (y)	Age Range, Mixed (y)	Mean Duration of Symptoms (Range)
Dental departments, Toronto	102	18	84	59.1 ± 10.2	36–84	52.2 ± 11.5	33–69	NR	NR	3.1 ± 2.9 y (3 mo–18 y)
Oral surgery, Association of BMS, The Netherlands	154	10%	9%	NR	NR	NR	NR	60 ± 11	30–84	4 ± 3.5 y (1–18 y)
Oral medicine, U.K.	25*	3	22	NR	NR	NR	NR	57	37–81	3 y 4 mo (3 mo–12 y)
Dental clinics, Sweden	32	6	26	55	40–69	46	38–57	NR	NR	NR
Special clinics, Israel	45	9	36	NR	NR	NR	NR	61 ± 10	NR	2.3 ± 2.27 y (0.2–10 y)
Oral medicine, U.K.	91	13	71	NR	NR	NR	NR	62	NR	NR

Abbreviations: NR = not recorded.
* 25 controls with painful chronic oral conditions.

in this review and the rest were rejected. The criteria for inclusion were clear diagnostic criteria that identified only those patients with no medical or odontological causes (except for the prevalence data), reports dealing exclusively with the condition defined above, and studies with a well-defined purpose and appropriate design. We used studies with observational data if randomized controlled or double-blind trials were lacking. Papers on the epidemiology of facial pain were found as detailed at the beginning of this chapter. To identify further references we searched several large review articles, the author's collection of papers, and the books *The Burning Mouth Syndrome* (van der Waal 1990), *Textbook of Pain* (Wall and Melzack 1989), and *Oral Manifestations of Systemic Disease* (Mason and Jones 1990).

DEFINITION AND DIAGNOSTIC CRITERIA

As other authors have noted in their reviews (Tourne and Fricton 1992; Bergdahl and Anneroth 1993), confusion surrounds the terminology of burning mouth as few authors define their diagnostic criteria. In many studies, burning mouth is a symptom of other diseases that are classified under three broad headings: local, systemic, and psychogenic diseases (Tourne and Fricton 1992; Bergdahl and Anneroth 1993). Local factors include bacterial and candidal in-fections, allergies, geographic tongue, mechanical and chemical irritation, oral habits (e.g., clenching and grinding), oral mucosal diseases, and xerostomia. Systemic factors include hematological deficiencies (e.g., folate, vitamin B12, iron), climacteric syndrome, and diabetes. Psychogenic factors include anxiety, depression, stress, life events, personality problems, and cancer phobia. Few investigators have used control data to validate their statements. In other studies a failure to identify medical or odontological factors leads to a diagnosis of BMS. Most studies include both types of patients but do not specify the number in each category.

The IASP classification of chronic pain defines "glossodynia and sore mouth (also known as burning tongue or oral dysesthesia)" as a "burning pain in the tongue or other oral mucous membranes" (code 051.x8) (Merskey and Bogduk 1994). The IHS classification does not include this syndrome. The IASP criteria do not specify clearly whether factors such as those mentioned above have been excluded. Some studies have defined selection criteria more clearly by stating that no medical or odontological factors were identified in patients diagnosed with BMS. This review includes only studies in which burning mouth, tongue, or oral mucosa were associated with no abnormalities other than dry mouth, dysgeusic taste, and altered taste perception. It excludes studies with pa-

Table II
Extended

Periodicity	Pain Severity	Pain Site	Other Oral Symptoms	Other General Symptoms	Reference
59% pain by mid-morning, 75% worse early evening	63.4 ± 27 (scale 0–100)	92% more than 1 site; tongue, hard palate, lower lip commonest	Dry mouth altered taste and heat pain tolerance	Headaches, sleep disturbance, menopausal symptoms more severe	Grushka 1987; Grushka et al. 1987
49% worse end of day, 28% continuous	NR	Most more than 1 site; tongue, lips, palate commonest; bilateral	43% taste disturbance	Sleep disturbance, anxiety, depression, neuroticism	Van der Ploeg et al. 1987
NR	NR	NR	NR	44% psychiatric disorder	Browning et al. 1987
Continuous	4.5 (scale 1–7)	77% tongue, lips, and palate	NR	NR	Bergdahl et al. 1995
88% all day, 89% every day	7.2 ± 2.5 (scale 1–10)	NR	NR	NR	Eli et al. 1994
NR	Over 50% 7–10 (scale 0–10)	NR	61% para-functional habits	NR	Paterson et al. 1995

tients reported to have geographic tongue, candidal infection, poorly fitting dentures, allergies, erosive lichen planus, or xerostomia due to Sjögren's disease. It is difficult to use these diagnostic criteria in population studies as the patients would require both an examination and possible investigations to exclude some of these associated factors. Population studies, therefore, have included any subjects who reported a burning sensation on the lips, tongue, or other intraoral site irrespective of cause.

Clinical features

Grushka (1987) is the only investigator to describe the clinical features of BMS in reference to a control group. Otherwise, the data quoted are from case series with clearly specified diagnostic criteria (Table II). Burning mouth has been reported in both sexes but is most frequent in women with a mean age of 50–60 years. The predominant feature is the symptom of burning pain, but subjects have used other descriptors including discomfort, tender, and annoying. The areas involved most frequently are the tongue, the anterior part of the hard palate, and the lower, inner aspect of the lower lip. The buccal mucosa is also often involved. In most patients the symptoms are bilateral (Grushka 1987).

The symptoms often continue for many months,

but studies give few details about duration and periodicity. Onset is gradual, and most patients have a constant pain that varies in intensity throughout the day but is most severe at the end of the day (Grushka 1987). The rare studies that measure intensity use the visual analogue scale and McGill Pain Questionnaire. Intensity varies from mild to severe, as shown in Tables II and III. Factors that appear to provoke symptoms in more than 50% of patients include tension, fatigue, speaking, hot and cold foods, eating, and working (Grushka 1987). Associated symptoms vary, and few studies define and compare subjects to an age- and sex-matched control group. Grushka (1987) showed a higher prevalence of dry mouth, persistent altered taste perception, and thirst, but no difference in other oral or dental features including candidiasis when compared to a control group. Patients had no greater prevalence of medical conditions such as diabetes, arthritis, and cardiovascular and gastrointestinal disorders (often linked to the syndrome) when compared to age- and sex-matched controls.

In general, burning mouth patients report more sleep disturbance, nonspecific health problems, pain complaints, and severe menopausal symptoms than do controls; headaches are the most common general symptoms. Anxiety, depression, personality disorders, and other psychiatric diseases are reported frequently in these patients. Many of these studies are unclear as to whether these symptoms are risk factors for development of BMS or a consequence of the syndrome; longitudinal cohort studies are lacking. The studies summarized in Table III use the same diagnostic criteria (no medical or odontological factors accounted for the burning mouth). All the studies used control groups or comparison data from other studies. Eli and colleagues (1994) compared 45 patients with BMS with carefully matched controls and found that the patients showed an increased tendency for somatization, obsession, compulsion, depression, anxiety, hostility, phobic anxiety, personal sensitivity, and psychosis as measured on the SCL-90 questionnaire.

Hampf and colleagues (1987) assessed 54 patients with orofacial dysesthesia, of whom 10 had BMS. They used age- and sex-matched controls, but only patients with symptoms proceeded to a semistructured psychiatric interview and assessment of DSM-III category. The control group was screened only with the Cornell Medical Index, which was not administered to the patients with burning mouth.

Miyaoka and colleagues (1996) assessed 50 women with glossodynia and found no differences on the general health questionnaire, but patients with BMS had more labile and anxious, premorbid personalities, which according to the authors probably predisposed them to the syndrome.

Signs and laboratory findings

Attempts have been made to assess burning mouth patients objectively and to look for etiological factors. The significance of some findings are unknown, even in studies with adequate control data. Cekic-Arambasin and colleagues (1990) reported that 50 patients with tongue symptoms had increased tongue temperature compared to a group of 50 age- and sex-matched subjects free of all oral symptoms. Grushka et al. (1987) showed that heat pain tolerance was altered in 72 patients with BMS compared to 43 age- and sex-matched controls. Other sensory modalities remained unchanged. Svensson and colleagues (1993) reported that pain and sensory thresholds were significantly lower in 23 patients with BMS as compared to controls. A study assessing salivary flow and content (Glick et al. 1976) revealed that protein, potassium, and phosphate concentrations were higher in 13 patients with BMS as compared to a control group of age- and sex-matched subjects. Tammiala-Salonen and Soderling (1993) assessed 18 patients with age- and sex-matched

controls and found no significant difference in the flow rates or the protein composition, adhesion, and agglutination properties of the saliva in the two groups.

Maragou and Ivanyi (1991) detected lower serum zinc levels in 30 patients with BMS as compared to 30 controls. However, the significance of these findings is unknown.

Grushka (1987) found that more than 58% of patients with burning mouth had one or more abnormal results for hematological or immunological factors, but these only differed marginally from the rate in normal controls and were probably of no significance.

Diagnostic difficulties

Theoretically, diagnosis is not difficult, as patients are clear in describing a burning sensation. The site is commonly the tongue, but it can involve almost any oral area. Patients usually report sensations of at least 3 months' duration, and symptoms can be constant or intermittent. Clinicians, however, recognize several conditions that may cause the symptoms. Identifying and treating these conditions often leads to a resolution of the burning. In these instances the burning mouth is a symptom rather than a disease entity. However, for a core of patients no causes can be found, and treatment of suspected factors has no effect on symptoms. Clinicians classify this group of patients as having BMS. Unfortunately, many studies do not clarify this distinction but group together all patients with burning mouths.

DEMOGRAPHIC FACTORS IN PREVALENCE

The epidemiological data on BMS are poor, and not a single study merits a high rating (Table IV). Only two studies deal exclusively with the epidemiology of burning mouth (Tammiala-Salonen et al. 1993; Locker and Grushka 1987). Further data are found in epidemiological studies dealing with facial pain in general. In all, we identified six studies that referred to burning mouth.

All studies simply aimed to identify patients who had symptoms of burning mouth; none assessed the causes. Only three studies were conducted in the community, and of these two (Tammiala-Salonen et al. 1993; Locker and Grushka 1987) assessed whether the subjects were representative of the population in the community. These three studies also described how they obtained their samples and the final response rate.

Table III
Psychological/psychiatric questionnaires and tests in case-control series of patients with burning mouth syndrome (BMS)
for which no medical or odontological causes were found

Reference	Questionnaire or Test	No. Patients	No. and Type of Controls	Psychological Features	Findings*
Grushka et al. 1987	MPQ, VAS, MMPI	72	43; age, sex matched	Personality changes	Personality changes same as other chronic pain
Eli et al. 1994	Recent life changes questionnaire, SCL-90	45	45; age, sex, ethnic group, socioeconomic status, education matched	Life events, psychopathological profile	No difference for life events; scored higher on SCL 90
Hampf et al. 1987	Psychiatric interview, CMI	54 (10 with BMS)	44; age, sex matched	Psychiatric illness	Severe personality disorder 7, mild personality disorder 3
van der Ploeg 1987	SSTI, Depression Adjective checklist, stress questionnaire, Dutch personality inventory	154	Previous studies	Anxiety, depression, neurosis	Patients scored higher on all tests
Zilli et al. 1989	GHQ 28, irritability, depression and anxiety scale	31	Previous study by same authors in pain clinics	Depression, anxiety, irritability	Depression increased, GHQ no different from other pain patients
Browning et al. 1989	GHQ 28, MADS	25	25; age sex organic oral pain matched	Depression, anxiety, cancer phobia	No psychiatric diagnosis 14 (21), major depression 2 (1), minor depression 7 (2), anxiety disorder 2 (1), cancer phobia 11(0)
Bergdahl et al. 1995	KSP, personality scale, psychological functioning scale, quality of life scale	32	32; age, sex matched	Personality, coping skills, quality of life	Lower socialization scale, anxiety, increased somatic symptoms, no quality of life differences
Paterson et al. 1995	HADS	91	69; age, sex matched	Anxiety, depression	Anxiety 26% (7%), depression 13% (1%)
Miyaoka et al. 1996	Psychiatric interview, Eysenck personality, GHQ 30, TAS	50 (all female)	24; age matched	Psychiatric illness, personality traits, neuroticism	Lower on extroversion and higher on TAS, decreased emotions, GHQ no difference, personality traits

Abbreviations: CMI = Cornell Medical Index; GHQ = General Health Questionnaire; HADS = Hospital Anxiety and Depression Scale; KSP = Karolinska Scale of Personality; MADS = Montgomery Asberg Depression Scale; MMPI = Minnesota Multiphasic Personality Inventory; MPQ = McGill Pain Questionnaire; SCL = symptom check list; SSTI = Spielberger State Trait Inventory; TAS = Toronto Alexithymia Scale; VAS = visual analogue scale.
* Findings in parentheses are for controls.

One study (Lipton et al. 1993) had a response rate of 93% and thus did not attempt to pursue nonresponders. Tammiala-Salonen and colleagues (1993) reported a response rate of 72% but did not discuss any attempt to contact nonresponders. Locker and Grushka (1987) assessed in detail the late responders and non-responders to their mail survey on oral and facial pain and published a separate report indicating that nonresponders were more likely to be male, over age 65, and born outside Canada. They estimated the prevalence of burning mouth at 4% in early responders but adjusted the rate upward to 5.3% after including late responders. These findings indicate that nonresponders probably had more symptoms. Only two studies (Tammiala-Salonen et al. 1993; Locker and Grushka 1987) provided details on the reliability of both the sampling method and examiners.

Three other studies report on burning mouth. One dealing exclusively with this condition (Basker et al. 1978) was conducted in general dental practices and in clinics treating diabetes and disorders of menopause. The other two studies, one in factory workers (Jaafar et al. 1989) and one in general dental practice (Richards and Scourfield 1996), were part of larger surveys to

Table IV
Prevalence of burning mouth syndrome (BMS)

Study Type	Source of Sample	Sample Size	Pain Severity	Duration of Symp-toms	Type of Prevalence Est.	Prevalence	Comments	Reference
CS population, Q, EX	Mini Finland project, Turku	600; R = 72%	Moder-ate	1–3 y	Period, 3 y	1–15% dependent on criteria	Included clinical examination	Tammiala-Salomen et al. 1993
CS population, mailed Q	City of Toronto	1014; R = 72%	NR	NR	Period, 1 mo	4.5% (5.3% incl. late respond-ers)	Assessed oral and facial pain	Locker and Grushka 1987, 1988
CS population, SCQ, interviewers	NHIS, USA (1989)	45,711; R = 93%	NR	NR	Period, 6 mo	0.7%; 0.8% F, 0.6% M	Patients had BMS with other pains; increased with age	Lipton et al. 1993
CS population, SCQ	[a]Five dental practices, [b]menopausal clinic, [c]diabetic clinic, UK	[a]392, [b]114, [c]110; R = NR	Over 50% mild to moderate	1–10 y	Lifetime and point	Lifetime 5.1%, point 2.6%	No details on sampling; 26% menopausal women had oral symptoms; 10% diabetics had BMS	Basker et al. 1978
Industrial population, SCQ, interviewers	Two factory populations, Malaysia	355; R = NR	NR	NR	Period, 1 mo	10.3%	No sample details; study assessed orofacial pain	Jaafar et al. 1989
CS population, SCQ	General dental practitioners, Wales	997; R = NR	NR	NR	Period, 1 mo	1.7%	No sample details; survey on oral health	Richards and Scourfield 1996

Abbreviations: CS = cross-sectional; EX = examination; F = female; M = male; NHIS = National Health Interview Survey; NR = not reported; Q = questionnaire; R = response; SCQ = self-completed questionnaire.

assess facial and dental pain and its social impact.

Studies by Locker and Grushka (1987), Richards and Scourfield (1996), and Basker et al. (1978) used self-report questionnaires, whereas Lipton et al. (1993) and Jaafar et al. (1989) used interviewers to complete the questionnaires. Only the study by Tammiala-Salonen et al. (1993) used both questionnaires and examination. No studies attempted a follow-up survey to assess how symptoms may change, especially with age.

All these studies specifically asked patients whether they had prolonged burning in the mouth or tongue. Three studies (Locker and Grushka 1987; Jaafar et al. 1989; Richards and Scourfield 1996) asked for symptoms in the previous month, one specified the last 6 months (Lipton et al. 1993), and two gave no indication of the time factor (Jaafar et al. 1989; Tammiala-Salonen et al. 1993).

Prevalence rates vary from 0.6% to 15% (Table IV). Tammiala-Salonen and colleagues (1993) present a range of prevalence rates dependent on the criteria used. The prevalence rate is 15% if all cases of prolonged burning are included, 11% for patients who have no lesions, 7.9% if candida is excluded, and 1% if the criteria are restricted to only subjects with continuous burning.

Only one study (Tammiala-Salonen et al. 1993) specifically inquired about other symptoms and found that 40% of patients reported altered taste and that 17% linked the start of symptoms with an illness or new therapies. Only this study attempted to assess the different sites affected by the burning. Locker and Grushka (1987) and Jaafar et al. (1989) attempted to assess the impact of symptoms on the lives of the sufferers, but they dealt with all forms of nondental facial pain rather than specifically with burning mouth.

Table V
Prevalence of burning mouth syndrome by
demographic group

Demographic Variable	Estimated Prevalence (per 100,000)	Prevalence (%)
Ethnicity		
White, non-Hispanic	693	19
Black, non-Hispanic	531	15
Hispanic	786	22
Other non-Hispanic	1598	44
Age Group		
18–34	609	19
35–54	696	21
55–74	757	23
75+	1184	36

Source: Lipton et al. (1993).

Two studies reported data on age and sex of patients with burning mouth. Tammiala-Salonen et al. (1993) gave a mean age of 55 years overall with a mean of 51 years for men and 57 years for women. Lipton et al. (1993) found that 0.8% of women and 0.6% of men complained of BMS, and estimated that the prevalence of burning mouth increases with age (Table V).

All studies reported a predominance of female subjects. Tammiala-Salonen et al. (1993) had a ratio of 3:1, whereas Basker et al. (1978) reported rates of 4.2% in women and 0.8% in men. The community studies by Lipton et al. (1993) found less difference, 0.8% in women and 0.6% in men. Biological, psychological, and sociocultural factors may explain these gender differences but they have not been assessed. In comparison with other facial pains, only BMS tends to increase with age (Lipton et al. 1993). Only Lipton and col-

leagues assessed ethnicity in burning mouth patients. The results of their analysis of four ethnic groups are shown in Table V.

No studies have reported prevalence of burning mouth by social, educational, or occupational groups. Also, the natural history of this syndrome is not known, and no longitudinal prospective cohort studies have been reported.

CONSEQUENCES

No studies have specifically evaluated the economic cost of BMS or cost to the patient in disability, handicap, and psychological problems. Bergdahl and colleagues. (1994) tried to estimate the economic cost in a study of 21 patients who had diverse types of burning mouth and often other systemic pains. They assessed the mean days of sickness benefit per insured person and reported considerably higher expenses for their patients compared to the age- and sex-matched controls in the Swedish population, 31,878 Skr versus 18,032 Skr, respectively.

CAUSATION AND PREVENTION

As noted in the discussion of clinical symptoms, psychological factors play a role in burning mouth, but it is not clear whether they are part of the syndrome or whether they are risk factors. No satisfactory randomized controlled trials and few good case-control studies have assessed risk factors for burning mouth (Table VI). Not a single study has considered whether smoking, alcohol, or dietary factors may be risk factors for this condition. Given this lack of knowledge, the literature offers no information about primary, secondary, or tertiary prevention.

Table VI
Risk factors for BMS in patients with no odontological or medical
causes in controlled studies with specified diagnostic criteria

Study Type	Risk Factor	Strength of Association	Likelihood of Causality	Reference
Case-control	Oral candidiasis, diabetes, arthritis, cardiovascular, gastrointestinal, menopause, iron deficiency anemia, nonspecific immunological deficiencies	None	Unlikely	Grushka 1987
Cohort	Lack of estrogen	Weak	May contribute	Ferguson et al. 1981

CHALLENGES FOR THE FUTURE

As others have also noted (Tourne and Fricton 1992; Bergdahl and Anneroth 1993), there is an urgent need for prospective collaborative studies that are carefully controlled, use strict diagnostic criteria, and randomly select subjects who are representative of the population of patients with burning mouth. Factors important for investigation include duration of symptoms, periodicity, severity, affected sites, associated oral and systemic symptoms, general health, drug history, and tobacco and alcohol use. Such studies may then resolve the issue of whether burning mouth is a symptom of a variety of known conditions or an entity in its own right, and may reveal etiological and risk factors.

Longitudinal cohort studies or case-control studies could give some indicator of natural history and risk factors and further elucidate the difference between burning mouth as a symptom and burning mouth as a condition.

ATYPICAL FACIAL PAIN/ATYPICAL FACIAL NEURALGIA

DEFINITION AND DIAGNOSTIC CRITERIA

Atypical facial pain (AFP) and atypical facial neuralgia are terms used to describe persistent facial pains that have no objective physiological signs or demonstrable organic lesions. The diagnosis of psychogenic pain is sometimes applied, but this approach appears to support a body-mind distinction for pain causation without acknowledging the interdependence of the two. *The Diagnostic and Statistical Manual of Mental Disorders* (DSM-IV) designates two types of somatoform disorders: those in which psychological factors are judged to have the major role in the onset, severity, exacerbation, or maintenance of the condition; and those in which both a medical condition and psychological factors are judged to have important roles. In either case, the pain is not better accounted for by mood disorder (e.g., depression), anxiety, or psychotic disorder. The IASP classification allows for a psychogenic pain diagnosis in the absence of physical symptoms.

Dworkin and Burgess (1987) have compared the DSM-III-R classification (the predecessor of DSM-IV) with that of the IASP for oral facial pain (see Table VII for a summary of their table plus the IHS classification). Dworkin and Burgess describe psychogenic headaches, atypical odontalgia, burning mouth syndrome, and atypical facial neuralgia as conditions that have distinct features and require separate classification.

The IHS (Headache Classification Committee 1988) under Section 12.8 classifies atypical facial pain and atypical odontalgia as "facial pain not fulfilling other criteria." Pfaffenrath and colleagues (1993) applied the IHS criteria to 35 patients with atypical facial pain and suggested that modifications are needed to this classification, which are discussed in a following section.

For this condition we used the literature search methods and the inclusion criteria described at the beginning of this chapter, and identified 25 articles.

Clinical features

Most of the clinical features identified for atypical facial pain are based on the following case series: Smith et al. (1969), 32 patients; Mock et al. (1985), 34 patients; Pfaffenrath et al. (1993), 35 patients; and Remick and Blasberg (1985), 121 patients. Some studies, but not all, used control groups. Melzack and colleagues (1986) used the McGill Pain Questionnaire to assess the character of the pain. Patients with atypical facial pain used words such as vicious, diffuse, and excruciating. In a similar study of 100 patients in the United Kingdom, 62% chose the word nagging; other common words chosen were throbbing, exhausting, tender, miserable, and tiring (Zakrzewska 1995). In a study of 32 patients, Smith et al. (1969) reported the following descriptors: boring, deep, and burning (12); sharp, jabbing, and striking (7); pulling and squeezing (4); steady ache (3); pressing (3); throbbing (2); and tingling (2). Pfaffenrath et al. (1993), in their study of 35 patients, reported words such as drawing, burning, stabbing, pressing, throbbing, toothache-like, pulsating, and drilling.

Pain varies from mild to severe, although in two placebo-controlled trials the pain was assessed initially as moderately severe (Seltzer et al. 1982; Feinmann et al. 1984). In a study of 70 patients, Holzberg and colleagues (1996) reported a mean pain rating index of 29.7 ± 15.1 (maximum 78).

The pain is often persistent, and several treatment trials used inclusion criteria of pain for 6 months or more. The periodicity of the pain varies, and all series

Table VII
Pain of psychological origin in the head and face

Nomenclature System	Delusional/Hallucinatory Orofacial Pain	Atypical Odontalgia, BMS, Atypical Facial Neuralgia
DSM-III-R	Profound thought disorder, psychosis	Stress, anxiety, depression, conversion reactions, and hypochondriacal concerns in absence of other major mental disturbance
DSM-III-R	Schizophrenia (when delusions and hallucinations are confirmed); somatoform pain disorder (if explanatory models are unconventional but not psychotic)	Somatoform pain disorder (307.80)
IASP	Pain of psychological origin in the head and face: delusional or hallucinatory pain (01x.x9a)	Pain of psychological origin in the head and face: hysterical or hypochondriacal (01x.x9b)
IHS	Facial pain not fulfilling criteria in groups 11 and 12 (not including BMS) (12.8)	

Source: Dworkin and Burgess (1987).
Note: Where a pathophysiological mechanism is strongly suspected, vascular and neural mechanisms may be involved. When a pathophysiological mechanism is known, DMS-III-R diagnosis is psychological factors affecting physical condition (316.00); the physical condition is listed in Axis III. An alternative IASP diagnosis may include: tension headache or chronic form, scalp-muscle contraction headache (033.x7b); alternative pain and dysfunction syndrome (034.x8a); osteoarthritis of the TMJ (033.x6); odontalgia (toothache-pulpitis) (031.x2c); periapical periodontitis and abscess (031.x2d); glossodynia and sore mouth (041.x5); or cracked tooth syndrome (034.x1).

report the pain as varying from constant daily pain to periods of no pain ranging from weeks to months (Mock et al. 1985; Pfaffenrath et al. 1993; see Table VIII). The Pfaffenrath team reported that 74% of patients had pain that radiated, 43% to the ipsilateral side and 31% to the contralateral. Mock and colleagues reported radiating pain in 83% of patients.

Stress is often considered a provoking factor and was reported by up to 86% of patients in the Pfaffenrath series. Other provoking features include cold, weather changes, chewing, and head movements. However, some patients reported no provoking factors. Although patients often state the pain is severe, work impairment seems to be minimal and was reported by only 14% of patients in the study by Feinmann et al. (1984) and by 28% in the series by Pfaffenrath. Feinmann, however, noted that over 75% of patients reported a life event 1–6 months before the onset of the pain; 28% of the patients in the series of Smith et al. (1969) reported such an event. Although some patients indicate that local warmth and pressure improve their facial pain (Pfaffenrath et al. 1993), few reports note any relieving factors apart from medications. Pfaffenrath and colleagues found that patients had consulted on average 7.5 different doctors (range 1–20), most often dentists, physicians, neurologists, and ear, nose, and throat (ENT) surgeons. Treatments ranged from surgery to antidepressant drugs, analgesics, homeopathy, and physical therapies.

Hampf et al. (1987) assessed 38 atypical facial pain patients by psychiatric interview using the DSM-III classification and compared them to age- and sex-matched controls seeking extraction of painless wisdom teeth. The control group were not interviewed but completed the Cornell Medical Index. Severe mental disturbance was found in 35% of cases and 7% of controls, whereas only 6% of cases (vs. 73% of controls) had no mental disturbance. Of the patients with atypical facial pain, 12 were psychotic, 16 had pathological personality disorders, and four had mild psychotic disorders.

Smith et al. (1969) and Remick and Blasberg (1985) investigated the psychiatric conditions found in patients with atypical facial pain, but neither study used controls. Smith and colleagues based their diagnosis on psychiatric interview and found that most patients had either depressive reaction, conversion reaction, or hysterical personality. Remick and Blasberg used the DSM-III classification and found that 16% had affective (depressive) disorders, 15% somatoform, 7% adjustment disorder, 6% psychosis, 5% anxiety, and 4% personality disorder. Patients scored higher on MMPI scores tending toward hysteria (Smith et al. 1969). Most studies report no physical abnormalities. Friedman (1995), however, evaluated 18 patients with AFP (IHS criteria) and found an area of tenderness and 0.2–1°C increased temperature (as compared to the opposite side) over the maxillary molar root api-

Table VIII

Prevalence of atypical facial pain (AFP) by age, gender, and social factors

Study Type	Disease Definition	Source of Sample	Sample Size	Pain Severity	Mean Symptom Duration (Range) (years)	Age (Range) (years)	Gender	Social Factors	Reference	Comments
Double-blind trial for treatment	44% facial arthromyalgia, 46% AFP	Oral and maxillo-facial clinic, UK	95	2 ± 0.6 (scale 1–4)	3.4 ± 4.3 (0.4–30)	42.7 ± 8.1 M, 45.7 ± 9.9 F (19–65) (facial pain)	14% M, 86% F (AFP only)	Social I & II 39%, Social III 46%, Social IV & V 14%	Feinmann et al. 1984	AFP and facial arthromyalgia patients only varied by age and gender
Retrospective case series	AFP	Facial pain clinic, Canada	34	—	50% pain >2 y	85% 31–60 y (21–63)	23% M, 76% F	—	Mock et al. 1985	
Prospective case series	AFP	Facial pain clinic, Germany	35	—	7 ± 5.9 y (1–30)	53.5 ± 14.9 (28–82)	11% M, 8% F	—	Pfaffenrath et al. 1993	
Prospective case series	AFP	Facial pain clinic, Italy	33	8.4 ± 1.34 (scale 0–10)	6.5 ± 6.4	40.9 ± 11.43	18% M, 81% F	—	Mongini et al. 1992	
Prospective case series	AFP, odontalgia	Oral and maxillo-facial clinic, Finland	34	—	—	46.1 (28–73)	30% M, 70% F	—	Hampf 1987	
Prospective case series	Mixed chronic facial pain	Facial pain clinic, USA	70	PRI on MPQ 30 ± 15.1	9.5 ±12.75	40 ± 13 (18-67)	11% M, 89% F	Education 14 ± 3 y (10–22 y)	Holzberg et al. 1996	
Prospective case series	86 AFP, 35 other	Facial pain clinic, Canada	121	—	—	52.4	17% M, 83% F	—	Remick and Blasberg 1985	29% found to have medical dental cause
Prospective	AFP	Neurology, dental clinics, USA	32	—	3.5 (0.6–10)	46.5 (28–79)	37% M, 62% F	50% M clerical; 40% F housewives	Smith et al. 1969	

Note: No data are presented on prevalence in the population or on racial groups.

Abbreviations: F = female; M = male; MPQ = McGill Pain Questionnaire; PRI = Pain Rating Index.

ces. Pfaffenrath et al. (1993) and Mock et al. (1985) both report that 38–63% of patients had altered sensations.

A small study involving six women with atypical facial pain and six healthy age- and sex-matched controls used positron emission tomography (PET) to assess changes in regional, cerebral blood flow (Derbyshire et al. 1994). Differences in blood flow in the prefrontal cortex and anterior, cingulate cortex were observed in the patients with atypical facial pain. Replication of his study in a larger group of patients with other chronic pain conditions and with controls is necessary to assess the significance of these findings.

Weddington and Blazer (1979) retrospectively compared the records of 87 patients discharged with a diagnosis of either trigeminal neuralgia (44) or atypical facial pain (43). They did not clearly define the diagnostic criteria, so it is not possible to ascertain whether the AFP group contained any patients with TMD pain or atypical odontalgia. The groups did not differ in sex, marital status, race, and occupation; both had a 2:1 ratio of women to men. Although trigeminal neuralgia patients were significantly older, both groups had patients with symptoms persisting more than 8 years. Psychiatric and psychosocial consultations were more common in patients with AFP, up to 67% compared to 5% in the trigeminal neuralgia group. The former were more frequently treated with psychotropic drugs. The authors, however, stressed the lack of high-quality data, especially for psychosocial factors.

DEMOGRAPHIC FACTORS IN PREVALENCE

Prevalence data for AFP are not available. Most studies do not clearly state the diagnostic criteria for atypical facial pain, and we suspect that data may include TMD and myofascial pain. Three papers attempted to characterize atypical facial pain (Mock et al. 1985; Mongini et al. 1992; Pfaffenrath et al. 1993), whereas two others specifically addressed psychological factors (Smith et al. 1969; Remick and Blasberg 1985). Only one study reporting on a clinical treatment trial clearly identified patients with atypical facial pain as opposed to facial arthromyalgia or TMD pain (Feinmann et al. 1984). Holzberg et al. (1996) did not clarify their criteria for chronic facial pain and most likely evaluated a mixed group of patients. Table VIII summarizes the findings.

NATURAL HISTORY, PROGNOSTIC FACTORS, AND PSYCHOLOGICAL CONSEQUENCES

Pfaffenrath et al. (1993) noted that up to 50% of patients may have symptom-free phases; in their study 23% of symptoms occurred spontaneously while 34% occurred during treatment. Pain-free intervals lasted for a few weeks in 40% of the patients and for several months in 17%.

Feinmann and Harris (1984) reported that 39% of patients were on medication after 1 year to prevent relapse, but of these 38% were pain free. An early response to drug treatment was a good predictor of freedom from pain after 1 year and also predicted relief of pain related to adverse life events (e.g., bereavement) if patients had received counseling. Feinmann (1993) then followed this same group of treatment trial patients. At 4 years she evaluated 71 of the original 84 patients and found that 57% had facial arthromyalgia and 43% atypical facial pain. The latter were more likely to develop intractable pain. Twenty-two patients (31%) were still in pain (intractable) and 49 (69%) were pain free. A comparison of the two groups showed no age or sex differences. Three of those in pain and six of those who were pain free were on regular medication. Seven patients had continuous pain (and also a long history of pain), whereas 15 had intermittent pain with a mean duration of 6.1 months that required treatment. Eleven (50%) of the intractable pain group had somatoform symptoms, similar to the findings noted by Speculand and colleagues (1979) in their mixed group of patients with intractable facial pain. Both groups had reported the same number of life events, but the intractable group had poorer psychological adjustment and became more neurotic.

CAUSATION AND PREVENTION

High-risk groups and risk factors

No risk factors have been assessed. Mongini et al. (1992) used the MMPI in a variety of pain syndromes and suggested that neuroticism and psychosis may predispose patients to developing atypical facial pain as these two features are often found in patients with this condition. Studies report that adverse life events such as bereavement, chronic illness in the family, or major financial problems may occur prior to the development of facial pain, a relationship noted in up to 20%

of patients in the series by Pfaffenrath et al. (1992) and more than 75% in the study by Feinmann et al. (1984).

Scope for prevention

In her 4-year follow-up review, Feinmann (1993) showed that if the intractable cases can be identified early by use of appropriate assessments, pain relief combined with counseling aimed at lifestyle changes may decrease chronicity.

Unnecessary dental treatment can be avoided through early evaluation by dentists to rule out medical and dental treatment as a cause of pain. In a study of 58 patients with AFP, Remick et al. (1983) found that 36% had submitted to 65 dental and surgical procedures in an attempt to treat the pain but only 14 (24%) had a specific medical or dental cause. They urge patients to seek a psychiatric assessment before dental and surgical treatments.

CHALLENGES FOR THE FUTURE

The literature reveals numerous remaining controversies with no unified, clearly defined diagnostic criteria. Much of the data relating to AFP includes TMD pain and perhaps atypical odontalgia. We need more data collected using strict diagnostic criteria, as done by the Pfaffenrath team, to establish whether this condition is a distinct entity or part of a psychiatric condition. Studies should compare this group of patients with those who have had clearly defined TMD pain, myofascial pain, and other chronic pain complaints. Once firm diagnostic criteria are determined for atypical facial pain, investigators can assess the prevalence of this condition through population studies using carefully designed questionnaires that must include psychological factors. Future clinical trials also require stricter diagnostic criteria.

ATYPICAL ODONTALGIA OR PHANTOM TOOTH SYNDROME

DEFINITION AND DIAGNOSTIC CRITERIA

IASP defines atypical odontalgia (034.x8b) as a pain in a tooth without major pathology related to endodontics or tooth extraction and that may be associated with psychological and emotional problems (1994). In 1978 Marbach coined the term "phantom tooth pain" and suggested that this pain is not atypical and has clear criteria. Marbach (1993a) later proposed that persistent pain or paresthesia in teeth and other oral tissues following dental and surgical procedures is a deafferentation pain similar to other phantom pains associated with amputations. He stressed that the onset of pain is associated with injury to a peripheral nerve that can occur either during routine dental or medical procedures such as endodontics and apicetomies or as a result of trauma to the face. A lag of several years may occur between the injury and the development of pain. The pain may be in the area of the injured tissues but could spread to adjacent healthy tissues as the injured afferent nerve attempts to regenerate. Radiological and laboratory tests are negative. Atypical odontalgia has also been referred to as idiopathic odontalgia, idiopathic periodontalgia, and even atypical facial pain. It is thus difficult to ascertain whether all cases described under atypical odontalgia are the same as phantom tooth pain because not all clinicians report that the onset of pain relates to peripheral nerve damage. Bates and Stewart (1991) suggest that atypical odontalgia and phantom tooth pain are the same, and they do not stress peripheral nerve damage as a prerequisite for this condition. Reik (1984), however, suggests that atypical odontalgia is a localized form of AFP. Some patients with dental pain have had endodontic treatment or extractions in an attempt to relieve pain, whereas others develop pain after a dental procedure that is different from the original type of pain. Marbach (1993a) suggests that lack of physical signs prior to endodontics may be a sign of phantom tooth pain.

For this condition we searched the MEDLINE and Cochrane databases from 1966 to June 1997 for the text words atypical odontalgia and phantom tooth pain. This search yielded 17 articles on atypical odontalgia and 11 on phantom tooth pain. After reading the abstracts on screen we rejected 18 of the 28 articles that were: reviews (10), a letter (1), a pilot study that was later repeated and incorporated into a larger series (1), or that reported mixed types of pain (2), theories on etiology (2), and investigations with no control data (3). We completely reviewed nine papers; a review of their literature yielded three more papers, of which we rejected one and used two. We included studies that had clear diagnostic criteria, dealt exclusively with atypical odontalgia, and used randomized controlled trials, double-blind trials, or observational data.

Table IX
Age and sex distribution of phantom tooth pain/atypical odontalgia

Study Type	Disease Definition	Source of Sample	Sample Size	Duration of Symptoms (Range)	Age (Range) (years)	Gender	Reference
Prospective	Atypical odontalgia	Facial pain clinic, Canada	120	3.1 y (0.1–20 y)	43 ± 13.9 (13–80)	81% F, 19% M	Schnurr and Brooke 1992
Prospective	Atypical odontalgia	Oral and maxillo-facial surgery, UK	44	0.2–20 y	43 ± 16 (20–70)	82% F, 18% M	Rees and Harris 1979
Prospective (mailed Q)	Phantom tooth pain	Endodontists, USA	732; R = 463 (30 with pain)	—	—	66% F, 33% M	Marbach et al. 1982
—	—	Clinic	8	4 y	45	86% F, 14% M	Reik 1984
Prospective	Atypical odontalgia	Dental college, USA	30	4.4 y (0.5–25 y)	584 (22–82)	90% F, 10% M	Bates et al. 1991
Retrospective (mailed Q)	Phantom tooth pain, post-traumatic dysesthesia	Endodontic patients, USA	206; R = 118	21 mo	—	4 F, 2 M	Campbell et al. 1990
Prospective	Phantom tooth pain	Facial pain clinic, USA	115*	—	38.8 ± 14.2	63% F, 37% M	Marbach 1993
Prospective	Atypical odontalgia	Orofacial pain clinic, USA	19	25.5 ± 5 mo	45.7 ± 3.19	79% F, 21% M	Graff-Radford and Solberg 1993
Prospective (Q)	Phantom tooth pain	Headache center, Italy	46 (matched controls)		47.6 ± 4.9	56% F, 43% M	Sicuteri et al. 1991

Note: No data are presented on prevalence in the population or by racial, occupational, educational, and social groups, or on pain severity.
Abbreviations: R = response; Q = questionnaire.
*72% of controls were employed, 68% married.

Clinical features

No studies compare the basic clinical features of atypical odontalgia to data from controls. Case series provide the best data, although many of these studies are poorly documented. The reports discussed in this section state the diagnostic criteria used. Only one report mentions use of the McGill Pain Questionnaire, but it does not present the results (Graff-Radford and Solberg 1993).

Marbach (1993a) characterizes phantom tooth pain as a dull, boring, and aching pain with occasional spontaneous, sharp pains. Intensity is moderate to severe but allows for normal sleep. Marbach (1993a) stresses that this pain is continuous. Many patients have experienced pain for several years, as summarized in Table IX. Stener and Brooke (1992) found that 30% of their patients with atypical odontalgia related the onset of pain to dental treatment. In a long-term follow-up of 28 patients they found that 63% described their pain as intermittent and 32% as continuous. The pain was located in the teeth, jaws, and gingiva of 93% of patients, and 22.5% reported pain in more than one site. Marbach reported similar findings. A local anesthetic may provide some relief; Bates et al. (1991) found it gave complete relief of pain in 46% of patients and partial relief in 31%. Graff-Radford and Solberg (1993) reported that somatic anesthetic blocks have equivocal results.

Two studies (Graff-Radford and Solberg 1993; Marbach 1993b) attempted to assess the psychological component of atypical odontalgia, and both concluded that psychiatric features are no greater than found in any patients suffering from chronic pain.

Marbach's study (1993b) focused on levels of distress or demoralization, personality factors, and coping mechanisms. He assessed 115 patients with phantom tooth pain, 151 with TMD pain, and 137 control subjects with no pain. This study showed that patients with both phantom tooth pain and TMD pain showed high levels of psychological distress or demoralization. The level of depression was higher in those with phantom tooth pain, which suggests that this condition is a physical expression of depression, although it is not clear which comes first. Personality measures and coping strategies were not significantly different, although patients with phantom tooth pain tended to have a higher external locus of control. Whether these changes are antecedents or consequences of phantom tooth pain could not be determined by this cross-sectional study.

Graff-Radford and Solberg (1993) assessed psychological functioning with the MMPI. They used a modified version of the IASP classification to establish their diagnosis, and did not stipulate that peripheral nerve damage should have occurred in association with pain. Their controls were patients with headaches matched for age, sex, and pain duration. The MMPI questionnaire produced mean profiles that were not elevated. Although 42% of atypical odontalgia patients had elevated depression, this finding was similar to control data from patient populations in general medical practice. The authors thus suggest that psychological factors are not implicated in atypical odontalgia.

Gratt and colleagues (1989) have noted that electronic thermography may be useful in the diagnosis of atypical odontalgia. Ten patients (selected according to strict criteria) and 10 controls with no history of facial pain or dental problems received electronic thermography on both sides of the face. In 84% of normal subjects both sides gave the same results, compared to only 66% in the atypical odontalgia group ($P > 0.01$). The thermographic results were assessed by numerous clinicians who were blind to the diagnosis, which guaranteed objectivity. This study needs to be repeated with larger groups of patients.

DEMOGRAPHIC FACTORS IN PREVALENCE

Only two studies have assessed the prevalence of phantom tooth pain (Marbach et al. 1982; Campbell et al. 1990). Marbach and colleagues asked 17 endodontists in New York City to mail a questionnaire to their patients to ascertain the prevalence of phantom tooth pain; one dentist agreed to do so. Seventy percent of the questionnaires were returned and 12% were undeliverable, and no attempts were made to contact nonresponders. Of the responders, 463 (63%) could be evaluated. In this group, 20 (9%) women and 10 (5%) men had pain 1 month after endodontics, and all except two women had had pain prior to treatment. Fifteen of these patients (4 men and 11 women) agreed to be examined more thoroughly, and eight of the women fulfilled the criteria of phantom tooth pain. Marbach (1982) estimated a 3–6% incidence of phantom tooth pain in this population.

Campbell and colleagues (1990) sent a questionnaire to 206 patients who received endodontic treatment at their dental institute. They reported a response rate of only 50% and identified three patients with phantom tooth pain according to Marbach's criteria and three with post-traumatic anesthesia. The latter diagnosis was made if no pain had been reported prior to endodontic treatment and if radiological examination revealed that treatment had been adequately performed. The authors postulate that this pain could be due to poor techniques during treatment, such as tissue trauma or trauma from local anesthesia, which would not show up radiologically. If we ignore this group of three patients, the prevalence of phantom tooth pain is approximately 2.5% in this population. These patients had experienced pain for an average of 21 months, but the study did not provide details on severity. A series of case-control studies offers some details on the age, sex, and duration of symptoms of these patients and the study results (Table IX).

CONSEQUENCES

No studies have assessed the economic costs of atypical odontalgia. They are potentially high, as these patients continue to seek diagnosis and treatment from a range of professionals (Stener and Brooke 1992).

NATURAL HISTORY

To evaluate long-term prognosis, Stener and Brooke (1992) attempted to contact 53 patients who had been assessed in their clinic 5 years previously. Only 28 patients responded, and of this sample 19 were still in pain and 7 had constant pain, while the rest had experienced quiescent periods.

CAUSATION AND PREVENTION

Marbach (1993a) cautions against endodontic procedures on teeth when the only symptom is pain that is not associated with physical signs or radiological changes. These patients may be predisposed to the development of phantom tooth pain. Sicuteri and colleagues (1991) postulate that patients who suffer from migraines and cluster headaches (idiopathic headaches) are at increased risk of developing phantom tooth pain and that prophylaxis for the former improves the latter. Their study included two groups of outpatients in a headache center and dental institute who had had two or more teeth extracted a year previously: 301 patients had idiopathic headaches and 280 were age- and sex-matched controls with no idiopathic headaches or phantom tooth pain. The report did not discuss other selection criteria and did not include the questionnaire used to obtain the data or response rates. The authors identified 46 patients (15%) with phantom tooth pain in the idiopathic headache group and none among the control group. Idiopathic headache preceded phantom tooth pain in most instances and was ipsilateral to the headache. Attacks of idiopathic headache led to worsening of phantom tooth pain. The study was reported again in 1993 (Nicolodi and Sicuteri 1993).

Marbach (1993a) states that it is impossible to predict which patients may develop phantom tooth pain but that clear diagnostic criteria may enable earlier diagnosis and initiation of treatment.

CHALLENGES FOR THE FUTURE

The diagnostic criteria for phantom tooth pain proposed by Marbach (1993a) need verification by controlled studies. It will be important to confirm previous peripheral nerve damage to provide evidence for Marbach's theory that phantom tooth pain is a de-afferentation pain and is not due to psychological problems.

Thousands of endodontists are performing root canal treatments and it is important to ascertain what percentage of patients develop phantom tooth pain and how they might be characterized either before or soon after this procedure so that effective treatments can be instituted earlier rather than later.

TRIGEMINAL NEURALGIA

Both the IASP and the IHS classifications recognize two forms of this condition. Trigeminal neuralgia or tic douloureux (IASP Code 006.x8a and IHS Code 12.2.1) is of unknown etiology. Secondary or symptomatic trigeminal neuralgia is related either to central nervous system lesions (tumor or aneurysm) or to local facial trauma. Most study data contain a mixture of both types, and secondary trigeminal neuralgia seems to account for about 1–2% of cases. No papers deal specifically with this form.

Although the literature contains more than 3000 articles on trigeminal neuralgia, McQuay and colleagues (1995) found only three randomized controlled trials exploring the value of anticonvulsants in managing neuropathic pain. There is only one randomized controlled trial of surgical treatments. No well-designed prospective studies with concurrent or even historical controls have been conducted, although some studies did report epidemiological data. The bulk of the data were obtained from descriptive case studies of surgical management by specialists in treating trigeminal neuralgia. Many studies failed to specify assumptions regarding diagnostic criteria, and most failed to assess data objectively.

We searched the literature using MEDLINE databases from 1966 to July 1997 and the Cochrane database 1996, Issue 3. We used the MeSH headings of trigeminal neuralgia and facial neuralgia and the text word tic douloureux. This search yielded 3285 articles, whereas using trigeminal neuralgia alone as a text word yielded 1616. We then applied the epidemiological terms described in the general section of this chapter and reduced the number of references to 364. We printed 63 articles and read the abstracts or full papers to identify 15 papers that met our criteria for evaluation. In addition, we had access to extensive literature obtained while writing an MD thesis and a book. We also searched two books on trigeminal neuralgia published in the United States (Rovit 1979; Fromm 1987) to identify further references. The criteria for inclusion were clear diagnostic criteria and randomized, controlled, or case-matched series. For surgical data we selected only studies assessing prognostic factors and case series of more than 10 patients.

DEFINITION AND DIAGNOSTIC CRITERIA

Most experts in trigeminal neuralgia would agree with the diagnostic criteria published by the IASP and IHS. However, patients often are not precise about their symptoms, and most experts encounter patients who describe other features that do not fit the classical description (Zakrzewska 1995). Some reports draw attention to this discrepancy and separately evaluate these groups of patients.

The diagnostic criteria for trigeminal neuralgia are too complex for inclusion in epidemiological surveys conducted by mailed questionnaires. Population-based studies are thus extremely rare; only one prospective epidemiological study is of sufficient sensitivity to definitively diagnose trigeminal neuralgia. This study (Munoz et al. 1988) supplemented the mailed questionnaire with an examination.

Clinical features

The clinical features of trigeminal neuralgia are well recognized and have been extensively described and referenced in three books (Rovit 1979; Fromm 1987; Zakrzewska 1995). The pain of trigeminal neuralgia is sharp, shooting, and similar to electric shock. However, many patients also describe a dull, throbbing, burning type of pain that occurs between attacks (Zakrzewska et al. 1999). Melzack and colleagues (1986) reported on the words chosen by trigeminal neuralgia patients who completed the McGill Pain Questionnaire (MPQ) and showed that the MPQ could discriminate well between trigeminal neuralgia and atypical facial pain. Pain severity can vary from mild to extremely severe. The MPQ and visual analogue scales can be used to assess severity, but studies rarely use these measures.

Trigeminal neuralgia, by definition, occurs within the distribution of the trigeminal nerve and is nearly always unilateral. Bilateral pain may occur several years after symptoms develop on one side of the face and is more frequently reported in patients with multiple sclerosis, as will be discussed later in this section.

Trigeminal neuralgia is paroxysmal, and the paroxysms may last only for a few minutes or seconds. They rarely occur at night. The pain spreads rapidly at the beginning of an attack and then recedes more slowly. The length of the refractory period is often related to the intensity and duration of the pain rather than to the stimulus. The length of remission is difficult to predict. An epidemiological study by Kurland (1958) noted that 58% of patients had long, spontaneous remissions that tended to occur soon after diagnosis. In Rasmussen's (1991) case series, 71–72% of both trigeminal neuralgia patients and those with facial pain due to other causes reported that pain was most frequent during the day, while only 18% reported the same frequency between day and night. Pronounced seasonal variations in pain frequency were reported by 31% of trigeminal neuralgia patients compared to 19% of those with other types of facial pain; 51% and 68%, respectively, reported no seasonal variations.

Touch, drafts of air, and facial movements can elicit outbursts of pain. Patients report that eating, talking, washing the face, or shaving provoke pain. Patients may lose considerable weight if they are unable to eat due to the pain. Rasmussen (1991) in his series of 229 patients with trigeminal neuralgia reported that only 4% of these patients had no precipitating factors. The precipitating factors identified were: chewing and talking (76%), touching (65%), cold (48%), heat (1%), movement of the head and bed rest (2%), stooping and abdominal contraction (1%), pressure by dentures (0.4%), and psychological factors (2%). A classic symptom is stimulation of pain by touching a trigger area. These areas vary in size from very small to large and diffuse. Fifty percent of Rasmussen's patients identified a trigger zone. Forty-three percent of patients with trigeminal neuralgia versus 30% of those with non-neuralgic facial pain reported associated symptoms such as lacrimation, rhinorrhea, salivation, swelling, and flushing. Rasmussen did not use a nonpain group to control for these associated factors. Patients in this study achieved pain relief only through drugs and surgery but could reduce the number of attack by avoiding light-touch sensations.

Clinical examination

Most patients show no abnormalities although more sophisticated testing may reveal some sensory deficit (Nurmikko 1991). Marbach and Lund (1981), using controls with and without pain, assessed patients for depression, anhedonia, and anxiety with a variety of well-validated questionnaires. They showed that patients with trigeminal neuralgia were more likely to suffer from anhedonia than diurnal depression.

Gordon and Hitchcock (1983) used the Illness Behavior Questionnaire and form A of the Eysenck Personality Inventory to assess 28 patients with non-neuralgic facial pain and 32 with trigeminal neuralgia. They reported that trigeminal neuralgia patients scored higher on denial compared to patients with other types of chronic, non-neuralgic facial pain and lower on irritability, but otherwise their illness behavior was similar to that of other chronic pain patients. They also were less convinced that their pain had a physical cause.

Diagnostic tools

In a controlled study, Hutchins and colleagues (1990) reported that magnetic resonance imaging (MRI) is useful in identifying masses or multiple sclerosis but is not helpful in predicting vascular compression. Another study (Baldwin et al. 1991) did find MRI useful for the latter. Magnetic resonance tomographic angiography (MRTA) has been proposed as the definitive investigation, but there are inadequate controlled, randomized trials to assess its sensitivity and specificity. Thermography has also been suggested, but specificity and sensitivity data are not available (Gratt et al. 1996).

Other findings

In a study of 16 patients with trigeminal neuralgia, Strittmatter and colleagues (1996) found that catecholamines and plasma cortisol were elevated in comparison to a control group, which suggests that the sympathetic nervous system may play a role in maintaining the condition. This observation supports the findings by Hampf and colleagues (1990) that sensory and autonomic changes can be detected in patients with trigeminal neuralgia and are reversed after surgery. Nurmikko (1991) has also discussed altered cutaneous sensations.

Difficulties of diagnosis

Although it would appear that the diagnostic criteria of trigeminal neuralgia were clear-cut as early as the 1920s, Frazier and Russell (1924) drew attention to a form that they called atypical facial neuralgia. Many studies do not make this distinction and have not carefully characterized patients according to the diagnostic criteria endorsed by the IASP or IHS. Furthermore, some patients describe clinical features that initially do not fit the classical definition of trigemi-

nal neuralgia but that later change in character to conform to this definition. Mitchell (1980) has called this condition pretrigeminal neuralgia, a designation supported by cases described by Fromm et al. (1990). Without clear diagnostic criteria, the incidence and prevalence of trigeminal neuralgia are difficult to estimate.

DEMOGRAPHIC FACTORS IN PREVALENCE

We identified only one report that attempted to estimate prevalence of trigeminal neuralgia (Munoz et al. 1988) (Table X). This study in a French village sought to determine the prevalence of neurological disease in an elderly population. Eighty-six percent of the 1144 inhabitants of the village responded to a questionnaire. Neurological conditions were identified on 304 questionnaires, but three patients died prior to the examinations conducted 3 months later and 40 refused to be examined. Neurological assessment revealed that 181 of the 261 subjects had some form of neurological disease and several had more than one diagnosis. In this population one man was diagnosed with trigeminal neuralgia for a prevalence of 0.1%. The report did not present confidence limits. Facial and head pain were diagnosed in 2.7% of the population, and trigeminal neuralgia was the least common diagnosis. However, the report did not state diagnostic criteria for the various conditions nor provide any further categorization of the diagnoses.

The remainder of the epidemiological data address incidence. Data have been collected in Rochester, Minnesota, USA, since 1945, with the most recent report published in 1990. Kurland (1958), Yoshimasu et al. (1972), and Katusic et al. (1990) all used the Rochester population, but this chapter describes only the latest report in detail. These studies used a hospital database to generate control groups when necessary. All data in the Rochester area are entered into a computerized diagnostic system that permits epidemiological studies of the community. All subjects had been patients at one of the hospitals in the Rochester area and had a diagnosis confirmed by a neurologist. The diagnostic criteria were clearly stated, and subjects were included in these studies only if they had been residents of Rochester for at least 1 year and had pain that began between 1945 and 1984 (Katusic et al. 1990). The investigators ascertained each subject's age at the time of the first episode of pain rather than at first clinical visit. The small number of cases may af-

Table X
Prevalence of trigeminal neuralgia

Study Type	Disease Definition	Source of Sample	Sample Size	Type of Prevalence	Prevalence	Reference
Prospective population (Q and EX)	Not defined	Village in France	1144; R = 993, EX = 261	Point	0.1%	Munoz et al. 1988
Retrospective cohort	Trigeminal neuralgia	Population of 60,000, Rochester, Minnesota, USA	75	Crude incidence, 1945–1984	4.3 per 100,000	Katusic et al. 1990
Retrospective cohort		Carlisle, UK	—	Crude incidence, 1955–1961	2.1 per 100,000	Brewis et al. 1996
Case-control	Not defined	Surgical cases of trigeminal neuralgia (cervical disk diseases used as controls), Massachusetts, USA	526; R = 90%	Crude incidence, 1955–1970	2.96 M, 3.47 F per 100,000	Rothman and Monson 1973

Note: No data are presented on pain severity of duration.
Abbreviations: EX = examination; F = female; M = male; Q = questionnaire; R = response.

fect the results, which are summarized in Table XI.

The crude annual incidence for women and men was 5.7 and 2.5 per 100,000 per year, respectively, and incidence rates increased with age, but the sex difference was not statistically significant. The annual incidence when adjusted to the 1980 age distribution of the U.S. population was 5.9 per 100,000 women and 3.4 per 100,000 men. The annual rates fluctuated somewhat from one decade to another during this study, although no particular time trend was evident. The average annual incidence increased with age and was highest in those over 80 years, especially for men. For a study covering the period 1945–1969, Yoshimasu and colleagues (1972) estimated an incidence rate of 4 per 100,000 (CI = 2.7–5.3), with 5 per 100,000 for women and 2.7 per 100,000 for men.

In 1966, Brewis and colleagues estimated the average annual incidence of 2.1 per 100,000 in the United Kingdom, based on a study of 70,000 inhabitants of Carlisle. However, the authors indicated this could be an underestimate because the local ENT hospitals had not been included in the survey.

Prevalence may be derived by multiplying the annual incidence by the median survival measured in years, providing that incidence does not change with time. If the incidence is high then an adjustment is required, although it probably is not appropriate in this cohort of patients. The prevalence of a current or recent attack of trigeminal neuralgia in a population aged 50–70 years would probably be less than 400 per 100,000 or 1 in 250, according to a 1990 study by Katusic and colleagues. They reported that the 10-year

survival of 45 patients with trigeminal neuralgia was 46% compared with an expected rate of 39%. The median age of onset was 67 years, with a range of 24–93 years. A generous estimate of the median survival of the population of 64-year-olds might be 20 years.

Rothman and Monson (1973a) conducted a case-control study with 526 patients first admitted for neurosurgical management of trigeminal neuralgia at Massachusetts General Hospital between 1955 and 1970, and 528 patients admitted for management of spondylosis, osteoarthritis, and ruptured disk of the cervical regions. They mailed a questionnaire to all patients and 6 weeks later sent a second questionnaire to nonrespondents, achieving a response rate of 90.7% for patients with trigeminal neuralgia and 86.8% for the controls. Of these, relatives completed the questionnaires for 10% of the trigeminal neuralgia cases and 6% of the controls. The authors found a high correlation between the data obtained from the medical records and the questionnaires, including those from relatives of deceased subjects. Nearly all patients were Massachusetts residents, so population data for the region were used to estimate sex ratios and age-specific rates. The authors presumably used the age at onset of symptoms as indicated in a table of results. The report did not state the diagnostic criteria for trigeminal neuralgia. For both men and women the rates rose with age and were highest in those aged 75 years and older; the rate was estimated at 11 per 100,000 in this oldest group. When adjusted to the age distribution of the U.S. population of 1950, the sex ratio of women to men was 1.17:1. The trigeminal neuralgia group had a greater proportion of women and a higher mean age than did the control group.

Given the scarcity of population-based data, Hamlyn (1999) attempted to derive prevalence, incidence, and patterns of case distribution from literature describing surgical management. An exhaustive review of cases published between 1935 and 1995 identified 86 publications covering 78 separate series and 16,727 cases. Three series totaling 1919 cases (11.4%) were from mainland China and Japan and the rest were almost exclusively from the United States, Australia, or Europe.

Several factors need to be considered in interpreting these data. Many series gave no diagnostic criteria, whereas others stated that the subjects included patients with atypical type trigeminal neuralgia, multiple sclerosis, or tumors. These studies tended to report either age at treatment, age at diagnosis, or age at first symptoms, but few series recorded age at onset. An important consideration is the potential for considerable delay in diagnosis, especially if a patient had long remission periods or brief early episodes. Some neurosurgeons will not perform microvascular decompression on patients older than 65, and other patients may be excluded from certain operations due to their medical history. Women seek health care more often than do men, and the data from surgical treatment samples may be biased toward female patients. The elderly seek and receive less health care than do the young. Patients receiving surgical treatment are also more likely to have intractable pain uncontrollable by medical therapies. These patients may thus constitute a different diagnostic category than those who respond to medical management. Although attempts were made to access all literature available, little is published from some continents, so geographic distribution of the disease is difficult to estimate. Data on the racial, educational, and occupational details of these patients are extremely rare.

Our analysis of the studies mentioned provided the following data. In 53 series of 7868 cases that had not had microvascular decompression (to reduce bias due to surgical selection of patients under age 65), the median of the mean ages of patients was 60 years, with a range of 50–72 years. The number of reported cases increased with each decade up to 70 years and then fell again. Just under 10% of patients sought care before the age of 40. Age-specific incidence is impossible to calculate from the data in these papers. An attempt was made to do so by looking at census surveys in England and Wales for the years 1935, 1965, and 1985, which represented the period covered by most reports. These data showed that the number of newly diagnosed cases by decade of life peaks at the seventh decade and is then maintained at the level found in the sixth decade.

In all but the data from Japan and mainland China, women predominate in the series with a mean of 59.5% of subjects (range 49–75%). These data were based on 77 series with 15,135 cases, the sex distribution of

Table XI
Age- and sex-specific average annual incidence rates per 100,000
population of first episode of trigeminal neuralgia

Age Group (years)	Women		Men		Total	
	No.	Rate	No.	Rate	No.	Rate
0–39	2	0.3	1	0.2	3	0.2
40–49	6	6.0	1	1.1	7	3.7
50–59	9	10.4	5	7.1	14	8.9
60–69	16	22.8	5	10.1	21	17.5
70–79	17	33.7	3	10.8	20	25.6
$\geq$80	5	18.2	5	45.2	10	25.9
Total	55	5.7	20	2.5	75	4.3
Age-adjusted rate* (95% CI)	5.9 (4.3–7.5)		3.4 (1.9–4.9)		4.8 (3.7–5.9)	
Age- and sex-adjusted rate (95% CI)*					4.7 (3.6–5.8)	

Source: Katusic et al. (1990), Rochester, Minnesota, 1945–1984.
* Adjusted to the 1980 U.S. total population.

Table XII
Treatment of patients with trigeminal neuralgia

Treatment	Total No. Episodes Treated	Total No. Times Treated*
Phenytoin (Dilantin)	33	52
Carbamazepine (Tegretol)	40	64
Phenytoin and carbamazepine	1	1
Alcohol block	31	95
Percutaneous radio frequency neurolysis	8	9
Microvascular decompression	8	9
Peripheral neurectomy	8	8
None	26	35

Source: Katusic et al. (1990), Rochester, Minnesota, 1945–1984.
*More than one treatment was used in some episodes.

cases was statistically significant from the England and Wales population census for 1985. In five reports on 1877 patients in mainland China and Japan, 56% of the patients were men.

Studies assessing the laterality of chronic pain (Campbell et al. 1985) found no predominance on one side of the body, although analysis of trigeminal neuralgia cases point to right-sided dominance (Rothman and Weeps 1974). Hamlyn (1999) found in his analysis of 57 series with 13,850 patients that 59% of cases were right-sided and only four series reported left-sided dominance. The side distribution did not vary in reports from different world regions. The number of bilateral cases was similar to the epidemiological data from Katusic et al. (1990). Hamlyn (1999) then attempted to look at the interdependence of sex, side, and age, but encountered difficulty because few series reported details by sex. The predominance of the right side was independent of sex, as was the affected side,

in seven studies totaling 775 cases. Rothman and Wepsic (1974) also attempted to link side of pain with handedness but found no correlation.

CONSEQUENCES

The economic costs of this condition have not been estimated but are likely to be high, given that many clinicians advocate computed tomography, MRI scans, or MRTA prior to treatment. Microvascular decompression is a major neurosurgical procedure with significant cost implications. Katusic et al. (1990) assessed the treatment received by patients in the Rochester study between 1945 and 1984 (Table XII).

NATURAL HISTORY AND PROGNOSTIC FACTORS

Trigeminal neuralgia is episodic. Katusic and colleagues (1990) in their epidemiological survey of 75 patients reported a median of three episodes, with a range of 1–11. They recorded a total of 220 episodes of which 194 had known beginning and ending dates. The median length of an episode was 49 days and the mean was 116 days, with a range of 1–1462 days. In 109 patients with trigeminal neuralgia, Rasmussen (1991) recorded pain-free intervals of years (6%), months (36%), weeks (16%), and days (16%). Diurnal constant pain occurred in 4% of patients, and 23% had no recordable pain-free intervals. Katusic et al. (1990) used Kaplan-Meier life table methods to estimate that 65% of patients would experience a second episode of pain within 5 years and 77% within 10 years. Of those 53 patients who had two or more episodes, 66% experienced a third episode within 5 years of the second episode and 79% had a third episode within 10 years. The proportion of patients with recurrences

Table XIII
Risk factors for trigeminal neuralgia

Study Type	Risk Factor	Strength of Association	Likelihood of Causality	Reference
Case-control	22 different factors: 1 = multiple sclerosis; 2 = religion (non-Jewish); 3 = country of birth (USA); 4 = smoking (non-smoking); 5 = alcohol (non-drinking); 6 = presence of tonsils	1–3 are strong; 4–5 may be linked	None	Rothman and Monson 1973
Cohort	Hypertension, multiple sclerosis	Borderline risk (significant for women) = 2.07 (95% CI = 1.2–3.4); RR = 20 (95% CI = 4.1–58.6)	Probably not causative	Katusic et al. 1990

after a second or third episode was similar to that after a first episode. Second episodes occurred in 82% of women by 10 years as compared to 64% of men, but this difference was not statistically significant. Age did not correlate with timing of the next episode. Based on the cases in Rochester, Rothman and Monson (1973b) showed that both men and women with trigeminal neuralgia exceeded the mean life span of the general population. They found no link with central nervous system disease but suggested a possible protective effect of smoking; patients smoked less compared to the general population.

Several surgical reports evaluate prognosis in relation to outcome; unfortunately, few give strict diagnostic criteria and no studies were controlled with age- and sex-matched patients who had other forms of surgical treatment. Prognostic features examined in the surgical cases include age, sex, duration of condition, previous surgery, preoperative sensory loss, type of pain and its distribution, i.e., number of involved divisions of the nerve, and previous response to anticonvulsant therapy. A variety of surgical findings have also been used as prognostic factors, for example, ease of operation, amount of compression, and the surgical site (Zakrzewska 1995). Good evidence of a correlation between these features and outcome is lacking. Neurosurgeons postulate that compression occurs at the root entry zone, but many do not define the exact area. Grooving of the trigeminal nerve is likely to be the best prognostic factor, but this has not yet been proven (Hamlyn and King 1992; Hamlyn 1999).

CAUSATION AND PREVENTION

The disease most frequently linked with trigeminal neuralgia is multiple sclerosis. Katusic and colleagues (1990) assessed the frequency of multiple sclerosis (MS) in their group of 75 patients. Three women had a history of MS prior to the diagnosis of trigeminal neuralgia compared to an expected number in all patients of 0.15. They estimated that the relative risk was 20 (95% CI = 4.1–58.6). Rothman and Monson (1973a) in their case-control study found nine cases of MS among patients with trigeminal neuralgia versus four in their control group. Thus, the proportion of patients with trigeminal neuralgia and MS is small. Other studies have linked trigeminal neuralgia and MS but none have attempted to conduct case-control studies.

Hypertension has also been considered a risk factor. The Katusic study (1990) reported a history of hy-

pertension in 19 patients in their cohort. The odds ratio for hypertension was 1.96 (95% CI = 1.2–3.1). An evaluation by sex found that hypertension was significant for women, who had a 2.07 relative risk (95% CI = 1.2–3.4), but not for men, who had a relative risk of 1.53 (95% CI = 0.3–4.5). Some investigators have suggested that some patients may have a familial history of trigeminal neuralgia, but no studies have included controls. A viral etiology has also been postulated, but no risk factor identified. Katusic and colleagues (1990) looked at the seasonality of onset and Rothman and Monson (1973a) looked at incidence of cold sores and sore throats, but neither found any association.

Only the two studies noted above have assessed risk factors for trigeminal neuralgia (Table XIII), the Katusic team (1990) in their longitudinal cohort of patients and Rothman and Monson (1973a) in their case-control group. Neither study provided reasons for the choice of factors. Rothman and Monson examined the following variables: age at diagnosis, sex, religion, race, marital status, handedness, socioeconomic status, country of birth, distance from Massachusetts, alcohol consumption, cigarette smoking, coffee consumption, stroke or heart attack, gallstones, asthma, stomach ulcer, tonsillectomy, MS, cold sores, and clinic of first visit. Relative to controls, trigeminal neuralgia patients smoked less, consumed less alcohol, had fewer tonsillectomies, and were less likely to be Jewish and less likely to be immigrants. Apart from religion, country of birth, and MS, other risk factors need further investigation.

Another possible risk factor is the anatomical division involved. In their analysis of the Rochester data, Rothman and Beckman (1974) showed that vertical location of the pain was associated with age at diagnosis; pain in the mandibular division occurred in patients with an earlier onset of disease. More right-sided cases were associated with upper face involvement.

Because no strong risk factors have been identified, there is currently no clear approach to prevention.

CHALLENGES FOR THE FUTURE

Although the diagnostic criteria are well-accepted and recognized, many studies do not specify diagnostic criteria and include cases that lack all the characteristics of trigeminal neuralgia. Population studies are needed to assess the true prevalence of trigeminal neuralgia and possible risk factors. All studies to date are based on hospital cases and in some instances only those treated surgically. This approach may exclude the less serious cases of trigeminal neuralgia and introduce sampling bias. No case-control studies have evaluated the role of behavioral and psychological factors. Longitudinal cohort or case-control studies are essential to establish risk factors and causality. Geographical differences may exist but can only be demonstrated through worldwide collaborative studies. The role of diagnostic tools needs to be assessed because MRI and MRTA are expensive and data on their specificity and sensitivity are lacking. Greater care with selection of cases based on sound diagnostic criteria and development of randomized controlled trials would lead to more effective treatment for patients with this condition. More detailed descriptions of surgical findings coupled with clear diagnostic criteria (e.g., grooving and compression) may permit better comparisons and give clues regarding causes. Longitudinal prospective studies on surgically treated cases, similar to that published by Zakrzewska et al. (1999), would provide clinicians with improved data on outcome based on physical and psychological morbidity over time.

GLOSSOPHARYNGEAL NEURALGIA

Glossopharyngeal neuralgia is a rare condition that has similar features to trigeminal neuralgia except that the pain occurs in the distribution of the glossopharyngeal nerve. The IASP defines it as "sudden, severe, brief, stabbing recurrent pains in the distribution of the glossopharyngeal nerve." The condition is recognized as a distinct entity by the IASP (006.x8b) and IHS (12.3).

DEFINITION AND DIAGNOSTIC CRITERIA

A search of the MEDLINE databases from 1966 to July 1997 and the Cochrane database using the MeSH headings of glossopharyngeal nerve and neuralgia produced 268 papers. Use of all the epidemiological terms outlined in the introduction produced six articles. We reviewed their reference lists and included reports relating to epidemiology that used clear diagnostic criteria.

Bruyn (1983) reviewed all the literature up to 1983 and summarized several case series with fewer than five patients, finding 314 cases. King (1987) reported

nine cases in Australia. Rushton et al. (1981) and Katusic et al. (1991a,b) analyzed population data from the Rochester area that included 12 incident cases and 207 referred cases from 1922 to 1991. One other article describes a familial case of trigeminal neuralgia and glossopharyngeal neuralgia (Knuckey and Gubbay 1979). The clinical description that follows is based on these studies.

Clinical features

The pain begins in the tonsillar fossa fauces or pharynx and then radiates either to the ear or throat, and is termed either pharyngeal or otalgic type depending on the region of predominance (Bruyn 1983; King 1987). Pain can radiate into the tongue and mandibular area, which can lead to misdiagnosis as trigeminal neuralgia of the mandibular division. Radiation to the eye, nose, and maxilla has been reported. In contrast to trigeminal neuralgia, the left side appeared to predominate in 78% of incident cases and 53% of referral cases (Katusic et al. 1991b). Pain was bilateral but not synchronous in 25% of the incident cases, whereas only 1.8% of referral cases had bilateral pain. Although patients describe the pain as sharp and shooting, they also report a dull, aching, burning "background" pain (Rushton et al. 1981; King 1987). Although pain can be extremely severe, in many cases it is mild, especially compared to that of trigeminal neuralgia (Katusic et al. 1991b). As with the latter, pain may occur several times daily and trigger episodes that may last from a few weeks to a month or two and then subside. In the series described by Katusic et al. (1991a) the interval between episodes ranged from 6 months to 9 years, but other reports indicate that the interval can be as long as 30 years. Patients with glossopharyngeal neuralgia report fewer recurrences (3.6%/year) than do patients with trigeminal neuralgia (21%/year) (Katusic et al. 1991b).

Provoking factors include swallowing, especially of cold liquids that cause pain when they contact the trigger area. Talking, moving the head, and yawning can be precipitating factors. Touching the trigger area can also set off pain. The pain is relieved by anticonvulsant drugs, but a 10% solution of cocaine applied to the trigger zone will give immediate relief in most cases (112 of 125 patients according to Rushton et al. 1981; Bruyn 1983). Syncope and cardiac arrhythmias have been associated with attacks of pain (Rushton et al. 1981).

DEMOGRAPHIC FACTORS IN PREVALENCE

Prevalence data are not available for this condition, and the only incidence data were collected by Katusic et al. (1991a) in the Rochester area. Between 1945 and 1984 they identified 12 cases for a crude incidence of 0.7 per 100,000. The age- and sex-adjusted annual incidence rate (using the 1980 U.S. population) was 0.8% per 100,000 (95% CI = 0.3–1.2). They found no significant differences between the sexes, although the age-adjusted male to female ratio was 2.2:1. Incidence begins to increase from age 59, with a peak occurring in the seventh decade. Bruyn's (1983) analysis of 314 cases found in the literature showed a peak incidence at around 50 years for both sexes but revealed no sex predominance. Rushton and colleagues (1981) reported that 57% of patients in their series were over 50 years of age. No attempt has been made to assess racial, social, educational, or occupational factors, although Bruyn (1983) reported two cases of glossopharyngeal neuralgia in blacks.

NATURAL HISTORY, PROGNOSTIC FACTORS, AND CONSEQUENCES

Not all cases are severe. The Rochester data on 12 incident cases revealed that three required surgical procedures, four required medications, and five only required intermittent topical cocaine (Katusic et al. 1991a). In this series 8 of the 12 patients had had only one episode of pain. The annual recurrence rate of pain appeared to be about 3.6%, and more than one episode per year is rare.

Neither the economic costs of this condition nor the cost to the patient have been assessed.

CAUSATION AND PREVENTION

Katusic and colleagues (1991a) examined season of onset and family history but found no pattern. Knuckey and Gubbay (1979) reported a family with three cases of trigeminal neuralgia in which one member had both trigeminal neuralgia and glossopharyngeal neuralgia. Rushton et al. (1986) reported 25 patients with combined trigeminal neuralgia and glossopharyngeal neuralgia. Katusic et al. (1991a) found one patient who had developed trigeminal neuralgia 28 years before the onset of glossopharyngeal neuralgia. These investigators also evaluated hypertension and MS as potential risk factors. The risk ratio for hypertension was 2 (95% CI = 0.79–7.42). None of the 12 patients in their series had a diagnosis of MS, nor did any in the series reported by Rushton et al. (1986).

Given the limited number of cases and lack of known etiological factors, prevention is not yet possible.

CHALLENGES FOR THE FUTURE

This disease is rare and more data will be forthcoming only if several centers collaborate on studies that use the diagnostic criteria in the IASP classification. The similarity to trigeminal neuralgia also means that studies focusing solely on glossopharyngeal neuralgia would not be cost effective. Comparisons between these two conditions may be useful in attempts to look for causes and risk factors.

CHRONIC MAXILLARY SINUSITIS

Maxillary sinusitis most frequently occurs as a brief, acute episode. It may, however, become chronic, which is the subject of this section. The IASP classification (1994) does not distinguish between chronic and acute and codes maxillary sinusitis under one group (031.x2a). It suggests that most patients with chronic maxillary sinusitis experience mild discomfort but not pain. The IHS classification (1988) includes a category called acute sinus headache in the Nose and Sinuses section (11.5.2), which states that "chronic sinusitis is not validated as a cause of headache or facial pain unless relapsing into an acute stage."

DEFINITION AND DIAGNOSTIC CRITERIA

A search of the MEDLINE databases from 1996 to July 1997 with the text words chronic, maxillary, and sinusitis yielded 197 references. Combining only the words maxillary and sinusitis produced 498 articles (the same as when maxillary sinusitis was used as a MeSH heading), whereas chronic sinusitis produced 783. Using all the epidemiological terms described at the beginning of this chapter, we identified 19 articles. We obtained and read six in full and rejected one for lack of diagnostic criteria. We rejected the others on screen because they related to treatment (3), investigations (3), epidemiology of respiratory infection or acute sinusitis (2), patients with asthma or sinusitis

(1), bacteriology (1), ethmoidal sinusitis (1), or were a review (1), or a study of medieval skulls (1). We used only articles that gave diagnostic criteria, dealt with chronic sinusitis, and addressed epidemiological or clinical factors.

Melen et al. (1986) emphasized the difficulty of diagnosis due to the lack of accepted definitions; most researchers believe that chronic maxillary sinusitis is the result of incompletely resolved acute sinusitis. In their study on 198 patients attending an ENT clinic, Melen and colleagues used three criteria to classify chronic maxillary sinusitis as of either rhinological or dental origin: (1) symptoms of facial pain, nasal congestion, or abnormal secretions that remain or reappear over at least 3 months; (2) sinus radiography or sinoscopy reveals persistent local or generalized mucosal swelling with or without secretion; (3a) chronic maxillary sinusitis of rhinological cause is considered when dental examination is normal but the sinusitis does not resolve; and (3b) chronic maxillary sinusitis of dental origin is diagnosed when dental causes such as oral antral fistula, inflammatory periapical lesions, or impacted teeth account for persistence.

Otten et al. (1991), in their long-term follow-up of chronic maxillary sinusitis in children, mention that the diagnostic criteria used were a history of purulent rhinitis lasting for at least 3 months and confirmed by anterior rhinoscopy and routine X-rays of the maxillary sinuses showing total or partial opacification. In evaluating functional endoscopic surgery in 24 cases of chronic sinusitis, Lund et al. (1991) stressed the importance of using a variety of symptoms and signs to objectively measure outcome based on firm criteria. They measured nasal obstruction, problems with the sense of smell, anterior rhinorrhoea, postnasal discharge, headache, and facial pain on a visual analogue scale of 0–10. They used objective measures to assess mucociliary function, olfaction (with the University of Pennsylvania Smell Identification Test), and extent of opacification (with CT scanning). The mean scores were 4.4 for facial pain and 6.5 for headache, but the authors do not state whether all patients reported pain.

Gliklich and Metson (1995a) have attempted to construct a questionnaire with criteria specific to chronic sinusitis as they found no studies that used specific outcome measures. Their survey questionnaire has two sections, one on "severity-based" and the other on "duration-based" symptoms. They validated this questionnaire on 125 consecutive patients who were defined as suffering from chronic sinusitis because their signs and symptoms had persisted for more than 3 months and either a CT scan showed evidence of disease or endoscopy showed active drainage in the middle meatus of the sinus. Most surveyed patients were due for ethmoid sinus surgery, and the test was also used as an outcome measure. They assessed the retest validity of the form at intervals of 2 weeks and 2 months after the initial survey and evaluated another 61 patients after surgery. The main symptoms assessed were pain or pressure, congestion or difficulty in breathing through the nose, nasal discharge or postnasal drip, and other symptoms identified by the patients. Of the 104 responses, 78% of patients reported sinus headache, pain, or pressure. Nasal drainage (postnasal drip) was reported in 88% and nasal congestion in 86%. Gliklich and Metson have now used this survey in thousands of patients and found it effective in discriminating chronic sinusitis from other facial pains (personal communication).

Clinical features

Based on the above reports, the following features may be considered indicative of chronic maxillary sinusitis. By definition, symptoms must be present for at least 3 months. In their study of 198 patients, Melen and colleagues (1986) reported a mean duration of symptoms of about 2 years but did not state the periodicity. Reports concur that the symptoms are similar to those of acute sinusitis and that patients may experience acute exacerbations. Pain is mild but can become severe during an acute episode. It occurs over the affected sinus and may be unilateral or bilateral, depending on pathology, and may radiate to the teeth. Reports do not specify provoking factors but indicate that a combination of antibiotics or surgery provide relief for most patients.

The most important features of chronic maxillary sinusitis are nasal discharge with or without congestion. Many cases are associated with dental problems. Nasal polyps are common and are a causal factor. In Melen's study (1986), nasal polyps were found in 13% of patients who had a dental cause for their maxillary sinusitis and in 23% of patients who had a rhinological cause. Both subjective and objective tests indicate that smell is affected (Lund et al. 1991). All clinicians use opacification of the sinus as a key criterion. Gliklich and Metson (1995a) have proposed a four-stage grading system. Other dental pathology may be identified on dental X-rays.

DEMOGRAPHIC FACTORS IN PREVALENCE

Prevalence of chronic maxillary sinusitis is impossible to estimate, and only one study has used clear diagnostic criteria to estimate incidence. Melen and colleagues (1986) analyzed all cases referred to an ENT clinic between 1978 and 1988 in a retrospective cohort study. From a clinic registration of 210,000 patients they identified 198 patients with 244 affected sinuses (a prevalence of 0.02%). Their age range was 17–73 years with a mean of 45.6. They specified that they only saw patients over 17 years. Subjects in the Gliklich and Metson (1995a) study of 104 patients had a mean age of 41 ± 13.6 (range 15–73) but they suffered from all forms of sinusitis. A study of chronic maxillary sinusitis in children reported an age range of 3–7 years (Otten et al. 1991).

In Melen et al.'s series (1986), the sex distribution was equal, but Gliklich and Metson's (1995a) patient population had a preponderance of women (64%). There are no prevalence data on racial, social, educational, or occupation groups.

CONSEQUENCES

We lack data on the economic costs of maxillary sinusitis. Gliklich and Metson (1995b) attempted to assess the effect of chronic sinusitis on patients using the SF-36 Health Survey. They evaluated 158 patients with all forms of chronic sinusitis (diagnostic criteria clearly specified) and found that although physical functioning remained intact, patients with chronic sinusitis reported poorer status than anticipated for bodily pain, general health, and social functioning. The scores were considerably lower than for other published data on chronic conditions such as angina, congestive heart disease, pulmonary disease, and back pain. It appears that chronic sinusitis affects health more than previously anticipated.

NATURAL HISTORY AND PROGNOSTIC FACTORS

Otten et al. (1991) assessed long-term outcome of chronic maxillary sinusitis in children. Their study methods were inadequate, but they suggest that a spontaneous cure occurs in most children by approximately the age of seven. Melen et al. (1986) found that in their clinic sample of adults, duration of symptoms averaged 1.9 years for dental causes and 2.3 years for

maxillary causes, but they did not report pain severity.

CAUSATION AND PREVENTION

Melen et al. (1986) drew attention to the high incidence of dental infections in these patients. They were unable to assess whether nasal polyps were the cause or consequence of chronic maxillary sinusitis. Identified dental causes include apical granuloma, marginal periodontitis, impacted teeth, and oral antral fistulae, which are most frequently associated with dental extractions. The literature includes no case-control studies or longitudinal cohort studies, so it is impossible to establish causality and relative risk.

The high association with dental pathology implies a potential to reduce the incidence of chronic maxillary sinusitis. All patients suffering from acute sinusitis that does not resolve immediately should be assessed both by dental and ENT surgeons to rule out causative pathology (Melen et al. 1986).

CHALLENGES FOR THE FUTURE

The primary challenge is to establish clear diagnostic criteria that include all forms of chronic sinusitis because it is difficult to distinguish between different sites. A questionnaire such as developed by Gliklich and Metson (1995a) would permit epidemiological surveys that could assess the extent of this disease and its economic impact. Preliminary studies indicate that patients with chronic sinusitis use considerably more health care resources and have greater disability than previously assumed, so it is important to assess risk factors and determine prevention strategies. Outcome measures for treatments can then be established as a basis for conducting randomized, controlled trials.

REFERENCES

American Psychiatric Association. *Diagnostic and Statistical Manual of Mental Disorders*, 3rd ed. Washington DC: American Psychiatric Association, 1987.

Baldwin NG, Sahni KS, Jensen ME, et al. Association of vascular compression in trigeminal neuralgia versus other "facial pain syndromes" by magnetic resonance imaging. *Surg Neurol* 1991; 36(6):447–452.

Basker RM, Sturdee DW, Davenport JC. Patients with burning mouths. A clinical investigation of causative factors, including the climacteric and diabetes. *Br Dent J* 1978; 145(1):9–16.

Bates RE, Jr, Stewart CM. Atypical odontalgia: phantom tooth pain.

Oral Surg Oral Med Oral Pathol 1991; 72(4):479–483.

Bergdahl J, Anneroth G. Burning mouth syndrome: literature review and model for research and management. *J Oral Pathol Med* 1993; 22(Suppl 10):433–438.

Bergdahl BJ, Anneroth G, Anneroth I. Clinical study of patients with burning mouth. *Scand J Dent Res* 1994; 102(5):299–305.

Bergdahl J, Anneroth G, Perris H. Cognitive therapy in the treatment of patients with resistant burning mouth syndrome: a controlled study. *J Oral Pathol Med* 1995a; 24(5):213–215.

Bergdahl J, Anneroth G, Perris H. Personality characteristics of patients with resistant burning mouth syndrome. *Acta Odontol Scand* 1995b; 53(1):7–11.

Bouckoms AJ, Sweet WH, Poletti C, et al. Monoamines in the brain cerebrospinal fluid of facial pain patients. *Anesth Prog* 1993; 39(6):201–208.

Brewis M, Poskanzer DC, Rolland C, Miller H. Neurological disease in an English city. *Acta Neurol Scand* 1966; 42(24):1–89.

Browning S, Hislop S, Scully C, Shirlaw P. The association between burning mouth syndrome and psychosocial disorders. *Oral Surg Oral Med Oral Pathol* 1987; 64(2):171–174.

Bruyn GW. Glossopharyngeal neuralgia. *Cephalalgia* 1983; 3(3):143–157.

Campbell JA, Lahuerta J, Bowsher D. Pain laterality in relation to site of pain and diagnosis. *Pain* 1985; 23(1):61–66.

Campbell RL, Parks KW, Dodds RN. Chronic facial pain associated with endodontic therapy. *Oral Surg Oral Med Oral Pathol* 1990; 69(3):287–290.

Cekic-Arambasin A, Vidas I, Stipetic-Mravak M. Clinical oral test for the assessment of oral symptoms of glossodynia and glossopyrosis. *J Oral Rehabil* 1990; 17(5):495–502.

Derbyshire SW, Jones AK, Devani P, et al. Cerebral responses to pain in patients with atypical facial pain measured by positron emission tomography. *J Neurol Neurosurg Psychiatry* 1994; 57(10):1166–1172.

Dworkin SF, Burgess JA. Orofacial pain of psychogenic origin: current concepts and classification. *J Am Dent Assoc* 1987; 115(4):565–571.

Eli I, Baht R, Littner MM, Kleinhauz M. Detection of psychopathologic trends in glossodynia patients. *Psychosom Med* 1994; 56(5):389–394.

Eversole LR, Stone CE, Matheson D, Kaplan H. Psychometric profiles and facial pain. *Oral Surg Oral Med Oral Pathol* 1985; 60(3):269–274.

Feinmann C. The long-term outcome of facial pain treatment. *J Psychosom Res* 1993; 37(4):381–387.

Feinmann C, Harris M, Cawley R. Psychogenic facial pain: presentation and treatment. *BMJ (Clin Res Ed)* 1984; 288(6415):436–438.

Ferguson MM, Carter J, Boyle P, Hart DM, Lindsay R. Oral complaints related to climacteric symptoms in oophorectomized women. *J R Soc Med* 1981; 74(7):492–498.

Frazier CH, Russell EC. Neuralgia of the face, an analysis of 754 cases with relation to pain and other sensory phenomena before and after operation. *Arch Neurol Psych* 1924; 11:557–563.

Friedman MH. Atypical facial pain: the consistency of ipsilateral. Maxillary area tenderness and elevated temperature. *J Am Dent Assoc* 1995; 126(7):855–860.

Fromm GH (Ed). *The Medical and Surgical Management of Trigeminal Neuralgia*. New York: Futura, 1987.

Fromm GH, Graff-Radford SB, Terrence CF, Sweet WH. Pretrigeminal neuralgia. *Neurology* 1990; 40(10):1493–1495.

Glick D, Ben-Aryeh H, Gutman D, Szargel R. Relation between idiopathic glossodynia and salivary flow rate and content. *Int J Oral Surg* 1976; 5(4):161–165.

Gliklich RE, Metson R. Techniques for outcomes research in chronic sinusitis. *Laryngoscope* 1995a; 105(4 Pt 1):387–390.

Gliklich RE, Metson R. The health impact of chronic sinusitis in patients seeking otolaryngologic care. *Otolaryngol Head Neck Surg* 1995b; 113(1):104–109.

Gordon A, Hitchcock ER. Illness behaviour and personality in intractable facial pain syndromes. *Pain* 1983; 17(3):267–276.

Graff-Radford SB, Ketelaer MC, Gratt BM, Solberg WK. Thermographic assessment of neuropathic facial pain. *J Orofac Pain* 1995; 9(2):138–146.

Gratt BM, Sickles EA, Graff-Radford SB, Solberg WK. Electronic thermography in the diagnosis of atypical odontalgia: a pilot study. *Oral Surg Oral Med Oral Pathol* 1989; 68(4):472–481.

Gratt BM, Graff-Radford SB, Shetty V, Solberg WK, Sickles EA. A 6-year clinical assessment of electronic facial thermography. *Dentomaxillofac Radiol* 1996; 25(5):247–255.

Grushka M, Sessle BJ, Howley TP. Psychophysical assessment of tactile, pain and thermal sensory functions in burning mouth syndrome. *Pain* 1987; 28(2):169–184.

Grushka M. Clinical features of burning mouth syndrome. *Oral Surg Oral Med Oral Pathol* 1987; 63(1):30–36.

Hamlyn PJ. *Neurovascular Compression of the Cranial Nerves in Neurological and Systemic Disease*. Amsterdam: Elsevier, 1999.

Hamlyn PJ, King TT. Neurovascular compression in trigeminal neuralgia: a clinical and anatomical study. *J Neurosurg* 1992; 76(6):948–954.

Hampf G. Dilemma in treatment of patients suffering from orofacial dysaesthesia. *Int J Oral Maxillofac Surg* 1987; 16(4):397–401.

Hampf G, Vikkula J, Ylipaavalniemi P, Aalberg V. Psychiatric disorders in orofacial dysaesthesia. *Int J Oral Maxillofac Surg* 1987; 16(4):402–407.

Hampf G, Bowsher D, Wells C, Miles J. Sensory and autonomic measurements in idiopathic trigeminal neuralgia before and after radiofrequency thermocoagulation: differentiation from some other causes of facial pain. *Pain* 1990; 40(3):241–248.

Harness DM, Peltier B. Comparison of MMPI scores with self-report of sleep disturbance and bruxism in the facial pain population. *Cranio* 1992; 10(1):70–74.

Harris M, Feinmann C, Jones JH, Mason DK (Eds). *Oral Manifestations of Systemic Disease*. Psychosomatic Disorders, 2nd ed. London: Bailliere Tindall, 1990, pp 30–60.

Headache Classification Committee of the International Headache Society. Classification and diagnostic criteria for headache disorders, cranial neuralgias and facial pain. *Cephalalgia* 1988; 7(8):1–96.

Holzberg AD, Robinson ME, Geisser ME, Gremillion HA. The effects of depression and chronic pain on psychosocial and physical functioning. *Clin J Pain* 1996; 12(2):118–125.

Hutchins LG, Harnsberger HR, Jacobs JM, Apfelbaum RI. Trigeminal neuralgia (tic douloureux): MR imaging assessment. *Radiology* 1990; 175(3):837–841.

Jaafar N, Razak IA, Zain RB. The social impact of oral and facial pain in an industrial population. *Ann Acad Med Singapore* 1989; 18(5):553–555.

Katusic S, Beard CM, Bergstralh E, Kurland LT. Incidence and clinical features of trigeminal neuralgia, Rochester, Minnesota, 1945–1984. *Ann Neurol* 1990; 27(1):89–95.

Katusic S, Williams DB, Beard CM, Bergstralh E, Kurland LT. Incidence and clinical features of glossopharyngeal neuralgia, Rochester, Minnesota, 1945–1984. *Neuroepidemiology* 1991a; 10(5-6):266–275.

Katusic S, Williams DB, Beard CM, Bergstralh EJ, Kurland LT. Epidemiology and clinical features of idiopathic trigeminal neuralgia and glossopharyngeal neuralgia: similarities and differences, Rochester, Minnesota, 1945–1984. *Neuroepi-*

demiology 1991b; 10(5–6):276–281.

Keefe FJ, Beckham JC. Behavioral assessment of chronic orofacial pain. *Anesth Prog* 1990; 37(2-3):76–81.

King J. Glossopharyngeal neuralgia. *Clin Exp Neurol* 1987; 24:113–1121.

Knuckey NW, Gubbay SS. Familial trigeminal and glossopharyngeal neuralgia. *Clin Exp Neurol* 1979; 16:315–319.

Kurland LT. Descriptive epidemiology of selected neurological and myopathic disorders with particular reference to a survey in Roch-ester, Minnesota. *J Chronic Dis* 1958; 8:378–418.

Lascelles RG. Atypical facial pain and depression. *Br J Psychiatry* 1966; 112(488):651–659.

LeResche L. Assessment of physical and behavioral outcomes of treatment. *Oral Surg Oral Med Oral Pathol Oral Radiol Endod* 1997; 83(1):82–86.

Lipton JA, Marbach JJ. Components of the response to pain and variables influencing the response in three groups of facial pain patients. *Pain* 1983; 16(4):343–359.

Lipton JA, Ship JA, Larach-Robinson D. Estimated prevalence and distribution of reported orofacial pain in the United States. *J Am Dent Assoc* 1993; 124(10):115–1121.

Locker D, Grushka M. Prevalence of oral and facial pain and discomfort: preliminary results of a mail survey. *Community Dent Oral Epidemiol* 1987; 15(3):169–172.

Locker D, Grushka M. Response trends and nonresponse bias in a mail survey of oral and facial pain. *J Public Health Dent* 1988; 48(1):20–25.

Lund VJ, Holmstrom M, Scadding GK. Functional endoscopic sinus surgery in the management of chronic rhinosinusitis. An objective assessment. *J Laryngol Otol* 1991; 105(10):832–835.

Lundeen TF, George JM, Toomey TC. Health care system utilization for chronic facial pain. *J Craniomandib Disord* 1991; 5(4):280–285.

Maragou P, Ivanyi L. Serum zinc levels in patients with burning mouth syndrome. *Oral Surg Oral Med Oral Pathol* 1991; 71(4):447–450.

Marbach JJ. Is phantom tooth pain a deafferentation (neuropathic) syndrome? Part I: Evidence derived from pathophysiology and treatment. *Oral Surg Oral Med Oral Pathol* 1993a; 75(1):95–105.

Marbach JJ. Is phantom tooth pain a deafferentation (neuropathic) syndrome? Part II: Psychosocial considerations. *Oral Surg Oral Med Oral Pathol* 1993b; 75(2):225–232.

Marbach JJ, Lund P. Depression, anhedonia and anxiety in temporomandibular joint and other facial pain syndromes. *Pain* 1981; (11):73–84.

Marbach JJ, Hulbrock J, Hohn C, Segal AG. Incidence of phantom tooth pain: an atypical facial neuralgia. *Oral Surg Oral Med Oral Pathol* 1982; 53(2):190–193.

Mason DK, Jones JH (Eds). *Oral Manifestations of Systemic Disease*, 2nd ed. London, 1990.

McQuay H, Carroll D, Jadad AR, Wiffen P, Moore A. Anticonvulsant drugs for management of pain: a systematic review. *BMJ* 1995; 311(7012):1047–1052.

McQuay HJ, Tramer M, Nye BA, et al. A systematic review of antidepressants in neuropathic pain. *Pain* 1996; 68(2–3):217–227.

Melen I, Lindahl L, Andreasson L, Rundcrantz H. Chronic maxillary sinusitis. Definition, diagnosis and relation to dental infections and nasal polyposis. *Acta Otolaryngol (Stockholm)* 1986; 101(3–4):320–327.

Melzack R, Terrence C, Fromm G, Amsel R. Trigeminal neuralgia and atypical facial pain: use of the McGill Pain Questionnaire for discrimination and diagnosis. *Pain* 1986; 27(3):297–302.

Merskey H, Bogduk N (Eds). *Classification of Chronic Pain. Descriptions of Chronic Pain Syndromes and Definitions of Pain Terms.* 2nd ed. Seattle: IASP Press, 1994.

Mitchell RG. Pre-trigeminal neuralgia. *Br Dent J* 1980; 149(6): 167–170.

Miyaoka H, Kamijima K, Katayama Y, Ebihara T, Nagai T. A psychiatric appraisal of "glossodynia." *Psychosomatics* 1996; 37(4):346–348.

Mock D, Frydman W, Gordon AS. Atypical facial pain. A retrospective study. *Oral Surg Oral Med Oral Pathol* 1985; 59:472–474.

Mongini F, Ferla E, Maccagnani C. MMPI profiles in patients with headache or craniofacial pain: a comparative study. *Cephalalgia* 1992; 12(2):91–98.

Munoz M, Dumas M, Boutros-Toni F, et al. [A neuro-epidemiological survey in a Limousin town]. [In French]. *Rev Neurol (Paris)* 1988; 144(4):266–271.

Nicolodi M, Sicuteri F. Phantom tooth diagnosis and an anamnestic focus on headache. *NY State Dent J* 1993; 59(10):35–37.

Nurmikko TJ. Altered cutaneous sensation in trigeminal neuralgia. *Arch Neurol* 1991; 48(5):523–527.

Otten FW, van Aarem A, Grote JJ. Long-term follow-up of chronic maxillary sinusitis in children. *Int J Pediatr Otorhinolaryngol* 1991; 22(1):81–84.

Paterson AJ, Lamb AB, Clifford TJ, Lamey PJ. Burning mouth syndrome: the relationship between the HAD scale and parafunctional habits. *J Oral Pathol Med* 1995; 24(7):289–292.

Pfaffenrath V, Rath M, Pollmann W, Keeser W. Atypical facial pain-application of the IHS criteria in a clinical sample. *Cephalalgia* 1993; 13(Suppl 12):84–88.

Rasmussen P. Facial pain. IV. A prospective study of 1052 patients with a view of: precipitating factors, associated symptoms, objective psychiatric and neurological symptoms. *Acta Neurochir (Wien)* 1991; 108(3–4):100–109.

Rees RT, Harris M. Atypical odontalgia. *Br J Oral Surg* 1979; 16(3):212–218.

Reik L, Jr. Atypical odontalgia: a localized form of atypical facial pain. *Headache* 1984; 24(2):222–224.

Remick RA, Blasberg B. Psychiatric aspects of atypical facial pain. *J Can Dent Assoc* 1985; 51(12):913–916.

Richards W, Scourfield S. Oral ill-health in a general dental practice in south Wales. *Prim Dent Care* 1996; 3(1):6–13.

Rothman KJ, Monson RR. Epidemiology of trigeminal neuralgia. *J Chronic Dis* 1973a; 26(1):3–12.

Rothman KJ, Monson RR. Survival in trigeminal neuralgia. *J Chronic Dis* 1973b; 26(5):303–309.

Rothman KJ, Beckman TM. Epidemiological evidence for two types of trigeminal neuralgia. *Lancet* 1974; 1(845):7–9.

Rothman KJ, Wepsic JG. Side of facial pain in trigeminal neuralgia. *J Neurosurg* 1974; 40(4):514–523.

Rovit RL, Murali R, Jannetta PJ (Eds). *Trigeminal Neuralgia.* Baltimore: Williams and Wilkins, 1990.

Rushton JG, Stevens JC, Miller RH. Glossopharyngeal (vago-glossopharyngeal) neuralgia: a study of 217 cases. *Arch Neurol* 1981; 38(4):201–205.

Stener RF, Brooke RI. Atypical odontalgia. Update and comment on long-term follow-up. *Oral Surg Oral Med Oral Pathol* 1992; 73(4):445–448.

Seltzer S, Dewart D, Pollack RL, Jackson E. The effects of dietary tryptophan on chronic maxillofacial pain and experimental pain tolerance. *J Psychiatr Res* 1982; 17(2):181–186.

Sicuteri F, Nicolodi M, Fusco BM, Orlando S. Idiopathic headache as a possible risk factor for phantom tooth pain. *Headache* 1991; 31(9):577–581.

Slade GD, Locker D, Leake JL, Wu AS, Dunkley G. The oral health status and treatment needs of adults aged 65+ living independently in Ottawa-Carleton. *Can J Public Health* 1990; 81(2):114–119.

Smith DP, Pilling LF, Pearson JS, et al. A psychiatric study of atypical facial pain. *Can Med Assoc J* 1969; 100(6):286–291.

Speculand B, Goss AN, Hallett E, Spence ND. Intractable facial pain. *Br J Oral Surg* 1979; 17(2):166–178.

Speculand B, Goss AN, Spence ND, Pilowsky I. Intractable facial pain and illness behaviour. *Pain* 1981; 11(2):213–219.

Strittmatter M, Grauer MT, Fischer C, et al. Autonomic nervous system and neuroendocrine changes in patients with idiopathic trigeminal neuralgia. *Cephalalgia* 1996; 16(7):476-480.

Svensson P, Bjerring P, Arendt-Nielsen L, Kaaber S. Sensory and pain thresholds to orofacial argon laser stimulation in patients with chronic burning mouth syndrome. *Clin J Pain* 1993; 9(3):207–215.

Tammiala-Salonen T, Hiidenkari T, Parvinen T. Burning mouth in a Finnish adult population. *Community Dent Oral Epidemiol* 1993; 21(2):67–71.

Tammiala-Salonen T, Soderling E. Protein composition, adhesion, and agglutination properties of saliva in burning mouth syndrome. *Scand J Dent Res* 1993; 101(4):215–218.

Tourne LP, Fricton JR. Burning mouth syndrome. Critical review and proposed clinical management. *Oral Surg Oral Med Oral Pathol* 1992; 74(2):158–167.

van der Ploeg HM, van der Waal N, Eijkman MA, van der Waal I. Psychological aspects of patients with burning mouth syndrome. *Oral Surg Oral Med Oral Pathol* 1987; 63(6):664–668.

van der Waal I. *The Burning Mouth Syndrome.* Copenhagen: Munksgaard, 1990.

Wall PD, Melzack R. *Textbook of Pain,* 2nd ed. Edinburgh: Churchill Livingstone, 1989.

Weddington WW, Jr, Blazer D. Atypical facial pain and trigeminal neuralgia: a comparison study. *Psychosomatics* 1936; 20(5):348–349.

Yoshimasu F, Kurland LT, Elveback LR. Tic douloureux in Rochester, Minnesota, 1945-1969. *Neurology* 1972; 22(9):952–956.

Zakrzewska JM. *Trigeminal Neuralgia.* London: W.B. Saunders; 1995.

Zakrzewska JM, Sawsan J, Bulman JS. A prospective, longitudinal study on patients with trigeminal neuralgia who underwent radiofrequency thermocoagulation of the Gasserian ganglion. *Pain* 1999; 79:51–58.

Zilli C, Brooke RI, Lau CL, Merskey H. Screening for psychiatric illness in patients with oral dysesthesia by means of the General Health Questionnaire–twenty-eight item version (GHQ-28) and the Irritability, Depression and Anxiety Scale (IDA). *Oral Surg Oral Med Oral Pathol* 1989; 67(4):384–389.

Correspondence to: Joanna M. Zakrzewska, Department of Oral Medicine, St Bartholomew's and the Royal London School of Medicine and Dentistry, Turner Street, London E1 2AD, United Kingdom. Fax: 0171-377-7627; email: J.M.Zak@mds.qmw.ac.uk.

Epidemiology of Pain, edited by
I.K. Crombie, IASP Press, Seattle, © 1999.

15

Temporomandibular Disorder Pain

Mark Drangsholt[a,b,c] and Linda LeResche[a]

Departments of [a]Oral Medicine and [b]Dental Public Health Sciences, School of Dentistry, and [c]School of Public Health and Community Medicine, University of Washington, Seattle, Washington, USA

Temporomandibular disorders (TMD) are a collection of common conditions affecting the temporomandibular joint (TMJ) and the muscles of mastication (National Institutes of Health 1996). These disorders have been principally characterized by (1) pain in the temporomandibular region or in the muscles of mastication, (2) limitations or deviations in mandibular range of motion, and (3) TMJ sounds during jaw function (American Dental Association 1983). Most patients with TMD seek care because of pain (Dworkin et al. 1990; Motegi et al. 1992). This chapter will focus on the epidemiology of pain resulting from the related conditions in this region, and will not specifically address nonpainful conditions of the TMJ, or "dysfunction," such as TMJ clicking, locking, or limitation of jaw opening without pain. Other authors have recently summarized the epidemiology of TMD, including LeResche (1997), Carlsson and LeResche (1995), Stohler (1997), de Bont et al. (1997), and Fricton and Schiffman (1995).

The use of epidemiological methods over the last 40 years has been refined and extended from the study of acute, infectious diseases to chronic conditions such as cancer and heart disease (Rothman and Greenland 1998b). More recently, these same methods have been applied to symptomatic conditions such as low back pain, behavioral disorders, migraine, and other headaches (Gordis 1988). These methods have the potential to help identify (1) how common the condition is, and any change in prevalence over time; (2) the natural history of the condition if left untreated; and (3) the risk factors for its onset and perpetuation. One of the characteristics of the epidemiological method is that it can help in the diagnosis, treatment, and prevention of a condition even if the biological mecha-

nisms are poorly understood. This property is especially helpful in pain conditions, where many of the mechanisms are only partly elucidated. Finally, epidemiological research is performed in human populations, so it is uniquely situated, compared to the basic sciences, to delineate the applicability of exposures to human populations, and ultimately it offers the prospect of altering risk through prevention (Hennekens and Buring 1987a).

BRIEF HISTORY OF THE STUDY OF TMD PAIN

Pain and dislocation in the jaw region were described and treated in humans as early as 3000 B.C. (McNeill 1997). In the 20th century, most of the interest in TMD has come from within dentistry because pain from these conditions is usually associated with jaw function and is located in the orofacial region. Early theories of cause and effect espoused by various clinicians and investigators in the 1930s to 1960s focused primarily on the structural and functional relationships between the upper and lower teeth and jaws, or dental occlusion (Costen 1934; Ramfjord and Ash 1966). Competing models of causation were proposed in the 1950s, first by Schwartz (1959), who saw stress or anxiety as a major etiological factor, and then by Laskin (1969), who extended Schwartz's psychophysiological model. These theories were based primarily on observations in the clinical setting, and not on epidemiological studies. Although basic and clinical research in the intervening 30 years has led to refinement of some of these etiological theories, controversy still exists among clinicians and researchers concerning the causes of these conditions.

Early clinical cross-sectional studies of TMD indicated that it was a relatively common, heterogeneous pain disorder that afflicted primarily women aged 20–45 (Campbell 1958). Helkimo (1974b) conducted a landmark cross-sectional study in Lapps of northern Finland in the early 1970s. It was the first moderately sized ($N = 321$), population-based epidemiological study of TMD, which was novel because it used a classification system of pain and dysfunction and reported age- and gender-specific estimates of dysfunction. Helkimo developed two separate indices that indicated severity of jaw pain and dysfunction: one depending on self-report, the "Anamnestic Dysfunction Index" or "A_i"; and one based on clinical examination, the "Clinical Dysfunction Index," or "D_i." He found that the signs and symptoms of TMD, as indicated by these indices, were common in this population (56–57%), but that a smaller percentage (21–31%) had what his "A" index would characterize as severe dysfunction. Many other similarly designed studies were conducted in the ensuing 20 years. In addition to describing prevalence, most of these cross-sectional studies also investigated possible risk factors, such as dental occlusion. Beyond these descriptive studies, analytic epidemiological investigations, such as case-control and cohort studies, have been performed only in the last 15 years. Scientific and professional groups in the United States, such as the National Institutes of Health and the American Dental Association, have sponsored and convened several conferences about TMD over the last decade and concluded that it is an important disorder in need of much more scientific study (Bryant and Sessle 1995).

In this chapter, we will discuss the classification of TMD, describe the prevalence and incidence of TMD pain, address the consequences of this disorder to the individual and society, summarize studies on the natural history and clinical course, and on risk factors and high-risk groups, comment on the gaps in knowledge, and finally, discuss possibilities for prevention and challenges for the future.

EPIDEMIOLOGY OF TMD

IDENTIFICATION AND SELECTION OF STUDIES

We searched multiple databases of the scientific literature using the following text words: temporoman-dibular, craniomandibular, and facial pain. The databases included MEDLINE 1965–August 1998, OLDMEDLINE 1962–1965, WORLDCAT 1960–present, Index to Scientific Book Contents 1986–March 1996, and BIOSIS 1991–present. To add to this list, we scanned reference sections from retrieved articles. These searches revealed 12,434 articles in MEDLINE, 1250 books, theses, and dissertations in WORLDCAT, 53 book chapters in Index to Scientific Book Contents, and 373 meeting abstracts in BIOSIS. We also searched using the following text words and MeSH subheadings: epidemiology, etiology, cohort, prevalence, incidence, risk factor, and odds ratio. We read all English-language article abstracts with these subheadings to determine eligibility. Inclusion criteria for descriptive epidemiological studies included a population-based sample with pain definition of either self-reported ambient or functional pain in or around the TMJ, and gender-specific estimates. Natural history studies were required to follow whole populations or persons with TMD over time with either no clinical treatment or a minimal level of conservative treatment. Analytic epidemiological studies were required to be either case-control, cohort, or cross-sectional designs with case definitions that included TMD pain for most cases and that addressed possible confounding by age and gender, at a minimum.

For comparison of similar studies, we compiled tables listing studies by type, sample size, and other methodological details. Studies often used dissimilar definitions and method, so that, in general, the data could not be quantitatively combined as would be done in a formal meta-analysis; instead, ranges of values are given where appropriate.

DEFINITION AND DIAGNOSTIC CRITERIA

Although many diseases may be associated with pain in the temporomandibular region, such as dental infection and malignant tumors, clinicians have assumed that almost all patients seeking treatment have pain of musculoskeletal origin (Fricton et al. 1985; Laskin and Block 1986; Schiffman et al. 1990; Lipton et al. 1993). A question that may be asked during history-taking to ascertain presence of musculoskeletal (TMD) pain is: "Do you have pain in or around your jaw joint, in the muscles of your face, or in your ear when at rest?" Common clinical signs of musculoskeletal problems in the temporomandibular region upon examination are: pain upon palpation of the TMJ or muscles of mastication, decreased ability to open the mouth or move the jaw from side to side, and clicking or grating sounds in the TMJ with jaw movement.

TMD pain conditions are similar to other musculoskeletal pain problems in that they lack objective diagnostic methods that can easily differentiate persons with the condition from those without it (Widmer 1995). There is no gold standard, such as tissue biopsy with cancer, against which a diagnostic test can be easily compared for accuracy and reliability. The best substitute is a comprehensive medical history, physical examination, and selective use of imaging for conditions affecting joint structures (Lund et al. 1995).

Historically, musculoskeletal signs and symptoms (including pain) in the temporomandibular region have been characterized as a syndrome. The presumed etiology and primary source of symptoms, however, have changed over time. Over the last 60 years, the focus of investigation and the assumed source of pain have oscillated from interest in the joint area, to interest in the muscles of mastication, and back to the joint region in the 1970s (Laskin 1998). Terminology has also differed depending on the presumed source of the problem (e.g., "TMJ syndrome" versus "myofascial pain-dysfunction syndrome"). In 1982, the American Dental Association President's Conference on the Examination, Diagnosis and Management of Temporomandibular Disorders (American Dental Association 1983) coined the term "temporomandibular disorders" (TMD), which articulates the idea that symptoms in the temporomandibular region are the result of a variety of disorders (including, for example, displacements of the temporomandibular joint disk and problems with the muscles of mastication), rather than a single syndrome with a single etiology. It was, however, recognized that many patients were best characterized as having multiple disorders.

During the 1960s and 1970s, when temporomandibular pain was considered part of a syndrome, measures used in epidemiological studies generally sought to characterize the severity of the syndrome. Thus, the measures developed combined pain with a range of joint and muscle symptoms. Symptoms indicating pathology presumed to be of greater severity (e.g., joint locking) were given more weight. The most widely used of such severity measures are the Helkimo Anamnestic and Clinical Indices (Helkimo 1974a), which have been employed in over 100 epidemiological studies.

During the 1980s and 1990s, several classifica-

tion schemes were developed based on the concept that pain and dysfunction in the temporomandibular region can be caused by a variety of different disorders. These include nonhierarchical classification schemes (Dworkin and LeResche 1992; Truelove et al. 1992; American Academy of Orofacial Pain 1996) that allow assigning subjects to multiple categories (for example, a subject might have both myofascial pain and disk displacement); hierarchical schemes that assign subjects with multiple disorders to the disorder of greatest presumed severity (Eversole et al. 1985); systems that use continuous scales to characterize the degree of severity in multiple domains, e.g., one index for palpation pain and one for dysfunction (Fricton and Schiffman 1986); or scales for pain report, joint dysfunction, palpation pain, stress, chronicity, psychological factors, and several others, all contributing to a global scale (Levitt et al. 1994). Although most of these classification schemes are based primarily on clinical findings and are aimed at classifying the physical pathology, some have explicitly attempted to classify or measure psychological factors and pain impact (Dworkin and LeResche 1992; Levitt et al. 1994). Only one of these systems (Dworkin and LeResche 1992) uses self-report of pain as an explicit criterion for some diagnoses.

Previous authors have identified development of a uniform classification system as a central issue in the study of temporomandibular disorders (Katz 1985; Rugh and Solberg 1985; Bryant and Sessle 1995; National Institutes of Health 1996). Diagnostic classification systems should possess at least some of the following characteristics: validity or accuracy, reliability or reproducibility among different clinicians at different times, and usefulness in helping to determine optimal treatment or prognosis (Sackett et al. 1991). Ideally, the system should be easy to use by clinicians and researchers and fit within the classification systems of other chronic pain conditions.

VALIDITY, RELIABILITY, AND CLINICAL UTILITY

Several classification systems have been used in epidemiological studies or have been designed with epidemiological research in mind. These measures by and large use clearly defined operational criteria and theoretically would produce reliable data. However, not all have been tested for reliability. Helkimo's indices, mentioned previously, are still widely used in epidemiological studies that are reported in scientific literature (De Kanter et al. 1993). However, the reliability, validity, and utility of these indices are untested (Van der Weele and Dibbets 1987). The Craniomandibular Index (CMI) was formulated by Fricton and Schiffman (1986), and includes both a muscle and dysfunction index, along with a total Symptom Severity Index (SSI). The TMJ scale, developed by Levitt and associates (1994), was designed for use in clinical dental practice and has seen a significant amount of psychometric development (Deardorff 1995). Reports of scale scores in large samples of patients from multiple dental practices have been published (Levitt and McKinney 1994). However, the TMJ scale is based solely on self-report, rather than examination findings, and scoring algorithms are not published. Importantly for epidemiological studies, both the TMJ scale and the CMI produce subject profiles rather than dichotomous classifications. The Research Diagnostic Criteria for TMD (RDC/TMD) were developed by a group of international investigators in the early 1990s (Dworkin and LeResche 1992). The RDC/TMD provides specifications for conducting a standardized clinical examination and uses algorithms to assign clinical (Axis I) diagnoses to subjects, based on examination findings and a few self-report questions that refer primarily to presence and location of pain. In addition, it allows classification of the subject's psychosocial status (Axis II) based on standardized psychometric instruments (c.f. Turk and Rudy [1990] for an alternative method of classifying the psychosocial status of chronic pain patients which has been applied to TMD in clinical settings). The RDC/TMD has been tested for reliability, and most recently, clinical utility of the multi-axial system (Garofalo et al. 1998; Ohrbach and Dworkin 1998), and appears to hold the most promise at this time. From the outset, however, the RDC/TMD was assumed by its developers to be a starting point, and modifications may need to be made as more studies investigating its validity and utility are reported.

One aspect of the validity of any diagnostic system is its ability to differentiate the condition in question from other conditions presumed to be unrelated. Data are not available concerning the ability of any of the classification systems described above to differentiate pain of musculoskeletal origin from the rare, life-threatening conditions that may mimic TMD pain, such as neoplastic tumors (Gobetti and Turp 1998). While this is clearly a concern from a clinical per-

spective, such differentiation may be impractical in epidemiological studies due to the low prevalence and variable presentation of the other conditions. Perhaps more important for epidemiological studies of TMD, most classification schemes have not been tested for their ability to rule out the more common and benign pain originating from teeth (Wright and Gullickson 1996). Criteria for differentiating TMD pain from other kinds of head pain have been proposed by researchers who helped create the International Headache Classification (IHC) in 1988 (Olesen 1988). Olesen proposed a minimum of five episodes of pain in the temporomandibular region, along with at least two of the following four clinical signs: (1) increased myofascial tenderness, (2) restricted opening, (3) disk displacement, and (4) signs of arthritis or arthrosis. The time course of TMD would be divided into episodic TMD—average pain frequency less than 6 of 12 months; or chronic TMD—pain frequency more than 6 of 12 months. The advantage of this system is that is fits within an accepted classification scheme for other cephalic pain diagnoses and gives a global diagnosis for each person; at this time, however, this system has not been tested for reliability, validity, or utility.

One of the aspects missing from most of the classification systems described above is a set of simple questions that could be asked in epidemiological studies over the telephone, in person, or on a written questionnaire that could classify a person as with or without TMD pain. For example, a question that was asked in an epidemiological study conducted in Seattle, Washington, USA, in 1986 using written questionnaires and telephone interviews to identify cases of TMD was compared with clinical examination findings and correctly classified 82% of persons screened (Widmer 1995). The same question with a different time frame is included in the RDC. Locker and Slade (1989) examined the validity of specific questions about TMD symptoms by examining a subset of patients. They found that sensitivity (75%) and specificity (78%) could be maximized by using two or more positive responses to nine questions about pain in the TM area at rest and with jaw function as compared with the standard of the Helkimo clinical index D-2 (most severe category). In future studies, it may be possible not only to ask about the presence or absence of TMD pain, but also about symptoms consistent with accepted TMD subgroups, such as TMJ disk displacement with reduction ("Do you have clicking in the jaw joint?") or osteoarthrosis ("Do you have grating or grinding in the jaw joint without pain?"). If such a set of questions could be proven reliable and valid compared with the standard of a thorough history, physical examination, and radiographic imaging, it would be a great boon to further epidemiological research. Collaboration and agreement among international investigators on a standard set of questions to ascertain the presence or absence of TMD pain (and potentially other symptoms) should be a high priority.

DIAGNOSTIC INSTRUMENTS AND TESTS

Many types of devices have been developed and advocated to aid in the diagnosis of TMD. These include jaw tracking devices, electromyography, electrical stimulation, sonography, thermography, and vibratography. However, none meets reliability, validity, and efficacy standards to assist in diagnostic classification (Lund et al. 1995; American Academy of Orofacial Pain 1996).

From the prior discussion, it is clear that much progress has recently occurred in the development of systems to classify temporomandibular disorders, but much work remains. Testing of the clinical utility of these systems should be a high priority for future longitudinal research studies, along with standardization of reliable and valid self-report questions for clinical and epidemiological research. Some of these systems are not mutually exclusive, and it may be that different systems will be used to address different aspects of the pain experience. For example, in a clinical epidemiological study, modifications of the IHS-type criteria could be used to initially differentiate TMD from other pains, Axis I of the RDC/TMD system could be used to provide a diagnosis of clinical subtypes, and Turk's MPI profiles or the current RDC Axis II could provide a psychosocial profile of the patients.

FREQUENCY

Investigations determining the frequency of a condition are typically the first step in epidemiological research. Studies of representative samples of the population are usually conducted to determine the *prevalence* of the problem, which is the number of persons with the condition at a specific time divided by the total size of that population. These studies are termed cross-sectional or prevalence investigations. Knowing the prevalence can help to determine the magnitude of a health problem, and the burden it places on society. Prevalence studies include persons who have just recently developed the disorder, or incident cases, along with others who may have had the condition for many years. *Incidence* is the number of persons developing the problem within a specific time divided by the total number of persons at risk. Incidence can only be determined by studying persons without the health problem over time within a defined population and then identifying those who develop the problem at specified points in the future. Studies of this type are commonly called cohort or longitudinal studies. Data on the prevalence and incidence of TMD pain will be summarized in this section.

A brief explanation of methodological problems and other threats to validity will clarify the criteria we used for deciding which cross-sectional studies could be included in this review. One common threat to the validity of prevalence studies involves using samples of persons who are not representative of the population, which produces a biased estimate of the proportion who have the condition. Samples that are population based, that is, subjects chosen from the population of an entire group, such as all adults with a telephone in a city, or all schoolchildren in a district, can generally yield unbiased prevalence estimates. Examples of selected and possibly biased samples are all persons visiting a dental office or university-based specialty clinic or volunteering for a health fair screening. Another threat to the accurate interpretation of data involves reporting the prevalence of a condition for an entire population with only one summary value. The age and gender mix of populations may differ, and most conditions vary in prevalence with these two demographic variables, so a common convention is to list both the age- and gender-specific estimates of the condition to permit fair comparisons between populations (Hennekens and Buring 1987b). Otherwise, differences in prevalence either between studies or within the same study could be due to the age-gender mix of the population studied.

Another complicating factor is the lack of standard questions used to assess presence of TMD pain. The 70 cross-sectional studies of TMD that estimated prevalence used over 40 different questions to ascertain the percentage of persons with self-reported TMD symptoms. Questions ranged from general assessments of pain or function such as: "Do you have pain in your jaw joint?" or "Do you feel pain in the muscles of your jaw or your jaw joint? Often or very often?" or

"Do you have tightness in your jaw muscles?" to functional measures, such as: "Do you have pain with chewing?" "pain in the ear region when opening wide?" "pain with biting?" These questions varied in content according to at least six factors: (1) type of sensation queried (e.g., tightness, discomfort, or pain); (2) area of the sensation (pain) in the face; (3) whether the sensation (pain) occurs at rest (ambient), with jaw movement (functional) or is unspecified; (4) applicable time period—unspecified, an explicit time interval (e.g., during the last 6 months), or lifetime (ever); (5) pain frequency (e.g., sometimes, often, or very often); and (6) pain severity (e.g., mild, moderate, or severe). Depending upon how the question is constructed, the prevalence for the condition even within the same study may vary by up to an order of magnitude; for example, in a prevalence study by Goulet et al. (1995), "jaw pain—quite often or very often" was reported by only 7% of the population, while jaw pain of any frequency was reported by 30% of the population. In the same study, jaw pain that was "severe" was reported by 10% of the population, but jaw pain of any intensity was reported by over a third of the population. The question "Does your jaw feel tired or stiff?" usually results in classifying a much higher proportion of persons with a TMD condition (e.g., 64% in one study) compared to the more familiar and meaningful term "pain" around the TMJ (10%) or jaw muscle pain (4%) (Pilley et al. 1992). Dworkin and LeResche (1993) estimated that the effect of the time interval on the population prevalence of TMD pain report ranged from 3.6% for pain experienced presently (point prevalence), to 12% for pain within the last 6 months (period prevalence), to 34% for lifetime prevalence of pain. Thus, the time frame of the question used to determine the frequency of the condition is critically important. Ideally, questions should be constructed that are reliable and accurately assess the same concept across different languages, and give prevalence estimates for a meaningful condition (such as pain) for a specific time interval, at a defined level of severity.

PREVALENCE

Over the last 50 years, several hundred studies have attempted to determine the prevalence of TMD. For this chapter, we used multiple searching methods of several databases to identify articles published from 1966 to August 1998. The searches identified 196 cross-sectional and cohort studies that reported the prevalence of TMD signs and symptoms and were published as original research in peer-reviewed journals in any language. After we excluded non-English articles, 133 studies remained. Studies that did not provide prevalence data on TMD pain report, such as those that assessed only the prevalence of TMD signs or of nonpainful TMD symptoms, e.g., difficulty opening wide, or combined pain with other symptoms, as determined by compound questions such as "Do you have pain *or* tightness in your jaw?" were excluded next; this left 71 studies. Next, we excluded studies of selected populations, leaving 43 population-based studies of TMD pain report in children and adolescents (9 studies) and adults (34 studies). Although the questions asked to assess pain in the temporomandibular region varied considerably, as discussed above, the questions could be grouped into two broad categories: ambient or unspecified TMD pain, that is, pain at rest (or at rest plus function), and functional pain, or pain with jaw opening or chewing.

TMD PAIN IN CHILDREN AND ADOLESCENTS

Table I lists nine studies that reported the prevalence of ambient TMD pain for children and adolescents up to the age of 18. Overall prevalence estimates for self-reported pain ranged from a low of 0.7% for "severe pain" in the TMJ in 11–16-year-olds (Sieber et al. 1997) to a high of 18.6% for "pain in the TMJ" in Finnish children aged 12 (Heikinheimo et al. 1989). Most estimates of the prevalence, however, centered around 2–6%. Nilner, for example, listed an overall prevalence proportion of "pain other than headache in the facial area" as 2% among 7–14-year-old Swedish schoolchildren, and 4% among 15–18-year-olds (Nilner 1981; Nilner and Lassing 1981). Four of these nine studies provided gender-specific prevalence estimates, so that the female-to-male prevalence ratio could be calculated. In general, the prevalence ratios varied between 0.5 and 2.0, indicating no consistent relationship in the report of TMD pain by gender.

Table II lists 12 studies that report the prevalence of TMD pain with jaw function in children and adolescents. The range of the overall prevalence of "pain with jaw opening" is from 0.2% to 12%, with 14 of 27 age-specific estimates between 3% and 8%. Only five of the 27 stratum-specific prevalence estimates were reported as gender-specific; these ranged from two to three females to every male, indicating a female predominance. The difference in the prevalence before

Table I
Prevalence of ambient TMD pain in children and adolescents

Reference	Study Type	Disease Definition	Source of Sample	Sample Size	Age Range (y)	Type of Prevalence	Overall Prevalence (%)	Prevalence in Males (%)	Prevalence in Females (%)	Prevalence Ratio
Nilner and Lassing 1981	CS	Pain other than head-ache in facial area	Swedish schoolchildren	440	7–14	point	2	n.r.	n.r.	n.c.
Nilner 1981	CS	Pain other than head-ache in facial area	Swedish schoolchildren	309	15–18	point?	4	n.r.	n.r.	n.c.
Wanman and Agerberg 1986	CS	Pain in face or jaws	Swedish schoolchildren	285	17	point	2.5	2.7	2.2	0.81
Kononen et al. 1987	CS	Pain (other than head-ache) in facial area	Finnish children	156	10–16	point	3	4	2	0.50
Heikinheimo et al. 1989	CS	Pain in area of TMJ	Finnish children	167	12 15	n.r. n.r.	18.6 12.6	16.9 8.4	20.2 16.7	1.20 1.99
Nielsen and Terp 1990	CS	TMJ pains	Danish 9th graders	706	14–16	n.r.	10.1	n.r.	n.r.	n.c.
Pilley et al. 1992	CS and cohort	Pain around TMJ	Welsh school-children	1018	15	period	8.8	6	11	1.83
Kononen and Nystrom 1993	CS and cohort	Pain other than head-ache in facial region	Finnish children	131	14 15 18	point? point? point?	4 6 1	n.r. n.r. n.r.	n.r. n.r. n.r.	n.c. n.r. n.r.
Sieber et al. 1997	CS	Pain in TMJ; "severe symptoms"	Swiss and Italian school-children	417	11–16	point?	0.01	n.r.	n.r.	n.c.

Abbreviations: CS = cross-sectional study design; n.c. = not calculable; n.r. = not reported.
Note: Pain severity was not noted in any studies except for Sieber et al. 1997.

Table II
Prevalence of functional TMD pain in children and adolescents

Reference	Study Type	Disease Definition	Source of Sample	Sample Size	Age Range (y)	Type of Prevalence	Overall Prevalence (%)	Prevalence in Males (%)	Prevalence in Females (%)	Prevalence Ratio
Nilner and Lassing 1981	CS	Painful when chewing Painful when opening wide	Swedish schoolchildren	440	7–14 7–14	point point	3.0 10.0	n.r. n.r.	n.r. n.r.	n.c. n.r.
Nilner 1981	CS	Painful when chewing Painful when opening wide	Swedish schoolchildren	309	15–18 15–18	point? point?	5.0 4.0	n.r. n.r.	n.r. n.r.	n.c. n.r.
Gazit et al. 1984	CS	Pain during normal opening of the mouth	Israeli schoolchildren	369	10–18	n.r.	3.0	n.r.	n.r.	n.a.
Kononen et al. 1987	CS	Pain when opening wide (currently) Pain when opening wide (currently and previously)	Finnish children	156 *	10–16 10–16	point 	6.0 8	4 5	8 11	2.00 2.20
Brandt 1985	CS	Pain on mandibular movement Pain in jaws and face during chewing	Canadian children	1342	6–17 6–8 9–10 11–12 13–14 15–17 6–17	point point	1.6 0 1.2 3 1.1 4.4 22.1	n.r. n.r. n.r. n.r. n.r. n.r.	n.r. n.r. n.r. n.r. n.r. n.r.	n.c. n.c. n.c. n.c. n.c. n.c.
Heikinheimo et al. 1989	CS	Pain on mouth opening			12 15 15		1.8 2.4 2.4	0 1.2 1.2	3.6 3.6 3.6	n.c. 3.00 3.00
Mohlin 1991	CS and cohort	Pain on mouth opening (sometimes/once per week) Pain upon mouth opening (once per week)	Welsh schoolchildren	1018	12 12	period period	12 0.6	n.r. n.r.	n.r. n.r.	n.c. n.r.
Pilley et al. 1992	CS and cohort	Pain on mouth opening (occasionally or often)	Welsh schoolchildren	1018	15	period	6	4	8	2.00
Motegi et al. 1992	CS	Pain with opening and closing of mouth, pain when chewing food, and any pain in TMJ	Japanese schoolchildren	7337	6–18 6–11 12–17	point?	1.3 0.2 1.9	n.r. n.r. n.r.	n.r. n.r. n.r.	n.c. n.c. n.c.
Kononen and Nystrom 1993	CS and cohort	Pain when opening wide	Finnish children	131	14 15 18	point?	8 3 3	n.r. n.r. n.r.	n.r. n.r. n.r.	n.c. n.c. n.c.
Kitai et al. 1997	CS and cohort	Do you have pain by active opening or lateral and forward movement of your jaw?	Japanese high school girls	361	12–17 12–13 13–14 14–15 15–16 16–17	point?	n.a.	n.a.	4.64 4.03 4.34 6.18 4.34	n.a.
Barone et al. 1997	CS	Pain on mandibular movement	Italian children	240	7, 11, 16	point	5.8	n.r.	n.r.	n.c.

Abbreviations: CS = cross-sectional study design; n.a. = not applicable; n.c. = not calculable; n.r. = not reported.
Note: No studies reported pain severity; only Molin et al. (1991) noted pain duration.
* Calculated by present authors.

and after puberty could not be compared because prevalence was not usually analyzed by age. The studies that did report prepubertal prevalence (below age 14) separately from postpubertal (age 14 and above) generally showed an increase (Brandt 1985; Heikinheimo et al. 1989; Motegi et al. 1992), although one study showed a decrease (Nilner and Lassing 1981), and others, such as Kitai et al. (1997), reported no discernible difference in the prevalence of functional TMD pain with age.

TMD PAIN IN ADULTS

We located 34 English-language articles published from 1965 to 1998 that were population-based studies of the prevalence of TMD pain in adults. Among these studies, 13 reported either ambient or unspecified TMD pain with separate gender-specific prevalence (Table III). Again, although the definitions and questions to assess pain varied considerably, the overall population prevalence of reported TMD pain was in a relatively narrow range of a low of 3.7% for "headaches in or near the ear" (Agerberg and Bergenholtz 1989) to 12% for "pain in the muscles of the face, the joint in front of the ear, or inside the ear" (Von Korff et al. 1988a) or facial and jaw pain (Helkimo 1974b). The prevalence appeared to systematically vary between men and women, with estimates to ranging from 0% to 10% for males and from 2% to 18% for females. The point estimates for women were roughly double the estimates for men, and, as shown previously, for children and adolescents. The female-to-male gender prevalence ratio ranged from 1.2 to 2.6, but most studies reported a ratio of about 2 to 1. The studies that reported the prevalence of TMD pain with age showed varying age-specific patterns, such as: declining with increasing age (Lipton et al. 1993; Matsuka et al. 1996); bell-shaped, with greatest prevalence around ages 25–54 (Dworkin et al. 1990; Goulet et al. (1995); increasing with age (Agerberg and Bergenholtz 1989); or little or no change with age (Helkimo 1974b). None of these age-specific prevalence curves, however, resembles the common exponential increase in prevalence with age of most chronic disabling conditions, such as rheumatoid arthritis or cardiovascular disease. Differing patterns in the male- female-specific proportions versus age may also be apparent, although few studies have the necessary detail to make any conclusions except that the proportion of males with pain is less at all ages for adults. It is tempting to compare these age- and gender-specific prevalence patterns of TMD pain with that of migraine (Lipton and Stewart 1997), another pain condition with a female predominance, especially from ages 15 to 50. However, only some of TMD studies (Von Korff et al. 1988a; Goulet et al. 1995) indicate an age- and gender-specific prevalence pattern similar to that of migraine.

Table IV shows 16 separate studies that were population based and reported gender-specific prevalence proportions for pain during jaw movement. The range of the overall population prevalence for functional TMD pain was 1.2–2%, with most of the prevalence estimates between 2% and 6%. The prevalence among males was again generally lower than among females, although the prevalence ratio of female to male ranged between 0.67 and 4.0. A comparison of these functional TMD pain proportions with ambient pain proportions within the same studies shows that, in general, ambient pain prevalence was higher by about 70%.

Thus, the information from these cross-sectional and cohort population studies shows that TMD pain is a relatively common condition that is reported, albeit rarely, early in life, becomes more prevalent in the teenage years, appears to be about twice as common in adult women as in men, and most likely declines into old age. It is important to note that these prevalence estimates of TMD pain are substantially lower than previous quantitative summaries of TMD-associated symptoms or signs (De Kanter et al. 1993), which were 34% for the Helkimo "*A*" index, and 46% for the "*D*" index. This is partly because the Helkimo index is a less stringent system that classifies persons with symptoms of dysfunction, such as a feeling of stiffness or fatigue in the jaws, or clicking in the jaw joint, but without pain, as cases with TMD.

METHODOLOGICAL WEAKNESSES AND LIMITATIONS OF PREVALENCE STUDIES

These prevalence estimates have some limitations and methodological weaknesses, as listed in the top half of Table V. Few studies reported the boundaries of time for the prevalence; for example, point prevalence, or pain experienced presently, was commonly mixed with period prevalence and lifetime prevalence, and this ambiguity probably explains some of the variation of the percentages. In addition, the severity or the frequency of the pain was not usually reported. Only two cross-sectional studies (Goulet et al. 1995; Riley

Table III
Prevalence of ambient TMD pain in adults

Reference	Disorder Definition	Source of Sample	Sample Size	Age Range (y)	Overall Prevalence (%)	Prevalence in Males (%)	Prevalence in Females (%)	Prevalence Ratio
Helkimo 1974b	Facial and jaw pain	Finnish Lapps	600	15–65	12	10	14	1.40
				15–24	10	n.r.	n.r.	n.c.
				25–34	2	n.r.	n.r.	n.c.
				45–54	14	n.r.	n.r.	n.c.
				55–65	15	n.r.	n.r.	n.c.
Molin et al. 1976	Frequent pain in front of ears	Swedish male military inductees	253	18–25	n.a.	5	n.r.	n.c.
Mohlin 1983	Pain in TMJ or muscles	Swedish women	272	20–45	n.r.	n.r.	6.3	n.c.
Szentpetery 1986	Recent pain in face, neck, or around ears	Hungarians	600	12–85	5.8	3.2	8.3	2.59
Wanman and Agerberg 1987	Pain in face or jaws	Swedish young adults	285	17	2.5	2.7	2.2	0.8
			275	18	2.5	1.4	3.8	2.7
			254	19	2.3	0	4.8	n.c.
Von Korff et al. 1988a	Pain in muscles of face, joint in front of ear, or inside ear (not infection) in the past 6 mo; not "fleeting" or "minor" pain	HMO enrollees in USA	1016	18–75	12	8	15	1.88
				18–24	n.r.	7	11	1.57
				25–44	n.r.	10	18	1.80
				45–64	n.r.	8	12	1.50
				65+	n.r.	0	2	n.c.
Locker and Slade 1988	Pain in face in front of ear	Canadian adults	677	18–65+	7.5	5	9.5	1.90
				<45	8.3	n.r.	n.r.	n.c.
				45+	7.2	n.r.	n.r.	n.c.
Agerberg and Bergenholtz 1989	"Headaches" in or near ear	Swedish adults	1578	25–65	3.7	2.5	4.9	1.96
				25	n.r.	0.5	4.5	9.00
				35	n.r.	1.5	3.4	2.27
				50	n.r.	2.6	3.5	1.35
				65	n.r.	5.4	7.9	1.46
Agerberg and Inkapool 1990	Pain in ear region	Swedish adults	637	18–64	7.9	6.7	9	1.34
Lipton et al. 1993	During the past 6 mo "more than once" pain in jaw joint or in front of ear	U.S. civilians	42370	18+	5.3	3.5	6.9	1.97
				18–34	6.5	n.r.	n.r.	n.c.
				35–54	5.0	n.r.	n.r.	n.c.
				55–74	4.0	n.r.	n.r.	n.c.
				75+	3.9	n.r.	n.r.	n.c.
Goulet et al. 1995	Do you feel pain in the muscles of your jaws or in your jaw joints often or very often?	French-speaking persons in Quebec	897	18–70+	n.r.	5	9	1.80
				18–34	n.r.	3.5	8.7	2.49
				35–54	n.r.	6.8	10.4	1.53
				>55		3.3	9.7	2.94
Matsuka et al. 1996	Facial pain, TMJ pain, jaw pain	Japanese adults	672	20–92	11	9.9	11.7	1.18
				20–39	15.2	n.r.	n.r.	n.c.
				40–59	11	n.r.	n.r.	n.c.
				60–92	5.7	n.r.	n.r.	n.c.
Riley et al. 1998	During the last 12 mo, did you have pain in the jaw joint or in front of the ear more than once?	Elder Floridians	1636	65+	7.1	4.7	9.3	1.98

Abbreviations: n.c. = not calculable; n.r. = not reported.
Note: Studies are cross-sectional unless noted. Only Von Korff et al. (1988a) reported pain severity.

et al. 1998) reported the spread or dispersion of the data, usually reported as a confidence interval. Although these intervals can often be calculated with the data presented, prevalence proportions given without such intervals do not allow readers to easily gauge the precision and stability of the estimates. This may be problematic, for example, with smaller studies, where authors and readers may pay undue attention to differences in the proportions that may be just the play of chance. Furthermore, if a sample is to be split up into at least 10-year age- and gender-specific prevalence groups, a common convention, relatively large samples (>1000 subjects) are needed to provide stable estimates. In addition, these studies are difficult to compare because they lack consistent definitions and terminology with which to describe TMD pain.

PREVALENCE OF SUBGROUPS OF TMD PAIN

Many authors have agreed that the symptoms of TMD are broad and probably encompass a series of related disorders that may be etiologically diverse, so interest in subdividing TMD into subgroups has grown (Bryant and Sessle 1995). As previously mentioned, separating masticatory muscle from temporomandibular joint disorders is a currently advocated approach. Most authors have relied upon the use of examination information for these subdivisions and not exclusively upon self-report data. Of the 43 population-based cross-sectional studies that had information on TMD pain self-report, however, only three reported data on self-report of TMD pain subgroups (Lipton et al. 1993; Locker and Miller 1994; Riley et al. 1998), and one reported on the subgroups of TMD pain according to the TMD/RDC (LeResche 1995). Lipton, in a large national study, showed that 5.3% of the U.S. population reported jaw joint pain (6.9% female, 3.5% male), versus 1.4% reporting facial pain in the last 6 months "more than once" (1.9% female, 0.91% male), and 0.18% with pain in both areas (Lipton et al. 1993). The coexistence of pain in multiple orofacial structures was common, such as the simultaneous report of jaw joint pain, toothache, and oral sores. Riley and colleagues (1998) in a population study of older (age 65+) residents in Florida, showed that 9.3% of women and 4.7% of men reported jaw joint pain, and 8.0% of women and 4.8% of men reported a dull aching pain in their face during the last year. However, the number of persons with both jaw joint and aching face pain was not discussed. In a post hoc application of the

TMD/RDC to examination data, LeResche found that 25% of the community cases met only the criteria for myalgia or myofascial pain, 3.3% with an internal derangement diagnosis and 4.2% with a joint diagnosis; most of these population-based cases had a diagnosis in more than one subgroup—muscle and disk, 8.3%; muscle and joint, 21.7%; muscle, joint, and disk, 7.5%. Thus, although subgroups of patients may be identified, most studies rely upon examination findings to subdivide the disorder into subgroups, which limits their application in epidemiological studies. It appears most common to have pain in both the joint and muscles of mastication.

Osteoarthritis (OA) of the temporomandibular joint, as indicated by pain and crepitation (grating sounds in the joint), and osteoarthrosis, indicated by crepitation alone, appear to display an epidemiological picture consistent with OA of other joints (Lawrence et al. 1998), including an increasing prevalence with age (Helkimo 1974b; Agerberg and Bergenholtz 1989; Dibbets and van der Weele 1992; Matsuka et al. 1996). Because OA often is not a painful condition, it is unclear how much OA contributes to the TMD pain experience in this older population. In summary, very few population-based studies have reported TMD pain subtypes, and larger cross-sectional and cohort studies are needed to quantify the size of these subgroups.

RACE

We could locate only two studies that reported the prevalence of TMD pain across racial categories. Lipton and colleagues (1993), in the large National Health Interview Survey, showed a slightly lower prevalence of jaw joint and facial pain among African Americans when compared to whites, although this estimate was not adjusted for socioeconomic status (SES), or gender. In contrast, a small cross-sectional study of 4–6-year-old children showed higher proportions of African American children reporting TMD pain, and also did not adjust by SES, among other methodological concerns, such as possible ethnic differences in the interpretation of questions about pain (Widmalm et al. 1995).

INCIDENCE

As previously mentioned, incidence refers to the number of new cases of disease that develop in a population of individuals at risk during a specific time

Table IV
Prevalence of functional TMD pain in adults

Reference	Disorder Definition	Source of Sample	Sample Size	Age Range (y)	Overall Prevalence (%)	Prevalence in Males (%)	Prevalence in Females (%)	Prevalence Ratio
Agerberg 1972	Does your face hurt when you gape [yawn]?	Swedish persons	1106	15–74	12	11	13	1.18
Molin 1976	Pain on wide opening of the mouth	Swedish men inductees	253	18–25	n.a.	3	n.r.	n.c.
Heloe and Heloe 1978	Have you during the last few years felt any pain in the mandibular joints on chewing, yawning, or opening your mouth wide?	Norwegians	241	65–79	8	3	12	4
Heloe and Heloe 1979	Pain when opening your mouth wide? Now or previously?	Northern Norwegians	246	25	5	3	7	2.33
					8	5	11	2.20
	Pain in the TMJ while chewing, yawning, or talking? Now or previously?		246	25	3	4	2	0.50
					5	6	4	0.67
Osterberg 1979	Does it hurt to open your mouth wide for a large bite?	Swedish elders	348	70	3	3	3	1
Norheim 1978	Pain upon gaping [yawning] or chewing in the last week?	Northern Norwegians	358	20–69	2.7	1	4	4.00
Mohlin 1983	Pain on movement	Swedish women	272	20–45	n.r.	n.a.	5	n.a.
Alanen 1982	Pain in jaw or jaw joint on chewing	Finnish male workers	853	18–57	n.a.	5.2	n.a.	n.c.
Szentpetery 1986	Recent pain in face, neck, or around ears	Hungarians	600	12–85	5.8	3.2	8.3	2.59
	Jaw pain on movement during exam				2.5	1.1	3.8	3.45
Locker and Slade 1988	Pain in TMJ while opening mouth wide	Canadian adults	677	18–65+	5.5	3.7	6.9	1.86
	Pain in TMJ while chewing				7.5	7.4	7.7	1.04
Tervonen and Knuuttila 1988	Pain during maximal opening of mouth	Finnish adults	1600	25–65	2.7	3	4	1.33
Salonen 1990	Pain at mandibular movement often	Swedish adults	920	20–80+	<1	<1	1	n.c.
	Pain at mandibular movement sometimes				4	4	4	1.00
	Pain with chewing often				2	3	2	0.67
	Pain with chewing sometimes				5	6	4	0.67
Agerberg and Inkapool 1990	Pain when opening wide?	Swedish adults	637	18–64	2.7	2.2	3.1	1.41
	Pain when chewing food?				0.1	0.2	0	0.00
Jensen 1993	Pain on jaw function	Danish adults	735	25–64	3.5	2.3	4.8	2.09
De Kanter 1993	Pain during jaw movement	Dutch	3468	15–74	1.2	0.7	1.7	2.43
	Pain in masticatory muscles during mastication			15–74	n.r.	0.2	0.4	2.00
	Pain in TMJ during mastication			15–74	n.r.	0.4	1.2	3.00
	Total			15–74	n.r.	1.3	3.3	2.54
Sato 1996	Does it hurt to open your mouth for a large bite?	Swedish adults	413	70	2	2	2	1.00

Abbreviations: n.a. = not applicable; n.c. = not calculable; n.r. = not reported.
Note: All studies are cross-sectional unless noted. Only Norheim (1978) noted pain severity; no studies reported duration of symptoms.

Table V
Methodological weaknesses and limitations of epidemiological studies of TMD pain

Study Type	Methodological Weakness or Limitation	Studies with Problem
Descriptive (*n* = 133)		
Prevalence	Inadequate sample size*	>80%
	Study is not performed on a representative sample of a defined population	>50%
	Case definition does not include pain or depends solely on physical assessment	>50%
	Case definition of pain is not explicit: does not include severity, duration	>95%
	Age- and gender-specific proportions are not given	>75%
	No mention of spread or dispersion of data; i.e., no confidence intervals	>95%
	Study does not report prevalence of TMD subgroups	>95%
Analytical (*n* = 253)†		
General and cross-sectional	Inadequate sample size*	>90%
	Case definition does not include pain or depends solely on physical assessment	>50%
	Case definition of pain is not explicit: does not include severity, duration	>95%
	Reliability and validity of main exposure measures are uncertain, e.g., bruxism, trauma, occlusion	>90%
	Potentially confounding variables (i.e., gender) are not addressed	>75%
	Study does not report risk of TMD subgroups	>95%
Cohort (*n* = 20)	Studies do not begin with an "inception cohort" of people without TMD pain	>75%
	Large (>40%) losses of subjects to follow-up occurred	>50%
	Data are analyzed as a cross-sectional study	>95%
	Incidence of new cases of TMD pain is not calculated	>95%
	Follow-up time is limited to 2 years or less	>50%
Case-control (*n* = 89)	Sample is subject to selection bias (e.g., clinical cases and controls)	>95%
	Inappropriate controls	>75%
	Prevalent and incident cases are not differentiated	>95%

* Statistical power less than 80% with a Type I error rate of 5%.
† Includes all cohort and case-control studies, plus 135 cross-sectional studies.

period (Hennekens and Buring 1987b). Calculation of incidence requires assembling a cohort of subjects without the disorder and following them over time until later assessment. Only 20 cohort studies of TMD have been published, and 13 do not report TMD pain as a measure (de Boever and van den Berghe 1987; Egermark-Eriksson et al. 1987; Osterberg et al. 1992; Kononen and Nystrom 1993; Magnusson et al. 1993; Wanman 1996). Several other studies list TMD pain report by subjects, but do not calculate the incidence or provide data to do so (Kampe and Hannerz 1991; Pilley et al. 1992; Nordstrom and Eriksson 1994; Onizawa and Yoshida 1996). Table VI shows three cohort studies that report the incidence of TMD pain or give enough data to calculate incidence. The incidence of new onset of TMD pain varies from 1.6 to 3.9 per 100 person-years, or from 1.6% to 3.9% per year. The incidence is probably higher in women, although only one study has reported data (Von Korff et al. 1993). Von Korff also reported the incidence of persistent TMD pain, defined as pain present on 90 or more of 180

days, at 1.2 per 1000 person-years, approximately an order of magnitude lower. The incidence over different ages is unknown, and needs to be investigated. Available prevalence and incidence data for TMD pain provide hints that the age- and gender-specific incidence curves may be similar to migraine—greater for females than males, with incidence peaking in the teens and declining slowly with increasing age (Lipton et al. 1997).

Incidence data have value because they can show not only how many persons develop the disorder, but also at what age. For example, if the pain first occurs during the teenage years, this finding should help to focus on exposures occurring just prior to or before this period. These exposures and putative risk factors could possibly include growth, hormones, or psychosocial changes. With cohort studies, we also can compare the incidence of other pain disorders and see how they are temporally related. Lastly, incidence or onset data can help to determine the induction period or latent period from the first occurrence of the exposure

Table VI
Longitudinal studies of TMD pain

Reference	Disorder Definition	Source of Sample	Years of Follow-up	Sample Size at Baseline	Incidence (%/y)		
					Overall	Males	Females
Kitai et al. 1997	Do you have any pain by active opening or lateral and forward movement of the lower jaw? (Subjects could really feel pain)	Japanese girls aged 12–13 aged 13–14 aged 14–15 aged 15–16	5	361	n.a.	n.r.	2.7 3.9 3.9 2.4
Von Korff et al. 1993	Pain in the TM region in the last 6 mo Persistent TMD pain (180 of 360 days)	HMO enrollees aged 18–65	3	1061	2.17 0.12	1.6	2.6
Heikenheimo et al. 1990	Pain on maximal opening	Finnish adolescents aged 12–15	3	167	1.8	n.s.	n.s.

Abbreviations: n.a. = not applicable; n.r. = not reported.

to the disorder's first manifestation.

Several authors, including Rugh and Solberg (1985) and Katz (1985), emphasized the need to study the incidence of TMD, yet only a few studies have been published in the ensuing 13 years. Why is this? There are several obstacles to this seemingly straightforward proposition. First, as the data available in Table VI show, the incidence of TMD pain appears to be on the order of two or three new cases per 100 persons per year. Thus, to allow for sufficient cases, an investigator needs to study and follow a large group of people without any initial history of TMD pain over a relatively long time interval with frequent queries. This is a time-consuming and expensive way to do research, and only one cohort study to date has had enough subjects—1016—to measure these low incidence rates (Von Korff et al. 1993). Second, the epidemiological methods for study of recurrent conditions like TMD are underdeveloped (Cumming et al. 1990). Epidemiology relies heavily on the identification of incident events of health problems, for example, acute diseases such as appendicitis or chronic diseases such as cancer, to help elucidate causal mechanisms. With acute or true chronic conditions, the person usually recovers or dies from the disease, and only a small fraction of acute cases develop a recurrence in the follow-up period. With pain conditions such as TMD and tension-type headache, recurrence is generally the norm. The first onset of facial pain may occur relatively early in life, and there easily could be many recurrent episodes that differ in pain location, intensity, character, and impact. The first onset of persistent pain, or an episodic type that is severe and disabling, may occur with or without a preceding period of less frequent

and intense pain. Thus, the case definition of TMD pain will likely be paramount in the interpretation of longitudinal studies of TMD onset, along with the further development of methods to study recurrent disorders.

Most longitudinal studies of TMD have shown that most persons who report signs and symptoms of TMD at baseline will not report them the next year. This fluctuation occurs in all studied age groups, and only a fraction have pain that is present at each point during the follow-up period (Kitai et al. 1997). For example, in a study of Japanese girls, although the incidence rate varied between two and four per 100 person-years, only one girl of 361 reported facial pain associated with function in each of four years, for a calculated pain incidence rate of 2.8 per 1000 person-years in four consecutive years, similar to Von Korff's previous estimate of persistent pain in adults of 1.2 per 1000 person-years. Thus, the incidence of TMD pain is low, and the incidence of persistent pain appears much lower. Interpretation of incidence rates for these episodic and recurring disorders is somewhat ambiguous, as recently noted for other chronic musculoskeletal disorders such as low back pain, migraine, and osteoarthritis (Lawrence et al. 1998).

TIME TRENDS

To our knowledge, no studies have been published that have specifically looked at trends in TMD incidence or prevalence over time. Recently Sato et al. (1996) compared the prevalence of "pain when opening the mouth wide" among two different cohorts of 70-year-olds 20 years apart, both in the same community. They used the same methods and many of the same investigators for both groups. Their data showed substantial decreases in the report of functional jaw pain for the most recent cohort. This difference could be due to the better dental health of the second group, to other selection factors associated with this cohort, or to chance. A longitudinal study of TMD patients showed small decreases in either the report of pain or pain apparent on clinical examination in successive birth cohorts 5 years apart (Osterberg et al. 1992). Locker conducted telephone surveys for TMD pain in 1987 (Locker and Slade 1988) and 1992 among the same population (Locker and Miller 1994). His studies found small differences in the prevalence of adults aged 18–65 who reported TMD pain ("pain in the face in front of the ear") in the last 4 weeks (7.5%, 1987; 5.8% in 1992). These studies of older patients may reflect pain associated with osteoarthritis. No studies could be located that look more specifically at masticatory muscle pain in children or younger and middle-aged adults. There is evidence that other head pain conditions, such as migraine (Lipton et al. 1997) and tension-type headache in children (Sillanpää and Anttila 1996), have increased in incidence or prevalence over the last few decades, while other serially conducted cross-sectional studies show decreases in reported musculoskeletal pain (Manninen et al. 1996). There is clearly a greater awareness of TMD, as evidenced by the dramatic increase in number of published studies (Antczak-Bouckoms 1995), funded research, number of clinicians reportedly treating these patients, and interest expressed in the lay press. However, the population most at risk for TMD in the United States—women aged 20–45 years—has increased substantially in the 1990s because of the "baby boom" after World War II, and so any increase seen may be simply a reflection of this population bulge (Rugh and Solberg 1985). Determining trends in the prevalence of TMD pain will not be easy; critical factors are the definition of the condition, the survey methods, and the characteristics of the population. Trends could be studied by using the same definitions and methods in a similar population years later, as illustrated above, or by studying the number of people seeking care within a defined population, such as a health maintenance organization (HMO), over time. Changes in the incidence over time are unknown, given the lack of longitudinal studies that report incidence.

An early study performed in Philadelphia in 1949 found that 11.6% of 700 unselected military person-nel and their dependents reported pain in the temporomandibular region. Only 5%, however, sought care for TMD (Markowitz and Gerry 1949, 1950). These figures are similar to data for prevalence and for those seeking care today. This finding, although limited because it comes from only a single study absent of methodological details, argues against any substantial change in the prevalence of either those reporting or demanding care for TMD-associated pain over the past 50 years.

DIURNAL OR LUNAR VARIATION

Few studies have investigated how TMD pain varies over a single day or a month. Both Goulet et al. (1995) and Dao et al. (1994) showed increases in pain symptoms for most of their subjects as the day progressed. More specifically, in a small case-control study, different daily pain patterns were found for bruxers and myofascial pain patients—the bruxers reported more pain in the morning, while the myofascial pain patients showed a general increase as the day progressed. A preliminary study by Dao et al. (1998) also shows differences during the 28-day menstrual cycle; women not taking oral contraceptives reported higher levels of TMD pain in the three days before menstruation.

SEASONALITY

Only one study has investigated the report of TMD pain over the seasons. Gallagher et al. (1995) and Raphael and Marbach (1992a,b), in a clinical study of 136 female TMD patients, showed a small but statistically significant increase in pain during the winter months. These issues of seasonality, although seemingly an arcane question for a chronic disorder such as TMD pain, should be investigated in both clinical and population-based studies, as new clues may surface regarding etiology. Such studies could be done within large clinical populations such as HMOs, which often have computer databases of patient care records.

Ecological or correlational studies are investigations where the unit of analysis is an entire population rather than the individual (International Epidemiological Association 1995). This type of study has the advantage that it can usually be conducted quickly and easily. We were unable to locate any ecological studies of TMD pain, and none are mentioned in the literature. This approach could be another strategy to

Table VII
Demand for TMD treatment

Reference	Subjects	Sample	Age (y)	Country	Time Period	Percentage Who Ever Sought Treatment for TMD			
						Males	Females	Total	F/M Ratio
0–12 Months									
Magnusson et al.1993	Persons	293	17, 21, 25	Sweden	now	0	2.4	n.r.	n.c.
Von Korff et al. 1988	HMO enrollees	1016	18–64	USA	6 mo	n.r.	n.r.	2.8	n.c.
Goulet et al. 1995	French speakers in Quebec	897	18+	Canada	9 mo	1.0	3.0	2.0	3
Wanman and Wigen 1995	Adults	~650	35	Sweden	1 y	n.r.	n.r.	3.0	n.c.
			50			n.r.	n.r.	3.0	n.c.
			65			n.r.	n.r.	1.0	n.c.
Mean								2.4	
10 Years to Lifetime									
Magnusson et al. 1993	Persons	293	17, 21, 25	Sweden	10 y	5	7.6	6.5	1.5
Norheim and Dahl 1978	Adults	358	20–69	Norway	lifetime	1.0	4.0	2.1	4
Locker and Slade 1988	Adults	677	18–65+	Canada	n.r.	n.r.	n.r.	2.8	n.c.
Swanljung and Ratanen 1979	Adults	579	18–64	Finland	lifetime	n.r.	n.r.	3.0	n.c.
Magnusson et al. 1991	Adults	119	20	Sweden	lifetime	n.r.	n.r.	3.0	n.c.
De Kanter et al. 1992	Probability sample	3468	15–74	Netherlands	lifetime	n.r.	n.r.	3.1	n.c.
Heloe and Heloe 1979	Adults	246	25	Norway	lifetime	2.0	5.0	4.0	2.5
Markowitz and Gerry 1949	U.S. military and dependents	700	18+	USA	lifetime?	n.r.	n.r.	6.4	n.c.
Agerberg and Carlsson 1972	Adults	1106	15–74	Sweden	lifetime	5.0	9.0	7.0	1.8
Von Korff et al. 1988a	HMO enrollees	1016	18–65	USA	lifetime	n.r.	n.r.	7.5	n.c.
Riley et al. 1998	Elder Floridians, face pain	1636	65–100	USA	lifetime	3.02	4.84	n.r.	1.60
	Elder Floridians, jaw pain					3.38	4.84	n.r.	1.43
Mean								4.5	2.6

Abbreviations: n.c. = not calculable; n.r. = not reported.
Note: All studies are population-based cross-sectional studies except for Markowitz. All studies are estimates of prior TMD treatment by self-report.

help identify new potential risk factors for pain. For example, studies might compare rates of TMD pain in developed versus developing countries. Khan (1990) has reported much lower proportions of persons reporting TMD pain in rural African countries than are generally found in Europe or North America, but the difference could be related to research methods and definition of TMD. Also, countries with social health care systems and others without the same support mechanisms could be compared, as could countries with different ethnic or racial groups. A universally accepted case definition for TMD pain along with studies to show that the meaning of the words is similar from language to language (Moore and Dworkin 1988) is needed for this type of study design to be fruitful.

CONSEQUENCES OF TMD PAIN

The consequences of TMD pain for the individual and society have been little studied. Multiple searches using the key words "costs," "burden," "consequences," "quality of life," and subheadings "economic" and "psychology" with temporomandibular disorders or dysfunction syndrome yielded fewer than 20 pertinent articles. Most of the work that has been done is limited to a handful of publications (Von Korff et al. 1988a, 1991; Reisine 1989; Dworkin 1995). Several of these authors have convincingly shown that TMD chronic pain appears to share many important features with other chronic pain conditions such as low back pain and headache, in terms of the psychological distress, individual burden, and other nonspecific features (Dworkin 1995). This next section will discuss the effect of TMD pain on the health care system, the economic costs of TMD pain, and, finally, the effect on the individual patient.

TMD AND HEALTH CARE SYSTEMS

TMD pain affects about 10% of women and 6% of men in any given year. Application of these percentages today's adult U.S. population would yield roughly 6,675,000 men and 13,350,000 women, or a total of 20 million adults in 1998. Further extension of the population prevalence for the world, assuming similar proportions across cultures, would give a rough estimate of 450 million adults afflicted worldwide. Furthermore, approximately one in three adults will develop TMD pain in his or her lifetime (Dworkin and

LeResche 1993). Thus, pain from temporomandibular disorders is a common condition.

Although TMD pain is common, for pain to have a direct impact on health care, those in pain must visit health care providers. What is the prevalence of persons seeking care for TMD pain? Table VII shows the studies that have asked, primarily in population surveys, "Have you ever sought care for TMD?" The upper part of the table shows four studies that limited this question to the previous 0–9 months; between 1% and 3% of respondents had sought care for their TMD during this period. A median estimate of 2% seeking treatment would correspond to 5,340,000 U.S. residents seeking care for TMD within a 6- to 12-month period in 1998. The lower part of the table shows that 2–7.5% of the populations in studies in North America and Scandinavia had sought care for TMD in their lifetime. These estimates show that approximately one-quarter to one-third of persons with TMD pain during a given year seek out and visit a practitioner. The female-to-male ratio, although calculable in only a few of the studies, was slightly larger than the population-based prevalence ratio, 2.5 women for every man.

A unique aspect of TMD pain is that patients often comment that they are not sure whom they should consult first for their symptoms—a physician, dentist, or other health care provider. Indeed, anywhere from 50% to 75% of patients will first visit a dentist, while the remainder seek a physician (Glaros et al. 1995; Turp et al. 1998). The first provider they see also has a strong effect on the next referral—physicians refer to other physicians, dentists to other dentists (Glaros et al. 1995; Turp et al. 1998). Because TMD pain may not be effectively resolved with traditional medicine, alternative health care is commonly sought (Eisenberg et al. 1993; Foreman et al. 1994; Turp et al. 1998) but is often not counted in surveys of cost.

Patients with TMD pain commonly consult physicians first, so it is somewhat surprising that so little time in medical school is spent on the diagnosis and management of the condition, even in institutions where the fundamental aspects of chronic pain diagnosis and management are part the curriculum. In addition, the medical research community appears to have had little interest in TMD pain. Of 12,400 scientific articles published about TMD and listed in MEDLINE in the last 33 years, fewer than 400 are in medical journals, and most of these are in otolaryngology journals. Fewer than five substantive articles on TMD appeared in a major medical journal in the last 30 years. Thus, these pain conditions, although commonly encountered in medical practice, appear to have been generally ignored in medical education and research. Delays in diagnosis and subsequent appropriate referral (Foreman et al. 1994), or incorrect diagnoses (Foreman et al. 1994; Glaros et al. 1995) were common findings in several recent studies of both dentists and physicians. Often, a correct diagnosis was not made until the third or fourth visit (Fricton et al. 1985; Foreman et al. 1994; Glaros et al. 1995). Controversy among different schools of thought, not necessarily lack of interest or training, may be an additional factor delaying diagnosis within dentistry (Von Korff et al. 1988). Inappropriate early care for TMD has also been identified among patients who eventually attended tertiary care pain clinics, although these studies may be biased because it is the patients who do not improve who are most likely to be referred for further care (Foreman et al. 1994). These preliminary findings indicate that current health care, staffing, and training for managing TMD pain may be inadequate, and more work needs to be done to better coordinate treatment for this condition.

ECONOMIC COSTS OF TMD PAIN

Economic costs to society for TMD pain include direct costs, such as the cost of providing care, and indirect costs, or those associated with work loss, decreased productivity of work, and economic consequences of other disruptions (Lipton and Stewart 1997). The direct costs of care for TMD have not been presented in the literature, but would need to include the medical, dental, and alternative health care systems. Only two estimates are available for the annual cost per patient of specialty care for TMD pain. The first estimate, U.S.$304, is probably low because it comes from an HMO where guidelines to provide cost-efficient care were in place, and it did not include the patient's other costs, including intraoral appliances (Von Korff 1995). The second study of TMD health care costs was conducted within a large East Coast U.S. HMO, and showed that both inpatient and outpatient costs per capita were almost double for members who sought care for TMD, compared to all other HMO members, adjusted for age and gender (Shimshak et al. 1997). These costs were substantial: inpatient claims, U.S.$935 versus $516 per year; outpatient claims, $1738 versus $870 per year, not including psychiatric care outside the HMO. Using the previous

estimates of the number of persons who annually present for TMD care in the traditional health care sector in the United States, and an estimate of the annual cost of the visits (i.e., approximately 5.3 million people with one or more visits multiplied by a conservative estimate of $400 per person-year for one or more visits) would result in a cost estimate of a little over $2 billion in 1998. A national survey of dentists about occlusal splint fabrication indicated that about $990 million a year was spent on occlusal splints alone in 1990, and most of these splints were used to treat TMD; this represented 2.9% of the total U.S. expenditure for dental services in 1990 (Pierce et al. 1995).

Indirect costs for TMD pain have not been published. Studies of related cephalic pain conditions, such as migraine, have estimated that the indirect costs of work loss and decreased productivity to be much greater than the direct costs (Lipton and Stewart 1997). Several TMD studies have shown unemployment and decreased work effectiveness among patients with TMD pain. Von Korff et al. (1992), for example, showed that 28.6% of TMD pain patients with high disability and severe limitations from pain (i.e., Grade IV) reported that they were unemployed, which is about five times higher than the regional average at that time. These unemployment levels were similar to those for Grade IV back pain (26.6%) and severe headache subjects (22.2%). In terms of work efficiency, Dao showed that 64% of a selected group of myofascial pain patients reported decreased efficiency at work, compared to 7.7% of subjects who were bruxers without pain (Dao et al. 1994). A similar proportion (26.1%) of people with reported work interference was found for patients referred to a craniofacial pain unit (Murray et al. 1996). No studies could be located that estimate the number of work days lost from absence or decreased productivity, or the monetary cost to society of TMD pain. As with migraine, the indirect costs are likely to be substantial, and larger than the direct costs of care, but are presently unknown for TMD pain.

COST TO THE PATIENT WITH TMD PAIN

One large population-based cross-sectional and cohort study of 1016 members of an HMO compared five different chronic pain conditions, including TMD pain, and showed that TMD chronic pain has similar individual impact and burden as back pain, severe headache, chest, and abdominal pain (Von Korff et al. 1988a). For example, for each of the five pain conditions, between 15% and 39% of persons reported "severe" pain; severe facial pain was reported by 16%. The usual duration of pain was 9 or more hours per day for 13–32% of persons with pain conditions, including 27% of those with facial pain. The percentage of persons unable to carry on some activities because of pain ranged from 14% for facial pain to 48% for severe headache. Measures of psychological distress, such as anxiety, depression, and somatization, were similar across all five pain conditions, including TMD. Subjects with possible major depression varied from 6% for abdominal pain to a high of 11% for facial pain. The societal costs of this comorbid condition are also great, including loss of life from suicide (Nemeroff 1998). Suicide and suicide attempts related to TMD pain are unstudied, but are important avenues for further research.

Other, nonpopulation studies of patients with TMD pain have reported how it can have dramatic negative consequences for the individual. A report of a TMD pain support group, for example, showed that some of those with pain had spent upwards of Can.$30,000 for treatment, had lost their jobs, houses, and belongings, and were still suffering significantly from the pain (Garro et al. 1994). Another study, previously cited, of patients at a TMD chronic pain center found that almost half reported difficulty chewing foods, and about one-third reported disturbed sleep and depression and felt that life was less satisfying (Murray et al. 1996). The proportion of all people with such severe impacts, however, can only be determined from population studies; for most conditions, studies can find and report groups of severely impacted individuals. Nevertheless, TMD pain clearly is associated with substantial burden for about one-quarter of those with the condition, and the pain predominately occurs during the peak productive years (ages 20–50).

NATURAL HISTORY OF TMD

"Natural history" typically has meant the course of a disorder from inception to resolution without therapy or formal intervention (International Epidemiological Association 1995). Other authors have indicated that this definition may be amended to include the outcome of a disorder without therapy that influences the rate of the disorder, or without effective therapy (Weiss 1996). Such studies can serve several important functions—first, to point out the need for

treatment of a condition, because some disorders, such as tension-type headache, resolve without formal intervention, while others, such as most malignant neoplasms, usually will result in death without treatment. Second, natural history studies that follow a disorder from its earliest inception may indicate if early detection is possible and can aid in primary prevention of the disease (Weiss 1996).

Searches of the scientific literature revealed 513 follow-up studies of patients with TMD; after excluding non-English studies, 402 remained. Exclusion of nonoriginal research yielded 390 studies. Most of these follow-up studies had small samples, generally fewer than 20 subjects. In addition, almost all studies treated the patients with an intervention. After the small studies and those with active treatments were excluded, two remained that were true natural history studies of TMD pain. Unfortunately, neither of these classified TMD with a pain measure (Sato et al. 1997; Kurita et al. 1998).

Since so few natural history studies of TMD pain have been published, we looked at other follow-up studies that included studies of entire populations with treatment of only a few individuals, and also follow-up studies of TMD pain patients treated conservatively, with minimal intervention. This first group of longitudinal studies, listed in Table VI, shows fluctuation in the symptoms of pain among those persons who report pain at any time point. Only a small fraction of the subjects deemed a case at any given time met criteria for a case one or more years later. This fluctuation of pain report over time has occurred in most population-based longitudinal studies of children and adults (Heikinheimo et al. 1990; Osterberg et al. 1992; LeResche 1995; Kitai et al. 1997; Ohrbach and Dworkin 1998). Less specifically, fluctuation of TMD symptoms, including pain, has been reported in several longitudinal studies (Nilner 1981; de Boever and van den Berghe 1987; Egermark-Eriksson et al. 1987; Kononen and Nystrom 1993; Magnusson et al. 1993; Wanman 1996). De Leeuw and colleagues (1995), in the longest follow-up study published to date, reported the status of a subset of patients conservatively treated for TMD pain and "permanent" TMJ disk displacement. At baseline, 93% had pain, and 30 years later, only 5% still reported pain (de Leeuw et al. 1995). In most longitudinal studies, only a small fraction of the population, or minority of the previously identified cases, consistently report pain. Thus, there is little information on the natural history of TMD pain, but the synthesis of the few available studies and other follow-up studies of minimally treated patient groups indicates that most persons with TMD pain will be pain free or have reduced pain at later follow-up. A small minority, usually less than 20%, have either continued or increased pain.

PROGNOSTIC FACTORS

A few longitudinal investigations have explored factors associated with the continued report of TMD pain (Von Korff et al. 1993; Fricton and Olsen 1996; Greco et al. 1997; Ohrbach and Dworkin 1998). The determination of predictive or prognostic factors does not necessarily indicate that these factors are causal. In general, most of these studies looking for predictors of chronic TMD pain have found few correlations with baseline physical signs or symptoms, such as magnitude of mandibular opening, TMD diagnostic subgroup, or number of joint sounds. Instead, some psychological factors have been associated with continued pain, such as correlates of depression (Fricton and Olsen 1996), score on the Beck Depression Inventory (Greco et al. 1997), characteristic pain intensity, nonspecific symptoms and depression (Garofalo et al. 1998), depression, anxiety and somatization (Ohrbach and Dworkin 1998), somatization (McCreary et al. 1992), and duration of initial symptoms (Wedel and Carlsson 1986). In addition, previous high levels of health care utilization have been predictive of continued TMD pain (Greco et al. 1997). Identification of a predictive factor may be a result of the unique characteristics of the studied population, so factors identified only in a single study should generally be discounted, unless the effect is very large or the study is large and methodologically strong. All the cited studies suffered from relatively small sample sizes, and many of the populations are from tertiary care centers, reflecting referral bias toward more difficult cases. Nevertheless, of the many variables studied so far, baseline depression, somatization, and other psychophysiological factors are the most promising predictors of continuing TMD pain.

HIGH-RISK GROUPS

Many previous articles have shown that adult women with TMD pain are vastly overrepresented in clinic populations (Carlsson and LeResche 1995), sometimes in ratios of up to 9:1 compared to men.

Although some of this discrepancy may be due to increased treatment-seeking behavior among women, population-based prevalence studies summarized above clearly show about 2:1 female-to-male ratios, while the proportion of women to men seeking care is at least 2.5:1. In a multivariate analysis of a population-based study, Von Korff et al. (1991) have shown that gender did not explain the difference in treatment seeking in their population; instead, women sought out care more often because they had more severe and persistent pain then did men. Thus, it appears that more women than men suffer from the disorder, and that women may seek care for TMD pain more often than men because their pain is more severe.

Early studies indicated that women of higher socioeconomic status (SES) sought care for TMD pain at higher rates than did those of low SES (Franks 1964; Heloe et al. 1977). However, given that much of TMD care in the United States is not covered by insurance, many persons of lesser economic means may not seek care because they can not afford it, which creates referral bias. The few population studies that have measured this variable have shown a slightly greater prevalence of low SES patients in population samples (Dworkin et al. 1990; Von Korff 1995) or in clinics that take patients with state-supported care (Smith and Syrop 1994). It appears that a clear relationship may not be seen until other population studies explore this relationship, or until subgroups of TMD pain, such as those with persistent pain, or mainly myofascial pain, are further evaluated.

Other risk factors investigated for TMD have included psychosocial stress, dental occlusal relationships, oral parafunction, and trauma, and a long list of other less well-accepted exposures (American Academy of Orofacial Pain 1996; LeResche 1997). These risk factors have generally been implicated through anecdotal observations of individual patients in clinic populations where clinicians have perceived higher-than-expected rates of these exposures among their patients with TMD. Unfortunately, current methods for measuring some of these exposures, such as occlusal relationships, can be unreliable (Keeling et al. 1996), and reliance upon past recall for trauma history (such as motor vehicle accidents) is often complicated by legal and financial incentives to obtain reimbursement for damages, besides the unknown effects of psychological trauma from the accident. Measuring oral parafunction with self-report (e.g., for sleep bruxism) may be inaccurate (Marbach et al. 1990), and requires expensive sleep laboratory studies for validation (Lavigne et al. 1996). The psychological measures are perhaps the most well-developed, reliable, and validated.

Inherent in studies of this condition are many other problems of clinical research, including lack of or inappropriate control groups; small sample sizes; no acknowledgment, assessment, or control for confounding variables; and absent or improper multivariate analyses. Furthermore, the associations of some factors with TMD pain have been interpreted as causation, even though few studies are longitudinal, the primary way to determine whether the exposure preceded the disorder.

Based on these premature assertions of causality, some clinicians have advocated specific therapies to both "cure" and prevent TMD pain. For example, alteration of occlusal relationships in patients with TMD pain by extensive dental rehabilitation, orthodontics, or surgery is widely practiced today, although we lack evidence that these relationships are either associated or causative (Pullinger et al. 1993). Reinforcement of almost any imaginable therapy has occurred, given that the natural history of TMD pain is generally improvement without formal medical intervention. Most risk factors assumed today for TMD and TMD pain are based on the opinions, anecdotes, and belief structures of a few influential clinicians in dentistry who have acquired an almost "guru-like" status (Greene 1992), rather than on evidence from epidemiological studies.

Thus, the only well-supported high-risk group from these descriptive epidemiological studies is women between the ages of 15 and about 50. Any putative risk factor that is not more prevalent in women than men is less likely to contribute much to the increased risk, unless a substantial biological synergism occurs between that risk factor and female gender.

DISORDERS ASSOCIATED WITH TMD PAIN

Several other disorders appear to occur more often among persons with TMD pain than among the general population. Both migraine and tension-type headache have been associated with TMD pain and other TMD symptoms in numerous cross-sectional and case-control studies (Molin et al. 1976; Wanman and Agerberg 1987). Migraine first occurs at relatively early ages (Lipton and Stewart 1997), so it is likely that the first onset of migraine precedes the first onset of TMD, although no studies have explored this rela-

tionship. Tension-type headache has been associated with TMD in multiple studies, although most are cross-sectional and often fail to differentiate TMD pain referred to pericranial structures from tension-type headache (Gerstner et al. 1994; Schiffman et al. 1995). Indeed, it is possible that what some patients and clinicians call tension-type headache is actually a type of TMD-associated pain, and vice versa. More work is needed to differentiate common headache types from TMD pain. Nevertheless, TMD pain and headache often appear together in the same patient, and may be caused by common risk factors.

Fibromyalgia, a chronic widespread pain of unknown origin, has been associated with TMD. Several studies have shown that approximately 75% of fibromyalgia patients fulfill criteria for TMD, and 12–25% of TMD patients meet diagnostic criteria for fibromyalgia (Plesh et al. 1996; Hedenberg-Magnusson et al. 1997; Cimino et al. 1998). Whether fibromyalgia increases risk for TMD, or TMD increases risk for fibromyalgia or is another manifestation of this syndrome, or whether both conditions are caused by common risk factors is not known (Wolfe 1995).

RISK FACTORS

Determining the risk factors and ultimately the factors that cause a disorder is a complex scientific endeavor. Epidemiological methods are now well developed to help to establish, first, whether an association exists between an exposure and the disorder, and second, to decide with the aid of accepted causal standards whether the observed association is likely to be one of cause and effect. Studies in the last 10 years have just begun to elucidate the risk factors for TMD pain.

For this review our inclusion criteria for studies investigating the risk factors for TMD pain included: controlled studies, such as a cohort, case-control, or cross-sectional study design; a case definition that included TMD pain as a major part of the case criteria; and control for potential confounding by at least age and gender.

COHORT STUDIES

Multiple search methods, previously described, revealed about 85 English-language longitudinal studies of TMD over the last 33 years; these were reduced to 20 by excluding studies that did not fit a strict definition of a cohort investigation (i.e., beginning with a population of non-cases, recording the exposure or risk factor at baseline before the onset of TMD pain, and then measuring the onset of pain at a later date (Hennekens and Buring 1987b). Other exclusions included studies that did not control for age and gender (5 studies), and finally, studies that did not have TMD pain as a predominant aspect of the case definition (13 studies). This left only two studies, which are listed in Table VIII. Von Korff et al. (1993), in the only cohort study with control for the possible confounding effects of age, gender and education, showed that high baseline depression scores (RR = 1.6) and multiple pains at the beginning of the study (RR = 3.7) were associated with the onset of TMD pain 3 years later in an adult population of HMO enrollees, although only the risk for multiple pains was statistically significant. Kitai et al. (1997) showed no association between several measures of malocclusion and the onset of TMD functional pain during a 5-year follow up of adolescent Japanese girls. All other longitudinal studies located that investigated putative risk factors for TMD pain failed to measure the association between the onset of the pain and the pre-existing exposure measure. Many of these studies essentially performed multiple cross-sectional analyses of the same cohort at different points over time, and then measured the association between pain and exposure *at that time only*. Unfortunately, such a study has only the strength of a cross-sectional study and is so grouped. The temporal sequence, a major criterion for demonstrating cause and effect, becomes ambiguous in this type of analysis.

CASE-CONTROL STUDIES

We identified about 110 case-control studies published from 1965 to 1998, and with the exclusion of 25 non-English studies, reduced these to 85. Studies that did not attempt to control for gender (30) and did not have pain as a major aspect of the case definition (50) were excluded. The remaining five studies are listed in Table VIII.

Molina et al. (1997), in a clinical study of 133 TMD cases and 133 controls, showed strong associations between TMD pain and self-reported bruxism, migraine, and mixed and tension-type headaches, while matching on age and gender with controls who were seeking dental care but did not have TMD. Unfortunately, Molina's team excluded the use of medi-

cations in the control group, which likely elevated associations of TMD and headache. LeResche et al. (1997b), in two large population-based case-control studies, investigated the effects of female exogenous hormone use, and found small but significant associations between seeking care for TMD pain and oral contraceptive (OC) use, after controlling for age, gender, and health care utilization (OR = 1.19). In a similar analysis, there was also a significant effect of postmenopausal hormone use among older women (OR = 1.32). A dose-response relationship was found between cumulative estrogen dose and risk of TMD. MacGregor and others (1996), in a small case-control study, found significant relationships with several novel exposures, including chronic respiratory infections, gastrointestinal infections, and chronic pain in long-term partners. Lee et al. (1995) and Hackney et al. (1993), in two small clinical case-control studies, investigated the relationship between forward head posture and TMD pain; one found a moderate association (OR = 1.9), while the other failed to find a relationship.

CROSS-SECTIONAL STUDIES

Cross-sectional studies, or cohort studies with cross-sectional analyses, were located next. About 200 studies have been published since 1966; 45 were excluded because they were not in English. Only 45 of the remaining 135 articles had pain as a major aspect of the case definition, and a further 42 were eliminated because they did not control for gender in the analyses, leaving only three studies, which are listed in Table VIII. Von Korff et al. (1988a), in a population-based cross-sectional study, showed associations between facial pain and self-rated fair to poor health status, major depression, and "a great deal" of family stress. Adjustment for potential confounders of age, gender, and education reduced all associations, so that only family stress remained a significantly increased risk. Sato and others, in cross-sectional analysis of a cohort study of older Swedish men and women, showed that both radiographic appearance of TMJ osteoarthritis and decreased number of supporting teeth were associated with pain upon mouth opening (Sato et al. 1996). Bibb, in a cross-sectional study of elders attending a health fair in California, showed nonsignificant associations of depression, arthritis, and reduced daily activities with jaw pain (Bibb et al. 1995).

None of the listed studies has specifically investi-

Table VIII

Risk factors for temporomandibular pain

Reference	Definition	Risk Factor	Sample Size	Magnitude of Association	Statistical Significance	Type of Measure	Adjustment for Potential Confounders	Likelihood of Causality
Cohort Studies								
Von Korff et al. 1993	Facial pain	Older age	1012	0.65	no	OR	Age, gender, education	**
		Gender	1012	1.49	no	OR	Age, gender, education	****
		College education	1012	0.83	no	OR	Age, gender, education	*
		Severe depression	1012	1.60	no	OR	Age, gender, education	****
		Number of pain conditions	1012	3.69	yes	OR	Age, gender, education	****
Kitai 1997	TMD pain	Malocclusion	361	~1.0†	n.r.	RR	All female	*
Case-control Studies								
LeResche 1997	TMD pain referrals	Exogenous hormone use	6455	1.32 (1.10–1.57)	yes	OR	Age, health service use	*
LeResche 1997	TMD pain referrals	Exogenous hormone use	7365	1.19 (1.01–1.40)	yes	OR	Age, health service use	*
Molina et al. 1997	TMD patients with pain	Self-reported bruxism	266	2.3†	yes	OR	Age, gender matched	**
		Any headache	266	3.2†	yes	OR	Age, gender matched	**
		Migraine headache	266	11.1†	n.r.	OR	Age, gender matched	**
		Tension headache	266	3.6†	n.r.	OR	Age, gender matched	**
		Mixed headache	266	2.2†	n.r.	OR	Age, gender matched	**
		Bruxism and tension headache	266	10.3†	n.r.	OR	Age, gender matched	**
		No bruxism and any headache	266	1.3†	n.r.	OR	Age, gender matched	
		Bruxism and any headache	266	4.5†	n.r.	OR	Age, gender matched	
McGregor et al. 1996	Orofacial muscle pain	Chronic recurrent upper resp. infections	83	positive	yes		Age, gender matched	*
		G.I. infections	83	positive	yes		Age, gender matched	*
		Previous appendectomy	83	positive	yes		Age, gender matched	*
		Somatization	83	positive	yes	means	Age, gender matched	*
		Obsessive-compulsive disorder	83	positive	yes	means	Age, gender matched	*
		Depression	83	positive	yes	means	Age, gender matched	****
		Pain in long-term partners	83	positive	yes		Age, gender matched	*
Lee et al.1995	TMD pain	Forward head posture	66	1.92†	yes	OR	Age, gender matched	*
Hackney et al.1993	TMD/ID with pain	Forward head posture	44	no assoc.	no	means	Age, gender matched	*
Cross-sectional Studies								
Von Korff et al. 1988a	Facial pain	Self-rated health status fair or poor	1016	1.9		PR	None	
		Self-rated health status fair or poor		n.s.	no		Age, gender, education	***
		Possible major depression		5.5†		PR	None	
		Possible major depression		n.s.	no		Age, gender, education	****
		Great deal of family stress		2.2†			None	
		Great deal of family stress		1.5	yes	OR	Age, gender, education	**
Sato 1996	Pain on opening mouth	Abnormal condyle on X-ray	643	2.5	yes	PR	Gender	***
Bibb 1995	Jaw pain	Eichner index of tooth support	429	positive	yes	?	Female only	**
		Depression		R = 0.09	no	CORR	Male only	***
		History of arthritis		R = 0.023	no	CORR	Female only	**
		Reduced activities of daily living		R = 0.029	no	CORR	Female only	**

Abbreviations: CORR = correlation; ID = internal TMJ disk replacement; n.r. = not reported; OR = odds ratio; PR = prevalence ratio; RR = risk ratio; TMD = temporomandibular disorder. † Magnitude of association was calculated by present authors. ‡ Each asterisk denotes a criterion for causation (see text).

gated genetic or familial factors associated with TMD pain. We located only two studies investigating familial factors, and both compared the occurrence of TMD in dizygotic (DZ) and monozygotic (MZ) twins. This design allows an estimation of the percentage of the disorder that can be explained by genetic versus environmental factors. Heiberg et al. (1980), in small study of 94 twins, did not show any genetic influence. A recent study of 146 MZ and 96 DZ twins showed a nonsignificant genetic influence of 24% for TMD pain (Michalowicz et al. 1998). One of the authors of this paper estimated that about 1200 twin pairs would be needed to demonstrate that the contribution from a genetic effect was not due to the play of chance alone because the prevalence of TMD pain was relatively low (8.7%) in their twin population (J. Hodges, personal communication, 1999). These two studies suggest that TMD pain does not appear to have a large heritable component, but much more work is needed in this area before solid conclusions can be made.

Notably absent from Table VIII are studies investigating trauma and occlusal factors, but all studies located that investigated these factors either did not include TMD pain as a major aspect of the case definition or did not attempt to control for confounding by at least gender. Other risk factors of interest but not included because they did not meet our criteria were generalized joint hypermobility, dental extractions, and orthodontic treatment. Some of these factors, such as generalized hypermobility, may be associated with specific TMD subtypes such as internal derangements but are not necessarily thought to be directly associated with TMD pain. None of the studies in Table VIII reported analyses by the TMD subtype, but such evaluation typically requires a large sample size or restriction of cases to that TMD subgroup.

Determining whether the risk factors in Table VIII may cause TMD pain can be viewed as a deductive process (Rothman and Greenland 1998a). First, is there an association that cannot be explained by the play of chance, selection and information biases, or confounding (Hennekens and Buring 1987c)? Either the confidence interval or statistical tests can tell us if the association could have occurred by happenstance. Most of the listed associations show statistical significance. All of the listed associations have also been adjusted by gender, a strong risk factor for TMD pain, and by age, decreasing the chance that confounding could explain the associations. Selection biases are possible, especially with the clinic-based case-control studies, but the articles generally provided insufficient information to tell if this bias is acting in any particular study. Information biases are also possible, including recall bias in the case-control studies, and bias from loss to follow-up in the cohort studies. Recall bias in case-control and cross-sectional studies is possible, especially for measures such as bruxism, because patients with TMD pain may be more cognizant of these oral parafunctions after visiting dental practitioners (Marbach 1990). The loss to follow-up in both cohort studies was relatively low (Kitai et al. 1997, 12% over 5 years; Von Korff et al. 1993, 21% over 3 years), which decreases this bias as an explanation for the findings. Thus, it appears that several factors are associated with an increased risk of TMD pain, including number of pain conditions, exogenous hormone use, self-reported bruxism, self-reported poor health, evidence of somatization, depression, and obsessive-compulsive disorder on standardized psychometric tests, and possibly forward head posture, loss of posterior tooth support, and radiographic appearance of osteoarthritis.

Which of these factors may also be causal? First, only the cohort studies can usually demonstrate a temporal association, and presence of other pains was the only statistically significant risk factor determined before the pain began, so it fulfills this criterion. Second, is the magnitude of the association large? "Large" is a subjective term, but associations greater than a ratio of two are less likely to be the result of residual confounding and add weight to the assessment. Odds ratios for several pain conditions—bruxism and evidence of osteoarthritis—are all greater than two. Third, is there evidence that increased exposure is associated the increased probability of pain? Exogenous estrogen shows this effect (LeResche et al. 1997), along with depression in the Von Korff cohort study. Fourth, is there consistency from study to study? Only a few of the studies in this table have looked at the same factors, and depression appears to be associated in varying degrees in all four of the studies that explored it (Von Korff et al. 1988a, 1993; Bibb et al. 1995; McGregor et al. 1996). Finally, are these risk factors biologically plausible, or are there examples of these risk factors associated with chronic pain in muscles or joints in other parts of the body? All would likely fulfill this criterion, except possibly forward head posture, and respiratory and gastrointestinal infections. Thus, factors associated with female gender, number of pre-existing pain conditions, and depression appear to fulfill the greatest number of causal criteria and should be regarded as the most likely to be associations of cause and effect. The other factors—bruxism, self-rated fair or poor health, and osteoarthritis—are suggestive of causation, but more studies are needed before these and the remaining listed factors can be thought of as causative factors. Given that depression appears to be associated with TMD pain, then the risk factors for depression, such as genetic predisposition, adverse childhood events, lack of physical exercise, etc. (Nemeroff 1998), should be considered as possible risk factors for TMD in future studies.

In summary, surprisingly few analytic studies of TMD pain fulfill basic epidemiological standards—most have uncontrolled confounding, are too small, include inadequate analyses, or have other problems, such as lack of validity or reliability of the measures.

RISK FACTORS FOR TMD PAIN: METHODOLOGICAL ISSUES

Establishing factors that cause a disorder requires extraordinary effort with regard to the design, conduct, and analysis of scientific studies. Although the foregoing discussion indicates substantial progress in identifying risk factors that may cause TMD pain, several issues are apparent after examining both the eligible and ineligible studies (see bottom half of Table V). First, many have samples too small to have a legitimate chance of finding an effect without making a Type II error; that is, finding no effect or association when an effect exists. In addition, with small sample sizes and many potential risk factors, there is a good chance that Type I errors (finding an association when none exists) are also occurring. Keeping track of the comparisons made within a study and reporting them in the manuscript is one way to identify or decrease this type of error. Corrections to statistical tests can also be applied formally, with so-called Bonferroni corrections with univariate analyses, or simply making the statistical criteria more stringent, for example, dropping from 0.05 to 0.01 for significance. Perhaps the best method to guard against these chance associations is to establish a priori risk factors that are of primary interest and report other observed relationships with caution. Investigations of occlusal factors and psychophysiological measures have appeared especially prone to these "multiple comparison" problems in the past literature.

We need a causal model of the role of hypoth-esized risk factors as a basis for developing targeted risk factor studies. The last widely disseminated etiological model of which we are aware was published in the late 1960s (Laskin 1969), and an updated model, however incomplete, is essential. Without such a model, an investigator may not be fully aware of the hypothesized direction of the proposed effects, if the factor is an intermediate, confounder, or effect modifier within a causal pathway, and may be uncertain how to handle that factor in the analysis. Causal models for other pain conditions (e.g., fibromyalgia; Yunus 1992) have recently been published, and may be good starting points.

Regarding the optimal designs to evaluate these risk factors, case-control studies are generally more efficient designs than cohort studies for disorders with low incidence rates and exposures that are relatively common, as shown with TMD, and they should be considered, especially if they can be nested within a known cohort of persons at risk for TMD pain. Cohort studies will still be needed to unequivocally demonstrate the temporal sequence between TMD pain and possible risk factors. Such large studies must be well-designed by collaborative research groups of epidemiologists, biostatisticians, and expert clinicians. They will be expensive, and researchers must convince funding agencies of their value.

SCOPE FOR PREVENTION

Prevention of TMD pain and suffering is a laudable goal that may result from the identification of causative factors that can be *modified* by action. Primary prevention, or removal of the risk factor before the onset of the disorder, is the ultimate goal, but, with the paucity of information about TMD risk factors, this task appears daunting. This type of prevention requires that a modifiable risk factor be known, and further requires a screening process to identify persons who are risk but without the disorder, and then a cost-effective method to remove or reduce the risk factor. No studies of primary prevention meeting these criteria were located for TMD pain, although two small randomized trials altered the dental occlusion of young adults and then followed these subjects for several years and observed the onset of signs and symptoms of TMD. The first, by Kirveskari et al. (1989), compared occlusal adjustment with placebo occlusal adjustment and did not find any significant differences in pain report among the subjects, although some of the multiple outcome measures did show a difference. The second, more recent, study by Karjalainen et al. (1997) also did not show differences in pain report between the placebo and active groups. (This study suffered from methodological problems in that the active group had an unspecified greater number of visits with the dentists, and the assessment process was not blind.) These two studies illustrate some of the difficulties of prevention trials: a large sample is usually needed for adequate statistical power; the primary outcome measures should be limited and listed a priori, blinding should be done to the extent possible; and the risk factor should be proven to be associated with the outcome in multiple nonexperimental studies before the expense of a trial is incurred.

Screening for persons at risk also needs to be addressed in a cost-effective manner. Although articles have been published discussing how to prevent TMD (e.g., Kirveskari et al. 1989; Karjalainen et al. 1997), there is no scientific basis for any such claims. Launching a primary prevention trial with the current limited knowledge seems ill advised. However, if we define the outcome measure more stringently, such as prevention of persistent and disabling TMD pain, this goal may be reachable in the near future, but the risk factors for progression to persistence need to be better defined.

Secondary prevention, or the early detection and treatment of TMD pain, may be practical at this point. For example, some of the risk factors for TMD in the psychosocial realm could be considered for a prevention trial, but it will likely require multiple large studies performed at different places and times before we will be convinced that secondary prevention is possible. Secondary prevention of persistent TMD pain may also be possible, and should be made a high priority, given the high cost and impact on the individual and society. For it to be feasible, we need to be able to accurately predict which patients are likely to develop persistent or disabling pain.

Tertiary prevention, or reducing complications by prompt diagnosis and effective treatment, is generally the starting point for most disorders, and should be the main focus for TMD pain at this time. Some methods of tertiary prevention include: (1) reduction of possible iatrogenic TMD pain by development of evidence-based treatment guidelines, and their dissemination to clinicians; (2) reduction of misdiagnoses and use of unnecessary diagnostic tests and in-

effective therapies among dentists and physicians through education and training; (3) effective management of comorbid conditions, such as depression; and (4) interventions that focus on fostering adaptive responses to pain. Other promising preventive strategies developed with other pain disorders could also be applied to TMD, given the overall similarity among chronic pain syndromes.

CHALLENGES FOR THE FUTURE

We have made substantial progress in understanding the epidemiology of TMD pain over the past 25 years, even though only a handful of published studies have fully employed modern epidemiological methods. It is likely that continued work using standard epidemiological methods will yield important advances in the knowledge of the causes, treatment, and prevention of these disorders. The main conclusions from this chapter are:

TMD pain is a common disorder experienced mainly by young and middle-aged women. We estimate 20 million adult Americans and 450 million adults worldwide suffer from this disorder.

Five TMD diagnostic systems are available, with differing levels of reliability, accuracy, and predictive ability. However, standardization on a single diagnostic system could greatly accelerate progress.

Descriptive epidemiological studies can be enhanced by following accepted methods in epidemiological research, such as reporting age- and gender-specific prevalence, and establishing standardized self-report definitions of TMD pain.

Although the data are limited, the proportion of persons complaining of TMD pain and seeking care for it appears to have changed little over the last 10–50 years.

Natural history studies reveal different clinical courses that usually result in the pain resolving, reducing, becoming episodic, or, in a few cases, persisting. The natural history can best be predicted by measures of depression and somatization, and not by clinical measures such as range of opening, type of clicking, or TMD pain subtype.

The societal burden of TMD pain is not well characterized, but the available data show that this pain has a substantial negative effect for about one-quarter of those with the condition. The personal impact can be great in some individuals, especially those with chronic persistent pain. Indirect costs of TMD pain, such as days of work missed and lost work effectiveness, are likely to be larger than the direct costs of health care for the condition.

Analytic epidemiological studies of TMD pain are still in their infancy. Both cohort and case-control studies are needed and should be of adequate size to have sufficient power to detect effects. Investigators and funding agencies alike need to acknowledge that these studies require substantial financial support. Investigators unfamiliar with these methods should consider collaboration with epidemiologists and biostatisticians.

Depression, multiple pain conditions, and factors related to female gender appear to be associated risk factors that are close to fulfilling the criteria for causation. Other risk factors, such as bruxism, exogenous reproductive hormones, trauma, and hypermobility, have insufficient evidence to support causality at this time.

Other risk factors need more quantitative work. Motor vehicle accidents, other trauma, and occlusal variables require more rigorous study to determine whether they are risk factors for TMD pain. In addition, some factors implicated in other pain conditions have not been thoroughly investigated for TMD and may hold promise as possible risk factors. These include: family history, physical, sexual and emotional abuse, adverse early life events, obesity/body fat, and physical inactivity.

Primary prevention of TMD pain, although an imporant goal, does not appear feasible at this time because neither screening tests nor strong evidence for preventive methods are yet available. Secondary and tertiary prevention of TMD pain may soon be possible by decreasing misdiagnoses, unnecessary tests and procedures, and unproven irreversible therapies that cause iatrogenic disorders, and by testing promising treatment methods, such as self-care and cognitive-behavioral therapy, through randomized controlled trials.

REFERENCES

Agerberg G, Carlsson GE. Functional disorders of the masticatory system: I. Distribution of symptoms according to age and sex as judged from investigation by questionnaire. *Acta Odontol Scand* 1972; 30:597–613.

Agerberg G, Bergenholtz A. Craniomandibular disorders in adult populations of West Bothnia, Sweden. *Acta Odontol Scand* 1989; 47:129–140.

Agerberg G, Inkapool I. Craniomandibular disorders in an urban Swedish population. *J Craniomandib Disord Facial Oral Pain* 1990; 4:154–164.

Alanen P, Kirveskari P. Stomatognathic dysfunction in a male Finnish working population. *Proc Finnish Dental Society* 1982; 78:184–188.

American Academy of Orofacial Pain. Differential diagnosis and management considerations of temporomandibular disorders. In: Okeson JP (Ed). *Orofacial Pain: Guidelines for Assessment, Diagnosis, and Management.* Chicago: Quintessence, 1996, pp 113–184.

American Dental Association. *The President's Conference on the Examination, Diagnosis and Management of Temporomandibular Disorders.* Chicago: American Dental Association, 1983.

Antczak-Bouckoms A. Epidemiology of research for temporomandibular disorders. *J Orofacial Pain* 1995; 9:226–234.

Barone A, Sbordone L, Ramaglia L. Craniomandibular disorders and orthodontic treatment need in children. *J Oral Rehab* 1997; 24(1):2–7.

Bibb CA, Atchison KA, Pullinger AG, Bittar GT. Jaw function status in an elderly community sample. *Community Dent Oral Epidemiol* 1995; 23:303–308.

Brandt D. Temporomandibular disorders and their association with morphologic malocclusion in children. In: Carlson DS, McNamara JA, Jr, Ribbens KA (Eds). *Developmental Aspects of Temporomandibular Joint Disorders,* Craniofacial Growth Series, Monograph 16. Ann Arbor: Center for Human Growth and Development, The University of Michigan, 1985, pp 279–298.

Bryant PS, Sessle BJ. Workshop recommendations on research needs and directions. In: Sessle BJ, Bryant PS, Dionne RA (Eds). *Temporomandibular Disorders and Related Pain Conditions.* Seattle: IASP Press, 1995, pp 467–478.

Campbell J. Distribution and treatment of pain in temporomandibular arthroses. *Br Dent J* 1958; 105(11):393–402.

Carlsson GE, LeResche L. *Epidemiology of Temporomandibular Disorders.* In: Sessle BJ, Bryant PS, Dionne RA (Eds). Progress in Pain Research and Management. Seattle: IASP Press, 1995, pp 211–226.

Cimino R, Michelotti A, Stradi R, Farinaro C. Comparison of clinical and psychologic features of fibromyalgia and masticatory myofascial pain. *J Orofacial Pain* 1998; 12:35–41.

Costen JB. A syndrome of ear and sinus symptoms dependent upon disturbed function of the temporomandibular joint. *Ann Otol Rhinol Laryngol* 1934; 43:1–15.

Cumming RG, Kelsey JL, Nevitt MC. Methodologic issues in the study of frequent and recurrent health problems: falls in the elderly. *Ann Epidemiol* 1990; 1:49–56.

Dao TTT, Lund JP, Lavigne GJ. Comparison of pain and quality of life in bruxers and patients with myofascial pain of the masticatory muscles. *J Orofacial Pain* 1994; 8:350–356.

Dao TTT, Knight K, Ton-That V. Modulation of myofascial pain by the reproductive hormones: a preliminary report. *J Prosthet Dent* 1998; 79:663–670.

de Boever JA, van den Berghe L. Longitudinal study of functional conditions in the masticatory system in Flemish children. *Community Dent Oral Epidemiol* 1987; 15:100–103.

de Bont LG, Dijkgraff LC, Stegenga B. Epidemiology and natural progression of articular temporomandibular disorders. *Oral Surg Oral Med Oral Pathol Oral Radiol Endod* 1997; 83:72–76.

De Kanter RJAM, Kayser AF, Battistuzzi PGFCM, Truin GJ, Van't Hof MA. Demand and need for treatment of craniomandibular dysfunction in the Dutch adult population. *J Dent Res* 1992; 71:1607–1612.

De Kanter RJAM, Truin GJ, Burgersdijk RCW, et al. Prevalence in the Dutch adult population and a meta-analysis of signs and symptoms of temporomandibular disorder. *J Dent Res* 1993; 72:1509–1518.

de Leeuw R, Boering G, Stegenga B, de Bont LG. Symptoms of temporomandibular joint osteoarthrosis and internal derangement 30 years after non-surgical treatment. *Cranio* 1995; 13:81–88.

Deardorff WH. TMJ scale. In: Conoley JC, Impara JC (Eds). *The Twelfth Mental Measurements Yearbook.* Lincoln, NE: The Buros Institute of Mental Measurements, The University of Nebraska-Lincoln, 1995, pp 1070–1071.

Dibbets JM, van der Weele LT. The prevalence of joint noises as related to age and gender. *J Craniomandib Disord* 1992; 6:157–160.

Dworkin SF. Personal and societal impact of orofacial pain. In: Fricton JR, Dubner RB (Eds). *Orofacial Pain and Temporomandibular Disorders.* New York: Raven Press, 1995, pp 15–32.

Dworkin SF, LeResche L. Research Diagnostic Criteria for Temporomandibular Disorders: review, criteria, examinations and specifications, critique. *J Craniomandib Disord Facial Oral Pain* 1992; 6:301–355.

Dworkin SF, LeResche L. Temporomandibular disorder pain: epidemiological data. *APS Bulletin* 1993; April/May:12–13.

Dworkin SF, Huggins KH, LeResche L, et al. Epidemiology of signs and symptoms in temporomandibular disorders: clinical signs in cases and controls. *J Am Dent Assoc* 1990; 120:273–281.

Egermark-Eriksson I, Carlsson GE, Magnusson T. A long-term epidemiologic study of the relationship between occlusal factors and mandibular dysfunction in children and adolescents. *J Dent Res* 1987; 66:67–71.

Eisenberg DM, Kessler RC, Foster C, et al. Unconventional medicine in the United States. Prevalence, costs, and patterns of use. *N Engl J Med* 1993; 328:246–252.

Eversole LR, Machado L. Temporomandibular joint internal derangements and associated neuromuscular disorders. *J Am Dent Assoc* 1985; 110:69–79.

Foreman PA, Harold PL, Hay KD. An evaluation of the diagnosis, treatment, and outcome of patients with chronic orofacial pain. *N Z Dent J* 1994; 90:44–48.

Franks AST. The social character of temporomandibular joint dysfunction. *Dent Practit* 1964; Nov:94–100.

Fricton JR, Olsen T. Predictors of outcome for treatment of temporomandibular disorders. *J Orofacial Pain* 1996; 10:54–65.

Fricton JR, Schiffman EL. Reliability of a craniomandibular index. *J Dent Res* 1986; 65(11):1359–1364.

Fricton JR, Schiffman EL. Epidemiology of temporomandibular disorders. In: Fricton JR, Dubner RB (Eds). *Orofacial Pain and Temporomandibular Disorders.* New York: Raven Press, 1995, pp 1–14.

Fricton JR, Kroening R, Haley D, Siegert R. Myofascial pain syndrome of the head and neck: A review of clinical characteristics of 164 patients. *Oral Surg Oral Med Oral Pathol* 1985; 60:615–623.

Gallagher RM, Marbach JJ, Raphael KG, Handte J, Dohrenwend BP. Myofascial face pain: seasonal variability in pain intensity and demoralization. *Pain* 1995; 61:113–120.

Garofalo JP, Gatchel RJ, Wesley AL, Ellis E. Predicting chronicity in acute temporomandibular joint disorders using the Research Diagnostic Criteria. *J Am Dent Assoc* 1998; 129:438–447.

Garro LC, Stephenson KA, Good BJ. Chronic illness of the temporomandibular joints as experienced by support-group members. *J Gen Intern Med* 1994; 9:372–378.

Gazit E, Lieberman M, Eini R, et al. Prevalence of mandibular

dysfunction in 10–18 year old Israeli schoolchildren. *J Oral Rehab* 1984; 11:307–317.

Gerstner GE, Clark GT, Goulet J-P. Validity of a brief questionnaire in screening asymptomatic subjects from subjects with tension-type headaches or temporomandibular disorders. *Community Dent Oral Epidemiol* 1994; 22:235–242.

Glaros AG, Glass EG, Hayden WJ. History of treatment received by patients with TMD: a preliminary investigation. *J Orofacial Pain* 1995; 9:147–151.

Gobetti JP, Turp JC. Fibrosarcoma misdiagnosed as a temporomandibular disorder: a cautionary tale. *Oral Surg Oral Med Oral Pathol Oral Radiol Endod* 1998; 85:404–409.

Gordis L. Challenges to epidemiology in the next decade. *Am J Epidemiol* 1988; 128:1–19.

Goulet J-P, Lavigne GJ, Lund JP. Jaw pain prevalence among French-speaking Canadians in Quebec and related symptoms of temporomandibular disorders. *J Dent Res* 1995; 74:1738–1744.

Greco CM, Rudy TE, Turk DC, Herlich A, Zaki HH. Traumatic onset of temporomandibular disorders: positive effects of a standardized conservative treatment program. *Clin J Pain* 1997; 13:337–347.

Greene CS. Temporomandibular disorders: the evolution of concepts. In: Sarnat BG, Laskin DM (Eds). *The Temporomandibular Joint: A Biological Basis for Clinical Practice.* Philadelphia: W.B. Saunders Company, 1992, pp 298–315.

Hackney J, Bade D, Clawson A. Relationship between forward head posture and diagnosed internal derangement of the temporomandibular joint. *J Orofacial Pain* 1993; 7:386–390.

Hedenberg-Magnusson B, Ernberg M, Kopp S. Symptoms and signs of temporomandibular disorders in patients with fibromyalgia and local myalgia of the temporomandibular system: a comparative study. *Acta Odontol Scand* 1997; 55:344–349.

Heiberg A, Heloe B, Heiberg AN, et al. Myofascial pain dysfunction (MPD) syndrome in twins. *Community Dent Oral Epidemiol* 1980; 8:434–436.

Heikinheimo K, Salmi K, Myllarniemi S, Kirveskari P. Symptoms of craniomandibular disorder in a sample of Finnish adolescents at the ages of 12 and 15 years. *Eur J Orthod* 1989; 11:325–331.

Heikinheimo K, Salmi K, Myllarniemi S, Kirveskari P. A longitudinal study of occlusal interferences and signs of craniomandibular disorder at the ages of 12 and 15 years. *Eur J Orthod* 1990; 12:190–197.

Helkimo M. Studies on function and dysfunction of the masticatory system: II. Index for anamnestic and clinical dysfunction and occlusal state. *Swed Dent J* 1974a; 67:101–121.

Helkimo M. Studies on function and dysfunction of the masticatory system: IV. Age and sex distribution of symptoms of dysfunction of the masticatory system in Lapps in the north of Finland. *Acta Odontol Scand* 1974b; 32:255–267.

Heloe B, Heloe LA. The occurrence of TMJ-disorders in an elderly population as evaluated by recording of "subjective" and "objective" symptoms. *Acta Odontol Scand* 1978; 36(1):3–9.

Heloe B, Heloe LA. Frequency and distribution of myofascial paindysfunction syndrome in a population of 25-year-olds. *Community Dent Oral Epidemiol* 1979; 7:357–360.

Heloe B, Heloe LA, Heiberg A. Relationship between sociomedical factors and TMJ symptoms in Norwegians with myofascial pain-dysfunction syndrome. *Community Dent Oral Epidemiol* 1977; 5:207–212.

Hennekens CH, Buring JE. Definition and background. In: Mayrent SL (Ed). *Epidemiology in Medicine.* Boston: Little, Brown and Company, 1987a, pp 3–15.

Hennekens CH, Buring JE. Measures of disease frequency and

association+. In: Mayrent SL (Ed). *Epidemiology in Medicine.* Boston: Little, Brown and Company, 1987b, pp 54–97.

Hennekens CH, Buring JE. Statistical association and cause-effect relationships. In: Mayrent SL (Ed). *Epidemiology in Medicine.* Boston: Little, Brown and Company, 1987c, pp 30–53.

International Epidemiological Association. *A Dictionary of Epidemiology.* 3rd ed. New York: Oxford University Press, 1995.

Jensen R, Rasmussen BK, Pedersen B, Lous I, Olesen J. Prevalence of oromandibular dysfunction in a general population. *J Orofacial Pain* 1993; 7:175–182.

Kampe T, Hannerz H. Five-year longitudinal study of adolescents with intact restored dentitions: Signs and symptoms of temporomandibular dysfunction and functional recordings. *J Oral Rehabil* 1991; 18:387–398.

Karjalainen M, Le Bell Y, Jamsa T, Karjalainen S. Prevention of temporomandibular disorder-related signs and symptoms in orthodontically treated adolescents: a 3-year follow-up of a prospective randomized trial. *Acta Odontol Scand* 1997; 55:319–324.

Katz RV. Response to oral health status in the United States: temporomandibular disorders. *J Dent Educ* 1985; 49:406–406.

Keeling SD, McGorray S, Wheeler TT, King GJ. Imprecision in orthodontic diagnosis: reliability of clinical measures of malocclusion. *Angle Orthod* 1996; 66:381–391.

Khan AA. The prevalence of myofacial pain dysfunction syndrome in a lower socio-economic group in Zimbabwe. *Community Dent Health* 1990; 7:189–192.

Kirveskari P, Le Bell Y, Salonen M, Forssell H. Effect of elimination of occlusal interferences on signs and symptoms of craniomandibular disorder in young adults. *J Oral Rehabil* 1989; 16:21–26.

Kitai N, Takada K, Yasuda Y, Verdonck A, Carels C. Pain and other cardinal TMJ dysfunction symptoms: a longitudinal survey of Japanese female adolescents. *J Oral Rehabil* 1997; 24:741–748.

Kononen M, Nystrom M. A longitudinal study of craniomandibular disorders in Finnish adolescents. *J Orofacial Pain* 1993; 7:329–336.

Kononen M, Nystrom M, Kleemola-Kujala E et al. Signs and symptoms of craniomandibular disorders in a series of Finnish children. *Acta Odontol Scand* 1987; 45:109–114.

Kurita K, Westesson P-L, Yuasa H, et al. Natural course of untreated symptomatic temporomandibular joint disc displacement without reduction. *J Dent Res* 1998; 77:361–365.

Laskin DM. Etiology of the pain-dysfunction syndrome. *J Am Dent Assoc* 1969; 79:147–153.

Laskin DM. Putting order into temporomandibular disorders. *J Oral Maxillofac Surg* 1998; 56:121–121.

Laskin DM, Block S. Diagnosis and treatment of myofacial pain-dysfunction (MPD) syndrome. *J Prosthet Dent* 1986; 56:75–84.

Lavigne GJ, Rompre PH, Montplaisir JY. Sleep bruxism: Validity of clinical research diagnostic criteria in a controlled polysomnographic study. *J Dent Res* 1996; 75:546–552.

Lawrence RC, Helmick CG, Arnett FC, et al. Estimates of the prevalence of arthritis and selected musculoskeletal disorders in the United States. *Arthritis Rheum* 1998; 41:778–799.

Lee W-Y, Okeson JP, Lindroth J. The relationship between forward head posture and temporomandibular disorders. *J Orofacial Pain* 1995; 9:161–167.

LeResche L. Research Diagnostic Criteria for Temporomandibular Disorders. In: Fricton JR, Dubner R (Eds). *Orofacial Pain and Temporomandibular Disorders.* New York: Raven Press, 1995, pp 189–203.

LeResche L. Epidemiology of temporomandibular disorders: Implications for the investigation of etiologic factors. *Crit Rev Oral Biol Med* 1997; 8:291–305.

LeResche L, Saunders K, Von Korff M, Barlow W, Dworkin SF. Use of exogenous hormones and risk of temporomandibular disorder pain. *Pain* 1997; 69:153–160.

Levitt SR, McKinney MW. Validating the TMJ scale in a national sample of 10,000 patients: Demographic and epidemiologic characteristics. *J Orofacial Pain* 1994; 8:25–35.

Levitt SR, Lundeen TF, McKinney MW. *The TMJ Scale Manual.* Durham, NC: Pain Resource Center, Inc., 1994.

Lipton JA, Ship JA, Larach-Robinson D. Estimated prevalence and distribution of reported orofacial pain in the United States. *J Am Dent Assoc* 1993; 124:115–121.

Lipton RB, Stewart WF. Prevalence and impact of migraine. *Neurol Clin* 1997; 15:1–13.

Lipton RB, Stewart WF, Von Korff M. Burden of migraine: societal costs and therapeutic opportunities. *Neurology* 1997; 48:S4–S9.

Locker D, Miller Y. Subjectively reported oral health status in an adult population. *Community Dent Oral Epidemiol* 1994; 22:425–430.

Locker D, Slade G. Prevalence of symptoms associated with temporomandibular disorders in a Canadian population. *Community Dent Oral Epidemiol* 1988; 16:310–313.

Locker D, Slade G. Association of symptoms and signs of TM disorders in an adult population. *Community Dent Oral Epidemiol* 1989; 17:150–153.

Lund JP, Widmer CG, Feine JS. Validity of diagnostic and monitoring tests used for temporomandibular disorders. *J Dent Res* 1995; 74:1133–1143.

Magnusson T, Carlsson GE, Egermark-Eriksson I. An evaluation of the need and demand for treatment of craniomandibular disorders in a young Swedish population. *J Craniomandib Disord Facial Oral Pain* 1991; 5:57–63.

Magnusson T, Carlsson G, Egermark I. Changes in subjective symptoms of craniomandibular disorders in children and adolescents during a 10-year period. *J Orofacial Pain* 1993; 7:76–82.

Manninen P, Riihimaki H, Heliovaara M. Has musculoskeletal pain become less prevalent? *Scand J Rheumatol* 1996; 25:37–41.

Marbach JJ, Raphael KG, Dohrenwend BP, Lennon MC. The validity of tooth grinding measures: etiology of pain dysfuntion syndrome revisited. *J Am Dent Assoc* 1990; 120:327–333.

Markowitz HA, Gerry RG. Temporomandibular joint disease: Section I. Statistical evaluation of temporomandibular disease. *Oral Surg Oral Med Oral Pathol* 1949; October:1309–1314.

Markowitz HA, Gerry RG. Temporomandibular joint disease (concluded): Section III. Clinical considerations of temporomandibular disease. *Oral Surg Oral Med Oral Pathol* 1950; January:75–117.

Matsuka Y, Yatani H, Kuboki T, Yamashita A. Temporomandibular disorders in the adult population of Okayama City, Japan. *J Craniomandibular Pract* 1996; 14:159–162.

McCreary CP, Clark GT, Oakley ME, Flack V. Predicting response to treatment for temporomandibular disorders. *J Craniomandib Disord Facial Oral Pain* 1992; 6(3):161–169.

McGregor NR, Butt HL, Zerbes M, et al. Assessment of pain (distribution and onset), symptoms, SCL-90-R Inventory responses, and the association with infectious events in patients with chronic orofacial pain. *J Orofacial Pain* 1996; 10:339–350.

McNeill C. History and evolution of TMD concepts. *Oral Surg Oral Med Oral Pathol Oral Radiol Endod* 1997; 83:51–60.

Michalowicz B, Pihlstrom B, Hodges J, Bouchard T, Jr. Genetic and environmental influences on signs and symptoms of TMD [Abstract]. *J Dent Res* 1998; 77:919–919.

Mohlin B. Prevalence of mandibular dysfunction and relation between malocclusion and mandibular dysfunction in a group of women in Sweden. *Eur J Orthod* 1983; 4:115–123.

Mohlin B, Pilley JR, Shaw WC. A survey of craniomandibular disorders in 1000 12-year-olds: Study design and baseline data in a follow-up study. *Eur J Orthodon* 1991; 13(2):111–123.

Molin C, Carlsson GE, Friling B, Hedegard B. Frequency of symptoms of mandibular dysfunction in young Swedish men. *J Oral Rehabil* 1976; 3:9–18.

Molina OF, dos Santos J, Jr, Nelson SJ, Grossman E. Prevalence of modalities of headaches and bruxism among patients with craniomandibular disorder. *J Craniomandibular Pract* 1997; 15:314–325.

Moore R, Dworkin SF. Ethnographic methodologic assessment of pain perceptions by verbal description. *Pain* 1988; 34:195–204.

Motegi E, Miyazaki H, Ogura I, Konishi H, Sebata M. An orthodontic study of temporomandibular joint disorders: Part I: Epidemiological research in Japanese 6–18 year olds. *Angle Orthod* 1992; 62:249–256.

Murray H, Locker D, Mock D, Tenenbaum HC. Pain and the quality of life in patients referred to a craniofacial pain unit. *J Orofacial Pain* 1996; 10:316–323.

National Institutes of Health. Management of temporomandibular disorders: National Institutes of Health Technology Assessment Conference statement. *J Am Dent Assoc* 1996; 127:1595–1606.

Nemeroff CB. The neurobiology of depression. *Scientific American* 1998; 278:42–49.

Nielsen L, Terp S. Screening for functional disorders of the masticatory system among teenagers. *Community Dent Oral Epidemiol* 1990; 18:281–287.

Nilner M. Prevalence of functional disturbances and diseases of the stomatognathic system in 15–18 year olds. *Swed Dent J* 1981; 5:189–197.

Nilner M, Lassing SA. Prevalence of functional disturbances and diseases of the stomatognathic system in 7–14 year olds. *Swed Dent J* 1981; 5:173–187.

Nordstrom G, Eriksson S. Longitudinal changes in craniomandibular dysfunction in an elderly population in northern Sweden. *Acta Odontol Scand* 1994; 52:271–279.

Norheim PW, Dahl BL. Some self-reported symptoms of temporomandibular joint dysfunction in a population in Northern Norway. *J Oral Rehab* 1978; 5:63–68.

Ohrbach R, Dworkin SF. Five-year outcomes in TMD: relationship of changes in pain to changes in physical and psychological variables. *Pain* 1998; 74:315–326.

Olesen J. *An International Journal of Headache.* Trondheim: Norwegian University Press, 1988.

Onizawa K, Yoshida H. Longitudinal changes of symptons of temporomandibular disorders in Japanese young adults. *J Orofacial Pain* 1996; 10:151–156.

Osterberg T, Carlsson GE. Symptoms and signs of mandibular dysfunction in 70-year-old men and women in Gothenburg, Sweden. *Community Dent Oral Epidemiol* 1979; 7:315–321.

Osterberg T, Carlsson GE, Wedel A, Johansson U. A cross-sectional and longitudinal study of craniomandibular dysfunction in an elderly population. *J Craniomandib Disord Facial Oral Pain* 1992; 6:237–246.

Pierce CJ, Weyant RJ, Block HM, Nemir DC. Dental splint prescription patterns: a survey. *J Am Dent Assoc* 1995; 126:248–254.

Pilley JR, Mohlin B, Shaw WC, Kingdon A. A survey of craniomandibular disorders in 800 15-year-olds: a follow-up study of children with malocclusion. *Eur J Orthod* 1992; 14:152–161.

Plesh O, Wolfe F, Lane N. The relationship between fibromyalgia and temporomandibular disorders: prevalence and symptom severity. *J Rheumatol* 1996; 23:1948–1952.

Pullinger AG, Seligman DA, Gornbein JA. A multiple logistic regression analysis of the risk and relative odds of temporomandibular disorders as a function of common occlusal features. *J Dent Res* 1993; 72(6):968–979.

Ramfjord SP, Ash M, Jr. Functional disturbances of temporomandibular joints and muscles. In: *Occlusion.* Philadelphia: W.B. Saunders Company, 1966, pp 160–178.

Raphael KG, Marbach JJ. A year of chronic TMPDS: evaluating patients' pain patterns. *J Am Dent Assoc* 1992a; 123:1–6.

Raphael KG, Marbach JJ. A year of chronic TMPDS: relating patient symptoms and pain intensity. *J Am Dent Assoc* 1992b; 123:49–55.

Reisine ST. The impact of temporomandibular dysfunction on patients' quality of life. *Community Dent Health* 1989; 6:257–270.

Riley JL, Gilbert GH, Heft MW. Orofacial pain symptom prevalence: selective sex differences in the elderly? *Pain* 1998; 76:97–104.

Rothman KJ, Greenland S. Causation and causal inference. In: Rothman KJ, Greenland S (Eds). *Modern Epidemiology.* Philadelphia: Lippincott-Raven, 1998a, pp 7–28.

Rothman KJ, Greenland S. The emergence of modern epidemiology. In: Rothman KJ, Greenland S (Eds). *Modern Epidemiology.* Philadelphia: Lippincott-Raven, 1998b, pp 3–6.

Rugh JD, Solberg WL. Oral health status in the United States: temporomandibular disorders. *J Dent Educ* 1985; 49:398–405.

Sackett DL, Haynes RB, Guyatt GH, Tugwell P. The selection of diagnostic tests. In: *Clinical Epidemiology: A Basic Science for Clinical Medicine.* Boston: Little, Brown and Company, 1991, pp 51–68.

Salonen L, Hellden L, Carlsson GE. Prevalence of sign and symptoms of dysfunction in the masticatory system: an epidemiologic study in an adult Swedish population. *J Craniomandib Disord Facial Oral Pain* 1990; 4:241–250.

Sato H, Osterberg T, Ahlqwist M, et al. Association between radiographic findings in the mandibular condyle and temporomandibular dysfunction in an elderly population. *Acta Odontol Scand* 1996; 54:384–390.

Sato S, Kawamura H, Nagasaka H, Motegi K. The natural course of anterior disc displacement without reduction in the temporomandibular joint: follow-up at 6, 12, and 18 months. *J Oral Maxillofac Surg* 1997; 55:234–238.

Schiffman EL, Fricton JR, Haley DP, Shapiro BL. The prevalence and treatment needs of subjects with temporomandibular disorders. *J Am Dent Assoc* 1990; 120:295–303.

Schiffman E, Haley D, Baker C, Lindgren B. Diagnostic criteria for screening headache patients for temporomandibular disorders. *Headache* 1995; 35:121–124.

Schwartz L. *Disorders of the Temporomandibular Joint: Diagnosis, Management, Relation to Occlusion of Teeth.* Philadelphia: Saunders, 1959.

Shimshak DG, Kent RL, DeFuria M. Medical claims profiles of subjects with temporomandibular joint disorders. *Cranio* 1997; 15:150–158.

Sieber M, Ruggia GM, Grubenmann E, Palla S. The functional status of the masticatory system of 11–16-year-old adolescents: classification and validity. *Community Dent Oral Epidemiol* 1997; 25:256–263.

Sillanpää M, Anttila P. Increasing prevalence of headache in 7-year-old schoolchildren. *Headache* 1996; 36:466–470.

Smith JA, Syrop S. TMD incidence and socioeconomic standing: eradicating the myth of the upper class patient. *NY State Dent J* 1994; 60:36–39.

Stohler CS. Phenomenology, epidemiology, and natural progression of the muscular temporomandibular disorders. *Oral Surg Oral Med Oral Pathol Oral Radiol Endod* 1997; 83:77–81.

Swanljung O, Rantanen T. Functional disorders of the masticatory system in southwest Finland. *Community Dent Oral Epidemiol* 1979; 7:177–182.

Szentpetery A, Huhn E, Fazekas A. Prevalence of mandibular dysfunction in an urban population in Hungary. *Community Dent Oral Epidemiol* 1986; 14:177–180.

Tervonen T, Knuuttila M. Prevalence of signs and symptoms of mandibular dysfunction among adults aged 25, 35, 50 and 65 years in Ostrobothnia, Finland. *J Oral Rehab* 1988; 15:455–463.

Truelove EL, Sommers E, LeResche L, Dworkin SF, Von Korff M. Clinical diagnostic criteria for TMD: new classification permits multiple diagnoses. *J Am Dent Assoc* 1992; 123:47–54.

Turk DC, Rudy TE. The robustness of an empirically derived taxonomy of chronic pain patients. *Pain* 1990; 43:27–35.

Turp JC, Kowalski CJ, Stohler CS. Treatment-seeking patterns of facial pain patients: many possibilities, limited satisfaction. *J Orofacial Pain* 1998; 12:61–66.

Van der Weele LTh, Dibbets JMH. Helkimo's index: A scale or just a set of symptoms? *J Oral Rehabil* 1987; 14:229–237.

Von Korff M. Health services research and temporomandibular pain. In: Sessle BJ, Bryant PS, Dionne RA (Eds). *Temporomandibular Disorders and Related Pain Conditions*. Seattle: IASP Press, 1995, pp 227–236.

Von Korff M, Dworkin SF, LeResche L, Kruger A. An epidemiologic comparison of pain complaints. *Pain* 1988a; 32:173–183.

Von Korff MR, Howard JA, Truelove EL, et al. Temporomandibular disorders: variation in clinical practice. *Medical Care* 1988b; 26(3):307–314.

Von Korff M, Wagner EH, Dworkin SF, Saunders KW. Chronic pain and use of ambulatory health care. *Psychosom Med* 1991; 53:61–79.

Von Korff M, Ormel J, Keefe FJ, Dworkin SF. Grading the severity of chronic pain. *Pain* 1992; 50:133–149.

Von Korff M, LeResche L, Dworkin SF. First onset of common pain symptoms: a prospective study of depression as a risk factor. *Pain* 1993; 55:251–258.

Wanman A. Longitudinal course of symptoms of craniomandibular disorders in men and women. A 10-year follow-up study of an epidemiologic sample. *Acta Odontol Scand* 1996; 54:337–342.

Wanman A, Agerberg G. Mandibular dysfunction in adolescents: I. Prevalence of symptoms. *Acta Odontol Scand* 1986; 44:47–54.

Wanman A, Agerberg G. Recurrent headaches and craniomandibular disorders in adolescents: a longitudinal study. *J Craniomandib Disord Facial Oral Pain* 1987; 1:229–236.

Wanman A, Wigren L. Need and demand for dental treatment: a comparison between an evaluation based on an epidemiologic study of 35-, 50-, and 65-year-olds and performed dental treatment of matched age groups. *Acta Odontol Scand* 1995; 53:318–324.

Wedel A, Carlsson GE. A four-year follow-up, by means of a questionnaire, of patients with functional disturbances of the masticatory system. *J Oral Rehabil* 1986; 13:105–113.

Weiss NS. Natural history of illness. In: *Clinical Epidemiology: The Study of the Outcome of Illness*. New York: Oxford University Press, 1996, pp 135–146.

Widmalm SE, Christiansen RL, Gunn SM. Race and gender as TMD risk factors in children. *Cranio* 1995; 13:163–166.

Widmer CG. Physical characteristics associated with temporomandibular disorders. In: Sessle BJ, Bryant PS, Dionne RA (Eds). *Temporomandibular Disorders and Related Pain Conditions*. Seattle: IASP Press, 1995, pp 161–174.

Wolfe F. Fibromyalgia. In: Sessle BJ, Bryant PS (Eds). *Temporomandibular Disorders and Related Pain Conditions*. Seattle: IASP Press, 1995, pp 31–46.

Wright EF, Gullickson DC. Identifying acute pulpalgia as a factor in TMD pain. *J Am Dent Assoc* 1996; 127:773–780.

Yunus MB. Towards a model of pathophysiology of fibromyalgia: aberrant central pain mechanisms with peripheral modulation [editorial]. *J Rheumatol* 1992; 19:846–850.

Correspondence to: Mark Drangsholt, DDS, MPH, Department of Oral Medicine, Box 356370, University of Washington, Seattle, WA 98195-6370, USA. Tel: 206-543-2034; Fax: 206-685-8024; email: drangs@u.washington. edu.

Epidemiology of Pain, edited by
I.K. Crombie, IASP Press, Seattle, © 1999.

16

Neck Pain

Geertje A.M. Ariëns, Jeroen A.J. Borghouts, and Bart W. Koes

*Institute for Research in Extramural Medicine, Department of Social Medicine,
Vrije Universiteit, Amsterdam, The Netherlands*

Neck pain occurs frequently in the West, but relatively little attention has been paid to the epidemiological aspects of this problem. Traditional epidemiological research has focused much more on low back pain, but neck pain and related disability account for many visits to general practitioners and other health care providers and often necessitate sick leave, creating a substantial burden to society.

Diagnosis of neck pain is problematic. Many different diagnostic labels describe different underlying pathologies. Various tissues and spinal structures may be affected, and regional syndromes have been reported. Terminology does not seem to be consistent, and definitions may not be presented, making it difficult to interpret the literature on the subject.

DEFINITION AND DIAGNOSTIC CRITERIA

The main feature of neck pain is self-reported pain in the cervical region, often accompanied by restriction of range of motion. In addition, functional limitations (restrictions in the activities of daily living) are usually associated with neck pain.

Pain may arise from several structures in the neck, including the spine and soft tissues. Pain researchers use a wide array of terms to describe populations of patients with neck pain and related disorders. Many terms describe regional syndromes such as occupational cervicobrachial disorders, upper extremity disorders, cervical osteoarthritis, tension neck syndrome, cervical spondylosis, and thoracic outlet syndrome. Labels incorporating a potential cause (such as "occupational") are common. The underlying pathophysiology of these diag-

nostic labels is not always clear, and most publications present no reproducible diagnostic criteria.

A relevant and simple distinction can be made between specific and nonspecific neck pain. Specific neck pain (an estimated 10% of cases) includes pathologies such as spinal tumors, systemic rheumatic disorders, infections, and fractures. Most cases of neck pain, however, can be labeled as nonspecific. In these cases no direct cause can be detected.

The validity and reproducibility of classification systems have rarely been investigated. In 1987, the Quebec Task Force on Spinal Related Disorders published a useful classification system with 11 categories, mainly based on a regional description of the pain, including pattern of radiation, duration of complaints (acute, subacute, and chronic), paraclinical findings, and response to treatment (Spitzer et al. 1987). This classification, although not yet systematically validated, has been frequently used in neck and back pain studies and in clinical care.

The literature has paid much attention to whiplash disorders, but a thorough summary falls outside the scope of this chapter. The Quebec Task Force on Whiplash Associated Disorders has published an extensive overview of this topic (Spitzer et al. 1995). Whiplash disorders are related to the occurrence, course, and prognosis of neck pain and of headache, but we will focus on neck pain as the primary symptom.

Definitions of neck pain in the epidemiological literature usually are based on the patient's subjective pain experience in the neck/cervical region. Patients are frequently asked to mark pain drawings to show the areas where they experience pain, stiffness, numbness, or other symptoms.

Table I
Results of cross-sectional studies on the frequency of neck pain in the general population or a general practice

Reference	Disease Definition	Study Population	Sample Size	Type of Prevalence Estimate	Prevalence*
Lau et al. 1996	Pain located in neck area using pain drawing	Residents of two housing blocks in Hong Kong, aged >30 y	Q: 1140, R = 70%	Lifetime and period (past year)	Men: 30–39 y: 38% (16%), 40–49 y: 38% (17%), 50–59 y: 21% (10%), 60–69 y: 29% (18%), >70 y: 25% (16%); women: 30–39 y: 34% (24%), 40–49 y 34% (21%), 50–59 y: 43% (24%), 60–69 y: 17% (11%), >70 y: 17% (10%)
Mäkelä et al. 1991	Current or previous neck pain for >3 mo with physical signs	Random sample in Finland, aged >30 y	Q + EX: 8000, R = 90%, *n* = 7217	Point	Men: 9.5%; women: 13.5%
Bovim et al. 1994	Neck pain	Random sample of general population, Norway, aged 18–67 y	Q: 10,000, R = 77%, *n* = 3914 men, 3734 women	Period (past year)	Men: 29%, >6 mo past year (10%); women: 40%, >6 mo past year (17%)
Westerling and Jonsson 1980	Neck pain, tenderness, stiffness	Random sample, county of Stockholm, Sweden	Q + EX: 3000, R = 90%, *n* = 1239 men, 1298 women	Period (past year)	10%
Andersson et al. 1993	Persistent/regularly recurrent pain for >3 mo in neck region (drawing)	Random sample of two primary health care districts, Sweden, aged 25–74 y	Q: 1806, R = 90% *n* = 799 men, 810 women	Point	Men: 14.5%; women: 19.1%; by age: 25–34 y: 9%, 35–44 y: 14%, 45–54 y: 35%, 55–64 y: 21%, 65–74 y: 15%
Brattberg et al. 1989	Any pain (short duration); obvious pain for >6 mo	Random sample, Sweden, aged 18–84 y	Q: 1009, R = 82%, *n* = 827	Point	"Any" pain: >6 mo: 19.3%, 1–6 mo: 2.3%, <1 mo: 4.6%; "obvious" pain: >6 mo: 12.7%, 1–6 mo: 1.3%
Jacobsson et al. 1989	Neck pain with or without brachialgia of >6 wk duration	Sample of elderly, Malmö, Sweden, aged 50–70 y	Q: 552 (responders of 1st survey), R = 81%, *n* = 230 men, 215 women	Period (past year)	Men: 3%; women: 10%
Takala et al. 1982	Rheumatic symptoms; neck ache, stiffness	Random sample, Finland, aged 40–64 y	R = 93%, *n* = 2268 (1045 men, 1223 women)	Period (past year)	Men: <50 y: 13%, >50 y: 20%; women: <50 y: 13%, >50 y: 22%

Abbreviations: EX = (physical) examination; Q = questionnaire; R = response.
* Items in parentheses are period prevalences (past year).

PREVALENCE

SEARCH STRATEGY

To identify relevant studies for estimating the incidence and prevalence of neck pain, we ran a MEDLINE search for 1966–1997 using the key words: neck, pain, cervical, incidence, prevalence, prognosis, survey, cross-sectional, cohort, and predictor. We checked the reference list of relevant studies identified by the MEDLINE search for additional studies, using the following selection criteria: (1) the paper was a full report (no letters or abstracts); (2) the study dealt with incidence or prevalence of neck pain (self-reported neck pain with or without physical signs) and presented these data separately from other co-morbidity; (3) the paper was written in English; (4) studies with fewer than 250 subjects were excluded; (5) papers dealing exclusively with whiplash trauma, headache, and specific (pathological) neck pain were excluded.

The MEDLINE search and the additional screening of references yielded 17 studies reporting on the frequency of neck pain. We categorized studies in two groups: general and primary care populations and occupational populations.

RESULTS

General populations

In general, relatively few data are available on the prevalence of patients with neck pain and none on incidence. Table I shows the prevalence data for studies conducted in general populations and primary care settings. All eight studies used cross-sectional designs.

Reported point prevalences range from 9.5% to 35%, although most studies reported figures ranging from 10% to 15%. Twelve-month period prevalences are reported as high as 40%. Table I also shows that the point prevalences and the 12-month period prevalences for women are somewhat higher than for men. Only one study reported data on lifetime prevalences; the highest was 43% for women in the 50–59 year age group.

The large variation in the prevalence estimates revealed by Table I may be largely explained by the variation in the definitions used in the various studies. In some studies acute and chronic neck pain were included, whereas other studies only considered chronic neck pain. In addition, although all studies were conducted in general populations or general practice settings, the source of the samples and their age distributions varied substantially.

Occupational populations

Table II shows prevalence data from studies in occupational settings. Again, no data on the incidence of neck pain were reported. All nine studies used cross-sectional designs, while two studies also included a longitudinal follow-up. A high proportion of studies on the occurrence of neck pain sampled occupational populations, possibly because of the presumed association between various aspects of work and the occurrence of the symptom. Three studies report point prevalences (pain in the previous week), with figures in one study ranging from 16% for severe symptoms to 48% for all neck pain; point prevalences in the other two studies were 32% and 33%, respectively.

Eight studies reported 12-month period prevalences; the highest figure was 76% among women in a random sample of salespeople in Denmark and the lowest was 5.7% for men reporting one or more attacks of neck pain lasting more than 12 hours in workers showing up for their annual medical examination in Bordeaux, France. Women had higher point and period prevalences than men. In general, 12-month pe-riod prevalences ranging from 30% to 60% were common in occupational populations.

CONSEQUENCES OF NECK PAIN

Neck pain is one of the major musculoskeletal complaints for which health care is sought. Although exact data are lacking, most patients seem to be managed in primary care settings. However, diagnostic interventions (imaging and neurological investigation) occur mostly in secondary care. Few data are available on the costs of neck pain to society; since neck pain often occurs in occupational settings, the costs related to sick leave and disability may be substantial. The nonmedical costs for neck pain are probably much higher than the direct medical costs related to the management of these problems, as is the case with low back pain (Tulder et al. 1995).

For the patients, neck pain is not usually life threatening, but it may cause pain, stiffness, and restriction in daily activities, and thus can have a major impact on quality of life. The socioeconomic consequences for those taking prolonged sick leave or receiving a disability pension may also lead to substantial personal suffering.

NATURAL HISTORY, PROGNOSTIC FACTORS, AND PSYCHOLOGICAL CONSEQUENCES

In general, an attack of neck pain or stiffness is usually defined as acute if it resolves within 1 or 2 weeks, although no systematic studies on the course of acute neck pain are available. To gain more insight regarding the clinical course and prognostic factors of nonspecific neck pain, Borghouts et al. (1998) conducted a systematic review.

LITERATURE SEARCH

We used the search strategy described by Dickersin et al. (1994) to search MEDLINE (1966) and Embase (1988–1996) for randomized clinical trials (RCTs). A second strategy focused on the identification of observational studies (Borghouts et al. 1998). In addition, we examined the references in relevant publications and selected a study for review if: (1) the study population consisted of patients suffering from nonspecific

Table II
Results of studies on the frequency of neck pain in an occupational setting

Reference	Study Type	Disease Definition	Source of Sample	Sample Size	Type of Prevalence Estimate	Prevalence
Kamwendo et al. 1991	CS	Neck pain and use of pain drawing	Medical secretaries	Q: 438, R = 96%, n = 420 women	Period (past year) and point (past week)	Period: 63%, point: 33%
Dartigues et al. 1988	CS	One or more attacks of neck/cervical pain in >12 h	Workers attending annual medical exam, Bordeaux, France	EX: 990, n = 990	Period (year)	Men: 5.7%, women: 15.1%
Schibye et al. 1995	CS, LGT	NQ: neck symptoms	Sewing machine operators (women), aged 17–64 y	Q: 327, R = 96% (CS) Q: 279, R = 86% (LGT)	Point (past week) and period (year)	Point: 32%, period: 56%
Viikari-Juntera et al. 1994	CS, LGT	Neck trouble (pain, ache, stiffness, numbness)	Machine operators, carpenters, office workers (men), aged 25–49 y	Q: 2222, R = 82%	Period (past year) in 1984 and 1987	1984: moderate: 22%, severe: 21%; 1987: moderate: 21%, severe: 28%
Bernard et al. 1994	CS	Neck symptoms (pain, numbness, tingling) for >1 wk	Random sample of newspaper employees using VDTs	Q: 1050, R = 93%, n = 973	Period (past year), >1 wk or >1 per mo	Period: 26%
Lagerström et al. 1995	CS	NQ: neck symptoms and severe symptoms	Swedish nursing personnel (women)	Q: 821, R = 84%, n = 688.	Point	Symptoms: 48%, severe symptoms: 16%.
Linton 1990	CS	Neck pain (requiring health care visit)	Employees, Sweden	Q: ?, R = 22.180	Period (past year)	Period: 31%, requiring help: 18%
Rosecrance et al. 1992	CS	Ache, pain, discomfort, numbness in neck area	Newspaper workers, USA	Q: 1250, R = 72%, n = 900	Period (12 mo)	Period: 46%
Skov et al. 1996	CS	NQ: pain, tenderness, discomfort	Random sample of salespeople, Denmark	Q: 1991, R = 66%, n = 1306	Period (12 mo)	Men: 54%, women: 76%

Abbreviations: CS = cross-sectional study design; EX = (physical) examination; LGT = longitudinal study design; NQ = Nordic Questionnaire; Q = questionnaire; R = response.

neck pain or musculoskeletal pain, of which a sub-group of patients with neck pain was presented separately; (2) the article was published in English, Dutch, or German; and (3) the study was observational (prospective or retrospective) or an RCT. A study was excluded if: (1) the study population comprised patients with specific underlying pathology such as tumors, trauma (fractures), infection, inflammatory disorders (rheumatoid arthritis), or osteoporosis; (2) it was cross-sectional (without follow-up); or (3) the total duration of the study was less than 3 weeks (including the intervention period).

Two reviewers assessed the methodological qual-ity of all identified publications using a standardized set of 13 criteria, divided into five categories: study population, study design, follow-up, outcome measures, and analysis and data presentation.

The prognosis of the patients was determined by calculating an overall percentage of recovery for the most important outcome measures: pain, general improvement, functional status, health care utilization, and lost days of work. Recovery was calculated using categories such as: "less or no more pain," "(slight) improvement," and "no symptoms." Prognostic factors were considered to be all factors influencing the clinical course as reported by the authors.

RESULTS

Twenty-three eligible publications were identified, which documented 6 observational studies (see Table III for details) and 17 RCTs (see Table IV). Only 7 of 23 studies contained 50% or more of the 13 quality items, indicating that methods used were generally poor. The most prevalent methodological shortcomings concerned the selection of the study population, the sample size, and the analysis techniques.

Clinical course

Twelve studies were conducted in a secondary care setting, eight in an occupational setting, and only one in a primary care setting. One study used patients recruited by a newspaper announcement, and another did not specify the setting. The main outcomes of the 23 studies are summarized in Table V, which shows the study populations clustered according to the duration of neck complaints. We defined the following populations: acute (complaints ≤ 3 months), subacute (≥ 3 months and ≤ 6 months), chronic (≥ 6 months), mixed (regardless of the duration of complaints), and unknown (duration of complaints not specified). Only two studies reported on acute patients, and no studies reported on subacute patients.

Pain. Twelve studies reported on pain, with a mean decrease ranging from 9% to 100% and a median of 34%. Two of these reported on improvement without presenting data to support the conclusions. Only two studies (Nordemar et al. 1981; Takala et al. 1994) used a follow-up of more than 6 months. Eight of 12 studies reported on chronic patients (range 26–63%; median 28%). One of these reported on improvement, again without presenting supporting data. Five studies reported on the proportion of patients with pain decrease (less pain or pain free) (range 22–79%; median 46%). Only two studies (Gore et al. 1987; Levoska and Keinänen-Kiukaanniemi 1993) used a follow-up period of more than 6 months.

General improvement. Twelve studies reported on the proportion of patients with general improvement (range 36–95%; median 47.5%). The nine studies that included chronic patients showed similar results (range 37–95%; median 47%). Two studies (Berg et al. 1988; Abbot et al. 1990) reported a follow-up period of more then 6 months.

Functional status. Three studies measured the proportion of patients who functionally improved (range 5–22%). All studies used a follow-up period of less than 6 months.

Health care utilization. Five studies reported a decreased intake of medication (mainly NSAIDs and analgesics) with a median decrease of 37% (range 32–80%). All studies used a follow-up period of less than 6 months. Two studies reported on treatments received previously (Gore et al. 1987; Abbot et al. 1990), and reported that 80% and 100% of the patients, respectively, had received some form of treatment in the past. Both studies used a retrospective follow-up period of at least 10 years.

Lost days of work. Abenhaim et al. (1988) and Rossignol et al. (1988) in a joint study reported that sick-listed patients took a mean of 25 sick days per year, and that 13% experienced recurrences, with a mean of 0.86 recurrences per year. Tellnes (1989) reported that 1.8% of sick-listed patients were still sick after 1 year of sickness certification, while a third study (Anonymous 1966) reported a 23% decrease in lost work time as a result of pain reduction. All studies used a mixed cohort of patients.

Most of the available information on the clinical course of neck pain concerns patients with complaints lasting more than 6 months who were treated in secondary care or in an occupational setting. Full recovery is not to be expected for all such patients. However, patients experienced a median reduction in pain of 46% (range = 22–79%) and a median general improvement of 47% (range = 37–95%). The median reduction in the use of analgesics was 37% (range = 32–80%). For most reported outcomes the median improvement (percentage of patients who had improved or mean improvement) ranged between 40% and 50%. A comparison of the outcomes (median and range) of all studies with those of only the "high-quality" studies detected no important differences.

Prognostic factors

Only six studies reported on prognostic factors (Table VI). The most frequently reported prognostic factors were age, sex, pain severity, localization, pain duration, occupation, and radiological findings. None of the studies reported the strength of the association (relative risk or odds ratio) between a prognostic factor and the outcome. Some studies failed to specify the direction of the association between a prognostic factor and the outcome, and three studies did not clarify whether a statistical test was used.

Table III
Details of observational studies on the clinical course of nonspecific neck pain

Reference*	Study Population	Case Definition	Study Design	Outcome Measures and Results
Abbott et al. 1990 (15)	Former patients of a pain clinic (Australia)	Patients with neck pain as presenting complaint, treated during 1972–1982 in pain clinic; 37% had a motor vehicle accident	Retrospective (lifetime?), $N = 55$	Treatment prior to pain clinic (PT, medication, alternative treatment, surgery): 100%, with 61% no improvement; treatment at the clinic (11.4 mo): 56% improvement
Berg et al. 1988 (15)	Male manual workers and office workers (Sweden)	Neck symptoms	Prospective, 3 y, $N = 21$ (retired men)	Retired men had fewer symptoms compared to before their retirement: manual 41% ($n = 15$); office 40% ($n = 6$); manual + office 41%
Gore et al. 1987 (31)	Former patients of an orthopedic surgeon (USA)	Patients with problems originating from the neck. No neck surgery, objective neurologic deficits, malignancies, or rheumatoid arthritis	Retrospective, ≥ 10 y, $N = 205$ (76 had a motor vehicle accident)	Percentage received treatment: 80%; change in pain (less or no more): 79%; change of jobs (quit or changed): 7%
Rossignol et al. 1988; Abenhaim et al. 1987† (23)	Occupational neck injuries compensated in 1981 in Quebec (Canada)	Any musculoskeletal complaint relating to the spine (cervical reported separately for a few outcome measures), compensated for work absenteeism for at least 1 d in 1981	Prospective, 3 y, $N = 2342$ (161 with cervical symptoms)	Mean cumulative duration of absence from work for 3 y: 74.5 d (SE = 12.6). Probability of being absent from work for 6 mo or more during 3 y compared with lumbar problems: RR = 0.76. Recurrence rate during 3 y: 38.5%. No. episodes among current cases: 2.58 (SE = 0.13). Recurrence in 3 y, compared with other back regions: RR = 1.00
Takala et al. 1992 (38)	Female bank tellers (Finland)	Non-cases retrospective; neck and shoulder symptoms prospective	Retrospective: 1 y (not analyzed), $N = 351$; Prospective: 5.5 mo, $N = 138$	Percentage who changed to a lower category: 36%. Symptoms: (0–7 d, 8–30 d, >30 d during previous 3 mo)
Tellnes 1989 (15)	Initial sickness certificates issued to residents of Buskerud during a 4-wk period (Norway)	ICHPPC-1 codes for several diagnoses registered during a 4-wk period including cervical spine syndromes (ICHPPC-1: 7200)	Prospective, 1 y, $N = 5042$ (57 with cervical spine syndromes)	Percentage still certified sick after 52 wk: 1.8%

Abbreviations: ICHPPC = International Classification of Health Problems in Primary Care; PT = physiotherapy; RR= relative risk; SE = standard error.
*Numbers in parentheses are method scores (maximum score = 100).
†Two papers reporting on one study.

Age. Sloop et al. (1982) and Loy (1983) reported no association between age and a worse prognosis, but Loy failed to specify whether a statistical test was used. A third study (Anonymous 1966) reported a statistically significant worse prognosis for women over 50 years old.

Gender. Three studies (Sloop et al. 1982; Loy 1983; Gore et al. 1987) reported no association between gender and a worse prognosis, but Loy did not

mention whether a statistical test was used. A fourth study (Anonymous 1966) found a statistically significant worse prognosis for women over 50 years old.

Pain. Three studies reported on the severity of pain as a prognostic factor. Gore et al. (1987) reported severe pain (at baseline) to have an unsatisfactory outcome that was statistically significant, except for a subgroup of patients without injuries. Sloop et al. (1982) reported a statistically significant worse

Table IV
Details of randomized clinical trials on the clinical course of nonspecific neck pain

Reference*	Study Population	Case Definition	Study Design	Treatment	Outcome Measures and Results
Anonymous 1966 (38)	Patients attending department of physical medicine (England)	Pain in neck and arm, with or without paresthesia, root distribution *Or:* Pain in neck and arm, full root distribution with paresthesia (without clinical evidence) *Or:* Pain or paresthesia in neck and arm, partial root distribution with abnormality in neck	RCT, 6 mo, N = 493	[a] Traction, instruction in posture, collar, aspirin [b] Positioning (for maximum relief of pain), instruction in posture, collar, aspirin [c] Collar, instruction in posture, aspirin [d] Placebo heat (SWD), aspirin [e] Placebo tablets, aspirin	*After 4 wk:* Proportion showing improvement: Physicians' assessment: 21%[a], 23%[b], 24%[c], 21%[d], 16%[e] Patients' assessment: 71%[a], 81%[b], 74%[c], 70%[d], 56%[e] Patients' and physicians' assessment: 46%[a], 52%[b], 49%[c], 46%[d], 36%[e] Increase in joint range (patients with initially restricted movements): flexion: 11°, extension: 9°, rotation: 7°, lateral flexion: 7° (all patients, groups not specified) Interference with work or stopping work (reduction): 30%[a], 23%[b], 18%[c], 24%[d], 20%[e] Sleep disturbed or seriously disturbed (reduction): 35%[a], 34%[b], 27%[c], 34%[d], 15%[e] *After 6 mo:* Proportion of patients with pain decrease since follow-up at 6 wk: 31% (all patients, groups not specified)
Ceccherelli et al. 1989 (46)	Females (Italy)	Painful myofascial syndromes in cervical region as result of mild cervical arthrosis or poor posture	RCT, 3 mo, N = 27	[a] Laser [b] Placebo laser	Mean pain decrease (MPQ): No. of words: 49% decrease[a], 2% increase[b] Total score: 55% decrease[a], 7% decrease[b] No. of words + total score: 52% decrease[a], 3% decrease[b]
Coan et al. 1982 (62)	Public service announcements in newspapers (Maryland, USA)	Neck pain or radicular arm and hand pain for at least 6 mo	RCT, 12 wk, N = 30	[a] Acupuncture [b] Control (no therapy)	Decrease in: Mean hours of pain: 68%[a], 0%[b] Mean pain score: 40%[a], 2%[b] Mean pain (hours + pain score): 54%[a], 1%[b] Mean no. pain pills: 54%[a], 10%[b] Mean limitation of activity: 32%[a], 12%[b] Proportion showing improvement: 80%[a], 13%[b]
Foley-Nolan et al. 1990 (54)	Rheumatology outpatients or physiotherapy department (Ireland), aged >18 y	Neck pain >8 wk, unresponsive to at least one course of NSAIDs	RCT, partial crossover, 6 wk, N = 20	[a] Neck collar connected with a unit of pulsed high frequency electromagnetic energy, continue NSAID use [b] Placebo neck collar (3 wk) and 3 wk as for (a), continue NSAID use	Mean decrease in: Pain (VAS): 71%[a], 55%[b] ROM: 33%[a], 39%[b] Pill count: 80%[a], 80%[b] Proportion showing improvement (patients' assessment on pain and ROM): 100%[a], 90%[b]
Goldie and Landquist 1970 (31)	Patients at department of orthopedic surgery (Sweden)	Cervical pain radiating down either of the upper extremities following a segmental pattern	RCT, 3 wk, N = 73	[a] Isometric exercises, analgesics, and muscle relaxant [b] Traction, analgesics, and muscle relaxant [c] No treatment; analgesics and muscle relaxant	Proportion showing improvement: Physicians' assessment: 46%[a], 69%[b], 69%[c] Patients' assessment: 70%[a], 65%[b], 30%[c] Patients' + physicians' assessment: 58%[a], 67%[b], 50%[c] Mean increase in ROM (patients with initially restricted movements): Rotation: 5°[a], 7°[b], 5°[c] Lateral flexion: 5°[a], 6°[b], 5°[c]

(continued)

Table IV
Continued

Reference*	Study Population	Case Definition	Study Design	Treatment	Outcome Measures and Results
Horvath and Fellmann 1969 (8)	Patients of rheumatology clinic (Switzerland)	Cervical syndrome	RCT, 3 wk, N = 40	[a] Nifluril [b] Placebo Both groups received sollux therapy, massage, and a thermal bath	Mean decrease (3-point scale) in: Pain (spontaneously): 54%[a], 35%[b] Pain (provoked): 37%[a], 32%[b] Pain (spontaneously + provoked): 45%[a], 34%[b] Tension: 33%[a], 33%[b] Increase in mobility of the neck: 35%[a], 18%[b]
Howe et al.1983 (15)	Patients attending the clinic of a two-man practice (England), aged 15–65 y	Pain in neck, arm, or hand from lesion in cervical spine; evidence of reduced movement in one or more cervical intervertebral joints or palpable asymmetry of the transverse processes of the atlas	RCT, 3 wk, N = 52	[a] Manipulation and/or injection and azapropazone [b] Azapropazone	Proportion showing improvement: Pain in neck: 76%[a], 58%[b] Stiff neck: 73%[a], 64%[b] Headache: 92%[a], 100%[b] Pain/paresthesia of shoulder: 75%[a], 69%[b] Pain/paresthesia of arm/hand: 82%[a], 80%[b] Increase in ROM: Rotation: 5°[a], not reported[b] Lateral flexion: 0°[a], not reported[b]
Jensen et al. 1995 (31)	Patients referred to an inpatient orthopedic department (Sweden), aged 20–55 y	Neck and shoulder pain without objective neurological signs; excluded comorbidity that could impair participation (e.g., heart condition, alcoholism)	RCT, 6 mo, N = 66	[a] Physical fitness, health behavior, plan for return to work [b] As for (a) plus cognitive behavioral intervention	Mean decrease in: Pain (VAS): 6%[a], 13%[b] Disability: 6%[a], 3%[b] Anxiety: 3%[a], 44%[b] Depression: 8%[a], 13%[b] Percentage of patients who noticed decrease in: Pain: 47%[a], 44%[b] Disability: 39%[a], 32%[b] Anxiety: 31%[a], 40%[b] Depression: 30%[a], 36[b]
Levoska and Keinänen-Kiukaan-niemi 1993 (46)	Female office workers employed by a bank or social insurance institution (Finland)	Neck or shoulder symptoms once a week or more, feeling of disturbance, muscle spasm, and tenderness in neck/shoulder on palpation	RCT, 1 y, N = 47	[a] Passive physiotherapy (surface heat, massage, stretching, exercises) [b] Active physiotherapy (stretching, dynamic muscle training, home exercises)	Percentage showing improvement in: Neck/shoulder pain: 14%[a], 18%[b] Cephalalgia or neck/shoulder pain: 18%[a], 36%[b] Neck/shoulder + cephalalgia or neck/shoulder pain: 16%[a], 27%[b]
Loy 1983 (15)	Consecutive patients of a general orthopedic clinic (Hong Kong)	Cervical spondylosis; excluded patients with acute symptoms for a few days	RCT, 6 wk, N = 60	[a] Traction and SWD [b] Electro-acupuncture	ROM: slight decrease [a], increase [b] Percentage of patients who noticed benefit: 54%[a], 87%[b]
Nordemar and Thörner 1981 (46)	Consecutive patients of dept. of physical medicine and medical rehabilitation (Sweden)	Patients with acute cervical pain, <3 d, without neurological symptoms	RCT, 3 mo, N = 30	[a] Collar, rest, analgesics [b] TENS, collar, rest, analgesics [c] Collar, rest, analgesics, MT	Mean pain decrease (VAS): 100%[a], 100%[b], 100%[c] Mean decrease in ROM: 100%[a], 100%[b], 100%[c]

(continued)

Table IV
Continued

Reference*	Study Population	Case Definition	Study Design	Treatment	Outcome Measures and Results
Petrie and Hazleman 1986 (62)	Outpatients at rheumatology clinic (England)	Chronic neck pain, arising from the neck with or without radiation to the shoulders or occiput, present on a daily basis for at least 6 mo	RCT, 2 mo, N = 26	[a] Acupuncture [b] Placebo TENS	Mean decrease in: Daily pain (VAS): 33%[a], 22%[b] Daily disability (VAS): 25%[a], 8% increase[b] Daily pill count: 23%[a], 9% increase[b] MPQ: 32%[a], 20%[b] Percentage of patients who noticed benefit: 77%[a], 50%[b]
Revel et al. 1994 (62)	Outpatients at department of rheumatology (France), aged ≥16 y	Chronic neck pain >3 mo, considered for a medical program	RCT, 10 wk, N = 60	[a] Rehabilitation (improve neck proprioception by active and passive motion) and medication (NSAID, analgesics) [b] Medication (NSAID, analgesics)	Mean pain decrease (VAS): 43%[a], 9%[b] Mean decrease in daily medication (NSAID, analgesics): 79%[a], 37%[b] Noticed benefit by patient: 60%[a], 27%[b] Mean decrease in ROM: Flexion/extension: 2%[a], 1%[b] Rotation: 0%[a], 0%[b]
Sloop et al. 1982 (54)	Patients referred to a department of medical rehabilitation (England)	Cervical spondylosis or nonspecific neck pain as described in standard texts, pain ≥1 mo	RCT, pseudo cross-over†, 3 wk, N = 39	[a] MT, diazepam [b] Diazepam	Percentage of patients who noticed benefit (pain, selected daily activities): 57%[a], 28%[b]
Takala et al. 1994 (15)	Women in a printing company (Finland)	Frequent neck symptoms without signs of cervical nerve root compression or tendinitis of the shoulder	RCT, cross-over design, 11 mo, N = 44	[a] Group gymnastics [b] Controls (no treatment)	Mean pressure pain threshold (bilaterally measured on four muscles (specified) with an algometer): First period[a,b] (spring): small increase Second period (autumn): no change
Thorsen et al. 1992 (62)	Female hospital laboratory technicians (Denmark), aged 18–65 y	Pain from neck and shoulder-girdle lasting at least 1 y, affecting the quality of work or daily living; 1–10 tender points	RCT, cross-over, 6 wk, N = 52	[a] Laser/placebo [b] Placebo/laser	Mean pain decrease at function (VAS): 27%[a], 50%[b] Mean pain decrease at rest (VAS): 39%[a], 50%[b] Mean pain decrease (function + rest): 33%[a], 50%[b] Mean decrease in analgesics: 33%[a], 40%[b] Percentage of patients who noticed benefit: 52% (all patients, groups not specified)
Vassljen et al. 1995 (54)	Female office workers (group 1). Female patients from local physio-therapists (group 2) (Norway)	*Group 1:* patients (n = 24) with shoulder and neck pain (≥3, scale 0–6) last 6 mo and previous 2 wk., and pain 3 d continuously past 2 wk. *Group 2:* patients (n = 9) with shoulder and neck pain past 2 wk, ≥1 trigger point upper trapezius, and pain on positive stretching	RCT (partial), 6 mo, N = 33	Group 1: [a]Individual physiotherapy, [b]Group exercise Group 2: [c]Individual physiotherapy	Mean pain decrease (VAS): 48%[a], 52%[b], 66%[c] Percentage of patients who noticed benefit: 83%[a], 42%[b], not reported[c]

Abbreviations: MPQ = McGill Pain Questionnaire; MT = manual treatment; RCT = randomized clinical trial; ROM = range of motion; SWD = short-wave diathermy; TENS = transcutaneous nerve stimulation; VAS = visual analogue scale.
* Numbers in parentheses are method scores (maximum score = 100).
† Patients who did not improve crossed over.

Table V
Outcome of studies on the clinical course of nonspecific neck pain

Outcome	Population (No. Studies)	Percentage (Range)	Median Percentage	Follow-up Time (Range, wk)	Median Follow-up Time (wk)
Mean pain decrease on VAS/numerical rating scale	Mixed (10)	9–100	34	3–52	11
	Chronic (7)	26–63	28	6–12	8
	Acute (1)	100	—	—	—
	Unknown (3)	9–49	—	—	—
Patients with pain decrease	Mixed (5)	22–79	46	24–520	38
	Chronic (1)	67	—	—	—
	Unknown (3)	22–79	—	—	—
Patients with general improvement (in patient's or therapist's opinion)	Mixed (12)	36–95	47.5	3–156	7
	Chronic (9)	37–95	47	3–46	6
	Acute (1)	36	—	—	—
	Unknown (2)	40–71	—	—	—
Patients with functional improvement (different scales)	Mixed (3)	5–22	9	8–24	12
	Chronic (2)	9–22	—	—	—
	Unknown (1)	5	—	—	—
Health care utilization					
Mean decrease in analgesic use	Chronic (5)	7–80	37	6–12	8
Patients who received treatment in the past	Mixed (2)	80–100	90	520–LT*	LT*

* LT = lifetime.

prognosis for patients with local tenderness on the initial examination, while Anonymous (1966) reported a statistically significant association between the severity of the attack and the prognosis but failed to specify the direction of the association.

Localization. Arm pain (mean duration of 6 years) and central nervous system symptoms were not associated with a worse prognosis, according to Sloop et al. (1982). Gore et al. (1987) reported no association between the localization of pain and a worse prognosis, while a third study (Anonymous 1966) reported a statistically significant worse prognosis for patients with bilateral paresthesia, but no worse prognosis for abnormal neurologic signs.

Duration and number of attacks. Loy (1983) reported no association between the duration of symptoms at baseline and a worse outcome, but did not clarify whether a statistical test was used. A second study reported both the average duration of symptoms in the previous attack and the number of previous attacks to be associated with improvement (Anonymous 1966); the direction of the association was not specified. The same study reported a statistically significant worse prognosis for a history of attacks of longer than 5 years or of having suffered more than three previous attacks.

Occupation. Berg et al. (1988) reported a statistically significant worse prognosis for manual workers

compared with office workers. After retirement both office and manual workers had fewer symptoms. Type of work (before retirement) was not associated with improvement, but it was not clear whether a statistical test was used to assess this association. A second study (Abbot et al. 1990) reported that change in occupation was not associated with improvement, and a third (Loy 1983) reported no association between type of occupation and prognosis. In the second and third studies, it was not clear whether a statistical test was used.

Radiological findings. Gore et al. (1987) reported no association between degenerative changes and the level of pain, and a second study (Anonymous 1966) reported no association between radiological findings and improvement. Two studies (Sloop et al. 1982; Loy 1983) reported that the severity of radiological findings was not associated with the prognosis, but Loy failed to clarify whether a statistical test was used.

In summary, only six studies reported on prognostic factors. Despite the limited number of studies and the low methodological quality, there are indications that localization (radiation to the arms and or neurological signs) and radiological findings (degenerative changes in the disks and joints) are not associated with prognosis. A higher severity of pain and a history of previous attacks seem to be associated with a worse prognosis.

Table VI
Prognostic factors for nonspecific neck pain

Reference	Prognostic Factors	Outcome	Association
Abbott et al. 1990	Financial compensation, change in occupation	Improvement	No*
Berg et al. 1988	Manual work (versus office work)	More symptoms	Yes
	After retirement (both manual/office workers)	Fewer symptoms	Yes
	Type of work (manual, office) before retirement	Fewer symptoms	No*
Gore et al. 1987	Sex	Worse outcome	No
	Initially severe pain:		
	Injured subgroup	Worse outcome	Yes
	Uninjured subgroup	Worse outcome	No
	Combined subgroups	Worse outcome	Yes
	Roentgenographic findings	Level of pain	No
	Localization of pain	Worse outcome	No
Sloop et al. 1982	Middlesex Hospital Questionnaire (emotional and situational factors), Social Readjustment Rating Scale (life changes), age, sex, history of trauma, pill count, presence of arm pain, radiographic grate, central nervous system symptoms	Improvement (VAS)	No
		Worse prognosis	
	Local tenderness on initial examination		Yes
Loy 1983	Duration of symptoms, age, sex, occupation, severity of radiological changes	Worse outcome	No*
Anonymous 1966	Age, severity of attack, number of previous attacks, average duration of symptoms in previous attack, whether symptoms were getting better or worse when the patient was first seen	Improvement (after 4 wk)	Yes†
	Range of neck movement, abnormal neurological signs, X-ray changes	Improvement (after 4 wk)	No
	History of attacks for >5 y, >3 previous attacks, bilateral paresthesia, women aged >50 y, symptoms that were getting better or worse when the patient was first seen	Worse outcome (after 6 mo)	Yes

* Not clear whether a statistical test was used.
† Direction of the association was not specified.

HIGH-RISK GROUPS

GENDER

Bovim et al. (1994) conducted a study on the prevalence of neck pain in the general Norwegian population. Of the 10,000 questionnaires they sent to a random sample drawn from the National Register of Norway, 7648 were returned. Two questions focused on neck pain: "Did you within the last year have troublesome neck pain?" (yes/no); and "If yes, for how long within the last year on the whole did you have these complaints?" (<1 month, 1–3 months, 3–6 months, >6 months). In total, 34% answered yes to the first question. If we compare men (n = 3914) to women (n = 3734), the latter reported significantly more neck pain than men (frequency was 40% for women and 29% for men), except for neck pain lasting for less than a month.

Dartigues et al. (1988) also found women to be more at risk (OR = 3.0, 95% CI = 1.9–4.6) than men in their study on risk factors for neck pain among the working population. Other studies confirm that the prevalence of neck pain in women is higher (Ursin et al. 1988; Mäkelä et al. 1991; Skov et al. 1996).

AGE

Mäkelä et al. (1991) studied the prevalence of neck pain in the adult population of Finland, sampling 7217 subjects (3637 men and 4363 women), whose age distribution corresponded closely to that of the Finnish population. Five percent of those aged 30–44, 14% of those aged 45–54, and as many as 22% of those aged 55–64 reported neck pain. Above the age of 65, the prevalence of neck pain decreased. Dartigues et al. (1988) looked at the relationship between age and neck pain in a working population of 990 men and women with a mean age of 35.8 years. The prevalence of neck pain was 4% in the lowest age group (<30 years) and increased significantly to 16% in the oldest (50–59 years). Lagerström et al. (1995) found similar results in their study of nursing personnel (aged 18–64). Age (as a continuous variable) showed a significant association with neck pain (OR = 1.31, 95% CI = 1.14–1.52). We can conclude that older people are more at risk of developing neck pain than younger people.

THE WORKING POPULATION

Hagberg and Wegman (1987) summarized the results of studies that compared neck trouble in different occupational groups, including miners, manual workers, farmers, typists, office workers, industrial workers, assembly line workers, dentists, and nurses. For many types of occupations, they reported an increased risk of neck trouble. Compared to assembly-line packers, slaughterhouse workers had a significantly greater risk for cervical syndrome (OR = 8.5, 95% CI = 1.0–71). The same was true for civil servants compared to iron foundry workers (OR = 4.8, 95% CI = 1.8–13). Compared to teachers and nurses of handicapped children, film-rolling workers (OR = 118, 95% CI = 6.9–1000) and lamp assemblers (OR = 5.1, 95% CI = 2.0–13) had a significantly increased risk of developing tension neck syndrome. Data entry operators (OR = 4.9, 95% CI = 1.8–13), typists (OR = 4.2, 95% CI = 1.6–11), and computer operators (OR = 3.2, 95% CI = 1.2–8.2) had an increased risk in comparison to office workers. Compared to shop assistants, workers at a scissors factory had an increased risk for tension neck syndrome (OR = 4.1, 95% CI = 2.3–7.2).

Different occupations are perceived to have different risks for the development of neck trouble. The literature appears to focus on certain occupations, for example office workers (with and without VDT use), assembly line workers, and industrial jobs, including heavy labor. Hence we lack a comprehensive overview of occupations associated with measured risk for neck pain.

CONCLUSION

Some specific populations have an increased risk for neck pain. First, women appear to have a higher chance of developing neck pain than do men. Second, the risk increases until age 65 and then seems to decrease. And finally, specific occupations have higher prevalences of neck pain. Prevention thus should primarily focus on these groups.

OTHER RISK FACTORS FOR NECK PAIN

Many studies have been conducted to identify various risk factors for neck pain. Most address only one or few risk factors, or a single type of risk factor, i.e., physical, psychosocial, or individual. Studies vary according to type and methodological quality, and not all studies achieve similar results.

METHODS

Literature search. To identify the most important risk factors for neck pain, we conducted a literature review to identify relevant studies and assessed their methodological quality to determine the most important risk factors for neck pain, including "work-related" and "non-work-related" factors. We performed online searches of MEDLINE, Embase, Psychlit, Sportdiscus, NIOSHtic, HSEline, and Cisdoc for studies that met the following criteria: (1) cross-sectional, case-control, or prospective cohort design; (2) the study population was community-based or working; (3) the outcome included one or more syndromes, signs, or symptoms related to the neck; (4) the outcome could be a self-reported or directly measured variable; (5) the outcome had to be reported separately for the neck region; (6) exposure assessment based only on job title was not allowed; (7) the publication must be a full report (peer reviewed), written in English, German, or Dutch.

In total, 46 studies fulfilled the criteria. Most of these (*n* = 43) were cross-sectional. One case-control study and two prospective cohort studies were also included. Other prospective cohort and case-control studies have been published on risk factors for musculoskeletal disorders, but they do not report their results separately for the neck region. Some studies (not included in our review) combine neck and shoulder pain as the outcome variable (Bjelle et al. 1981; Jonsson et al. 1988; Ekberg et al. 1994; Viikari-Juntura 1991).

Methodological quality. For the 46 studies identified, we assessed methodological quality using a checklist based on quality assessment tools used in systematic reviews of RCTs on the effectiveness of treatment, but adapted to assess the methodological quality of observational studies. Different tools were developed for cross-sectional, case-control, and prospective cohort studies. The quality assessment evaluated information, validity, and precision in five categories: (1) Purpose must be specific and well defined. (2) Study population must be described as to main

Table VII
Descriptives of all studies that had a total quality score of at least 7 points

Reference*	Study Type	Study Population	Outcome Measure(s)	Physical Risk Factor(s) and Strength of Association
Ahlberg-Hultén et al. 1995 (7)	CS	Female nurses and nurse's aides; participation rate = 79% (n = 90)	Self-reported neck pain	*Work-related factors:* Poor relations with superiors (–0.14, P = 0.40); conflicts (0.11, P = 0.52); stress (0.08, P = 0.72); intensity of authority over decisions (0.05, P = 0.71); psychological demands (0.00, P = 0.97); skill utilization (–0.03, P = 0.73)
Bernard et al. 1994 (9)	CS	Newspaper employees using video display terminals; response at baseline 93% (n = 973)	Self-reported neck symptoms	*Work-related factors:* Time spent on telephone (OR = 1.4, CI = 1.0–1.8); number of hours spent under a deadline per week (OR = 1.7, CI = 1.4–3.0); work variance (OR = 1.7, CI = 1.2–2.5); number of breaks (n.s.); job control (n.s.); job security (n.s.); interaction with co-workers or customers (n.s.); group conflict (n.s.) *Non-work-related factors:* Lack of social support from spouses and friends (n.s.); height (n.s.); use of eye-glasses (n.s.); existing medical conditions (n.s.); hours spent typing away from work (n.s.)
Bovenzi et al. 1991 (8)	CS	Cases: male forestry workers using chain-saws (n = 65); controls: male hospital maintenance workers not exposed to vibration (n = 31)	Self-reported persisting neck pain	*Work-related factors:* Vibration >7.5 m/s^2 (OR = 3.8, P = 0.03); vibration <7.5 m/s^2 (OR = 0.9, n.s.)
			Tension neck syndrome	Vibration >7.5 m/s^2 (OR = 3.8, P = 0.03); vibration <7.5 m/s^2 (OR = 0.9, n.s.)
			Cervical syndrome	Vibration >7.5 m/s^2 (OR = 10.7, P < 0.005); vibration <7.5 m/s^2 (OR = 2.8, n.s.)
Dartigues et al. 1988 (7)	CS	A working population (n = 990)	Self-reported recurrent cervical pain syndrome	*Work-related factors:* Sitting posture (n.s.); cervical spine rotation (OR = 2.4, CI = 1.5–3.8); cervical spine flexion (OR = 1.7, CI = 1.0–3.0); cervical spine extension (OR = 2.3, CI = 1.5–3.7); permanent posture (n.s.); muscular activity (n.s.); conflict related to work (OR = 3.1, CI = 2.0–4.8) *Non-work-related factors:* Strenuous muscular activity during leisure time (OR = 0.4, CI = 0.2–0.7); anxiety (OR = 3.4, CI = 2.2–5.1); insomnia (OR = 3.6, CI = 2.4–5.6); depression (OR = 4.0, CI = 2.5–6.4); conflict related to family (OR = 1.8, CI = 1.1–3.0)
Hales et al. 1994 (10)	CS	Telecommunication employees utilizing video display terminals for at least 6 h/d; response at baseline = 96% (n = 512)	Self-reported neck disorders	*Work-related factors:* Routine work lacking decision-making opportunities (OR = 4.2, CI = 2.1–8.6); lack of productivity standard (OR = 3.5, CI = 1.5–8.3); fear of being replaced by computers (OR = 3.0, CI = 1.5–6.1); high information-processing demands (OR = 3.0, CI = 1.4–6.2); job requires a variety of tasks (OR = 2.9, CI = 1.5–5.8); increasing work pressure (OR = 2.4, CI = 1.1–5.5) *Non-work-related factors:* Hours per week spent on recreational activities or hobbies (n.s.)

(continued)

Table VII
Continued

Reference*	Study Type	Study Population	Outcome Measure(s)	Physical Risk Factor(s) and Strength of Association
Kamwendo et al. 1991 (9)	CS	Female medical secretaries and office personnel; response at baseline = 96% (*n* = 420)	Self-reported neck pain	*Work-related factors:* Sitting 5 h/d or more (OR = 1.49, CI = 0.86–2.61); work with office machines >5 h/d (OR = 1.65, 1.02–2.67); interesting and stimulating work (n.s.); work variation (n.s.); friendly spirit of cooperation with fellow workers (*P* = 0.013); help and support with difficulties at work (n.s.); ability to influence working conditions (*P* = 0.001); too much to do (*P* = 0.010); good contact and concert with superiors (n.s.); demands of work too great (n.s.); anxiety about possible reorganization or new techniques at work (n.s.)
Lagerström et al. 1995 (7)	CS	Female nursing personnel of a hospital; response at baseline = 84% (*n* = 688)	Self-reported ongoing neck symptoms	*Work-related factors:* Low support from superiors (OR = 2.08, CI = 1.32–3.26; OR = 2.03, CI = 1.28–3.16)†; high work demand (n.s.); lack of stimulation (n.s.); low work control (n.s.) *Non-work-related factors:* BMI (n.s.); low physical fitness (OR = 1.43, CI = 1.02–2.01; OR = 1.42, CI = 1.00–2.02); smoking (n.s.)
			Self-reported severe ongoing neck symptoms (>6 on a 10-point scale from "not at all" to "very much")	*Work-related factors:* Low support from superiors (n.s.); high work demand (OR = 1.82, CI = 1.14–2.92; OR = 1.82, CI = 1.14–2.92); lack of stimulation (n.s.); low work control (n.s.) *Non-work-related factors:* BMI (n.s.); low physical fitness (OR = 1.82, CI = 1.18–2.80; OR = 1.68, CI = 1.09–2.59); smoking (n.s.)
Linton 1990 (8)	CS	Full-time employees working during day (*n* = 22,180)	Self-reported neck pain	*Work-related factors:* Heavy lifting (OR = 1.41–1.83)‡; monotonous work (OR = 2.25–2.95); sitting (OR = 0.94–1.33); uncomfortable posture (OR = 1.59–2.42); overall psychosocial score (OR = 1.89–2.57); work content (OR = 1.94–2.47); social support (OR = 1.38–2.57); psychosocial work load (OR = 1.24–1.49) *Non-work-related factors:* Exercise (OR = 0.91–1.06); eating regularly (OR = 1.20–1.36); alcohol consumption (OR = 0.80–1.05); smoking (OR = 1.18–1.77)
Mäkelä et al. 1991 (11)	CS	Finnish adults drawn from the population register, representing the Finnish adult population of 30 y and older; response at baseline = 90% (*n* = 7217)	Chronic neck syndrome	*Work-related factors (age 30–64 y):* Physical stress at work (OR = 1.35, CI = 1.27–1.42; OR = 1.26, CI = 1.18–1.33); mental stress at work (OR = 1.20, CI = 1.12–1.28) *Non-work-related factors (age 30–64 y):* Injury to the back, neck, or shoulder (OR = 1.97, CI = 1.62–2.38); former smoker (n.s.); current smoker (n.s.); BMI (<23 is referent level) 23–25.9 (OR = 1.46, CI = 1.13–1.89); BMI 26–28.9 (OR = 1.36, CI = 1.03–1.78); BMI 29–31.9 (OR = 1.37, CI = 1.00–1.87); BMI 32–34.9 (OR = 1.51, CI = 1.01–2.26); BMI >35 (n.s.); parity per each additional birth (OR = 1.10, CI = 1.04–1.16)

(continued)

Table VII
Continued

Reference*	Study Type	Study Population	Outcome Measure(s)	Physical Risk Factor(s) and Strength of Association
Mäkelä et al. 1991 (continued)				*Work-related factors (age >64 y):* Physical stress at work (OR = 1.21, CI = 1.08–1.34; OR = 1.12, CI = 1.00–1.26); mental stress at work (OR = 1.27, CI = 1.11–1.46)
				Non-work-related factors (age >64 y): Injury to the back, neck, or shoulder (OR = 1.58, CI = 1.12–2.22.); former smoker (n.s.); current smoker (n.s.); BMI (<23 is referent level) 23–25.9 (n.s.); BMI 26–28.9 (n.s.); BMI 29–31.9 (OR = 1.96, CI = 1.19–3.24); BMI 32–34.9 (n.s.); BMI >35 (n.s.); parity per each additional birth (n.s.)
Skov et al. 1996 (8)	CS	Random 8% sample of the members of the association Danish Active Salespeople; response at baseline = 66% (*n* = 1306)	Self-reported neck symptoms	*Work-related factors:* 25% of work time sitting (OR = 2.68, CI = 1.31–5.49); 50% of work time sitting (OR = 1.92, CI = 0.98–3.79); 75% of work time sitting (OR = 2.18, CI = 1.11–4.29); 100% of work time sitting (OR = 2.80, CI = 1.40–5.59); lifting heavy loads (n.s.); demands in the work (n.s.); variation in work (highest quartile is referent value), next to highest quartile (OR = 1.78, CI = 1.16–2.73), next to lowest quartile (n.s.), lowest quartile (OR = 1.82, CI = 1.23–2.69); control over time, low compared to high control (OR = 1.4, CI = 1.07–1.93), medium compared to high control (n.s.); perceived competition, high compared to low competition (OR = 1.44, CI = 1.08–1.91), medium compared to low perceived competition (n.s.)
				Non-work-related factors: Annual driving distance 5–10,000 km (OR = 0.99, CI = 0.45–1.76); annual driving distance 10–15,000 km (OR = 1.48, CI = 0.75–2.93); annual driving distance 15–30,000 km (OR = 1.74, CI = 1.01–2.99); annual driving distance 30–50,000 km (OR = 2.10, CI = 1.24–3.54); annual driving distance >50,000 km (OR = 2.43, CI = 1.36–4.34); leisure-time sports activities (n.s.)
Tharr 1995 (8)	CS	Representatives from two teleservice centers (response at baseline = 95% (*n* = 108)	Self-reported neck symptoms	*Work-related factors:* Chair discomfort (OR = 3.5, CI = 1.4–8.9); hours spent typing at VDT work station (n.s.); hours spent on telephone (n.s.); time continuously sitting on a chair (n.s.); work-load variability (OR = 1.2, CI = 1.0–1.4)
Johansson 1995 (8)	CS	Home care workers (*n* = 305)	Self-reported neck symptoms	*Work-related factors:* Lifting heavy loads (RR = 1.21, CI = 0.92–1.59); monotonous movements (RR = 1.33, CI = 1.04–1.69); twisted postures (RR = 1.26, CI = 0.97–1.63); deeply forward-flexed torso (RR = 1.33, CI = 1.06–1.68; *P* < 0.15); hands above shoulder level (RR = 1.17, CI = 0.96–1.44); low influence and control over work (RR = 1.27, CI = 1.00–1.62); poor supervisory climate (RR = 1.23, CI = 0.99–1.53); low stimulus from the work itself (RR = 1.33, CI = 1.05–1.67); poor relationships with fellow workers (RR = 1.19, CI = 0.94–1.50); low psychological work load (RR = 1.52, CI = 1.20–1.94; *P* < 0.001)

(continued)

Table VII
Continued

Reference*	Study Type	Study Population	Outcome Measure(s)	Physical Risk Factor(s) and Strength of Association
Johansson 1995 (continued)			Self-reported work-related neck symptoms	*Work-related factors:* Lifting heavy loads (RR = 1.74, CI = 1.09–2.77); monotonous movements (RR = 1.73, CI = 1.22–2.47); twisted postures (RR = 1.69, CI = 1.09–2.63; $P < 0.15$); deeply forward-flexed torso (RR = 1.68, CI = 1.20–2.34; $P < 0.01$); hands above shoulder level (RR = 1.38, CI = 1.03–1.84); low influence and control over work (RR = 1.30, CI = 0.93–1.81); poor supervisory climate (RR = 1.29, CI = 0.93–1.79); low stimulus from the work itself (RR = 1.52, CI = 1.10–2.11); poor relationships with fellow workers (RR = 1.20, CI = 0.87–1.65); low psychological work load (RR = 1.83, CI = 1.28–2.61; $P < 0.001$)
Kilbom et al. 1986 (7)	CS	Female assembly-line workers of two electronic manufacturing companies; response at baseline = 77% ($n = 106$)	Severity of self-reported neck symptoms	*Work-related factors:* Increased average time per work cycle in neck flexion ($P < 0.01$); increased average time per work cycle with upper arm abducted 0–30° ($P < 0.05$); overtime work (n.s.); perceived psychological stress at work (n.s.); work satisfaction (n.s.); number of breaks and rest pauses at work (n.s.) *Non-work-related factors:* Leisure-time physical activity (n.s.)
Bergqvist et al. 1995 (7)	CS	Office workers ($n = 353$); response: Q = 92%, PE = 91%, WA = 82%	Tension neck syndrome	*Work-related factors:* Keyboard too high (OR = 4.4, CI = 1.1–17.6); limited rest-break opportunities (OR = 7.4, CI = 3.1–17.4)
Ignatius et al. 1993 (8)	CS	Female typists working in the Government Housing Department; response at baseline = 52% ($n = 170$)	Self-reported neck pain	*Work-related factors:* Mismatch of desk and chair heights (OR = 3.0, $P = 0.021$; OR = 2.98); bending neck at work (OR = 3.4, $P = 0.012$; OR = 2.62); daily typing hours (n.s.); bending back at work (n.s.); no rest other than lunch breaks (n.s.)
Lau et al. 1996 (7)	CS	All adults >30 y living in two housing blocks in Shatin, Hong Kong	Self-reported neck pain	*Non-work-related factors:* Sports activity (n.s.)
Bru et al. 1996 (7)	CS	Female hospital staff; response at baseline 85% ($n = 586$)	Neck pain index (based on self-reported data)	*Work-related factors:* Perceived ergonomic load (n.s.); work overload ($P = 0.004$); social relations ($P = 0.005$); work content ($P = 0.03$)
Andersen and Gaardboe 1993 (7)	CS	Female sewing machine operators ($n = 424$); response of total cohort = 78.2% ($n = 896$)	Self-reported chronic neck pain	*Non-work-related factors:* Leisure-time exercise (OR = 0.89, CI = 0.63–1.25)
Schibye et al. 1995 (7)	CS	Female sewing machine operators; response at baseline = 94% ($n = 306$)	Self-reported neck symptoms	*Work-related factors:* Individual adjustment of table and chair (n.s.)

(continued)

Table VII
Continued

Reference*	Study Type	Study Population	Outcome Measure(s)	Physical Risk Factor(s) and Strength of Association
Rundcrantz et al. 1991 (7)	PR	Official dentists in Malmö; response at baseline = 90% (*n* = 359); response at follow-up = 92% (*n* = 315)	Self-reported neck symptoms	*Work-related factors:* Changing own position to the patient to obtain a direct view (n.s.); alter the position of the patient to obtain a direct view (n.s.)
Mundt et al. 1993 (8)	CC	Cases: patients with cervical disk herniation (*n* = 68); controls: persons free of disk herniation (*n* = 63); *N* = 63 cases matched to a control (93%)	Herniated cervical disk	*Non-work-related factors:* Baseball (RR = 1.05, CI = 0.40–2.75); golf (RR = 0.59, CI = 0.21–2.61); bowling (RR = 1.63, CI = 0.70–3.83); swimming (RR = 0.71, CI = 0.31–1.63); diving (RR = 0.96, CI = 0.36–2.52); jogging (RR = 0.86, CI = 0.41–1.81); aerobics (RR = 0.94, CI = 0.39–2.29); racket sports (RR = 1.14, CI = 0.50–2.60); any of these sports (RR = 0.39, CI = 0.12–1.30); use of free weights (RR = 1.87, CI = 0.74–4.74); weightlifting (RR = 0.75, CI = 0.31–1.78)
Viikari-Juntura et al. 1994 (11)	PR	Male machine operators, carpenters, and office workers; response at baseline = 69% (*n* = 2222); response at follow-up 82% (*n* = 1832)	Self-reported neck pain, change from 1984 to 1987:	*Work-related factors:* Twisting or bending at work (OR = 1.8; CI = 1.2–2.7); job satisfaction (n.s.)
			None to moderate	*Non-work-related factors:* Physical exercise (n.s.); car driving (n.s.); ex-smoker (n.s.); current smoker (OR = 1.5, CI = 1.0–2.4)
			None to severe	*Work-related factors:* Twisting or bending at work (OR = 1.9, CI = 1.2–3.2); job satisfaction (OR = 1.7, CI = 1.1–2.6)
				Non-work-related factors: Physical exercise (n.s.); car driving (n.s.), ex-smoker (n.s.); current smoker (OR = 2.2, CI = 1.3–3.7; OR = 1.8, CI = 1.0–3.2)
			Persistent severe	*Work-related factors:* Twisting or bending at work (n.s.); job satisfaction (n.s.)
				Non-work-related factors Physical exercise (n.s.); car driving (n.s.); ex-smoker (n.s.); current smoker (OR = 1.9, CI = 1.0–3.5)
Zettenberg et al. 1997 (8)	CS	*N* = 564 car assembly workers	Self reported neck complaints	*Work-related factors:* Good relation with co-workers/foreman (*P* < 0.01; *P* < 0.01); work satisfaction (*P* < 0.04); stress at work (*P* < 0.001)

Abbreviations: BMI = body mass index; CC = case-control study design; CI = 95% confidence interval; CS = cross-sectional study design; n.s. = not significant; OR = odds ratio; PE = physical examination; PR = prospective study design; Q = questionnaire; RR = risk ratio; WA = workplace assessment.

*Numbers in parentheses are method scores.

†If two analyses were carried out for a specific exposure and outcome, both results are presented.

‡Several age-specific odds ratios ranging from 1.41 to 1.83 are presented in this study.

features, and response at baseline and follow-up (only for prospective cohort studies) must be at least 80% or there must be evidence that the nonresponse is not selective. (3) Exposure measurements must include measurement of physical and psychosocial factors at work and during leisure time, historical exposure at work, and history of neck pain, and exposure assessment must be blinded to disease status (only for cross-sectional studies). (4) Outcome measurements must be standardized methods of acceptable quality; data must be collected for at least 1 year and 3 months (only for prospective cohort studies). (5) Analysis and data presentation must include appropriate statistical model with measures of association controlled for confounding, and the number of cases must be at least 10 times the number of independent variables in the analysis.

On every item in each category, a study was rated "positive," "negative," or "don't know." All scores were added to reach a final "method" score. If all items were rated "positive," the maximum score was 15 for cross-sectional studies, 17 for prospective cohort studies, and 19 for case-control studies. Only studies with a method score of 7 or higher will be described. Extensive information on the identification of studies, methodological quality assessment, and results are reported elsewhere (Ariëns et al., submitted).

RESULTS

Table VII shows the 23 studies with a method score of 7 or higher, and groups the different risk factors for neck pain into work-related and non-work-related factors. Twenty of these studies included work-related risk factors in their analysis, and 10 studies included non-work-related risk factors.

Not all studies used the same type of outcome measure and instruments. Most studies used neck symptoms as an outcome measure (neck pain in the past 12 months), while others used neck syndromes (tension neck syndrome, cervical syndrome) or neck signs (neck movement restriction, neck tenderness). Most studies analyzed working populations; only Mäkelä et al. (1991) and Lau et al. (1996) used a general population.

Work-related risk factors for neck pain

Within work-related risk factors, physical and psychosocial factors can be distinguished. Mäkelä et al. (1991) found significant associations with neck

pain for both physical and mental stress at work. Linton (1990) also found a significant association between an overall psychosocial score and neck pain. Other studies investigated more specific aspects of physical and psychosocial load at the workplace.

Physical risk factors. Dartigues et al. (1988) reported that twisting, flexion, and extension of the neck were associated with neck pain. Kilbom et al. (1986) and Ignatius et al. (1993) also found significant association between neck flexion and self-reported neck pain. Three studies looked at heavy lifting in relation to neck pain: Linton (1990) showed odds ratios varying between 1.41 and 1.83 and Johansson (1995) reported odds ratios of 1.21 and 1.74, while Skov et al. (1996) did not find a significant association between heavy lifting and neck pain. Bovenzi et al. (1991) investigated vibration as a risk factor. They directly measured the amount of vibration and for all outcome measures they reported a significant association with neck pain.

Researchers have often studied time spent sitting at work using office machines, with mixed results. Skov et al. (1996) found a significant association with neck pain. Bernard et al. (1994) showed an odds ratio of 1.4 for the relationship between increased time spent on the telephone and neck pain. Linton (1990) reported odds ratios varying between 0.94 and 1.33 for the relationship between sitting posture and self-reported neck pain, and Kamwendo et al. (1991) showed odds ratios of 1.49 and 1.65 for this relationship. Dartigues et al. (1988), Tharr (1995), and Ignatius et al. (1993) stated that the relationship between sitting posture while using office machines and self-reported neck pain was not significant.

Other physical load factors associated with neck pain were adverse workplace design factors (Bergqvist et al. 1995; Ignatius et al. 1993; Tharr 1995), twisting and bending of the torso (Ignatius et al. 1993; Viikari-Juntera et al. 1994; Johansson 1995), working with the hands above shoulder level (Johansson 1995), upper arm abduction (Kilbom et al. 1986), and work involving monotonous movements (Linton 1990; Johansson 1995).

Psychosocial risk factors. Three studies looked at psychosocial work load in relation to neck pain. Ahlberg-Hultén et al. (1995) and Kilbom et al. (1986) reported that this relationship was not significant, but Johansson (1995) reported odds ratios of 1.52 and 1.83 for the relationship between low psychological work load and neck pain. Skov et al. (1996) and Kamwendo et al. (1991) looked at psychosocial work load in relation to neck pain, but could find no significant relationship. Bru et al. (1996) did find a significant association between work overload and neck pain, as did Lagerström et al. (1995) and Linton (1990).

Interpersonal relationships are another psychosocial risk factor that is related to neck pain. Poor relationships with superiors and co-workers, conflicts at work, and poor social support at work are all related to an increase in the occurrence of neck pain (Dartigues et al. 1988; Linton 1990; Kamwendo et al. 1991; Johansson 1995; Lagerström et al. 1995; Bru et al. 1996; Zettenberg et al. 1997). However, Ahlberg-Hultén et al. (1995), Bernard et al. (1994), and Kamwendo et al. (1991) failed to confirm all of these results.

Viikari-Juntera et al. (1994) found an odds ratio of 1.7 for the relationship between low job satisfaction and the development of severe neck pain, but could not confirm this relationship for other neck-related outcome measures. Zettenberg et al. (1997) reported a significant association between low job satisfaction and self-reported neck symptoms, but Kilbom et al. (1986) did not find a significant association between job satisfaction and neck pain.

Another psychosocial factor investigated in several studies is influence and control over one's work. Bernard et al. (1994) failed to find a significant association between this factor and neck pain, as did Lagerström et al. (1995) and Ahlberg-Hultén et al. (1995). On the other hand, Kamwendo et al. (1991) did report a significant association between the ability to influence work conditions and the occurrence of neck pain. Skov et al. (1996) and Johansson (1995) reported odds ratios of 1.44 and 1.27, respectively, indicating an association between low influence and control over one's work and neck pain.

Mixed results have been reported for the relationship between diversity of work tasks and neck pain. While Bernard et al. (1994), Hales et al. (1994), and Tharr (1995) reported a positive relationship between increased diversity and neck pain, Skov et al. (1996) showed the opposite result. According to Skov and colleagues, low diversity of tasks is related to a higher incidence of neck pain. Kamwendo et al. (1991) found no significant association. Results were also mixed for other psychosocial factors including work content, qualitative demands, job security, work pressure, and rest-break opportunities. To summarize, the literature addresses many work-related risk factors, but the re-

sults are varied. However, it is clear that both physical and psychosocial factors play a role in the development of neck pain.

Non-work-related risk factors for neck pain

Dartigues et al. (1988) showed an odds ratio of 0.4 for strenuous activity during leisure time in relation to neck pain. Linton (1990), Skov et al. (1996), Kilbom et al. (1986), Lau et al. (1996), Andersen and Gaardboe (1993), and Viikari-Juntera et al. (1994) could find no significant association between neck pain and physical activity during leisure time. Mundt et al. (1993) reported odds ratios varying between 0.59 and 1.87 for the relationship between participating in different sports and herniated cervical disk, and measured an overall score for sports participation, reporting an odds ratio of 0.39 for the relationship between this factor and the occurrence of herniated cervical disk. Lagerström et al. (1995) found that low physical fitness is significantly associated with neck pain.

Other non-work-related factors that were significantly associated with neck pain according to at least one study were: smoking, alcohol consumption, anxiety, depression, insomnia, conflicts related to friends and family, eating habits, annual driving distance, parity, and body mass index. Most of these risk factors were examined in other studies with sometimes contradictory results. For example, Lagerström et al. (1995) and Mäkelä et al. (1991) both found no significant relationship between smoking and neck pain, in contrast to Linton (1990) and Viikari-Juntera et al. (1994), who found an association between current smoking and neck pain.

CONCLUSIONS

The literature describes many potential risk factors for neck pain. We reviewed the studies with the highest method scores, including 3 longitudinal studies and 20 cross-sectional studies. It is difficult to conclude from cross-sectional studies whether there is a causal relationship between risk factors and the occurrence of neck pain. In summarizing work-related risk factors, we may conclude that physical load factors (for example vibration, twisting and flexion of the neck, sitting posture, and heavy lifting) are important predictors of neck pain, and that psychosocial factors at work are also important (for example work variance, work pressure, and lack of decision-making possibilities). Results concerning the relationship between neck pain and non-work-related risk factors are mostly inconclusive.

SCOPE FOR PREVENTION

Prevention of neck pain should in theory primarily focus on the populations at risk (women, older persons, and certain occupational groups). While certain work-related physical factors are inevitable, other factors can certainly be modified (for example, by adjusting ergonomic factors in the workplace). By changing the work environment of an individual, psychosocial factors at work may also change. Furthermore, many non-work-related risk factors for neck pain are modifiable and may offer the possibility of prevention.

At the same time, the profile of persons at risk for neck pain is still far from clear. The development of effective prevention programs is therefore still in its early phase.

CHALLENGES FOR THE FUTURE

Only three prospective cohort studies met the criteria for inclusion in this review. To identify the causal relationships between predictors and outcome (neck pain), prospective study designs are clearly needed. Furthermore, most of the studies described in this chapter used subjective measures for the exposure assessment. Few researchers described the quality of the methods used to estimate exposure. Most studies were based on questionnaires.

In summary, future research on risk factors for neck pain should be prospective, with objective, standardized, high-quality measurements to estimate exposure, and must address not only physical factors at the workplace, but also psychosocial factors at work and non-work-related factors.

REFERENCES

Abbot P, Rounsefell B, Fraser R, Goss A. Intractable neck pain. *Clin J Pain* 1990; 6:26–31.

Abenhaim L, Suissa S, Rossignol M. Risk of recurrence of occupational back pain over three years follow-up. *Occup Environ Med* 1988; 45:829–833.

Ahlberg-Hultén GK, Theorell T, Sigala F. Social support, job strain and musculoskeletal pain among health care personnel. *Scand J Work Environ Health* 1995; 21:435–439.

Andersen JH, Gaardboe O. Prevalence of persistent neck and upper limb pain in a historical cohort of sewing machine operators. *Am J Ind Med* 1993; 24:677–687.

Andersson HI, Ejlertsson G, Leden I, Rosenberg C. Chronic pain in a geographically defined general population: studies of differences in age, gender, social class, and pain localization. *Clin J Pain* 1993; 9:174–182.

Anonymous. Pain in the neck and arm: a multi centre trial of the effects of physiotherapy. *BMJ* 1966; 1:253–258.

Ariëns GAM, Van Mechelen W, Bongers PB, Bouter LM, Van der Wal G. Physical risk factors for neck pain: a systematic review. Submitted.

Berg M, Sandén Å, Torell G, Järvholm B. Persistence of musculoskeletal symptoms: a longitudinal study. *Ergonomics* 1988; 1:1281–1285.

Bergqvist U, Wolgast E, Nilsson B, Voss M. The influence of VDT work on musculoskeletal disorders. *Ergonomics* 1995; 38:754–762.

Bernard B, Sauter S, Fine L, Petersen M, Hales T. Job task and psychosocial risk factors for work-related musculoskeletal disorders among newspaper employees. *Scand J Work Environ Health* 1994; 20:417–426.

Bjelle A, Hagberg M, Michaelsson G. Occupational and individual factors in acute shoulder-neck disorders among industrial workers. *Br J Ind Med* 1981; 38:356–363.

Borghouts JAJ, Koes BW, Bouter LM. The clinical course and prognostic factors of non-specific neck pain: a systematic review. *Pain* 1998; 77:1–13.

Bovenzi M, Zadini A, Franzinelli A, Borgogni F. Occupational musculoskeletal disorders in the neck and upper limbs of forestry workers exposed to hand-arm vibration. *Ergonomics* 1991; 34:547–562.

Bovim G, Schrader H, Sand T. Neck pain in the general population. *Spine* 1994; 19:1307–1309.

Brattberg G, Thorslund M, Wikman A. The prevalence of pain in a general population. The results of a postal survey in a county of Sweden. *Pain* 1989; 37:215–222.

Bru E, Mykletun RJ, Svebak S. Work-related stress and musculoskeletal pain among female hospital staff. *Work Stress* 1996; 10:309–321.

Ceccherelli F, Altafini L, Lo Castro G, et al. Diode laser in cervical myofascial pain: a double-blind study versus placebo. *Clin J Pain* 1989; 5:301–304.

Coan RM, Wong G, Coan PL. The acupuncture treatment of neck pain: a randomized controlled study. *Am J Chin Med* 1982; 4:326–332.

Dartigues JF, Henry P, Puymirat E, et al. Prevalence and risk factors of recurrent cervical pain syndrome in a working population. *Neuroepidemiology* 1988; 7:99–105.

Ekberg K, Bjorkqvist B, Malm P, et al. Case-control study of risk factors for disease in the neck and shoulder area. *Occup Environ Med* 1994; 51:262–266.

Foley-Nolan D, Barry C, Coughlan RJ, O'Connor P, Roden D. Pulsed high frequency (27 MHz) electromagnetic therapy for persistent neck pain: a double blind, placebo-controlled study of 20 patients. *Orthopedics* 1990; 13:445–451.

Goldie I, Landquist A. Evaluation of the effects of different forms of physiotherapy in cervical pain. *Scand J Rehabil Med* 1970; 2–3:117–121.

Gore DR, Sepic SB, Gardner GM, Murray MP. Neck pain: a long-term follow-up of 205 patients. *Spine* 1987; 12:1–5.

Hagberg M, Wegman DH. Prevalence rates and odds ratios of shoulder-neck diseases in different occupational groups. *Br J Ind Med* 1987; 44:602–610.

Hales TR, Sauter SL, Peterson MR, et al. Musculoskeletal disorders among visual display terminal users in a telecommunications company. *Ergonomics* 1994; 37:1603–1621.

Horvath J, Fellmann N. Behandlungsergebnisse mit Nifluril im doppelten Blindversuch bei degenerativen zervikalen Veränderungen mit oder ohne Zervikalsyndrom. *Praxis* 1969; 42:1342–1345.

Howe DH, Newcombe RG, Wade MT. Manipulation of the cervical spine: a pilot study. *J Roy Coll Gen Pract* 1983; 33:574–579.

Ignatius YTS, Yee TY, Yan LT. Self–reported musculoskeletal problems amongst typist and possible risk factors. *J Hum Ergol* 1993; 22:83–93.

Jacobsson L, Lindgarde F, Manthorpe R. The commonest rheumatic complaints of over six weeks' duration in a twelve-month period in a defined Swedish population. *Scand J Rheumatology* 1989; 18:353–360.

Jensen I, Nygren Å, Gamberale F, Goldie I, et al. The role of the psychologist in multidisciplinary treatments for chronic neck and shoulder pain: a controlled cost–effectiveness study. *Scand J Rehabil Med* 1995; 27:19–26.

Johansson JÅ. Psychosocial work factors, physical work load and associated musculoskeletal symptoms among home care workers. *Scand J Psych* 1995; 36:113–129.

Jonsson BG, Persson J, Kilbom A. Disorders of the cervicobrachial region among female workers in the electronics industry: a two-year follow-up. *Int J Ind Ergonomics* 1988; 3:1–12.

Kamwendo K, Linton S, Mororits U. Neck and shoulder disorders in medical secretaries. *Scand J Rehab Med* 1991; 23:127–133.

Kilbom Å, Persson J, Jonsson BG. Disorders of the cervicobrachial region among female workers in the electronics industry. *Int J Ind Ergonomics* 1986;1:37–47.

Lagerström M, Wenemark M, Hagberg M, Hjelm EW, The Moses Study Group. Occupational and individual factors related to musculoskeletal symptoms in five body regions among Swedish nursing personnel. *Int Arch Occup Environ Health* 1995; 68:27–35.

Lau EMC, Sham A, Wong KC. The prevalence and risk factors for neck pain in Hong Kong Chinese. *J Public Health Med* 1996; 18:396–399.

Levoska S, Keinänen-Kiukaanniemi S. Active or passive physiotherapy for occupational cervicobrachial disorders? A comparison of two treatment methods with 1-year follow-up. *Arch Phys Med Rehabil* 1993; 74:425–430.

Linton S. Risk factors for neck and back pain in a working population in Sweden. *Work and Stress* 1990; 4:41–49.

Loy TT. Treatment of cervical spondylosis. Electro acupuncture versus physiotherapy. *Med J Austr* 1983; 2:32–34.

Mäkelä M, Heliövaara M, Sievers K, et al. Prevalence, determinants, and consequences of chronic neck pain in Finland. *Am J Epidemiol* 1991; 134:1356–1367.

Mundt DJ, Kelsey JL, Golden AL, et al. An epidemiologic study of sports and weight lifting as possible risk factors for herniated lumbar and cervical discs. *Am J Sports Med* 1993; 21:854–860.

Nordemar R, Thörner C. Treatment of acute cervical pain. A comparative group study. *Pain* 1981; 10:93–101.

Petrie JP, Hazleman BL. A controlled study of acupuncture in neck pain. *Br J Rheumatol* 1986; 25:271–275.

Revel M, Minguet M, Gergoy P, Vaillant P, Manuel J. Changes in cervicocephalic kinesthesia after a proprioceptive rehabilitation program in patients with neck pain: a randomized controlled study. *Arch Phys Med Rehabil* 1994; 75:895–899.

Rosecrance JC, Cook TM, Wadsworth CT. Prevalence of musculoskeletal disorders and related job factors in 900 newspaper workers. In: Kumar S (Ed). *Advances in Industrial Ergonomics and Safety*. Taylor and Frances, 1992.

Rossignol M, Suissa S, Abeheim L. Working disability due to occupational back pain: Three-year follow-up of 2,300 compensated

workers in Quebec. *J Occup Environ Med* 1988; 30:502–505.

Rundcrantz B-L, Johnsson B, Moritz U. Pain and discomfort in the musculoskeletal system among dentists. A prospective study. *Swed Dent J* 1991; 15:219–228.

Schibye B, Skov T, Ekner D, Christiansen JU, Sjogaard G. Musculoskeletal symptoms among sewing machine operators. *Scand J Environ Health* 1995; 21:427–434.

Skov T, Borg V, Orhede E. Psychosocial and physical risk factors for musculoskeletal disorders of the neck, shoulders, and lower back in salespeople. *Occup Environ Med* 1996; 53:351–356.

Sloop PR, Smith DS, Goldenberg E, Doré C. Manipulation for chronic neck pain. A double-blind controlled study. *Spine* 1982; 7:532–535.

Spitzer WO, Leblanc F, Dupuis (Eds). Scientific approach to the assessment and management of activity-related spinal disorders. *Spine* 1987; 7(Suppl):1–59.

Spitzer WO, et al. Scientific monograph of the Quebec task force on whiplash-associated disorders: redefining "whiplash" and its management. *Spine* 1995; 20(Suppl).

Takala J, Sievers K, Klaukka T. Rheumatic symptoms in the middle-aged population in southwestern Finland. *Scand J Rheumatology* 1982; 47(Suppl):15–29.

Takala E-P, Viikari-Juntura E, Tynkkynen E-M. Does group gymnastics at the workplace help in neck pain? *Scand J Rehabil Med* 1994; 26:17–20.

Takala E-P, Viikari-Juntura E, Moneta GB, Saarenmaa K, Kaivanto K. Seasonal variation in neck and shoulder symptoms. *Scand J Work Environ Health* 1992; 18:257–261.

Tellnes G. Duration of episodes of sickness Certification. *Scand J Prim Health Care* 1989; 7:237–244.

Tharr D. Evaluation of work-related musculoskeletal disorders and job stress among teleservice center representatives. *Appl Occup Environ Hyg* 1995; 10:812–817.

Thorsen H, Gam AM, Svensson BH, et al. Low level laser therapy for myofacial pain in the neck and shoulder girdle. A double-blind, cross-over study. *Scand J Rheumatol* 1992; 21:139–142.

Van Tulder MW, Koes BW, Bouter LM. A cost-of-illness study of back pain in the Netherlands. *Pain* 1995; 62:233–240.

Ursin H, Endresen IM, Ursin G. Psychological factors and self-reports of muscle pain. *Eur J Appl Physiol* 1988; 57:282–290.

Vasseljen O, Johansen BM, Westgaard RH. The effect of pain reduction on perceived tension and EMG-recorded trapezius muscle activity in workers with shoulder and neck pain. *Scand J Rehabil Med* 1995; 27:243–252.

Viikari-Juntera EJ, Vuori J, Silverstein B, et al. A life-long prospective study on the role of psychosocial factors in neck-shoulder and low-back pain. *Spine* 1991; 16:1056–1061.

Viikari-Juntura E, Riihimaki H, Videman T, Mutanen P. Neck trouble in machine operating, dynamic physical work and sedentary work: a prospective study on occupational and individual risk factors. *J Clin Epidemiol* 1994; 47:1411–1422.

Westerling D, Jonsson B. Pain from the neck-shoulder region and sick leave. *Scand J Soc Med* 1980; 8:131–136.

Zettenberg C, Forsberg A, Hansson E, et al. Neck and upper extremity problems in car assembly workers. A comparison of subjective complaints, work satisfaction, physical examination and gender. *Int J Ind Erg* 1997; 19:277–289.

Correspondence to: Geertje A. M. Ariëns, MSc, Institute for Research in Extramural Medicine, Department of Social Medicine, Vrije Universiteit, Van der Boechorststraat 7, 1081 BT Amsterdam, The Netherlands. Tel: +31-20-4445986; Fax: +31-20-4448387; email: g.ariens.emgo@ med.vu.nl.

Epidemiology of Pain, edited by
I.K. Crombie, IASP Press, Seattle, © 1999.

17

Shoulder Pain

Daniëlle A.W.M. van der Windt[a] and Peter R. Croft[b]

[a]*Institute for Research in Extramural Medicine, Vrije Universiteit, Amsterdam, The Netherlands; and*
[b]*Primary Care Sciences Research Centre, School of Postgraduate Medicine, Keele University, Hartshill,
Stoke-on-Trent, United Kingdom*

EPIDEMIOLOGICAL STUDIES OF SHOULDER PAIN

Shoulder pain is a common and disabling problem. Pain and loss of motion often result in functional disability and loss of productivity at work. Insurance data from Sweden show that neck–shoulder pain has become a considerable health problem (Nygren et al. 1995). In 1994 approximately 18% of total paid sick leave for musculoskeletal disorders was used for neck and shoulder problems.

The number of epidemiological studies reporting on the occurrence of shoulder pain and on potential risk factors has greatly increased in the last decade. This chapter provides an overview of studies on the prevalence of shoulder pain in the general population, in primary health care, and in the workplace. It evaluates the literature on risk factors for shoulder pain, including studies conducted in an occupational setting and studies of individual risk factors (such as age, gender, and education) and psychosocial factors (such as personality characteristics, stress, job satisfaction, and social support).

CASE DEFINITION

Defining shoulder pain for epidemiological studies presents a number of difficulties. Shoulder pain may be the result of many disorders within the shoulder complex, but it can also be caused by referred pain from internal organs and from the cervical or thoracic spine. The lack of generally accepted criteria for the diagnostic classification of shoulder pain adds to the confusion. Several methods have been proposed for classifying shoulder pain into specific patho-anatomical diagnostic categories, but there is little evidence to show that such groupings are reliable or valid (Cyriax 1981; Neer 1983; Hedtmann and Fett 1989; Uhthoff and Sarkar 1990). Indeed, some studies have questioned whether some of these classifications can be repeated (Bamji et al. 1996; Buchbinder et al. 1996; Liesdek et al. 1997).

Few epidemiological surveys have attempted to distinguish between specific shoulder disorders (rotator cuff tendinitis, biceps tendinitis, impingement syndromes, and adhesive capsulitis, for example). Researchers usually establish the presence of shoulder pain by asking study participants directly about pain in the shoulder area. However, pain arising from the shoulder complex may be felt in a wide area, including the neck and arm, and may be misinterpreted. Pope and colleagues (1997a) demonstrated that the occurrence of shoulder pain in a general population may range between 31% and 48% across four case definitions, using different combinations of direct questions and pain drawings. They also showed that the prevalence of shoulder pain decreased to 20% when the case definition included at least some associated disability as measured by a standardized shoulder disability questionnaire.

This chapter presents the case definition of shoulder pain along with the results of the studies, as the definition varies considerably among studies. Information is restricted to data presented for shoulder pain only, although many studies, particularly those conducted in an occupational setting, have been aimed at combined neck and shoulder symptoms. Some of these studies are of relatively good quality in terms of methods used, and provide highly relevant data on risk factors. The references of relevant studies on combined shoulder–neck pain are listed in Appendix I.

SEARCH STRATEGY

A MEDLINE literature search of the period January 1, 1966, to November 30, 1997, was conducted, using the following key words: shoulder, shoulder joint, pain, incidence, prognosis, prevalence, incidence, survey, cross-sectional, cohort, case-control, case-referent, determinant, predictor, risk factor, etiology, aetiology, causative, and prevention. All relevant MEDLINE citations were retrieved and examined. The references of all retrieved articles were screened for additional publications. A paper was included in the review if it had been written as a full report (i.e., not as an abstract or a letter to the editor), if it had been published in the English language, and if it described a study on the frequency of shoulder pain or on risk factors for the development of shoulder pain (other pain syndromes could have been included, but data on shoulder pain had to have been presented separately). Papers reporting on acute trauma-related injuries (fractures, dislocations, and ruptures) were excluded.

A total of 131 relevant citations were retrieved. Screening of the references resulted in an additional 84 citations. Of the 215 papers, 132 did not meet the selection criteria: 53 appeared to be reviews, 12 referred to patient series or studies in laboratory conditions, 4 reported on the prognosis of shoulder pain, 3 reported on acute injuries, 45 did not report data on shoulder pain separately, and 15 were excluded for more than one reason. A total of 83 papers were selected for review in this chapter.

FREQUENCY OF SHOULDER PAIN

CRITICAL APPRAISAL

Many lists of criteria are available for the critical appraisal of intervention studies (randomized trials), but only a few have been designed for observational studies. The criteria used in this chapter were based on textbooks on epidemiology and review articles on the etiology of musculoskeletal disorders (Rothman 1986; Stock 1991; Wacholder et al. 1992; Bongers et al. 1993; Sommerich et al. 1993; Hales and Bernard 1996).

Table I
Criteria for the critical appraisal of studies on the frequency of shoulder pain

A) Well-defined study purpose (1).

B) Adequate description of the study population: setting, selection criteria, age/gender, and size (1).

C) Definition of pain: shoulder pain is diagnosed according to well-defined explicit criteria, using a standardized questionnaire (1), interview (1), or physical examination (2). Registers in which diagnosis is recorded using a nonstandardized procedure are considered inadequate.

D) Appropriate study design: all patients of the target population, random sample, representative sample, or check for generalizability (2).

E) Adequacy of sample size: > 250 (2).

F) Appropriateness of analysis: prevalence rates (point prevalence, period prevalence, or lifetime prevalence) or incidence rates are presented with adequate time frame (1). Response rates should be reported (1).

G) Validity of interpretation of findings: discussion of the results in light of potential drawbacks of the study (selection bias, nonresponse, etc.) (1).

Note: Numbers in parentheses are method scores.

All papers reporting on the frequency of shoulder pain were critically reviewed according to a standardized set of methodological criteria, referring to the formulation of the study objective, definition of pain, appropriate study design, adequacy of sample size, appropriateness of analyses, and validity of the interpretation of findings. These criteria are described in detail in Table I.

Each study was assigned a total method score by summing the weighting scores for all criteria. Most criteria received a weighting score of 1, but three criteria received a score of 2. An appropriate sampling procedure was considered important, so as to provide a representative sample of the target population (D in Table I). Physical examinations were preferred to evaluation by standardized questionnaires (C), and an adequate sample size was considered to be important to obtain a precise estimate of the frequency of shoulder pain (E). Defining an adequate sample size depends on variables such as the expected proportion of cases in the target population, the degree of precision required, and the practical limitations of the study setting. We decided arbitrarily that a sample size of at least 250 was adequate to obtain a sufficiently precise estimate (standard error not exceeding approximately 15% of the estimated proportion). The maximum attainable score for studies on the frequency of shoulder pain was 11 points.

RESULTS

Of the selected papers, 68 present data on the frequency of shoulder pain. The designs and results of these studies are presented separately for studies conducted in the general population or in primary care (Table II), an occupational setting (Table III), a specific patient population or hospital setting (Table IV), and in athletics (Table V). The most frequent shortcomings concerned an assessment of shoulder pain limited to questionnaires or consultation of records (criterion C, 39 of 68 studies), inadequate sample size (F, 30 studies), and inadequate discussion of potential selection bias or consequences of nonresponse (G, 27 studies). The results of the quality assessment for each study in the review are presented in Appendix II.

The median method score was quite high (9 points of a maximum score of 11) for studies conducted in general population samples. Point prevalences in samples from Western populations under 65 years of age range between 1.9% in a sample of Finnish residents (Mäkelä 1993) and between 6% and 26% in a random sample of Stockholm residents (Allander 1974). Studies in the elderly report higher estimates, between 5% (Mäkelä et al. 1993) and 34% (Chakravarty and Webley 1993). Period prevalences (over the past year) vary between 6.7% (Jacobsson et al. 1989) and 61% (Westerling and Jonsson 1980). The results of the studies are difficult to compare because of the wide variation in study setting, target population, case definition, and response rate. However, nearly all studies reported a higher frequency of shoulder pain with increasing age, and a somewhat higher frequency in women. Finally, relatively low estimates were reported for the Philippines (1–2%, Manahan et al. 1985) and for Pima Indians (6%, Jacobsson et al. 1996), whereas a study conducted in South Africa resulted in a relatively high estimate of point prevalence (22%, Meyers et al. 1982).

Much attention has been directed toward shoulder pain in occupational settings (38 of 68 studies). The results of the studies are difficult to compare because of widely varying case definitions and study settings. Studies with a relatively high method score (a median score of at least 9) report a higher frequency of shoulder pain for women compared to men (Dimberg et al. 1989), for a heavy work load (Dimberg et

al. 1989; Johansson and Rubenowitz 1994), for the use of vibrating tools (Dimberg et al. 1989), and for certain job types—dentists and dental hygienists (Rundcrantz et al. 1990; Liss et al. 1995), secretaries (Kamwendo et al. 1991), clerical workers (Rossignol et al. 1987), professional drivers (Backman 1983), employees in fish-processing plants (Ohlsson et al. 1994), and construction workers (Stenlund et al. 1992, 1993).

Studies conducted in specific patient populations (Table IV) show the frequency of shoulder pain to be considerably higher in diabetics and stroke patients (hemiplegic shoulder). Studies of athletes report frequent occurrence of shoulder pain in swimmers (Table V).

CONSEQUENCES

Most patients (90%) who consult a physician or therapist for shoulder pain are treated in primary care (van der Windt et al. 1996). Nevertheless, the incidence of shoulder pain in primary care, 6.6–11.2 cases per 1000 registered patients per year (Croft 1993; van der Windt et al. 1995), appears to be much lower than the prevalence in the general population or in occupational settings. This means that many episodes may go unreported or that patients with chronic shoulder problems may stop visiting their doctor. Considering the high prevalence of shoulder pain in occupational settings, the economic costs caused by loss of productivity (so-called indirect costs) are probably much higher than the direct costs of medical care. So far, little information is available on the economic costs of shoulder pain. Data based on Swedish insurance registers, provided by Nygren and colleagues (1995), suggest that the percentage of paid sick leave for neck–shoulder pain is approaching that for low back pain. Pain and restriction of mobility caused by shoulder problems often cause sleep disturbances and functional disability. Inability to work, loss of productivity, and incapacity to carry out household activities can be a considerable burden to the patient and to society.

PROGNOSIS

Studies from primary care show that 40–50% of patients report persisting or recurrent symptoms 1 year after first consulting a general practitioner (Croft et al. 1996; Sobel and Winters 1996; van der Windt et al. 1996). These observations confirm reports of poor

Table II
Results of studies on the prevalence of shoulder pain in the general population or in a general practice

Reference	Study Type*	Disease Definition	Source of Sample	Sample Size	Type of Prevalence Estimate	Prevalence
Allander 1974	CS (11)	Painful shoulder (pain and restricted ROM)	Random sample of Stockholm residents	Q: 15268, R = 97.8%; EX: 4195, R = 90.5%	Point (annual incidence)	Men: 31–35 y, 8% (0.9); 42–46 y, 15% (2.5); 56–60 y, 26% (1.1); 70–74 y, 20% (1.6). Women: 31–35 y, 6% (0.8); 42–46 y, 15% (2.1); 56–60 y, 18% (1.1); 70–74 y, 15% (0.9)
Jacobsson et al. 1989	CS (11)	Subacromial shoulder pain >6 wk	Random sample of Malmö residents	Q: 900, R = 77%, n = 696; EX: R = 61%, n = 552	Period (past year) (95% CI)	Q: 6.7% (4.4–9.1); men 4.3%, women 9.3%
Takala et al. 1982	CS (11)	Ache, stiffness, numbness or pain in the shoulder	Random sample of general population, Finland, 40–64 y	Q + EX: R = 93.3%, n = 1045 men, 1223 women	Period (past year)	<50 y 11%, >50 y 22%; women: left 15%, right 19%; men 17%
Ekberg et al. 1995	CS (10)	Subjective shoulder symptoms	Random sample of semi-rural community, Sweden	NQ: 900, R = 73%, 18 excluded, n = 637	Period (6 mo)	Men 35%, women 40%
Jacobsson et al. 1996	CS (10)	Shoulder pain and restricted ROM	Pima Indians >20 y	4719, EX: 4230	Point, sex and age adjusted (95% CI)	Pain 5.9% (5.1–6.6); restricted ROM 8.5 % (7.7–9.4); both 4.4% (3.8–5.0)
Pope et al. 1997a	CS (10)	Shoulder pain; 4 case definitions	Random sample from general practice, UK	Q: 500, R = 66%; EX: 74%, n = 232	Period (past month)	34%; shoulder pain with any disability 20%
Bergenudd et al. 1988; Bergenudd and Johnell 1991; Bergenudd and Nilsson 1994	PC (9)	>24 h of shoulder pain in last month, ROM <145° abduction	Malmö residents, all elementary school third graders, 1938	1983; Q: 1362, R = 91%, n = 1070; EX: 830, R = 69%, n = 574	Period (month)	14%; men 13%, women 15%
Chard et al. 1991	CS (9)	Specific shoulder disorders	Random sample from general practices, >70 y, UK	Q + EX: 644	Point	Complaints 26%; confirmed diagnosis 21%
Cunningham and Kelsey 1984	CS (9)	Self-reported shoulder symptoms	HANES I: random sample 25–74 y, USA	6913	Point	Q 6.7%; EX 3.0%
Mäkelä et al. 1993	CS (9)	Shoulder disorder	Representative sample of residents, Finland	Q + EX: 8000, R = 90%, n = 7217	Point	30–64 y, 1.9%; ≥ 65 y, 4.6%
Westerling and Jonsson 1980	CS (9)	Pain, tenderness, stiffness in shoulders	Sample of residents, Stockholm, 18–65 y	Q: 2537, R = 85%	Period (past year)	61%

(continued)

Table II
Continued

Reference	Study Type*	Disease Definition	Source of Sample	Sample Size	Type of Prevalence Estimate	Prevalence
Van der Windt et al. 1995	PC (9)	Specific shoulder disorders, GP diagnosis	All incident cases from 11 general practices, The Netherlands	35,150 in practice population, 392 cases	Cumulative incidence (95% CI)	11.2/1000/y (1.1–12.3); men 8.4/1000/y, women 11.1/1000/y
Bergström et al. 1985	PC (8)	Shoulder complaints	Sample of 70-year olds, Göteborg (born 1901–1902)	1980; Q: 134, R = 96%, n = 129; EX: n = 99	Period (?)	16%; men 15%, women 16%; only 31% restricted ROM
Chakra-varty and Webley 1993	CS (8)	Specific shoulder disorders	Random sample from general practice >65 y, UK	EX: 65–74 y, 50; > 75 y, 50	Point (?)	34%; 9% severe, 30% disability
Manahan et al. 1985	CS (7)	Present shoulder pain	Sample of residents, Philippines	Q: 2000, R = 84%, n = 1685	Point	Men 0.9%, women 1.6%; ≥ 15 y: men 1.7%, women 2.8%
Meyers et al. 1982	CS (7)	Specific shoulder disorders	Census in rural and urban South Africa	Q + EX: rural, R = 88.1%, n = 127; urban, R = 85.3%, n = 35	Point Lifetime	Point: rural 22%, urban 22.8%; lifetime: rural 71%, urban 51.4%

Abbreviations: CS = cross-sectional; EX = physical examination; GP = general practitioner; NQ = Nordic Questionnaire; PC = prospective cohort; Q = questionnaire; R = response; ROM = range of motion.
*Numbers in parentheses are method scores.

long-term outcome of shoulder disorders in hospital studies (Reeves 1975; Binder et al. 1984; Chard et al. 1988; Shaffer et al. 1992) and in two population surveys in the elderly (Chard et al. 1991; Vecchio et al. 1995). Various patient characteristics can modify recovery from shoulder disorders. Diabetes mellitus (Loew 1994; Pollock et al. 1994), shoulder pain accompanied by neck pain (van der Windt et al. 1996), increasing age (Mulcahy et al. 1994; Yamanaka and Matsumoto 1994), severe symptoms at presentation (Bartolozzi et al. 1994; Croft et al. 1996), and involvement of the dominant side (Binder et al. 1984; Chard et al. 1988) have all been implicated in a poor prognosis. Mild trauma preceding the onset of symptoms (Yamanaka and Matsumoto 1994; van der Windt et al. 1996), early presentation to health care professionals (Hazleman 1972; Chard et al. 1988; Bartolozzi et al. 1994; Croft et al. 1996; van der Windt et al. 1996), overuse through practicing sports or hobbies (Chard et al. 1988; van der Windt et al. 1996), and acute onset (Hazleman 1972) seem to predict a favorable outcome.

The reasons for persistence and recurrence of shoulder pain can also include psychosocial or work-related factors. Increasing evidence shows that levels of distress are related to recovery from low back pain in primary care (Waddell 1987; Klenerman et al. 1995). This finding may also apply to chronic pain in general, including shoulder pain (Linton 1992). An occupational study of neck, shoulder, and arm problems has shown that long-term sick leave depended mostly on the work situation, rather than on individual patient characteristics (Ekberg and Wildhagen 1996). Patients on long-term sick leave perceived their work tasks to be monotonous, and complained of uncomfortable sitting positions, high demands for precision, high job constraints, few opportunities for stimulation and development in their jobs, and limited ability to exert their own influence on their work.

In conclusion, the risk of developing chronic shoulder pain warrants further investigation, but it seems to be related to multiple factors, including individual patient and disease characteristics and work-related and psychosocial factors.

Table III
Results of studies on the prevalence of shoulder pain in an occupational setting

Reference	Study Type*	Disease Definition	Source of Sample	Sample Size	Type of Prevalence Estimate	Prevalence
Hales et al. 1994	CS (11)	Specific shoulder disorders	Telephone companies, random sample of 5 job titles, USA	Q + EX: 573, R = 93%, n = 533, 13 excluded, n = 518	Point	Rotator cuff tendinitis 15%, bicipital tendinitis 6%, thoracic outlet syndrome 0.4%
Bernard et al. 1994	CS (10)	Work-related shoulder symptoms	Random sample, 3000 full-time newspaper employees, USA	Q: 1050, R = 93%, n = 973	Period (year)	17%
Dimberg et al. 1989	CS (10)	Shoulder symptoms, specific diagnoses	Volvo Flygmotor, all employees, Sweden	NQ: 2933, R = 96%, n = 2814	Point	13%; men 12%, women 20%; light work 11%, heavy work 17%, vibrating tools 19%
Johansson and Rubeno-witz 1994	CS (10)	(Work-related) shoulder pain	Random sample, metal industry, Sweden	NQ: 241 blue collar, 209 white collar, R ± 90%	Period (past year) 95% CI	Any shoulder pain: blue collar 44% (38–50), white collar 39% (32–46). Work-related: blue collar 36% (29–42), white collar 26% (19–32)
Kamwendo et al. 1991	CS (10)	Shoulder pain	Female secretaries, Sweden	NQ: 438, R = 96%, n = 420	Point (past 7 d); period (past year)	Point 34%, period 62%; 13% prevents work in past year
Lagerström et al. 1995	CS (10)	Shoulder symptoms	All nursing personnel, hospital, Sweden	Q: 821, R = 84%, n = 688	Point	31%; severe symptoms 11%
Liss et al. 1995	CS (10)	Shoulder symptoms	Dental hygienists (DH) and dental assistants (DA), Canada	NQ: 2142 DH, R = 50%, n = 941; 304 DA, R = 50.5%, n = 109	Period (past year) Point (past week) OR (95% CI)	Period: DH 49.8%, DA 26.9% (OR = 2.4; 1.4–4.2): point: DH 24.7%, DA 11.1% (OR = 2.5; 1.3–4.7)
McCor-mack et al. 1990	CS (10)	Miscellaneous shoulder conditions	Random sample manufacturing industry, USA	Q: 2261, R = 90.5%, n = 2047; Q + EX: n = 956, R = 94%, n = 895	Point	Q + EX: 5%
Näyhä et al. 1994	CS (10)	Shoulder pain on movement, due to snowmobile driving	Male reindeer herders, Finland	Q: 3720, R = 73%, n = 2705; 16–64 y: 1793	Period (lifetime, past year)	Lifetime 38% (20–60%), increasing with use; past year 22% (18–29%), adjusted for age
Mackay-Rossignol et al. 1987	CS (10)	Almost always stiffness or soreness/missed work	Random sample of worksites, clerical workers	Q: 1545, R = 67–100%	Period (past 2 mo)	39–43%
Sauter et al. 1991	CS (10)	Shoulder discomfort, almost constant	Two government agencies, USA	Q: n = 992, R = 91%, n = 902; 539 VDT users	Point	Right 15%, left 10%
Shugars et al. 1987	CS (10)	Shoulder pain	Sample of American Dental Association	Q: 2000, R = 66%, 64 excluded, n = 1253	Period (past year)	16%
Skov et al. 1996	CS (10)	Shoulder symptoms	Random sample of salespeople, Denmark	NQ: 1991, R = 66%, n = 1306	Period (past year)	Men 35%, women 47%

(continued)

Table III
Continued

Reference	Study Type*	Disease Definition	Source of Sample	Sample Size	Type of Prevalence Estimate	Prevalence
Backman 1983	CS (9)	Shoulder pain	Male professional drivers, Finland	Q: 1453, R = 80%; EX: 633 males	Period (past month)	70%; ages 30–34 y: 65%, 25–29 y: 63%, 40–44 y: 69%, 45–49 y: 74%, 50–54 y: 78%
Van der Beek et al. 1993	CS (9)	Regular pain/stiffness shoulder	Random sample of truck drivers, The Netherlands	Q: 1000, R = 55%	Point (?)	26%
Ohlsson et al. 1994	CS (9)	Shoulder symptoms	Fish-processing plants, Sweden	EX: 172 current + 208 former employees	Point	55% current employees, 33% former employees
Rund-crantz et al. 1990	CS (9)	Pain/discomfort shoulders	All dentists, Malmö, Sweden	Q: 395, R = 90.8%, n = 359	Period (past year)	Right 20%, left 10%, both shoulders 23%
Rund-crantz et al. 1991	PC (9)	Pain/discomfort shoulders	All dentists, Malmö, Sweden	Q: 315, R = 92%, n = 311	Period (1990); incidence (1987–1990)	Men 49%, women 73%; 17/100/2.5 y = 6.8/100/y
Punnett et al. 1985	CS (9)	Persistent pain for 1 mo during past year	Garment workers (G) and hospital employees (H), USA	G: 214, R = 84%, Q + EX: 179; H: R = 40%, Q + EX: 73	Period (past year) RR (95% CI)	G 19.6%, H 8.8%; RR = 2.2 (1.0–4.9)
Stenlund et al. 1992	CS (9)	Acromio-clavicular osteoarthritis	Random sample of construction workers, Sweden	EX: 54 bricklayers, 55 rock blasters, 98 foremen; R = 75–89%	Point	Bricklayers: right 59.3%, left 40.7%. Rock blasters: right 61.8%, left 23.4%. Foremen: right 61.8%, left 56.4%
Stenlund et al. 1993	CS (9)	Shoulder tendinitis	Random sample of construction workers, Sweden	EX: 54 bricklayers, 55 rock blasters, 98 foremen, R = 75–89%	Point	Bricklayers: right 14.8, left 11.1. Rock blasters: right 40%, left 33%. Foremen: right 17.1%, left 8.2%
Luopa-jarvi et al. 1979	CS (8)	Specific shoulder disorders	Female assembly line packers, shop assistants, Finland	Packers: 163, Q + EX: 152; assistants: 143, Q + EX:133	Point	Packers 11.8%, assistants 3.7%
Osborn et al. 1990	CS (8)	Shoulder pain	Random sample of dental hygienists, USA	Q: 493, R = 89%, n = 385	Period (past year)	19%
Palmer 1996	CS (8)	Shoulder complaints	Tomato trainers and tomato pickers, UK	NQ: 114, R = 94.7%	Point (past week); period (past year); OR (95% CI)	Point: 25.0%; trainers 35.7%, pickers 13.5%; OR = 3.6 (1.2–11.1). Period: 44.4%; trainers 64.3%, pickers 23.1%; OR = 5.9 (2.4–16.7)
Herberts et al. 1981	CS (7)	Supraspinatus tendinitis	Arendal shipyard Göteborg, all welders, all office workers aged >40 y	Q + EX: 131 welders, 561 office workers	Period (past year)	Welders: 27% (subsample verified by EX 12%); office: 2%
Milerad and Ekenvall 1990	CS (7)	Shoulder symptoms	Random sample dentists (D) and pharmacists (P), Sweden	NQ: 100 D, R = 99%; NQ: 100 P, R = 100%	Lifetime, RR (95% CI)	D 15%, P 4%; RR = 3.8 (1.2–10.3)

(continued)

Table III
Continued

Reference	Study Type*	Disease Definition	Source of Sample	Sample Size	Type of Prevalence Estimate	Prevalence
Wells et al. 1983	CS (7)	Current shoulder pain	Random sample of letter carriers (LCa/b), meter readers (MR), postal clerks (PCl), USA	LCa: 104 increased load, LCb: 92 no increase, MR: 76, PCl: 127 (Q)	Point	LCa 23%, LCb 13%, MR 7%, PCl 5% (adjusted for age, years on the job, Quetelet index, previous work)
Yu and Wong 1996	CS (7)	Discomfort or ache since start of current job	Employees Hong Kong bank, frequent/infrequent VDT users	90 frequent, R = 90%; 61 infrequent, R = 66%; Q: 121	Period (job duration)	16.5%; frequent VDT users 25%, infrequent VDT users 4%
Flodmark and Aase 1992	CS (6)	Shoulder symptoms	All blue-collar workers, ventilation shaft manufacturer, Sweden	NQ: 67, R = 87% n = 58	Period (past year)	40%
Jonsson et al. 1988	PC (6)	Moderate to severe symptoms/ change of symptoms	Female employees, assembly departments, Sweden	Q + EX: 96	Point	Baseline: 10%, 1 y: 16%, 2 y: 20% (10% at 2 y following job change)
Christen-sen 1986	CS (5)	Pain/discomfort in neck and shoulders, 8 d	Assembly plant, Denmark	Q: 36, R = 67%, n = 25	Period (past year)	40%; men 11%, women 56%
Magnus-sen et al. 1996	CS (5)	Shoulder pain	Random sample of male truck drivers, bus drivers, sedentary workers, USA/Sweden	NQ: truck drivers 117, bus drivers 111, sedentary 137	Period (?)	USA: bus 42%, truck 29%, sedentary 15%; Sweden: truck 33%, bus 41%, sedentary 14%
Sakibara et al. 1995	CS (5)	Shoulder stiffness, almost every day	Apple and pear farmers, Japan	65; EX: pears 65, apples 56	Point	Apples: 15–20%, pears: ±30%; tenderness: apples 28.8%, pears: 48.1%
Sokas et al. 1989	CS (5)	Shoulder ache during >6 wk	Participants in health promotion convention, garment workers, USA	517, R = 63%, n = 144 following exclusions	Period (?)	13.1%; comparison with general population (n = 6913): POR = 2.10 (1.30–3.40)
Viikari-Juntura 1983	CS (5)	Specific shoulder disorders	Slaughterhouse workers, Finland	EX: 113	Point	3.5%
Buckle 1987	CS (4)	Regular shoulder pain at least once a week	Chicken-proces-sing factory, UK	Q: 235, R = 61.3%, n = 144	Point; lifetime	Point 15%, lifetime 42%, medical treatment 14%
Sakibara et al. 1987	CS (4)	Shoulder stiffness, almost every day	Apple and pear farmers, Japan	62, R = 77%, Q: 48	Point	Thinning pears: men 45%, women 50% ; bagging pears: men 20%, women 35%; bagging apples: men –, women 20%
Hünting et al. 1981	CS (3)	Shoulder symptoms: tendomyotic pressure points on EX	Data entry, VDT use, typing, traditional office work, Switzerland	EX: n = 53, n = 109, n = 78, n = 54	Point	38%, 28%, 35%, 11%

Abbreviations: EX = physical examination; NQ = Nordic Questionnaire; PC = prospective cohort; POR = prevalence odds ratio; Q = questionnaire; R = response; RR = relative risk; VDT = video display terminal.

* Numbers in parentheses are method scores.

Table IV
Results of studies on the prevalence of shoulder pain in specific patient populations

Reference	Study Type*	Disease Definition	Source of Sample	Sample Size	Type of Prevalence Estimate	Prevalence
Mavrikakis et al. 1989	CS (9)	Calcific shoulder tendinitis	Inpatients, internal medicine department, Greece	EX (radiography): 824 diabetics type II, 320 nondiabetics	Point	Diabetics 31.8%, nondiabetics 10.3%
Sattar and Luqman 1985	CS (9)	Shoulder pain ≥3 mo, ROM <50%	Consecutive diabetics and nondiabetics in hospital, Kuwait	Q + EX: 100 diabetics, 100 controls	Point	Diabetics 19%, controls 3%
Nichols et al. 1979	CS (8)	Shoulder pain	UK wheelchair users; spinal cord injured	Q: 708, R = 73%, n = 517	Lifetime	51.4%; >1 mo duration, 42%
Bohannon et al. 1986	Retro-spective (6)	Hemiplegic shoulder, positive Fugl-Meyer test	Consecutive records of stroke patients, USA	Records: 50	Period (?)	72%
Brocklehurst et al. 1978	PC (6)	Other report	Surviving stroke patients, UK	135	Annual incidence	32%
Chard and Hazleman 1987	CS (5)	Shoulder disorders	Aged >70 y, admitted to emergency ward for other reasons	Q + EX: 100	Incidence (?) Point (?)	Men 16%, women 26%

Abbreviations: CS = cross-sectional; EX = physical examination, PC = prospective cohort; Q = questionnaire, R = response.
* Numbers in parentheses are method scores.

Table V
Results of studies on the prevalence of shoulder pain among athletes

Reference	Study Type*	Disease Definition	Source of Sample	Sample Size	Type of Prevalence Estimate	Prevalence
McMaster and Troup 1993	CS (10)	Shoulder pain interfering with training	Competitive swimmers, USA	Q: 13–14 y, 993; 15–16 y, 198; USA team, 71	Point	13–14 y, 10%; 15–16 y, 13%; team 26%
Stocker et al. 1995	CS (9)	Swimming-related shoulder pain ≥3 wk	Random sample collegiate/masters swimmers, USA	Q: R = 18%, collegiate 532, masters 395	Period (swimming career)	Collegiate 47%, masters 48%
Winge et al. 1989	PC (7)	Shoulder overuse/strain (no acute trauma)	Randomly sampled tennis team, Denmark	R = 86%, Q: 89	Incidence	17.4% of players per season
Beach et al. 1992	CS (5)	Shoulder pain	Swimmers, Pittsburgh University team, USA	± 46, R = 70% EX: n = 32	Lifetime Point	87%; 69% some pain, 31% pain affecting swimming
Lo et al. 1990	CS (5)	Shoulder impingement syndrome	Competitive and regular recreational athletes, Hong Kong	Q: 372, R = 100%	Point (?)	29%; any shoulder problems 44%
Richard-son et al. 1980	CS (5)	Shoulder pain	Competitive swimmers, USA	EX: 137	Period (swimming career)	42%, men 46%, women 40%; elite group: men 47%, women 57%

Abbreviations: CS = cross-sectional; EX = physical examination, PC = prospective cohort; Q = questionnaire, R = response.
* Numbers in parentheses are method scores.

CAUSES OF SHOULDER PAIN

CRITICAL APPRAISAL

Papers reporting on risk factors for shoulder pain were critically evaluated according to a standardized set of methodological criteria. As shown in Table VI, three types of designs can be distinguished in the studies of risk factors: cross-sectional (0 points), case-referent (1 point), and prospective cohort designs (2 points). Selection bias, information bias, and confounding variables can occur in all three designs, but they have less influence in prospective studies. However, because of demands on time, personnel, and financial resources, prospective designs are rare.

The risk of selection bias is high in cross-sectional studies because of health-related selection (the healthy worker effect). Furthermore, these designs generally do not describe the temporal relationship between exposure (risk factors) and disease. Evidence on risk factors is somewhat stronger when obtained from case-referent designs. Selection bias in case-referent designs can be prevented by selecting controls randomly from a subset of the general population, although this can be quite difficult to achieve. In case-referent designs an additional quality point was assigned when appropriate controls were selected (C).

Information bias may result in misclassification and an incorrect estimate of the strength of the association between risk factors and shoulder pain. Prevention of information bias is difficult, particularly in cross-sectional designs, but additional points were given to reward an attempt to obtain an objective assessment of either risk factors or shoulder pain by employing an independent observer or by using a blinded procedure (F).

Researchers should adjust for potential confounding variables by performing a stratified or multivariate analysis (H), and should select a sample large enough to evaluate several risk factors simultaneously with sufficient precision. Although sample-size calculations for etiological studies depend on a number of factors that may differ among study settings, approximately 100 cases should be sufficient to detect an odds ratio (OR) of 3.0, assuming a frequency of 20% of the exposure variable in the control group (G). The maximum attainable score for studies on risk factors for shoulder pain was 16 points.

Nonexperimental studies cannot establish a direct link between risk factors and shoulder pain. However,

Table VI
Criteria for the critical appraisal of studies on risk factors
for shoulder pain

A) Well-defined study purpose (1).

B) Adequate description of the study population: setting, selection criteria, age/gender, and size (1).

C) Appropriate study design: prospective cohort studies (2), case-referent studies (1), cross-sectional studies (0). (Case-referent designs are assigned an additional point if adequate referents are selected: random sample from source population or matched controls.)

D) Definition of pain: shoulder pain is diagnosed according to explicit criteria, using a standardized questionnaire (1), interview (1), or physical examination (2). Registers in which diagnosis is recorded using a nonstandardized procedure are considered inadequate (0).

E) Exposure: assessment of exposure variables (risk factors) in all participants according to explicit criteria, using a standardized procedure: questionnaire or interview (1), camera recordings (2), or observations (2).

F) Prevention of information bias: e.g., assessment of exposure variables (risk factors) or shoulder pain by an independent or blinded observer (2), who is unaware of the exposure or disease status.

G) Adequacy of sample size: at least 100 cases (sufficient to establish an odds ratio of 3.0 assuming a frequency of 20% of the exposure variable in the controls).

H) Appropriateness of analyses: control for exposure duration (if adequate) (1), potential confounders (1), and nonresponse or drop-out rate (1).

I) Validity of interpretation of findings: discussion of the results in light of potential drawbacks of the study (selection bias, information bias, nonresponse, etc.) (1).

using the results of studies with relatively high method scores, we evaluated the causality of risk factors according to the following criteria (Sommerich et al. 1993; Hales and Bernard 1996): the strength of the association (OR or relative risk ≥ 3), the consistency of the association across studies, the dose–response relationship between the exposure level and the frequency or severity of shoulder pain, the temporal relationship between risk factor and occurrence of shoulder pain, and the biological plausibility of the association.

RESULTS

The literature search identified 32 papers reporting on risk factors for shoulder pain: 24 cross-sectional studies, 7 case-referent designs, and 1 prospective cohort study. Unfortunately, case-referent studies and prospective cohort studies were scarce. Restricting our review to these studies would have limited this chap-

Table VII
Results of studies on risk factors for shoulder pain in the general population, including evaluation of psychosocial factors

Reference	Study Type*	Disease Definition	Source of Sample	Sample Size	Risk Factors and Strength of Association (95% CI)
Pope et al. 1997b	CR (10)	Shoulder pain > 24 h in past month, some disability	Random sample of patients registered with general practice, UK	39 cases; controls: random selection 1:5/1:6	Women: n.s.; men (logistic regression): occupational activity: weight one shoulder: RR = 5.5 (1.8–17.4), work above shoulder level: RR = 2.1 (0.8–5.8), require rests or breaks: RR = 3.0 (0.9–9.6); work conditions: damp: RR = 5.4 (1.6–19), cold: RR = 6.4 (1.5–27); psychosocial factors: monotonous: 2.7 (1.3–5.4), work stress: RR = 1.9 (0.9–4.1)
Wright and Haq 1976	CR (9)	Shoulder pain >3 wk plus limitation of ROM	Outpatient department, UK	EX: 186 cases, 69 controls (eye patients)	Psychological factors: n.s.; Maudsley personality inventory: n.s.
Bergenudd et al. 1988; Bergenudd and Nilsson 1994	Prospective/ CS (mean score = 7)	>24 h of shoulder pain in last month, ROM <145° abduction	Malmö residents, all elementary school third graders, 1938	EX: 574	Individual factors: low intelligence: $P < 0.05$ in men; income: n.s.; psychosocial factors: low job satisfaction: $P < 0.05$ in women; work load: women $P <0.01$, men $P <0.05$
Takala 1982	CS (7)	Ache, stiffness, numbness of pain in the shoulder	Random sample of general population, Finland, aged 40–64 y	Q + EX: 1045 men, 1223 women	BMI $\geq$ 30: women 21%, men 13%; BMI < 30: women 18%, men 17%; psychiatric symptoms: women 33%, men 29%; no psychiatric symptoms: women 13%, men 17%; job groups: office work: 10–13%, agriculture: 19–21%

Abbreviations: BMI = body mass index; CR = case-referent; CS = cross-sectional; EX = physical examination; n.s. = not significant; Q = questionnaire; ROM = range of motion; RR = risk ratio.

ter considerably and would have meant discarding all information from cross-sectional studies, some of which appeared to use relatively well-considered methods.

The designs and results of all 32 studies are summarized in Table VII, presented separately for studies conducted in the general population and in occupational settings. The table presents separately those studies that include an evaluation of psychosocial risk factors. The method scores range between 4 and 12 points out of a maximal attainable score of 16, with a median score of 8. The critical appraisal suggests the following frequent shortcomings: assessment of exposure by questionnaire or interview only, with no observations or recordings (criterion E, 27 studies), no attempt to prevent information bias (F, 24 studies), inadequate sample size (G, 15 studies), and inadequate analysis (H, 11 studies). Details regarding the critical appraisal of each study are summarized in Appendix III.

Several studies included adjustments for confounding variables, but the methods of analysis varied considerably, from adjustment for age and sex only to the use of a multivariate model that adjusted for the influence of all other potential risk factors for shoulder pain. This variation in methods makes it difficult to interpret the magnitude of the reported associations. The tables in this chapter present univariate estimates, where available, and indicate when only the results of a multivariate model have been presented. An additional problem of statistical analysis relates to the use of the odds ratio in cross-sectional studies. The high prevalence of shoulder pain, particularly in some occupational settings, reduces the reliability of the odds ratio as an estimate of the relative risk, resulting in overestimation of the magnitude of the association (Axelson et al. 1994; Lagerström et al. 1995; Skov et al. 1996; Pope et al. 1997b). The use of the odds ratio also assumes equal duration of the disorder in the exposed and unexposed populations, which may not be true for work-related musculoskeletal disorders (Axelson et al. 1994; Skov et al. 1996). Only a few studies have considered these difficulties and have presented risk or prevalence ratios instead of, or in addition to, odds ratios (Skov et al. 1996; Pope et al. 1997b).

Table VIII
Results of studies on risk factors for shoulder pain in an occupational setting, including evaluation of psychosocial factors

Reference	Study Type*	Disease Definition	Source of Sample	Sample Size	Risk Factors and Strength of Association (95% CI)
Bernard et al. 1994	CS (12)	Work-related symptoms	Random sample, 3000 full-time newspaper employees, USA	Q: 973	Multiple logistic regression: women: OR = 2.2 (1.5–3.3); high job pressure: OR = 1.5 (1.0–2.2); number of years employed: OR = 1.4 (1.2–1.8); lack of participation in job decision making: OR = 1.6 (1.2–2.1)
Hales et al. 1994	CS (12)	Specific shoulder disorders	Telephone companies, random sample of 5 job titles, USA	Ex: 518	Multiple logistic regression: work factors (number of times rising from chair): OR = 1.9 (1.2–3.2); individual factors: n.s.; psychosocial factors (fear of being replaced by computers): OR = 2.7 (1.3–5.8); electronic performance monitoring: n.s.; no. keystrokes/day: n.s.
Kvarn-ström and Halldén 1983	CR (12)	Occupa-tional cervical brachial disorder	11000 employees, engineering company, Sweden	Cases 112 Controls: random sample	Work load factors (subjective work load): $P < 0.05$; work environment (work load at home): $P < 0.05$; well-being: n.s.; job content: $P < 0.05$; monotonous/ repetitive work; social/ethnic factors (education outside Sweden): $P < 0.05$: low muscle strength: $P < 0.05$
Dimberg 1989	CS (9)	Shoulder symptoms, specific diagnoses	Volvo Flygmotor, all employees, Sweden	Q: 548	Multivariable analysis: individual factors (short stature, age): $P < 0.05$; work load factors (high physical stress, vibrating hand tools): $P < 0.05$: psychosocial factors (mental stress): $P < 0.05$
Lager-ström et al. 1995	CS (9)	Shoulder symptoms	All nursing personnel hospital, Sweden	Q: $n = 688$	Multiple logistic regression (severe shoulder symptoms): individual factors: age: OR = 1.22 per 10 y (1.02–1.46), body mass index: n.s., smoking: n.s.;low fitness: OR = 2.22 (1.47–3.36); work conditions: n.s.; psychosocial factors (high work demand): OR = 1.65 (1.05–2.59)
Johansson and Rubeno-witz 1994	CS (8)	Work-related shoulder pain	Random sample metal industry, Sweden	NQ: 241 blue-collar, 209 white-collar, $R \pm 90\%$	Multiple regression, adjusted for age and sex: blue/white collar: years of employment: n.s.; psychosocial factors: low control over work: $R = 0.018/0.17$, poor supervisor climate: $R = 0.16/0.20$, low stimulus from work: $R = 0.26/0.22$, poor relationships among workers: $R = 0.09/0.21$, high psychological load: $R = 0.27/0.24$; subjective work load: monotonous work: $R = 0.15/0.32$, extreme work posture: $R = 0.14/-$, light materials handling: $R = 0.04 / 0.18$, twisted work postures: $R = -/0.16$
Kamwen-do et al. 1991	CS (8)	Shoulder pain	Female secretaries, hospital, Sweden	NQ: $n = 420$	Psychosocial factors: no friendly spirit of cooperation ($P = 0.028$), unable to influence work conditions ($P = 0.003$), too much to do ($n = 0.054$); length of employment (adjusted for age): OR = 1.94 (1.13–3.36)/5 y; sitting >5 h/d: n.s.; hours at terminals/typewriters: OR = 1.87 (1.18–2.98); part time/full time: n.s.
Skov et al. 1996	CS (8)	Shoulder symptoms	Random sample of salespeople, Denmark	NQ: $n = 1306$	Multiple logistic regression (PPRs also presented and slightly lower): work factors: 10–19 y in car (vs. <10): OR = 1.64 (1.19–2.27); psychosocial factors: high work demand: OR = 1.47 (1.05–2.07), uncertainty of employment: OR = 1.52 (1.01–2.29); individual factors: sex (female): OR = 1.77 (1.20–2.62), smoking (OR = 1.46 (1.08–1.96)
Linton and Kamwen-do 1989	CS (7)	Shoulder pain	Female secretaries, hospital, Sweden	NQ: $n = 420$	Poor social work environment: OR = 3.32 (1.53–7.23); poor work content OR = 2.51 (1.27–4.88); high work demands: n.s.; poor social support: 1.62 (0.95–2.78)

(continued)

Table VIII
Continued

Reference	Study Type*	Disease Definition	Source of Sample	Sample Size	Risk Factors and Strength of Association (95% CI)
Bru et al. 1993	CS (5)	Shoulder pain (combined score of intensity during past 30 d and past year)	3000 female hospital employees, Norway	Q: 586	Multiple regression: personality traits: neuroticism R^2 = 0.06, $P < 0.0001$; in midwives/children's wards: neuroticism R^2 = 0.17, $P = 0.006$; in orthopedic wards/auxiliary nurses: anxiety R^2 = 0.17, $P = 0.0011$, extraversion R^2 = 0.34, $P = 0.0003$
Flodmark and Aase 1992	CS (4)	Shoulder symptoms	All blue-collar workers, ventilation shaft manufacturer, Sweden	NQ: 58	Type A behavior (Borner Questionnaire): Borner scores higher in cases, $P < 0.01$

Abbreviations: CR = case-referent; CS = cross-sectional; EX = physical examination; NQ = Nordic Questionnaire; n.s. = not significant; Q = questionnaire; OR = odds ratio, PPR = prevalence proportion ratio.

Table IX
Results of studies on risk factors for shoulder pain in the general population (no evaluation of psychosocial risk factors)

Reference	Study Type*	Disease Definition	Source of Sample	Sample Size	Risk Factors and Strength of Association (95% CI)
English et al. 1995	CR (12)	Specific shoulder disorders	Patients aged 16–65 y, orthopedic clinics	EX: 72 cases, 996 controls	Age: RR = 1.37 per 5 y (1.23–1.53). Adjusted for age: repeated elbow flexion: RR = 0.38 (0.17–0.83); total daily elbow flexion: RR = 1.10 per hour (0.9–1.23); static work above shoulder level, range of motion, etc.: n.s.
Epstein et al. 1993	CR (10)	Shoulder impinge-ment, rotator cuff tear (surgery)	Departments of radiology and orthopedics, USA	EX: 30 cases, 47 controls	Hooked acromion on MRI: impingement: $P = 0.17$; rotator cuff tear: $P < 0.001$
Jacobsson et al. 1992	CR (9)	Subacromial shoulder pain > 6 wk	Random sample of Malmö residents, aged 50–70 y	Q + EX: 36 cases, controls: 5:1, $n = 180$	Multiple logistic regression: individual factors: sleep disturbances, living conditions, education: n.s.; physical activity at work: n.s.; occupational work load: self-rated heavy load, OR = 5.4 (3.4–8.6)
Griegel-Morris et al. 1992	CS (5)	Shoulder pain	Healthy volunteers, USA	Q: 88	Postural abnormalities: n.s.

Abbreviations: CR = case-referent; CS = cross-sectional; EX = physical examination; MRI = magnetic resonance imaging; n.s. = not significant; OR = odds ratio; Q = questionnaire; RR = risk ratio.
* Numbers in parentheses are method scores.

Table X
Results of studies on risk factors for shoulder pain: occupational setting (no evaluation of psychosocial risk factors)

Reference	Study Type*	Disease Definition	Source of Sample	Sample Size	Risk Factors and Strength of Association (95% CI)
Stenlund et al. 1992	CS (10)	Acromio-clavicular osteoarthritis	Random sample of construction workers, Sweden	EX: 54 bricklayers, 55 rock blasters, 98 foremen	Multiple logistic regression, adjusted for age (right side): job title: brick OR = 2.21 (1.03–4.72), rock OR = 2.13 (0.98–4.64); sum of load lifted: >25000 metric tons, OR = 3.18 (1.09–9.24); years of manual work: >28 y, OR = 2.91 (1.15–7.35); sum of vibration: >25000 h, OR = 2.18 (1.04–4.56)
Stenlund et al. 1993	CS (10)	Shoulder tendinitis	Random sample of construction workers, Sweden	EX: 54 bricklayers, 55 rock blasters, 98 foremen	Adjusted for age, dexterity, smoking, sports activities (right side): job title: brick OR = 0.44 (0.16–1.25), rock OR = 1.71 (0.71–4.17); sum of load lifted: >25000 metric tons, OR = 1.02 (0.59–1.76); years of manual work: >28 y, OR = 1.10 (0.68–1.79); sum of vibration: >25000 h, OR = 1.66 (1.06–2.61)
Van der Beek et al. 1993	CS (9)	Regular pain/stiffness shoulder	Random sample of truck drivers, The Netherlands	Q: 534	Multiple logistic regression, adjusted for age (90% CI): pallets (n = 125): OR = 2.1 (1.3–3.6); wheeled cages (n = 66): OR = 2.0 (1.1–3.7); packed goods (n = 109): OR = 2.3 (1.3–3.9); bulk cargo (n = 99): OR = 1.1
Kilbom et al. 1986	CS (9)	Slight, moderate or severe shoulder symptoms	All female employees, electronics factory, Sweden	n = 138, n = 96 after exclusions	Multiple regression (R^2 = 0.16): maximum voluntary contraction, HR, perceived exertion (n.s.); workload factors: years of employment ($P < 0.05$); small stature ($P < 0.05$); work posture: low rate of arm flexions ($P < 0.05$); high percentage of work cycle with arm in 0–30° abduction ($P < 0.05$)
Liss et al. 1995	CS (9)	Shoulder symptoms	Dental hygienists, dental assistants, Canada	NQ: n = 941; n = 109 dental assistants	Multiple logistic regression (95% CI): individual factors: age, handedness, activities/hobbies: n.s.; previous shoulder pain: OR = 2.1 (1.2–3.8); length of employment: OR = 3.9 (1.9–7.9) for 1–19 y vs < 1 y; work conditions: trunk rotated: OR = 3.1 (1.9–4.9), 5–6 d/wk: OR = 1.8 (1.1–3.2), type of practice: OR = 1.8 (1.2–2.8)
Ohlsson et al. 1989	CS (9)	Shoulder pain during last 7 d	Female assembly workers, previous and current, plus random sample of residents, Sweden	Current: n = 148, previous: n = 76, controls: n = 60	Assembly work: OR = 3.4 (1.6–7.1), adjusted for age; length of employment: OR increases, but is dependent on age; work pace: $P < 0.001$ (graphical display)
Kvarn-ström 1983	CS (8)	>4 wk sick leave due to shoulder pain	17251 person-years wage earners, 16539 person-years salaried staff, engineering company, Sweden	112 cases (controls: expected numbers based on man years)	Sex: $P < 0.01$ (women), age: $P < 0.01$ (>25 y in women); immigrant: RR = 3.09; job type: significant differences, e.g., assembly-line workers, RR = 4.5
Punnett et al. 1985	CS (8)	Persistent pain for 1 mo during past year	Garment factory and hospital employees, USA	Garment: Q + EX, 179; hospital: Q + EX, 73	Job title: $P < 0.05$; non-native speaker (immigrants): $P < 0.05$

(continued)

Table X
Continued

Reference	Study Type*	Disease Definition	Source of Sample	Sample Size	Risk Factors and Strength of Association (95% CI)
Westgaard and Jansen 1992	CS (7)	Work-related shoulder pain	Clothing company, Norway	Q: 210 production workers, 35 other	Work task variables: n.s.; individual variables: previous symptoms, adjusted $R^2 = 0.02$, $P = 0.04$
Bjelle et al. 1979	CR (6)	Shoulder pain > 3 mo	Manual workers, Sweden	EX: 20 cases, 40 controls	Work load: n.s.; work above shoulder level: $P < 0.05$
Rundcrantz et al. 1990	CS (6)	Pain/discomfort in shoulders	All dentists, Malmö, Sweden	Q: $n = 359$	Working posture: $P < 0.05$; position of patient: n.s.; working hours: n.s.; age: $P < 0.001$; years of employment: $P < 0.05$; mirror use: $P < 0.05$
Yu and Wong 1996	CS (6)	Discomfort or ache since starting current job	Employees of Hong Kong bank, frequent/ infrequent VDU users	90 frequent, $R = 90\%$; 61 infrequent, $R = 66\%$; Q: 121	Multiple logistic regression, adjusted for age and sex: fixed keyboard height: OR = 8.7 (2.4–32.4); frequent user: OR = 18.8 (2.2–164.7); bending back: OR = 5.1 (1.5–17.2)
Herberts et al. 1981	CS (5)	Supraspinatus tendinitis	Arendal shipyard, Göteborg, Sweden, all welders, all office workers aged >40 y	Q + EX: 11 cases, 11 controls	Welding years: n.s.; shoulder load: n.s.

Abbreviations: CS = cross-sectional; CR = case-referent; EX = physical examination; n.s. = not significant; Q = questionnaire; NQ = Nordic Questionnaire; OR = odds ratio; RR = relative risk.
* Numbers in parentheses are method scores.

INDIVIDUAL AND LIFESTYLE FACTORS

A wide variety of individual factors have been considered as potential risk factors for the development of shoulder pain. No significant associations have been found for level of education, living conditions, sleep disturbances (Hales et al. 1994), recreational activities (Hales et al. 1994; Liss et al. 1995), left- versus right-handedness (Liss et al. 1995), income (Bergenudd et al. 1988, Bergenudd and Nilsson 1994), postural abnormalities (Griegel-Morris et al. 1992), or body mass index (Takala et al. 1982; Lagerström et al. 1995).

Contradictory results have been reported for a few potential individual risk factors. Lagerström and colleagues (1995) failed to detect a significant association for smoking in a cross-sectional survey of nursing personnel, yet a random sample of salespeople found a small but statistically significant association between smoking and shoulder symptoms (OR = 1.46, Skov et al. 1996). Low muscle strength was a risk fac-

tor for shoulder symptoms in employees of a Swedish engineering company (Kvarnström and Halldén 1983), but there was no significant association for female employees of a Swedish electronics factory (Kilbom et al. 1986). Kilbom and colleagues' multivariate model adjusted the strength of the association for potential confounding by other individual factors, work conditions, and psychosocial factors.

Various studies have confirmed the association between age and the frequency of shoulder pain (Kvarnström 1983; Rundcrantz et al. 1990; English et al. 1995; Lagerström et al. 1995). Two studies that obtained relatively good method scores (9 and 12 points) reported a relative risk of 1.37 per 5 years (English et al. 1995) and an odds ratio of 1.22 per 10 years (Lagerström et al. 1995). Studies using a multivariate analysis (Bernard et al. 1994; Skov et al. 1996) confirmed a higher frequency of shoulder pain in women, as reported in earlier epidemiological surveys. Bernard and colleagues, whose 1994 study received a high method score (12 points), reported an odds ratio of

2.2 for female gender in a random sample of newspaper employees.

Three studies report an association between immigrant status and a high frequency of shoulder pain (Kvarnström 1983; Kvarnström and Halldén 1983; Punnett et al. 1985). However, sample sizes were small (Punnett 1985) or the results had not been adjusted for potential confounding by other factors (Kvarnström 1983; Kvarnström and Halldén 1983). Other factors found to be significantly associated with shoulder pain were previous episodes of shoulder pain (OR = 2.1, Liss et al. 1995), low physical fitness (OR = 2.2, Lagerström et al. 1995), and small stature (Kilbom et al. 1986; Dimberg et al. 1989).

Likelihood of causality

For most individual risk factors, the likelihood that their association with shoulder pain represents causality is rather small. Consistent positive associations that were statistically significant and were based on studies using relatively good methods have been reported for age and gender only. Three studies reported a dose–response relationship for the association between age and the occurrence of shoulder pain (Allander 1974; Backman 1983; Näyhä et al. 1994; see Table II). A temporal relationship for most individual and lifestyle risk factors has not yet been established, because of the lack of well-conducted long-term prospective studies.

Diagnostic imaging studies have shown that tears of the rotator cuff are more frequent at older ages, regardless of the presence of shoulder pain (Sher et al. 1995). Degeneration of the rotator cuff over the years, caused by impairment of perfusion and nutrition, added to cumulative mechanical stress, is a biologically plausible explanation for the association between age and shoulder pain (Armstrong et al. 1993).

In conclusion, there is reasonably strong evidence that shoulder pain is an age-related phenomenon, implicating both aging of the joint structure and cumulative stress.

WORK-LOAD FACTORS

Epidemiological studies on shoulder pain have directed much attention toward the possible association between work-load factors and shoulder pain. Most studies have estimated work load by job title or by using structured interviews or questionnaires. Job titles are an inadequate indicator of occupational exposure, however, as specific characteristics vary across work sites (Croft 1993; Sommerich et al. 1993). Direct assessment of work load, for example by observations or analysis of video recordings, is preferred, but involves expensive and time-consuming methods that have only rarely been attempted (Herberts et al. 1981; Kilbom et al. 1986; Bernard et al. 1994).

A significant association between job titles and the occurrence of shoulder pain has been reported by a few studies with relatively good methods (median method score of at least 8). A random sample of Swedish construction workers found that bricklayers had a relatively high risk of developing acromioclavicular osteoarthritis compared to foremen (OR = 2.21, Stenlund et al. 1992), whereas shoulder tendinitis was frequently diagnosed in rock blasters (OR = 3.33, Stenlund et al. 1993). Shoulder pain was more prevalent among female assembly workers than in a random sample of Swedish residents (OR = 3.4, Ohlsson 1989). Furthermore, Kvarnström (1983) reported significant associations for several job titles in an engineering industry, as did Punnett and colleagues (1985) for several job titles at a garment factory.

Various work-load factors and other job characteristics were reported to be significantly related to a high occurrence of shoulder pain. In studies with a median method score of at least 8, these factors were: self-rated handling of heavy loads (OR = 2.0–5.4; Kvarnström and Halldén 1983; Dimberg et al. 1989; Jacobsson et al. 1992; Stenlund et al. 1992; Van der Beek et al. 1993), length of employment (OR = 1.4–3.9; Kilbom et al. 1986; Dimberg et al. 1989; Stenlund et al. 1992; Kamwendo et al. 1991; Bernard et al. 1994; Liss et al. 1995; Skov et al. 1996), work posture (OR= 2.1–5.5; Johansson and Rubenowitz 1994; Pope et al. 1997b), damp or cold work conditions (OR = 5.4–6.4, Pope et al. 1997b), monotonous work (OR = 2.7, Pope et al. 1997b; $P < 0.05$, Kvarnström and Halldén 1983), number of times rising from one's chair (OR = 1.9, Hales et al. 1994), and use of vibrating tools (OR = 1.66, Stenlund et al. 1993; OR = 2.18, Stenlund et al. 1992; $P < 0.05$, Dimberg et al. 1989).

Stenlund showed that risk factors may differ among specific shoulder conditions. Work load and length of employment were related to the occurrence of acromioclavicular arthritis, but not to tendinitis. Other studies did not address specific shoulder conditions.

Likelihood of causality

Consistent positive associations between work-load factors and shoulder pain were reported for self-rated work load and for length of employment. The association was quite strong in many studies, with odds ratios of 3.0 or higher (Table VII). Although infrequently studied, damp or cold working conditions, monotonous work, and the use of vibrating tools do show consistent associations with shoulder pain. A dose–response relationship was reported for length of employment (Kamwendo et al. 1991; Liss et al. 1995) and work load (Stenlund et al. 1992; Skov et al. 1996). Again, a temporal relationship for work-load factors is difficult to establish because of the shortage of long-term prospective studies. In addition, the importance of length of employment as a causative factor is obscured by some researchers' failure to define whether the association was adjusted for age.

Evidence of biological plausibility backs up the epidemiological observations. The circulation to tendon tissue may be impaired if the humeral head compresses the tendon against the coracoacromial arch or if the tension in the tendon increases. This may be the case in work tasks requiring the sustained elevation of the hands and involving static work postures. Furthermore, repetitive shoulder movements may produce a metabolic depletion in muscle cells, causing muscular pain (Hagberg 1984). Biomechanical studies using electromyography have demonstrated that increased levels of muscle activity during awkward and static work postures are associated with shoulder pain, as are fewer occurrences of low activity levels (micropauses in muscular activity) (Erdelyi et al. 1988; Veijersted et al. 1993; Hägg and Åström 1997). The affected muscles and tendons are more susceptible to microtears and inflammatory changes, which may result in pain and impairment (Hagberg 1984; Armstrong et al. 1993).

In conclusion, long-term prospective cohort studies have not yet established a temporal relationship, but considerable evidence indicates that length of employment, work posture, and work load are causative factors in the development of shoulder pain.

PSYCHOSOCIAL FACTORS

Tables VII and VIII summarize the results of studies that evaluated the association between psychosocial factors and the occurrence of shoulder pain. Sig-nificant associations were reported for several psychosocial factors, including work stress (Lagerström et al. 1995; Pope et al. 1997b), lack of participation in job decision making (Kamwendo et al. 1991; Bernard et al. 1994; Johansson and Rubenowitz 1994), fear of being replaced by computers (Hales et al. 1994), mental stress (Dimberg et al. 1989; Kamwendo et al. 1991), high work demand (Lagerström et al. 1995; Skov et al. 1996), monotonous work (Linton and Kamwendo 1989), and a poor social work environment (Linton and Kamwendo 1989; Kamwendo et al. 1991; Johansson and Rubenowitz 1994). The associations are not particularly strong; odds ratios presented by studies with relatively high method scores vary between 1.5 for a high work demand (Skov et al. 1996) and 2.7 for fear of being replaced by computers (Hales et al. 1994).

Conflicting results have been reported for personality characteristics or traits. Two studies with relatively low method scores report increased neuroticism, anxiety, and type A behavior in patients with shoulder pain. However, using a case-referent design, Wright and Haq (1976) could not establish differences on the Maudsley Personality Inventory between shoulder patients and patients with eye problems.

Likelihood of causality

Estimates reported for the association between psychosocial risk factors and shoulder pain were not particularly strong, but the findings were consistent. Nearly all studies evaluating psychosocial factors reported statistically significant associations (Tables VII and VIII). The lack of prospective studies is once again evident. However, in a longitudinal study of a sample of the general population, Leino and Magni (1993) observed that depression and distress predicted the development of neck and shoulder symptoms. Some reciprocity of effect was demonstrated; for example, musculoskeletal symptoms at baseline predicted future increased stress in men.

Shoulder pain is most likely the result of many factors, including individual differences, work-load factors, and psychosocial variables. Several authors have proposed multifactorial models to explain the causes of musculoskeletal symptoms such as shoulder pain (Maeda 1977; Kilbom 1988; Linton 1992; Bongers et al. 1993; Hales and Bernard 1996). Psychological factors appear to be important in the development and maintenance of subacute and chronic problems. Psychosocial factors at work, such as a poor social work environment, a high work demand, or job dissatisfaction, together with an inadequate personal capacity to cope with these factors, may increase work-related stress. The increase in stress may increase muscle tone directly, or it may moderate the relationship between mechanical work load and musculoskeletal symptoms. Such a sequence might influence the perception or reporting of symptoms or cause a reduced capacity to cope (Bongers et al. 1993; Hales and Bernard 1996).

STRATEGIES FOR PREVENTION

The objectives of prevention are perceived differently by individual sufferers, employers, and insurance companies. The individual will be interested in improved health and less discomfort or pain, whereas the employer hopes for an increase in productivity, and the insurer for a reduction in paid sick leave (Harms-Ringdahl 1995). Complete health and high productivity may be constrained by several factors, some of which are difficult to modify, such as gender, age, employment level, and lifestyle factors. Preventive measures will therefore tend to focus on external factors in the work environment. Sommerich and colleagues (1993) used the available evidence on the importance of work-load factors to formulate preventive measures relating to repetition (avoiding repetitive arm movements), posture (minimizing shoulder flexion and abduction, and avoiding static postures), force (reducing or eliminating forceful or heavy work and handheld weight), and rest (requiring frequent rest breaks).

Despite these attempts to modify the work environment ergonomically, many workers still experience work-related shoulder pain. Several studies have shown that, because the problem is multifactorial, its solution may require more than the modification of workload factors alone. Additional measures might include attention to the organization of work, including variation in work tasks, an adequate work pace, a stimulating social environment, and good opportunities for development and for influencing one's work.

Various psychologically oriented programs have been suggested as a means of preventing neck or shoulder problems, such as education and therapy programs, efforts to adapt the psychosocial work environment, and health promotion programs (Linton 1992). As yet, there is limited evidence to show whether these preventive measures are effective or applicable. Secondary intervention programs for work-related shoulder pain, aimed at workstation redesign, work reorganization, and worker education, may also be effective, but the cost-effectiveness of these potentially large-scale interventions has received little attention (Kilbom 1988). Psychosocial and behavioral factors may demonstrate their potency when employed in a multidisciplinary package. Some cognitive behavioral methods adapted for shoulder or neck pain are activity training, relaxation as a coping strategy, improvement of adherence to treatment regimes, and the involvement of management (Linton 1992). Management involvement may facilitate the process of returning to work and ensure co-operation between managers and workers to improve job design and work environment, including both work-load and psychosocial factors (Rowe 1987).

CHALLENGES FOR THE FUTURE

The search for the causes of shoulder pain still faces many challenges. Further studies are needed to assess exposure and to improve case definition. Longitudinal studies of risk factors must be designed to evaluate the onset and chronicity of symptoms and to determine appropriate time frames for sick leave.

The studies reviewed in this chapter frequently classify the level of exposure in terms of job titles or job characteristics. Job titles often imply an unknown combination of several physical risk factors but do not offer information about specific exposures that may cause shoulder pain and that should be avoided to prevent it. Researchers must quantify the postures to be avoided, the number of repetitions that may be harmful, or the maximum loads that should be carried (Stock 1991; Sommerich et al. 1993). Criteria should be developed not only to assess exposure (for example by using video recordings, observations, or validated questionnaires), but also to facilitate case definition (through standardized questionnaires or physical examinations), as no consensus exists regarding the definitions of shoulder pain or specific shoulder disorders. Standardized criteria may be useful within epidemiological study designs.

Most studies included in this chapter are cross-sectional. These studies are subject to survivor bias (the healthy worker effect); workers who develop shoulder pain may leave the workplace or select different jobs (Stock 1991), which will tend to underestimate the magnitude of an association. However, longitudinal studies are costly and may not be feasible in the workplace. Work conditions and exposures may be altered during the study, complicating the interpretation of results. Furthermore, a longitudinal design does not entirely avoid the risk of survivor bias. Monotonous jobs with a high work load or repetitive movements may have a high turnover of personnel, and it can be difficult to trace workers who have quit their jobs. Nevertheless, longitudinal studies that evaluate new employees for musculoskeletal symptoms and provide periodic follow-up assessments will provide valuable information on temporal and dose–response relationships. To establish the relative contribution of each factor and the role of potential confounding variables, studies should evaluate not only physical workload factors, but also psychosocial factors (including work stress, participation in decision making, work content, and a social work environment). Such studies will provide the information needed to set priorities in the prevention of shoulder pain.

REFERENCES

Allander E. Prevalence, incidence, and remission rates of some common rheumatic diseases or syndromes. *Scand J Rheumatol* 1974; 3:145–153.

Armstrong TJ, Buckle P, Fine LJ, et al. A conceptual model for work-related neck and upper-limb musculoskeletal disorders. *Scand J Work Environ Health* 1993; 19:73–84.

Axelson O, Fredriksson M, Ekberg K. Use of the prevalence ratio *vs* the prevalence odds ratio as a measure of risk in cross-sectional studies. *Occup Environ Med* 1994; 51:574.

Backman AL. Health survey of professional drivers. *Scand J Work Environ Health* 1983; 9:30–35.

Bak K, Magnusson SP. Shoulder strength and range of motion in symptomatic and pain-free elite swimmers. *Am J Sports Med* 1997; 25:454–459.

Bamji AN, Erhardt CC, Price TR, Williams PL. The painful shoulder: can consultants agree? *Br J Rheumatol* 1996; 35:1172–1174.

Bartolozzi A, Andreychik D, Ahmad S. Determinants of outcome in the treatment of rotator cuff disease. *Clin Orthop* 1994; 308:90–97.

Beach ML, Whitney SL, Dickoff-Hoffman SA. Relationship of shoulder flexibility, strength, and endurance to shoulder pain in competitive swimmers. *J Orthop Sports Phys Ther* 1992; 16:262–268.

Bergenudd H, Johnell O. Somatic versus nonsomatic shoulder and back pain experience in middle age in relation to body build, physical fitness, bone mineral content, gamma-glutamyl-transferase, occupational work load, and psychosocial factors. *Spine* 1991; 16:1051–1055.

Bergenudd H, Nilsson B. The prevalence of locomotor complaints in middle age and their relationship to health and socioeconomic factors. *Clin Orthop* 1994; 308:264–270.

Bergenudd H, Lindgärde F, Nilsson B, Petersson CJ. Shoulder pain in middle age. A study of prevalence and relation to occupational, work load and psychosocial factors. *Clin Orthop* 1988; 231:234–238.

Bergström G, Bjelle A, Sorensen LB, Sundh V, Svanborg A. Prevalence of symptoms and signs of joint impairment at age 79. *Scand J Rehabil Med* 1985; 17:173–182.

Bernard B, Sauter S, Fine L, Petersen M, Hales T. Job task and psychosocial risk factors for work-related musculoskeletal disorders among newspaper employees. *Scand J Work Environ Health* 1994; 20:417–426.

Binder AI, Bulgen DY, Hazleman BL, Roberts S. Frozen shoulder: a long-term prospective study. *Ann Rheum Dis* 1984; 43:361–364.

Bjelle A, Hagberg M, Michaelsson G. Clinical and ergonomic factors in prolonged shoulder pain among industrial workers. *Scand J Work Environ Health* 1979; 5:205–210.

Bohannon RW, Larkin PA, Smith MB, Horton MG. Shoulder pain in hemiplegia: statistical relationship with five variables. *Arch Phys Med Rehabil* 1986; 67:514–516.

Bongers PM, De Winter CR, Kompier MAJ, Hildebrandt VH. Psychosocial factors at work and musculoskeletal disease. *Scand J Work Environ Health* 1993; 19:297–312.

Brocklehurst JC, Andrews K, Richards B, Laycock PJ. How much physical therapy for patients with stroke? *BMJ* 1978; 1:1307–1310.

Bru E, Mykletun RJ, Svebak S. Neuroticism, extraversion, anxiety and type A behaviour as mediators of neck, shoulder and lower back pain in female hospital staff. *Person Individ Diff* 1993; 15:485–492.

Buchbinder R, Goel V, Bombardier C, Hogg-Johnsson S. Classification systems of soft tissue disorders of the neck and upper limb: Do they satisfy methodological guidelines? *J Clin Epidemiol* 1996; 49:141–149.

Buckle P. Musculoskeletal disorders of the upper extremities: the use of epidemiologic approaches in industrial settings. *J Hand Surg* 1987; 12A:885–889.

Chakravarty K, Webley M. Shoulder joint movement and its relationship to disability in the elderly. *J Rheumatol* 1993; 20:1359–1361.

Chard MD, Hazleman BL. Shoulder disorders in the elderly (a hospital study). *Ann Rheum Dis* 1987; 46:684–687.

Chard MD, Satelle LM, Hazleman BL. The long-term outcome of rotator cuff tendinitis—a review study. *Br J Rheumatol* 1988; 27:385–389.

Chard MD, Hazleman R, Hazleman BL, King RH, Reiss BB. Shoulder disorders in the elderly: a community survey. *Arthr Rheum* 1991; 34:766–769.

Christensen H. Muscle activity and fatigue in the shoulder muscles of assembly-plant employees. *Scand J Work Environ Health* 1986; 12:582–587.

Croft P. Soft tissue rheumatism. In: Silman AJ, Hochberg MC (Eds). *Epidemiology of the Rheumatic Diseases*. Oxford: Oxford Medical Publications, 1993, pp 375–421.

Croft P, Pope D, Silman A. The clinical course of shoulder pain: prospective cohort study in primary care. *BMJ* 1996; 313:601–602.

Cunningham LS, Kelsey JL. Epidemiology of musculoskeletal impairments and associated disability. *Am J Public Health* 1984; 74:574–579.

Cyriax J. *Textbook of Orthopaedic Medicine*. London: Baillière Tindal, 1981.

Dimberg L, Olafsson A, Stefansson E, et al. The correlation between work environment and the occurrence of cervicobrachial symptoms. *J Occup Med* 1989; 31:447–453.

Ekberg K, Karlsson M, Axelson O, Björkqvist B, Bjerre-Kiely B. Cross-sectional study of risk factors for symptoms in the neck and shoulder area. *Ergonomics* 1995; 38:971–980.

Ekberg K, Wildhagen I. Long-term sickness absence due to musculoskeletal disorders: the necessary interventions of work conditions. *Scand J Rehabil Med* 1996; 28:39–47.

English CJ, Maclaren WM, Court-Brown C, et al. Relations between upper limb soft tissue disorders and repetitive movements at work. *Am J Industr Med.* 1995; 27:75–90.

Epstein RE, Schweitzer ME, Frieman BG, Fenlin JM, Mitchell DG. Hooked acromion: prevalence on MR images of painful shoulders. *Radiology* 1993; 187:479–481.

Erdelyi A, Sihvonen T, Helin P, Hänninen O. Shoulder strain in keyboard workers and its alleviation by arm supports. *Int Arch Occup Environ Health* 1988; 60:119–124.

Flodmark BT, Aase G. Musculoskeletal symptoms and type A behaviour in blue collar workers. *Br J Industr Med* 1992; 49:683–687.

Griegel-Morris P, Larson K, Mueller-Klaus K, Oatis CA. Incidence of common postural abnormalities in the cervical, shoulder, and thoracic regions and their association with pain in two age groups of healthy subjects. *Phys Ther* 1992; 72:425–431.

Hagberg M. Occupational musculoskeletal stress and disorders of the neck and shoulder: a review of possible pathophysiology. *Int Arch Occup Environ Health* 1984; 53:269–278.

Hägg GM, Åström A. Load pattern and pressure pain threshold in the upper trapezius muscle and psychosocial factors in medical secretaries with and without shoulder/neck disorders. *Int Arch Occup Environ Health* 1997; 69:423–432.

Hales TR, Sauter SL, Peterson MR, et al. Musculoskeletal disorders among visual display terminal users in a telecommunications company. *Ergonomics* 1994; 37:1603–1621.

Hales TR, Bernard BP. Epidemiology of work-related musculoskeletal disorders. *Orthop Clin North Am* 1996; 27:679–709.

Harms-Ringdahl K, Schüldt K, Ekholm J. Principles of prevention of neck-and-shoulder pain. *Scand J Rehabil Med* 1995; 32(Suppl):87–96.

Hazleman BL. The painful stiff shoulder. *Rheumatol Phys Med* 1972; 11:413–420.

Hedtmann A, Fett H. The so-called periarthropathia humeroscapularis: classification and analysis of 1266 cases. *Z Orthop Ihre Grenzgeb* 1989; 127:643–649.

Herberts P, Kadefors R, Andersson G, Petersén I. Shoulder pain in industry: an epidemiological study on welders. *Acta Orthop Scand* 1981; 52:299–306.

Hünting W, Läubli Th, Grandjean E. Postural and visual loads at VDT workplaces. I. constrained postures. *Ergonomics* 1981: 24:917–931.

Jacobsson L, Lindgärde F, Manthorpe R. The commonest rheumatic complaints of over six weeks' duration in a twelve-month period in a defined Swedish population. *Scand J Rheumatol* 1989; 18:353–360.

Jacobsson L, Lindgärde F, Manthorpe R, Ohlsson K. Effect of education, occupation and some lifestyle factors on common rheumatic complaints in a Swedish group aged 50–70 years. *Ann Rheum Dis* 1992; 51:835–843.

Jacobsson L, Nagi DK, Pillemer SR, et al. Low prevalences of chronic widespread pain and shoulder disorders among Pima Indians. *J Rheumatol* 1996; 23:907–909.

Johansson JA, Rubenowitz S. Risk indicators in the psychosocial and physical work environment for work-related neck, shoulder and low back symptoms: a study among blue- and white collar workers in eight companies. *Scand J Rehabil Med* 1994; 26:131–142.

Jonsson BG, Persson J, Kilbom A. Disorders of the cervicobrachial

region among female workers in the electronics industry. A two year follow up. *Int J Ind Ergonomics* 1988:3:1–12.

Kamwendo K, Linton SJ, Moritz U. Neck and shoulder disorders in medical secretaries. Part I. Pain prevalence and risk factors. *Scand J Rehabil Med* 1991; 23:127–133.

Kilbom A. Intervention programmes for work-related neck and upper limb disorders: strategies and evaluation. *Ergonomics* 1988; 31:735–747.

Kilbom A, Persson J, Jonnson BG. Disorders of the cervicobrachial region among female workers in the electronic industry. *Int J Ind Ergonomics* 1986; 1:37–47.

Klenerman L, Slade PD, Stanley IM, et al. The prediction of chronicity in patients with an acute attack of low back pain in a general practice setting. *Spine* 1995; 20:478–484.

Kvarnström S. Occupational cervicobrachial disorders in an engineering company. *Scand J Rehabil Med* 1983, 8(Suppl):77–100.

Kvarnström S, Halldén M. Occupational cervicobrachial disorders: a case-control study. *Scand J Rehabil Med* 1983, 8(Suppl):101–114.

Lagerström M, Wenemark M, Hagberg M, Wigaeus Hjelm EW. Occupational and individual factors related to musculoskeletal symptoms in five body regions among Swedish nursing personnel. *Int Arch Occup Environ Health* 1995; 68:27–35.

Leino P, Magni G. Depressive and distress symptoms as predictors of low back pain, neck-shoulder pain, and other musculoskeletal morbidity: a 10-year follow-up of metal industry employees. *Pain* 1993; 53:89–94.

Liesdek C, van der Windt DAWM, Koes BW, Bouter LM. Soft-tissue disorders of the shoulder: a study of inter-observer agreement between general practitioners and physiotherapists and an overview of physiotherapeutic treatment. *Physiotherapy* 1997; 83:12–17.

Linton SJ. An overview of psychosocial and behavioral factors in neck-and-shoulder pain. *Scand J Rehabil Med* 1992; 32(Suppl):67–78.

Linton SJ, Kamwendo K. Risk factors in the psychosocial work environment for neck and shoulder pain in secretaries. *J Occup Med* 1989; 31:609–613.

Liss GM, Jesin E, Kusiak RA, White P. Musculoskeletal problems among Ontario dental hygienists. *Am J Ind Med* 1995; 28:521–540.

Lo YPC, Hsu YCS, Chan KM. Epidemiology of shoulder impingement in upper arm sport events. *Br J Sports Med* 1990; 24:173–177.

Loew M. Über den Spontanverlauf der Schultersteife. *Krankengymnastik* 1994; 46:432–438.

Luopajarvi T, Kuorinka I, Virolainen M, Holmberg M. Prevalence of tenosynovitis and other injuries of the upper extremities in repetitive work. *Scand J Work Environ Health* 1979; 5(Suppl 3):48–55.

Mackay Rossignol A, Pechter Morse E, Summers VM, Pagnotto LD. Video display terminal use and reported health symptoms among Massachusetts clerical workers. *J Occup Med* 1987; 29:112–118.

Maeda K. Occupational cervicobrachial disorder and its causative factors. *J Human Ergol* 1977; 6:193–302.

Magnusson ML, Pope MH, Wilder DG, Areskoug B. Are occupational drivers at an increased risk for developing musculoskeletal disorders? *Spine* 1996; 21:710–717.

Mäkelä M, Heliövaara M, Sievers K, et al. Musculoskeletal disorders as determinants of disability in Finns aged 30 years or older. *J Clin Epidemiol* 1993; 46:549–559.

Manahan L, Caragay R, Muirden KD, et al. Rheumatic pain in a Philippine village. *Rheumatol Int* 1985; 5:149–153.

Mavrikakis ME, Drimis S, Kontoyannis DA, et al. Calcific shoulder periarthritis (tendinitis) in adult onset diabetes mellitus: a controlled study. *Ann Rheum Dis* 1989; 48:211–214.

McCormack RR, Inman RD, Wells A, Berntsen C, Imbus HR. Prevalence of tendinitis and related disorders of the upper extremity in a manufacturing workforce. *J Rheumatol* 1990; 17:958–964.

McMaster WC, Troup J. A survey of interfering shoulder pain in United States competitive swimmers. *Am J Sports Med* 1993; 21:67–70.

Meyers OL, Jessop S, Klemp P. The epidemiology of rheumatic disease in a rural and an urban population over the age of 65 years. *South African Med J* 1982; 62:403–405.

Miettinen OS. *Theoretical Epidemiology: Principles of Occurrence Research in Medicine.* New York: John Wiley & Sons, 1985.

Milerad E, Ekenvall L. Symptoms of the neck and upper extremities in dentists. *Scand J Work Environ Health* 1990; 16:129–134.

Mulcahy KA, Baxter AD, Oni OOA, Finlay D. The value of shoulder distension arthrography with intraarticular injection of steroid and local anaesthetic: a follow-up study. *Br J Radiol* 1994; 67:263–266.

Näyhä S, Anttonen H, Hassi J. Snowmobile driving and symptoms of the locomotive organs. *Arct Med Res* 1994; 53(Suppl 3):41–44.

Neer CS. Impingement lesions. *Clin Orthop* 1983; 173: 70–77.

Nichols PJR, Norman PA, Ennis JR. Wheelchair user's shoulder? *Scand J Rehabil Med* 1979; 11:29–32.

Nygren A, Berglund A, Von Koch M. Neck-and-shoulder pain, an increasing problem: strategies for using insurance material to follow trends. *Scand J Rehabil Med* 1995; 32(Suppl):107–112.

Ohlsson K, Attewell R, Skerfving S. Self-reported symptoms in the neck and upper limbs of female assembly workers. *Scand J Work Environ Med* 1989; 15:75–80.

Ohlsson K, Hansson G-A, Balogh I, et al. Disorders of the neck and upper limbs in women in the fish processing industry. *Occup Environ Med* 1994; 51:826–828.

Osborn JB, Newell KJ, Rudney JD, Stoltenberg JL. Musculoskeletal pain among Minnesota dental hygienists. *J Dental Health* 1990; 63:132–138.

Palmer KT. Musculoskeletal problems in the tomato growing industry: tomato trainer's shoulder? *Occup Med* 1996; 46:428–431.

Pollock RG, Duralde XA, Flatow EL, Bigliani LU. The use of arthroscopy in the treatment of resistant frozen shoulder. *Clin Orthop* 1994; 304:30–36.

Pope DP, Croft PR, Pritchard CM, Silman AJ. Prevalence of shoulder pain in the community: the influence of case definition. *Ann Rheum Dis* 1997a; 56:308–312.

Pope DP, Croft PR, Pritchard CM, Silman AJ, Macfarlane GJ. Occupational factors related to shoulder pain and disability. *Occup Environ Med* 1997b; 54:316–321.

Punnett L, Robins JM, Wegman DH, Keyserling WM. Soft tissue disorders in the upper limbs of female garment workers. *Scand J Work Environ Health* 1985; 11:417–425.

Reeves B. The natural history of the frozen shoulder syndrome. *Scand J Rheumatol* 1975; 4:193–196.

Richardson AB, Jobe FW, Collins HR. The shoulder in competitive swimming. *Am J Sports Med* 1980; 8:159–163.

Rothman KJ. *Modern Epidemiology.* Boston: Little, Brown & Co, 1986.

Rowe SA. Management involvement—a key element in preventing musculoskeletal problems in visual display unit users in Australia. *Ergonomics* 1987; 30:367–372.

Rundcrantz B-L, Johnsson B, Moritz U. Cervical pain and discomfort among dentists: epidemiological, clinical and therapeutic aspects. *Swed Dent J* 1990; 14:71–80.

Rundcrantz B-L, Johnsson B, Moritz U. Pain and discomfort in the musculoskeletal system among dentists. *Swed Dent J* 1991; 15:219–228.

Sakibara H, Miyao M, Kondo T, et al. Relation between overhead work and complaints of pear and apple orchard workers. *Ergonomics* 1987; 30:805–815.

Sakibara H, Miyao M, Kondo T, Yamada S. Overhead work and shoulder-neck pain in orchard farmers harvesting pears and apples. *Ergonomics* 1995; 38:700–706.

Sattar MA, Luqman WA. Periarthritis: another duration-related complication of diabetes mellitus. *Diabetes Care* 1985; 8:507–510.

Sauter SL, Schleifer LM, Knutson SJ. Work posture, workstation design, and musculoskeletal discomfort in a VDT data entry task. *Human Factors* 1991; 33:151–167.

Shaffer B, Tibone JE, Kerlan RK. Frozen shoulder: a long term follow-up. *J Bone Joint Surg Am* 1992; 74:738–746.

Sher JS, Uribe JW, Posada A, Murphy BJ, Zlatkin MB. Abnormal findings on magnetic resonance images of the asymptomatic shoulder. *J Bone Joint Surg Am* 1995; 77A:10–15.

Shugars D, Miller D, Williams D, Fishburne C, Strickland D. Musculoskeletal pain among general dentists. *Gen Dent* 1987; 35:272–276.

Skov T, Borg V, Ørhede E. Psychosocial and physical risk factors for musculoskeletal disorders of the neck, shoulders, and lower back in salespeople. *Occup Environ Med* 1996; 53:351–356.

Sobel JS, Winters JC. The long-term course of shoulder complaints as seen in general practice. In: *Shoulder Complaints in General Practice.* Amsterdam: Meditekst, 1996, pp 105–112.

Sokas RK, Spiegelman D, Wegman DH. Self-reported musculoskeletal complaints among garment workers. *Am J Ind Med* 1989; 15:197–206.

Sommerich CM, McGlothlin JD, Marras WS. Occupational risk factors associated with soft tissue disorders of the shoulder: a review of recent investigations in the literature. *Ergonomics* 1993; 36:697–717.

Stenlund B, Goldie I, Hagberg M, Hogstedt C, Marions O. Radiographic osteoarthrosis in the acromioclavicular joint resulting from manual work or exposure to vibration. *Br J Ind Med* 1992; 49:588–593.

Stenlund B, Goldie I, Hagberg M, Hogstedt C. Shoulder tendinitis and its relation to heavy manual work and exposure to vibration. *Scand J Work Environ Health* 1993; 19:43–49.

Stock SR. Workplace ergonomic factors and the development of musculoskeletal disorders or the neck and upper limbs: a meta-analysis. *Am J Ind Med* 1991; 19:87–107.

Stocker D, Pink M, Jobe FW. Comparison of shoulder injury in collegiate- and master's-level swimmers. *Clin J Sports Med* 1995; 5:4–8.

Takala J, Sievers K, Klaukka T. Rheumatic symptoms in the middle-aged population in Southwestern Finland. *Scand J Rheumatol* 1982; 47(Suppl):15–29.

Uhthoff HK, Sarkar K. An algorithm for shoulder pain caused by soft-tissue disorders. *Clin Orthop* 1990; 254:121–127.

van der Beek AJ, Frings-Dresen MHW, van Dijk FJH, Kemper HCG, Meijman TF. Loading and unloading by lorry drivers and musculoskeletal complaints. *Int J Industr Ergon* 1993; 12:13–23.

van der Windt DAWM, Koes BW, Jong BA de, Bouter LM. Shoulder disorders in general practice: incidence, patient characteristics and management. *Ann Rheum Dis* 1995; 54:959–964.

van der Windt DAWM, Koes BW, Boeke AJP, et al. Shoulder disorders in general practice: prognostic indicators of outcome. *Br J Gen Pract* 1996; 46:519–523.

van Ouwenaller C, Laplace PM, Chantraine A. Painful shoulder in hemiplegia. *Arch Phys Med Rehabil* 1986; 67:23–36.

Vecchio PC, Kavanagh RT, Hazleman BL, King RH. Community survey of shoulder disorders in the elderly to assess the natural history and effects of treatment. *Ann Rheum Dis* 1995; 54:152–154.

Veiersted KB, Westgaard RH, Andersen P. Electromyographic evaluation of muscular work pattern as a predictor of trapezius myalgia. *Scand J Work Environ Health* 1993; 19:284–290.

Viikari-Juntura E. Neck and upper limb disorders among slaughterhouse workers. *Scand J Work Environ Health* 1983; 9:283–290.

Wacholder S, McLaughlin JK, Silverman DT, Mandel JS. Selection of controls in case-control studies. I. Principles. *Am J Epidemiol* 1992; 135:1019–1028.

Waddell G. A new clinical model for the treatment of low back pain. *Spine* 1987; 12:632–644.

Warner JJP, Micheli LJ, Arslanian LE, Kennedy J, Kennedy R. Patterns of flexibility, laxity, and strength in normal shoulders and shoulders with instability and impingement. *Am J Sports Med* 1990; 18:366–375.

Wells JA, Zipp JF, Schuette PT, McEleney J. Musculoskeletal disorders among letter carriers. *J Occup Med* 1983; 25:814–820.

Westerling D, Jonsson BG. Pain from the neck-shoulder region and sick leave. *Scand J Soc Med* 1980; 8:131–136.

Westgaard RH, Jansen T. Individual and work-related factors associated with symptoms of musculoskeletal complaints. II. Different risk factors among sewing machine operators. *Br J Ind Med* 1992; 49:154–162.

Winge S, Jørgensen U, Lassen Nielsen A. Epidemiology of injuries in Danish championship tennis. *Int J Sports Med* 1989; 10:368–371.

Wright V, Haq AMMM. Periarthritis of the shoulder. I. Aetiological considerations with particular reference to personality factors. *Ann Rheum Dis* 1976; 35:213–219.

Yamanaka K, Matsumoto T. The joint side tear of the rotator cuff: a follow-up study by arthrography. *Clin Orthop* 1994; 304:68–73.

Yu ITS, Wong TW. Musculoskeletal problems among VDU workers in a Hong Kong bank. *Occup Med* 1996; 46:275–280.

Correspondence to: Daniëlle van der Windt, PhD, Institute for Research in Extramural Medicine, Vrije Universiteit, Van der Boechorststraat 7, 1081 BT Amsterdam, The Netherlands.

APPENDIX I

Studies on combined shoulder–neck pain

Anderson HL, Ejlertsson G, Leden I, Rosenberg C. Chronic pain in a geographically defined general population: studies of differences in age, gender, social class, and pain localisation. *Clin J Pain* 1993; 9:174–182.

Bjelle A, Hagberg M, Michaelson G. Occupational and individual factors in acute shoulder-neck disorders among industrial workers. *Br J Ind Med* 1981; 38: 356–363.

Bjelle A, Hagberg M, Michaelson G. Work-related shoulder-neck complaints in industry: a pilot study. *Br J Rheumatol* 1987; 26:365–369.

Carlson CR, Wynn KT, Edwards J, Okeson JP, Nitz AJ, Workman DE, Cassisi J. Ambulatory electromyogram activity in the upper trapezius region. *Spine* 1996; 21:595–599.

Chiang FIC, Ko YC, Chen SS, Yu HS, Wu TN, Chang PY. Prevalence of shoulder and upper-limb disorders among workers in the fish processing industry. *Scand J Work Environ Health* 1993; 19:126–131.

Ekberg K, Björkqvist B, Malm P, et al. Case-control study of risk factors for disease in the neck and shoulder area. *Occup Environ Med* 1994; 51:262–266.

Hägg GM, Åström A. Load pattern and pressure pain threshold in the upper trapezius muscle and psychosocial factors in medical secretaries with and without shoulder/neck disorders. *Int Arch Occup Environ Health* 1997; 69:423–432.

Hasvold T, Johnsen R. Headache and neck or shoulder pain—frequent and disabling complaints in the general population. *Scand J Prim Health Care* 1993; 11:219–224.

Hasvold T, Johnsen R, Førde OH. Non-migrainous headache, neck or shoulder pain, and migraine differences in association with background factors in a city population. *Scand J Prim Health Care* 1996; 14:92–99.

Hedberg G, Björkstén M, Ouchterlony-Jonnson E, Jonnson B. Rheumatic complaints among Swedish engine drivers in relation to the dimensions of the driver's cab in the Rc engine. *Appl Ergonomics* 1981; 12:93–97.

Holmström EB, Lindell J, Moritz U. Low back and neck/shoulder pain in construction workers: occupational workload and psychosocial risk factors. Part 2: Relationship to neck and shoulder pain. *Spine* 1992; 17:672–677.

Jensen K, Nilsen K, Hansen K, Westgaard RH. Trapezius muscle load as a risk indicator of occupational shoulder-neck complaints. *Int Arch Environ Health* 1993; 64:415–423.

Kvarnström S. 1983. Diseases of the musculoskeletal system in an engineering company. *Scand J Rehabil Med* 1983; 8(Suppl):61–76.

Leino P, Magni G. Depressive and distress symptoms as predictors of low back pain, neck-shoulder pain, and other musculoskeletal morbidity: a 10-year follow-up of metal industry employees. *Pain* 1993; 53:89–94.

Levoska S, Keinänen-Kiukaanniemi SM. Psychosocial stress and job satisfaction in female office employees with and without neck-shoulder symptoms. *Work & Stress* 1994; 8:255–262.

Manninen P, Riihimdki H, Heliövaara M. Has muskuloskeletal pain become less prevalent? *Scand J Rheumatol* 1996; 25:37–41.

Marcus M, Gerr F. Upper extremity musculoskeletal symptoms among female office workers: associations with video display terminal use and occupational psychosocial stressors. *Am J Ind Med* 1996; 29:161–170.

Niemi SM, Levoska S, Rekola KE, Keindnen-Kiukaanniemi SM. Neck and shoulder symptoms of high school students and associated psychosocial factors. *J Adolescent Health* 1997; 20:238–242.

Ryan GA, Bampton M. Comparison of data process operators with and without upper limb symptoms. *Community Health Studies* 1988; 12:63–68.

Salminen JJ, Pentti J, Wickström G. Tenderness and pain in neck and shoulders in relation to type A behaviour. *Scand J Rheumatol* 1991; 20:344–350.

Schierhout G, Meyers JE, Bridger RS. Work related musculoskeletal disorders and ergonomic stressors in the South African workforce. *Occup Environ Med* 1995; 52:46–50.

Takala E-P, Viikari-Juntura E, Moneta GB, Saarenmaa K, Kaivanto K. Seasonal variation in neck and shoulder symptoms. *Scand J Work Environ Health* 1992; 18:257–261.

Tola S, Riihimäki H, Videman T, Viikari-Juntura E, Hänninen K. Neck and shoulder symptoms among men in machine operating, dynamic physical work and sedentary work. *Scand J Work Environ Health* 1988; 14:299–305.

Vasseljen O, Westgaard RH. A case-control study of trapezius muscle activity in office and manual workers with shoulder and nack pain. *Int Arch Occup Environ Health* 1995a; 67:11–18.

Vasseljen O, Westgaard RH, Larsen S. A case-control study of psychological and psychosocial risk factors for shoulder and neck pain at the work place. *Int Arch Occup Environ Health* 1995b; 66:375–382.

Veiersted KB, Westgaard RH. Development of trapezius myalgia among female workers performing light manual work. *Scand J Work Environ Health* 1993a; 19:277–283.

Veiersted KB, Westgaard RH, Andersen P. Electromyographic evaluation of muscular work pattern as a predictor of trapezius myalgia. *Scand J Work Environ Health* 1993b; 19:284–290.

Viikari-Juntura E, Vuori J, Silverstein BA, Kalimo R, Kuosma E, Videman T. A life-long prospective study on the role of psychosocial factors in neck-shoulder and low-back pain. *Spine* 1991; 16:1056–1061.

Westerling D, Jonsson BG. Pain from the neck-shoulder region and sick leave. *Scand J Soc Med* 1980; 8:131–136.

Westgaard RH, Jesnen C, Hansen K. Individual and work-related risk factors associated with symptoms of musculoskeletal complaints. *Int Arch Occup Environ Health* 1993; 64:405–413.

APPENDIX II
Critical appraisal of studies on the frequency of shoulder pain

Reference	A	B	C	D	E	F	F2	G	Final Score
Allander 1974	1	1	2	2	2	1	1	1	11
Backman et al. 1983	1	1	1	2	2	1	1	0	9
Beach et al.1992	1	1	1	0	0	1	1	0	5
Bergenudd et al. 1988	0	0	2	2	2	1	1	0	8
Bergenudd et al. 1991	1	1	2	2	2	1	1	0	10
Bergenudd and Nilsson 1994	1	1	2	2	2	1	1	0	10
Bergström et al. 1985	1	1	2	2	0	0	1	1	8
Bernard et al. 1994	1	1	1	2	2	1	1	1	10
Bohannon et al. 1986	1	1	1	2	0	0	0	1	6
Brocklehurst et al. 1978	1	1	0	2	0	1	1	0	6
Buckle et al. 1987	1	0	1	0	0	1	1	0	4
Chakravarty and Webley 1993	1	1	2	2	0	0	1	1	8
Chard et al. 1991	1	1	2	2	2	1	0	0	9
Chard and Hazleman 1987	1	1	2	0	0	0	0	1	5
Christensen et al. 1986	1	1	1	0	0	1	1	0	5
Cunningham and Kelsey 1984	1	0	2	2	2	1	0	1	9
Dimberg et al. 1989	1	1	1	2	2	1	1	1	10
Ekberg et al. 1995	1	1	1	2	2	1	1	1	10
Flodmark and Aase 1992	1	0	1	2	0	1	1	0	6
Hales et al. 1994	1	1	2	2	2	1	1	1	11
Herberts et al. 1981	1	1	2	2	0	1	0	0	7
Hunting et al. 1981	1	0	2	0	0	0	0	0	3
Jacobsson et al. 1989	1	1	2	2	2	1	1	1	11
Jacobsson et al. 1996	1	1	2	2	2	1	0	1	10
Johansson and Rubenowitz 1994	1	1	1	2	2	1	1	1	10
Jonsson et al. 1988	0	1	2	0	0	1	1	1	6
Kamwendo et al. 1991	1	1	1	2	2	1	1	1	10
Lagerström et al. 1995	1	1	1	2	2	1	1	1	10
Liss et al. 1995	1	1	1	2	2	1	1	1	10
Lo et al.1990	1	0	1	0	2	0	1	0	5
Luopajarvi et al. 1979	1	1	2	2	0	1	1	0	8
Mackay-Rossignol et al. 1987	1	1	1	2	2	1	1	1	10
Magnussen et al. 1996	1	0	1	2	0	0	1	0	5
Mäkelä et al. 1993	1	0	2	2	2	1	1	0	9
Manahan et al. 1985	0	1	1	0	2	1	1	1	7
Mavrikakis et al. 1989	0	1	2	2	2	1	1	0	9
McCormack et al. 1990	1	0	2	2	2	1	1	1	10
McMaster and Troup 1993	1	1	1	2	2	1	1	1	10
Meyers et al. 1982	1	0	2	2	0	1	1	0	7
Milerad and Ekenvall 1990	1	1	1	2	0	0	1	1	7
Näyhä et al.1994	1	1	1	2	2	1	1	1	10
Nichols et al. 1979	1	1	1	0	2	1	1	1	8
Ohesson et al. 1994	1	1	2	2	0	1	1	1	9
Osborn et al. 1990	1	0	1	2	2	1	1	0	8
Palmer et al. 1996	1	1	1	2	0	1	1	1	8
Pope et al. 1997a	1	1	1	2	2	1	1	1	10
Punnett et al. 1985	1	1	2	2	0	1	1	1	9
Richardson et al. 1980	0	0	2	2	0	0	1	0	5
Rundcrantz et al. 1990	1	1	1	2	2	1	1	0	9
Rundcrantz et al. 1991	1	1	1	2	2	1	1	0	9
Sakibara et al. 1987	1	0	1	0	0	1	1	0	4
Sakibara et al. 1995	1	0	2	0	0	1	1	0	5
Sattar and Lugman 1985	1	1	2	2	0	1	1	1	9
Sauter et al. 1991	1	1	1	2	2	1	1	1	10
Shugars et al. 1987	1	1	1	2	2	1	1	1	10
Skov et al. 1996	1	1	1	2	2	1	1	1	10

(continued)

APPENDIX II
Continued

Reference	A	B	C	D	E	F	F2	G	Final Score
Sokas et al. 1989	1	1	1	0	0	0	1	1	5
Stenlund et al. 1992	1	1	2	2	0	1	1	1	9
Stenlund et al. 1993	1	1	2	2	0	1	1	1	9
Stocker et al. 1995	1	1	1	2	2	1	1	0	9
Takala et al. 1982	1	1	2	2	2	1	1	1	11
Viikari-Juntura 1983	1	0	2	0	0	1	0	1	5
Wells et al. 1983	1	1	1	2	0	1	0	1	7
Westerling and Jonsson 1980	0	1	1	2	2	1	1	1	9
Winge et al. 1989	1	1	1	2	0	1	1	0	7
van der Beek et al. 1993	1	1	1	2	2	0	1	1	9
Van der Windt et al. 1995	1	1	1	2	2	1	0	1	9
Yu and Wong 1996	1	1	1	2	0	1	1	0	7

Note: A = purpose; B = description of population; C = assessment of pain; D = representative sample; E = sample size; F = analysis; F2 = response rate; G = discussion. All numbers are method scores.

APPENDIX III
Quality assessment of studies on risk factors for shoulder pain

Reference	A	B	C	D	E	F	G	H	I	Final Score
Bergenudd et al. 1988	0	0	2	2	1	0	0	0	0	5
Bergenudd et al. 1994	1	1	2	2	1	0	0	2	0	9
Bernard and Nilsson 1994	1	1	0	1	2	2	2	2	1	12
Bjelle et al. 1979	0	1	1/1	2	1	0	0	0	0	6
Bru et al. 1993	1	1	0	1	1	0	?	1	0	5
Dimberg et al. 1989	1	1	0	1	1	0	2	2	1	9
English et al. 1995	1	1	1/1	2	1	2	0	2	1	12
Epstein et al. 1993	1	0	1/1	2	2	2	0	0	1	10
Flodmark and Aase 1992	1	0	0	1	1	0	0	0	1	4
Griegel-Morris 1992	1	0	0	1	2	0	0	0	1	5
Hales et al. 1994	1	1	0	2	1	2	2	2	1	12
Herberts et al. 1981	1	0	0	2	2	0	0	0	0	5
Jacobsson et al. 1992	1	1	1/1	2	1	0	0	1	1	9
Johansson and Rubenowitz 1994	1	1	0	1	1	0	2	1	1	8
Kamwendo et al. 1991	1	1	0	1	1	0	2	1	1	8
Kilbom et al. 1986	1	1	0	2	2	0	0	2	1	9
Kvarnström 1983	1	1	0	2	1	0	2	1	0	8
Kvarnström and Halldén 1983	1	1	1/1	2	1	2	2	0	1	12
Lagerström et al. 1995	1	1	0	1	1	0	2	2	1	9
Linton and Kamwendo 1989	1	1	0	1	1	0	2	0	1	7
Liss et al. 1995	1	1	0	1	1	0	2	2	1	9
Ohlsson et al. 1989	1	1	0	1	1	0	2	2	1	9
Pope et al. 1997b	1	1	1/1	1	1	2	0	1	1	10
Punnett et al. 1985	1	1	0	2	1	0	0	2	1	8
Rundcrantz et al. 1990	1	1	0	1	1	0	2	0	0	6
Skov et al. 1996	1	1	0	1	1	0	2	1	1	8
Stenlund et al. 1992	1	1	0	2	1	2	0	2	1	10
Stenlund et al. 1993	1	1	0	2	1	2	t	2	1	10
Takala et al. 1982	1	1	0	2	1	0	1	0	1	7
van der Beek et al. 1993	1	1	0	1	1	0	2	2	1	9
Westgaard and Jansen 1992	1	0	0	1	1	0	2	1	1	7
Wright and Haq 1976	1	1	1/0	2	1	0	2	0	1	9
Yu and Wong 1996	1	1	0	1	1	0	0	1	1	6

Note: A = purpose; B = description of population; C = design; D = assessment of pain; E = assessment of exposure; F = information bias; G = sample size; H = analysis; I = discussion. All numbers are method scores.

Epidemiology of Pain, edited by
I.K. Crombie, IASP Press, Seattle, © 1999.

18

Low Back Pain

Clermont E. Dionne

*Department of Rehabilitation, Faculty of Medicine, Laval University, Sainte-Foy, Quebec, Canada;
and Quebec Rehabilitation Research Institute, Quebec City, Canada*

Low back pain (LBP) is among the most frequent health problems and has a significant effect on quality of life. The literature on LBP is vast, and many statistics have been published in heterogeneous studies, so that it can be difficult to recognize the full extent of the problem.

This chapter summarizes the epidemiological evidence on adult mechanical LBP, with a special emphasis on its frequency, causes, and consequences. Only studies that met the following scientific criteria were reviewed: (1) well-defined purpose, (2) definition of LBP provided, (3) appropriate study design, (4) adequate statistical power, (5) appropriate analyses, and (6) valid interpretation of findings. These criteria were interpreted as suggested by Bombardier et al. (1994).

DEFINITION AND DIAGNOSTIC CRITERIA

Low back pain is thought to arise from several anatomical structures, including ligaments, muscles and fascia, outer fibers of the annulus fibrosus, facet joints, the vertebral periosteum, blood vessels, and spinal nerve roots (Deyo 1992). However, only rarely can a specific cause be identified (Dillane et al. 1966; White and Gordon 1982; Spitzer et al. 1987; Waddell 1987). Furthermore, modern imaging techniques have shown that some spinal abnormalities, such as disk herniation, are common in persons with no back pain (Riihimaki 1991). The absence of objective findings in almost all cases of LBP has forced clinicians and investigators to rely on the symptoms of LBP, which are quite diverse. This situation has engendered numerous definitions and diagnostic classifications of

LBP that render the comparison of study results difficult. For instance, Fardon et al. (1993) asked orthopedic surgeons at two major spine meetings to write down their four most common diagnoses of LBP; they collected 50 different terms altogether from 51 respondents.

In this chapter, we will consider low back pain as "any report of pain that occurs between the gluteal folds inferiorly and the line of the 12th rib superiorly, plus sciatica and cruralgia even if there are no concurrent symptoms in the back" (adapted from Anderson 1986), excluding LBP due to pregnancy, menstruation, viral infection, or cancer (McKinnon et al. 1997). This definition could be applied quite easily with drawing manikins such as the one displayed in Fig. 1.

FREQUENCY OF LOW BACK PAIN

ESTIMATES OF FREQUENCY

The frequency of an episodic disease can be defined as a function of its incidence, prevalence, and recurrence. The often insidious onset of LBP, its variability over time, and its episodic character are the source of important methodological difficulties in estimating the frequency of this problem (Leboeuf-Yde and Lauritsen 1995). For example, some investigators of LBP incidence included patients who had previously experienced back pain but were free of symptoms at the beginning of follow-up (thus considering recurrent episodes as incident ones), while others selected patients who had never had LBP previously ("true" incident cases). Also, since the prevalence of an episodic disease is determined by its rate of occur-

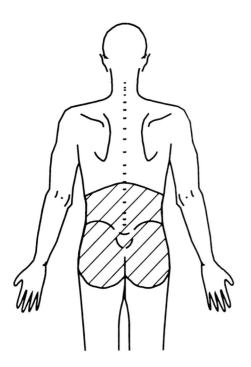

Fig. 1. Manikin showing spatial definition of low back pain (Papageorgiou et al. 1995, reprinted with permission).

rence (incidence rate), the average episode duration, and the average number of episodes (Von Korff and Parker 1980), differences in prevalence could reflect differences in any of the above factors. Unfortunately, many reports on LBP focus on prevalence measures.

The concept of recurrence as it relates to episodic LBP is also poorly defined. Five different uses of the term "recurrence" were found in published reports on LBP: (1) the occurrence of relapsing symptoms reported as being related to a previous injury, (2) any further episode reported as being related or not to a previous back injury, (3) therapeutic failure after back injury, (4) administrative decisions that generally have little or nothing to do with the problem itself (Abenhaim et al. 1988), and (5) persistence of back pain over time (Biering-Sørensen and Thomsen 1986). Again, the disease is defined by different sets of symptoms, most frequently "pain in the lower back with at least 1 day of absence from work." These different approaches, given the heterogeneous populations studied and the use of different types of estimates, yield widely varying results that are often difficult to compare. The statistics presented in this chapter should be considered with this in mind.

Among spinal pain problems, pain in the low back is clearly the most prevalent, representing 70–80% of

all cases (Rossignol et al. 1988; Guo et al. 1995). This problem is very common in the general population, affecting 58–84% of all adults at some point of their life (lifetime prevalence) (Andersson 1981; Svensson et al. 1983; Biering-Sørensen and Thomsen 1986; Svensson et al. 1990; Walsh et al. 1992; Von Korff et al. 1993a; Skovron et al. 1994; Papageorgiou et al. 1995; Harreby et al. 1996; Hillman et al. 1996; McKinnon et al. 1997; Cassidy et al. 1998). When a stringent definition of LBP is used, however, the lifetime prevalence is much lower. The U.S. second National Health and Nutrition Examination Survey (NHANES II), for example, reported a lifetime prevalence of 13.8% for "pain in the lower back on most days for at least two weeks" (Deyo and Tsui-Wu 1987). More recently, Cassidy et al. (1998) reported an 84.1% lifetime prevalence estimate of LBP in Saskatchewan, Canada. The 6-month period prevalence was also quite high (men 68.8%; women 73.6%). However, when LBP problems in the past 6 months were graded on pain intensity and disability with the Chronic Pain Questionnaire (Von Korff et al. 1992), most episodes appeared not to be disabling, with 11% of subjects overall having significant levels of disability. Similarly, the 1-year cumulative incidence estimates vary between 17% (Biering-Sørensen and Thomsen 1986) and 34% (Croft et al. 1995), but drop to 4.0–7.5% when only problems severe enough to require a medical consultation are considered (Dillane et al. 1966; Croft et al. 1995). These results shed some light on the reasons for the large variation in prevalence estimates, and show that although LBP as such is common, it has severe consequences only in a small proportion of those affected.

At any given time (point prevalence), 4.4–33.0% of the adult population suffers from LBP. Again, higher figures correspond to more general definitions (Svensson et al. 1983; Cunningham and Kelsey 1984; Lee et al. 1985; Deyo and Tsui-Wu 1987; Bergenudd and Nilsson 1988; Heliövaara et al. 1991; Skovron et al. 1994; Harreby et al. 1996; Hillman et al. 1996; Liira et al. 1996; McKinnon et al. 1997; Cassidy et al. 1998).

In studies conducted among workers, definitions of back pain often include a criterion related to work absenteeism (generally at least 1 day of absence) or to compensation claims. With such criteria, statistics are much more conservative: the 1-year cumulative incidence of compensation claims for back pain (70% in the low back) with at least 1 day of absence from work has been estimated at 1.4% in Canada (Abenhaim and

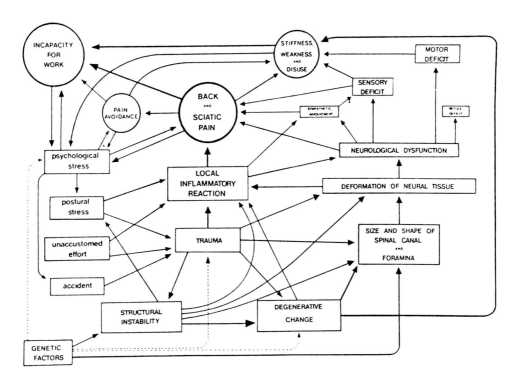

Fig. 2. Lloyd and Troup's (1983) multifactorial etiological model of back pain (reprinted with permission).

Suissa 1987).

Quite low figures have been obtained in Japan, where the 2-year cumulative incidence of compensable backache causing more than 4 days of absenteeism among workers is 0.01% (Kuwashima et al. 1997). However, this result cannot be generalized to other countries because of the particularities of the workers' compensation system in Japan (Hadler 1994).

Although the lower figures of frequency obtained by using more stringent definitions of LBP may seem reassuring, they are still dramatic, because even a low percentage of persistent problems creates a large number of cases (Steinberg 1982). More than 26 million of Americans of working age (20–64 years) have frequent back pain, and almost 6 million among those aged 65 years and more (Lawrence et al. 1998).

Analyses conducted by Deyo and Tsui-Wu (1987) on NHANES II data showed important regional variations in lifetime prevalence of LBP in the United States: the lowest prevalence was found in the northeastern states (10.9%) and the highest in the western states (15.0%). There is no clear explanation for this variation.

In Japan, LBP caused by accidents at work is more frequent at the beginning of the week and immediately after starting the day's work (most cases occur at 9 A.M., followed by 10 A.M.); no important monthly variations were observed (Kuwashima et al. 1997).

Evidence does not support an increase in the frequency of LBP over the past decades as such, but rather a major increase in reporting low-back-related disability (Cunningham and Kelsey 1984; Waddell 1987, 1991, 1996). For instance, recent studies on trends in the prevalence of low back in Finland in the past two decades reported quite stable figures that could not explain the increase in the societal costs of LBP during this period (Leino et al. 1994; Heistaro et al. 1998).

DETERMINANTS OF FREQUENCY

Low back pain is considered to have a multifactorial etiology involving a complex web of factors. Several models have attempted to conceptualize the relations between postulated contributory factors, but none has been scientifically validated. As an example, Fig. 2 presents the model developed by Lloyd and Troup (1983).

In general, studies on risk factors for LBP suffer from the same methodological difficulties stated previously. Investigators often aim to estimate the frequency of LBP and to identify risk factors concurrently in the same study. Apart from other differences in the methods, the heterogeneity in the types of outcome variables used would alone explain conflicting results. But it is the reliance on bivariate analyses (i.e., with no account taken of potential confounders) that probably most complicates the comparison of study results on risk factors. Consequently, this chapter reports only the results of studies that have used multivariate methods.

Sociodemographic factors

The effect of age on the frequency of LBP is still unclear. The risk of LBP is high during the most productive years (25–55), with a peak between 30 and 39 years (Steinberg 1982; Bergquist-Ullman and Larsson 1977; Lawrence et al. 1998), and decreases after the fifth decade of age (Battie et al. 1990; Liira et al. 1996; Heistaro et al. 1998). However, this decrease could be the result of a "healthy worker effect," where those in jobs at high risk of back pain tend to change jobs after this age (Anderson 1986; Abenhaim and Suissa 1987).

Similarly, the effect of gender on the onset and the prevalence of LBP is not well understood. Although LBP is found more often among men, many arguments support the hypothesis that this is because more men perform tasks with a high risk of back pain (Abenhaim and Suissa 1987). However, in a study by Abenhaim et al. (1988), which controlled for age, site of symptoms, and occupation, men were almost twice as likely as women to have a recurrence. Among recurrent cases, in contrast, men and women had on average the same number of episodes. This suggests that the difference between sexes might arise early in the evolution of a back condition, before the onset of a first recurrence. Conversely, some studies have found higher prevalence rates among women (Skovron et al. 1994; Heistaro et al. 1998).

Persons with low educational status tend to have more low back problems (Viikari-Juntura et al. 1991; Heistaro et al. 1998), although this association is, again, not well understood. Education could act as a proxy for socioeconomic status and be a marker for occupational, physical, environmental, and behavioral risk factors for LBP or for back-related disability (Dionne et al. 1995). A similar association has been reported for family income (Croft and Rigby 1994; Liira et al. 1996; Heistaro et al. 1998).

Clinical factors

A history of previous back problems is a strong predictor of future episodes of LBP. The Boeing study associated recent episodes with a history of back prob-

lems during the past 10 years (Battie et al. 1990; Bigos et al. 1991). A Finnish study (Heliövaara et al. 1991) also identified a history of traumatic back injury as a predictor of nonspecific LBP (OR = 2.5; 95% CI = 2.0–3.0) and sciatica (OR = 2.4; 95% CI = 1.9–3.2).

Obesity has been linked with the incidence of LBP only among women, in a prospective study conducted in the United States (Battie et al. 1990). However, several reports describe an association between obesity and prevalence measures among both men and women (Deyo and Bass 1989; Orvieto et al. 1994; Liira et al. 1996; Heistaro et al. 1998).

A positive association between body height and the prevalence of LBP has been reported in some studies (Heliövaara et al. 1991; Croft and Rigby 1994). Heliövaara and colleagues (1991) reported that among 50–64-year-old subjects, the odds ratio for LBP with each increase of 10 cm in body height was 1.5 (95% CI = 1.5–2.0).

Musculoskeletal abnormalities have long been thought to be the main cause of LBP, and are still part of the "myths" that surround this problem. No evidence supports this idea, except in the case of extreme deformities. For example, Soukka et al. (1991) found no significant association between leg-length inequality up to 20 mm (as measured by radiologic examination) and the prevalence of LBP.

Other health problems that have been associated with LBP are osteoarthritis of the knee, hip, or hand (OR = 5.3; 95% CI = 4.1–6.9), other musculoskeletal diseases (excluding osteoarthritis and inflammatory polyarthritis) (OR = 3.8; 95% CI = 3.1–4.7), mental disorders (OR = 1.3; 95% CI = 1.1–1.6), and diabetes (OR = 0.4; 95% CI = 0.3–0.8) (Heliövaara et al. 1991).

Occupational factors

Burdorf (1992, 1993), in papers on exposure assessment of risk factors for back pain, concluded that in most epidemiological studies on back pain in occupational groups the quality of exposure data is poor. This might explain why the effects of occupational exposure on back pain, despite extensive study, are still controversial. In fact, most of the evidence on the impact of occupational factors on LBP comes from empirical findings and the consistency of the results across many studies.

The physical workload of a job (Heliövaara et al. 1991; Heistaro et al. 1998), frequent bending and lifting at work (Liira et al. 1996), working with the back in awkward positions (flexion, twist, or lateral bend) (Punnett et al. 1991; Liira et al. 1996), and operating vibrating equipment (Liira et al. 1996) are the best documented occupational risk factors. These factors certainly explain part of the high frequency of LBP that is often identified in specific occupations, especially among drivers, construction workers, and nurses (Abenhaim et al. 1988; Liira et al. 1996).

Mental stress at work may play a role in LBP (Leino 1989; Heliövaara et al. 1991; Bongers et al. 1993; Houtman et al. 1994) and has been measured as a single variable (dull or monotonous work, high perceived work load, hurried or tight work schedule, and being worried about making mistakes), or (as proposed by Karasek and Theorell 1990) as a combination of high psychological demands and low decision latitude modified by social support at work. Bongers and colleagues (1993) reviewed the studies on psychosocial factors at work and musculoskeletal disease and summarized the possible mechanisms by which psychosocial factors at work (demands, job control, and social support) may affect musculoskeletal disease. First, psychological factors at work would directly influence the mechanical load through changes in posture, movement, and exerted forces. Second, psychosocial factors at work, together with personal capacity to cope with such factors, may increase work-related stress and the accompanying symptoms. This increase in stress may increase muscle tone, which in the long term could lead to the development of musculoskeletal symptoms due to some unknown but specific physiological mechanism. It also may moderate the relationship between mechanical load and musculoskeletal symptoms due to enhancement of the perception of symptoms or the reduction of the capacity to deal with them. From their review, Bongers and colleagues concluded that, in spite of contradictory or inconsistent results, monotonous work, high perceived work load, and time pressure are related to musculoskeletal symptoms. Their data also suggest that low control over one's work and lack of social support by colleagues are positively associated with musculoskeletal disease.

Job satisfaction is one of the few factors that has been clearly and consistently shown to affect the frequency of LBP (or its report) (Bergenudd and Nilsson 1988; Bigos et al. 1991; Linton and Warg 1993; Skovron et al. 1994). This variable probably acts by reflecting the worker's perception of the physical and psychosocial environment at work.

Although not as common as one might think, spe-cific injuries at work still are responsible for a significant proportion of low back problems. Heliövaara et al. (1991) estimated the proportion of the prevalence of sciatica related to back injuries (population attributable fraction) at 16.5% and that of unspecified LBP at 13.7%.

Psychological factors

Psychological factors, namely depression (Åkerlind et al. 1992; Croft et al. 1995), self-confidence (Viikari-Juntura et al. 1991), and a propensity to somatization (Gilchrist 1976; Bigos et al. 1991; Bacon et al. 1994) are clearly associated with LBP. Because most reports are from cross-sectional studies, it is unclear whether these psychological conditions precede or follow the onset of back problems (Von Korff et al. 1993b); some evidence supports each mechanism (Leino 1989; Croft et al. 1995; Mannion et al. 1996). While there is still much to learn about the role of psychological factors in the natural history of LBP, their importance is difficult to deny.

Behavioral factors

The association of cigarette smoking with back pain frequency measures has been reported in several papers and has passed tests of several criteria of causality (Deyo and Bass 1989; Heliövaara et al. 1991; Ernst 1993; Leboeuf-Yde et al. 1996; Liira et al. 1996; Heistaro et al. 1998). The association persists after adjustment for confounders and appears to reflect an independent effect of smoking on back pain (Ernst 1993). In a study of NHANES II data, Deyo and Bass (1989) found a significant dose-response relationship with the 1-year prevalence of LBP. Although several hypotheses have been advanced to explain this association, the most attractive assumes that smoking reduces vertebral blood flow by mechanisms working in concert: carboxyhemoglobin, vasoconstriction, atheroma, fibrinolytic defect, and hematological defect. As a result, tissue would receive less blood supply and be more vulnerable to other causes of back pain, such as mechanical stress (Jayson et al. 1984; Hambly and Mooney 1992; Ernst 1993). Although more research is needed on cigarette smoking as a risk factor for LBP, this is one determinant for which the scientific evidence is relatively clear. However, the contribution of cigarette smoking to LBP appears to be small (OR = 1.0–2.0).

Few reports of good scientific quality describe the impact of physical activity on LBP. Recent evidence comes from the study of Heistaro et al. (1998), who found a cross-sectional association between leisure-time physical activity and the prevalence of LBP. Subjects with high level of physical activity were less likely than others to suffer from LBP. The association was not very strong, however (OR = 0.88; 95% CI = 0.85–0.92). In a 25-year prospective cohort study of 640 Danish schoolchildren, Harreby et al. (1997) reported lower lifetime, 1-year, and point prevalence estimates among subjects who were physically active during their leisure time (at least 3 hours/week). Interestingly, being physically active was significantly associated with higher education and social class.

Other factors

Obstetric and gynecological factors seem to play a part in the natural history of LBP among women, other than during pregnancy. A cross-sectional study conducted in Sweden found that the number of live births and the number of abortions were significantly associated with the prevalence of LBP in multivariate analyses (Svensson et al. 1990). The same study also identified a significant association of LBP with higher frequency of menopausal symptoms. Adera et al. (1994) also found significant relationships between premature menopause and lifetime prevalence of LBP lasting at least 2 weeks. Mechanisms that could explain these associations include osteoporosis associated with hormonal changes.

Parenthood is another factor that has been linked with the prevalence of LBP. The odds ratio comparing men and women with at least four children to those without children reached 1.9 among men (95% CI = 1.2–2.8) and 1.6 among women (95% CI = 1.1–2.2) in the study of Silman et al. (1995). This relationship could reflect the physical demands associated with child rearing.

Surprisingly, few studies have focused on seasonal variation in LBP incidence. Such investigations might reveal important associations with changing environmental factors.

CONSEQUENCES OF LOW BACK PAIN

Apart from psychological distress, which will be discussed later in this chapter under "Natural history,"

the consequences of LBP for the patient and the society are fourfold: activity limitation (or functional limitations), work absenteeism, use of health services, and costs. These consequences are obviously intimately interwoven, though not equivalent, and are often not clearly distinguished in the literature.

FUNCTIONAL LIMITATIONS

Reports on back-related functional limitations confirm the self-limited character of most LBP episodes. Hence, the lifetime prevalence of LBP lasting for more than 24 hours, during which it was impossible to put on socks, stockings, or tights, was established at 5.3–16.7% (depending on gender and age) in a 5% random sample of men and women aged 20–59 years in the general population in Britain (Walsh et al. 1992). This prevalence closely resembles the most conservative estimates of the lifetime prevalence of LBP presented earlier. Other studies in Canada and Finland that have used different measures of low back-related functional limitations have reached similar conclusions (Mäkelä et al. 1993; Cassidy et al. 1998). Still, LBP is the most frequent cause of activity limitation among adults younger than 45 (Kelsey and White 1980) and is second only to arthritis in those aged 45–65 (Colvez and Blanchet 1981).

In a singular study design, Mäkelä et al. (1993) examined the determinants of disability for all causes among Finns aged 30 years or more. They found that chronic LBP was the determinant having the highest impact on reduced working capacity and occasional need for help in activities of daily living among those aged 30–64 when they controlled for other illnesses, age, sex, and social determinants of disability.

Lower educational achievement has been strongly associated with back-related functional limitations (Cunningham and Kelsey 1984; Lee et al. 1989; Mäkelä et al. 1993; Von Korff et al. 1993a; Badley and Ibañez 1994; Hurwitz and Morgenstern 1997). A close examination of this association among 1213 enrollees of a large health maintenance organization in Washington State suggested that this relationship could be explained by several (intervening) factors, the most important being a propensity to report diffuse physical symptoms (somatization), symptoms of depression, occupational factors (strength requirements and frequent handling), and cigarette smoking (Dionne et al. 1995). This information may have important implications for etiological studies on low-back-related func-

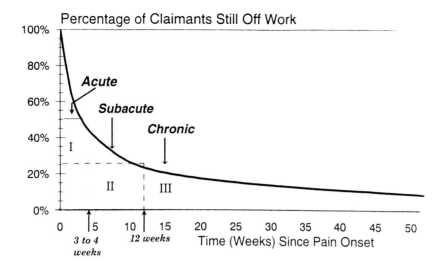

Fig. 3. Return to work among compensated workers with low back pain as a function of time, and the three-phase model of the natural history of low back pain (Frank et al. 1996, reprinted with permission).

tional limitations: adjusting for education could lead to underestimation of the effect of a variable that education is a proxy for, e.g., cigarette smoking.

WORK ABSENTEEISM

Work absenteeism is certainly one of the most deleterious effects of LBP and incurs enormous expenses for employers and society. The 1-year period prevalence estimates of time off work because of LBP vary between 5.1% and 13.5% (Walsh et al. 1992; Hillman et al. 1996). Back pain problems constitute the leading cause of work disability in the United States (Lawrence et al. 1998), and significantly affect all sectors of the economy. For instance, among military recruits in basic training in the U.S. Air Force, LBP is the third most frequent cause of discharge after patellofemoral syndrome and pes planus (Anderson and Charlesworth 1993). Similarly, in a prospective study of all army conscripts aged 18–30 years in Norway during 1990–91 (military service is mandatory for males in Norway), Heir and Glomsaker (1996) identified LBP as the most frequent diagnosis group for all medical consultations and the first reason for sick leave and discharge.

In 1981, in Quebec, 7.4% of workers compensated for a back problem (those with more than 6 months' duration) explained 68.2% of lost days (Abenhaim and Suissa 1987; Spitzer et al. 1987). The mean cumulative duration of absence from work for LBP during a 3-year period among all workers studied was 82.2 calendar days (Rossignol et al. 1988).

The Quebec Task Force on Spinal Disorders (Spitzer et al. 1987), among others, has shown that the longer the worker with back pain is away from work, the less likely he or she is to return. As illustrated in Fig. 3, after 3 months of work absenteeism the slope of the curve flattens markedly, as the probability of returning to work decreases significantly.

There appears to be a strong association between the attribution of a specific initial medical diagnosis and long-term absence from work (6 months or more) among compensated patients with LBP (OR = 4.9; 95% CI = 2.8–8.4). This factor would act through labeling: a "specific" diagnosis at the beginning of a compensation episode could signify, for the treating physician as well as for the worker, that the condition is serious and calls for a "specific" clinical treatment (Abenhaim et al. 1995). Similarly, older age (for each 10-year increase OR = 1.4; 95% CI = 1.2–1.6) and the amount of daily compensation (OR comparing Canadian $50 to less than $40 = 1.8; 95% CI = 1.0–3.4) are associated with a higher risk of long-term absence from work (Rossignol et al. 1988; Abenhaim et al. 1995). Other determinants include the presence of previous chronic episodes, disability status at entry, compensation status, job satisfaction, initial pain worse when standing or lying down, and gender (worst outcome for men) (Coste et al. 1994).

Work status in general is determined not only by medical factors, but also by psychosocial and socioeconomic variables. According to Waddell, return to work for LBP patients is determined more by psychosocial factors than by physical disease (Waddell 1987).

USE OF HEALTH SERVICES

Studies that have addressed the use of health services for LBP have considered mainly the number of visits to a health professional, bed rest, medication use, spinal radiographs, spinal surgery, and hospitalizations. An estimated 2.8–4.5% of all adult ambulatory visits to physicians are motivated by LBP (Hart et al. 1995), which ranks it among the five leading reasons for medical consultations, along with upper respiratory infections, hypertension, pregnancy care, and general medical exams (Cypress 1983; Hart et al. 1995). In the general population, the 1-year period prevalence of medical consultation for LBP varies from 6.5% to 19.1% (Walsh et al. 1992; Hillman et al. 1996; McKinnon et al. 1997), while the 1-year cumulative incidence has been estimated at 6.4% (Papageorgiou et al. 1995).

A British study on LBP prevalence found important geographical differences in general practice consultation rates despite homogeneous prevalence of symptoms (Walsh et al. 1992). Subjects in northern areas were three to four times more likely to consult a doctor than were those living in the south. These differences were not explained by age, sex, social class, or severity of symptoms.

Most back pain visits are made to generalist physicians (family physicians and general internists). However, back pain accounts for the largest percentage of caseload for some specialists, namely neurosurgeons and orthopedic surgeons (Hart et al. 1995).

In the United States, 150 of 100,000 nonsurgical hospitalizations (265,500 in 1990) and 158 of 100,000 surgical hospitalizations (279,000 in 1990) are attributable to LBP each year. Although the rate of nonsurgical hospitalization for LBP decreased between 1979 and 1990 in this country, that of surgical procedures increased by 55% (Davis 1994; Taylor et al. 1994). An analysis of data from the U.S. National Hospital Discharge Survey by Taylor et al. (1994) uncovered a wide geographical variation in hospitalization and surgery rates, far greater than might be explained by differences in the prevalence of back problems. Similarly, in a small-area analysis of surgery for LBP in Washington State, the rate of surgery for LBP varied from 11.5 in 100,000 to 172.1 in 100,000, nearly a 15-fold difference between counties. Much of this difference could not be explained by the variables considered in the study. The authors concluded that the surgeons' practice styles (determined by variable diffusion of medical innovations, preconceptualization [i.e., degree of conservatism], tolerance for uncertainty, and reaction to patient expectations) may be responsible for this wide variation (Volinn et al. 1992).

In 2660 subjects with a history of LBP from a population survey conducted on a probability sample of about 5000 Belgian adults stratified by gender, age, social class, and habitat, Szpalski et al. (1995) identified health beliefs (belief that LBP would be a life-long problem), increasing age, and the frequency of symptoms (daily versus non-daily) as the most important determinants for use of health services (visits to a health professional, bed rest, taking medication, and X-rays). The authors hypothesized that, in accordance with the fear avoidance model of Waddell, negative health beliefs may reflect a more disabling behavior leading to labeling.

Other predictors of health services utilization are depression score, disability score, disability payments, duration of the pain problem, disk or arthritis diagnosis (Walsh et al. 1992; Engel et al. 1996), gender (more consultations among women), and social class (Walsh et al. 1992; Szpalski et al. 1995).

COSTS

In Quebec, 7.4% of workers compensated for a back problem in 1981 (those with more than 6 months' duration) were responsible for 73.2% of medical costs and 76% of compensation and indemnity payments (Can. $45,000 per case per year in 1985); in contrast, the average direct cost per case of back pain was Can. $4650 per year (Abenhaim and Suissa 1987).

Other studies have confirmed that most of the costs of LBP are incurred by a minority of cases. This knowledge has important implications for the development of preventive strategies (Leavitt et al. 1971; Spengler et al. 1986; Frymoyer and Cats-Baril 1987; Spitzer et al. 1987; Volinn et al. 1991; Weinstein and Scheer 1992; Engel et al. 1996).

The literature offers several estimates of direct and indirect costs from which it is difficult to generalize. However, this information provides a sense of the financial burden attached to LBP. For instance, in the U.S. Air Force Basic Military Training Station at Lackland, it costs an estimated $446,320 per year simply to train new Airmen Basics to replace those discharged for LBP (Anderson and Charlesworth 1993). From this example, it is easy to understand the importance of similar costs for employers in different industries. Other cost estimates are presented in Table I.

Costs incurred for LBP are likely to be heavily determined by physicians' practices, given the wide variation in diagnostic procedures used among and even within medical specialties. According to Cherkin et al. (1994), this variation could explain many of the geographical differences in medical care for LBP.

While factors associated with use of health services are also linked to the costs attributed to LBP, a large proportion of expenses associated with this problem derives from diminished productivity and disability payments. Thus, other determinants of LBP-related costs include duration of absence from work (Spitzer et al. 1987), chronic pain grade, duration of pain, initial diagnosis (disk or arthritis) (Engel et al. 1996), older age, and gender (more expensive claims for women) (Bigos et al. 1986; Snook 1988).

NATURAL HISTORY

The natural history of LBP is often described in three phases: acute (onset to 3–4 weeks), subacute (3–4 to 12 weeks), and chronic (more than 12 weeks) (Frank et al. 1996). This model, defined according to time until return to work, is presented in Fig. 3. While it certainly has some utility, especially in providing a structure for timing of interventions, it becomes increasingly obvious that this model does not capture the full reality of the natural history of LBP. Although most patients (80–90%) with LBP will return to work in a few weeks regardless of treatment provided (Dillane et al. 1966; Vallförs 1985; Spitzer et al. 1987), recurrences are frequent (up to 62% of patients in the following year) (Bergquist-Ullman and Larsson 1977; Troup et al. 1981; Abenhaim et al. 1988; Rossignol et al. 1992). Some authors have shown that the recurrent character of the disease is linked with a less favorable long-term prognosis (Bergquist-Ullman and Larsson 1977; Abenhaim et al. 1988; Von Korff et al. 1993a).

The picture of the natural history of LBP looks different when we shift outcome variables from "time until return to work" to "pain and functional limitations." Among primary care patients with back pain, Von Korff has shown, based on his own and other studies, that 1 month after the initial episode of back pain has resolved, about 33% of patients continue to experience pain of at least moderate intensity and functional limitations, while 20–25% report substantial activity limitations. At 12 months, more than 25% experience pain during more than half the days and 15–20% have moderate to severe activity limitations (Von Korff and Saunders 1996). These results highlight the variable nature of LBP and remind us that absence from work is not the only deleterious effect for the patient.

Psychological disturbances (particularly symptoms of anxiety and depression) have long been described as part of the LBP problem (Sargent 1946; Fulcher 1962; Westrin et al. 1972; Sternbach et al. 1973; Gentry et al. 1974; Gilchrist 1976; Blumer and Heilbronn 1982; Von Korff et al. 1988; Philips and Grant 1991; Åkerlind et al. 1992; Waddell 1993;

Table I
Estimates of costs related to low back pain (in U.S. or Canadian dollars)

Type of Costs (Country)	Estimated Annual Cost	Reference
Total cost of low back pain to society, 1996 (USA).	>U.S.$\$100 \times 10^9$	Waddell 1996
Total cost of low back pain to society, 1996 (UK)	U.S.$\$9 \times 10^9$	Waddell 1996
National Workers' Compensation Boards aggregate for low back injury and disability, 1995 (Canada)	Can.$\$1.875\text{–}2.25 \times 10^9$	Liberty International Canada 1995
Compensation expenses for low back pain paid by the Quebec Workers' Compensation Board, 1993 (Canada)	Can.$\$420 \times 10^6$	CSST 1994
Cost of training new Airmen Basics to replace those discharged for low back pain in the U.S. Air Force Basic Military Training Station at Lackland, 1993 (USA)	U.S.$446,320	Anderson and Charlesworth 1993
Workers' compensation estimated costs for low back pain (medical and indemnity costs), 1989 (USA)	U.S.$\$11.4 \times 10^9$	Webster and Snook 1990
Direct costs of personal medical care for back pain, 1988 (USA)	U.S.$\$17.9 \times 10^9$	Snook 1988
Costs of treatment and compensation for low back pain, 1976 (USA)	U.S.$\$14 \times 10^9$	Akeson and Murphy 1977

Bacon et al. 1994; Pietri-Taleb et al. 1995). Again, whether these symptoms precede or follow the occurrence of LBP or disability is still unclear, but the distress experienced by persons affected by LBP is real and requires attention (Åkerlind et al. 1992).

Studies on prognostic factors for LBP provide numerous predictors of outcome. However, their results are inconsistent and have rarely been replicated. Factors that appear to help in establishing a prognosis, based on the limited available scientific evidence, are pain-related disability (Von Korff et al. 1993a; Coste et al. 1994), number of days in pain (Von Korff et al. 1993a), educational status (Von Korff et al. 1993a), psychological distress (Main et al. 1992; Dionne et al. 1997), and gender (worst prognosis for women) (Von Korff et al. 1993a).

PREVENTION

HIGHER RISK GROUPS

Current knowledge indicates that workers in occupations involving frequent bending and lifting, prolonged awkward positions (bending and twisting), or exposure to vibrations, are at higher risk, especially if they also experience a high level of mental stress in the work environment. Primary prevention efforts should thus be directed toward such occupational groups.

As for secondary and tertiary prevention, the picture and the importance of the problem suggest focusing on two populations: (1) LBP patients with delayed recovery after 3–4 weeks, especially if they experience high levels of pain and distress; and (2) health care providers, particularly those who are less actively involved in continuing education.

SCOPE FOR PREVENTION

Back pain is extremely common and spares few. Ultimately, all adults are at risk. Videman (1991) asks: "Can (low back pain) be prevented if the cause is unknown?" Regardless, we must face the fact that the complete eradication of LBP is impossible (Hadler 1986; Dwyer 1987; Waddell 1987, 1991). However, the enormous burden LBP presents to society calls at the least for preventive strategies aimed at stopping the epidemic of chronic disability related to LBP. Given current knowledge, we have no other choice than to use the limited scientific and empirical evidence available to define prevention strategies.

In the general population, education on proper working techniques and body mechanics appears to be crucial to the prevention of LBP. However, changing the behaviors of adults who have not been affected by the health condition we want to prevent is not an easy task, and it might be more efficient, at least in the long term, to direct efforts toward children and adolescents in the hope of reducing their risk level when they reach adulthood. Prevention programs focused on cigarette smoking and obesity have many other health benefits and might be worthwhile.

The four major approaches to preventing LBP at work overlap to some extent: preemployment selection, safety training, ergonomics, and treatment, including rehabilitation (Troup 1984). Preemployment selection methods (medical evaluation, strength testing, and X-rays, bone scans, and ultrasonography of the low back) are ineffective and bear the risk of labeling prospective employees as "handicapped," with possible ethical and legal consequences (Gibson 1988; Himmelstein and Andersson 1988; Deyo et al. 1991; Bigos et al. 1992a,b; Battie et al. 1993; Dueker et al. 1994).

Available studies on the effectiveness of safety training have provided mixed results. In a meta-analysis conducted on six studies, Gebhardt (1994) found a modest decrease in the occurrence of back pain and back-related work absenteeism and suggested that safety training should be combined with organizational and ergonomic adjustments. Shi (1993) conducted a cost–benefit analysis of such a program. Over 1 year, 205 employees of a Northern California county were exposed to a back injury prevention program that combined education, training, physical fitness activities, and ergonomic improvement. The author reported a modest reduction in the prevalence of back pain over 1 year but significant improvement in job satisfaction and risky behaviors and a return on investment of 179%. More evaluative studies of such programs are needed.

If we recognize the importance of occupational factors in LBP, ergonomic interventions appear to be crucial in prevention. However, the scientific evidence supporting the efficiency of this approach is limited (Garg and Owen 1992; Shi 1993), and this may be explained by the complexity involved in the implementation and evaluation of ergonomic interventions in the work environment. More research is thus needed to document the impact of ergonomic interventions as a strategy for the prevention of LBP in the workplace. Citing recent findings suggesting that psychosocial factors might be more important than work load as risk factors for back problems among nurses, Burton et al. (1997) argued that ergonomic interventions might be suboptimal and should be accompanied by psychosocial interventions.

Several investigators have suggested that, considering the scope of LBP in the general population and the difficulty of identifying efficient primary prevention interventions, research efforts directed toward the prevention of back-related disability would be more cost-effective (Nachemson 1983; Hadler 1986; Waddell 1987; Deyo et al. 1991; Spitzer 1993). We need a set of markers that would allow early identification of patients who are at higher risk of chronicity so we can pursue more aggressive early intervention and reduce the cost of treating patients who are more likely to recover. Such sets of predictors need not necessarily be causally related to LBP disability, as is sometimes implied in the literature. At worst, they would constitute a screening tool but still help to improve the clinical management of low back problems. Such theoretical predictive models already exist, but none has yet been validated (Leavitt et al. 1971; Murphy and Cornish 1984; Frymoyer and Cats-Baril 1987; Burton et al. 1989; Lee et al. 1989; Goertz 1990; Burton and Tillotson 1991; Cats-Baril and Frymoyer 1991; Frymoyer 1992; Lancourt and Kettelhut 1992; Main et al. 1992; Leino and Magni 1993; Klenerman et al. 1995; Cherkin et al. 1996; Nordin et al. 1996; Dionne et al. 1997).

One important aspect of the prevention of low-back-related disability is the need to minimize iatrogenic adverse consequences (Dwyer 1987; Deyo et al. 1991; Deyo 1993; Spitzer 1993). Although we still have much to learn about LBP and how to treat it, we have considerable information on what *not* to do (Waddell 1991). It is crucial to educate health care professionals on deleterious interventions and the best available treatment strategies. Tremendous efforts have been made in recent years to that end, especially in the United States (Bigos et al. 1994), the United Kingdom (Clinical Standards Advisory Group 1994), and Canada (Spitzer et al. 1987; Spitzer 1993). It is important to continue the diffusion of this information to health care professionals in general, but above all to make sure it also reaches health care providers who are less actively involved in continuing education.

CHALLENGES FOR THE FUTURE

Numerous authors have stressed the importance of reaching consensus about definitions and methods of data collection in back pain research (Dwyer 1987; Burdorf 1992; Leboeuf-Yde and Lauritsen 1995; Borkan and Cherkin 1996). This goal appears to be a significant challenge to back pain investigators. Some efforts in that direction have already been made, but more are needed (Spitzer et al. 1987; Frymoyer et al. 1991; Nelson 1991). In the long term, achieving such consensus will not only improve the quality of individual studies, but also allow the conducting of formal

Classification	Symptoms	Duration of symptoms from onset	Working status at time of evaluation
1	Pain without radiation		
2	Pain + radiation to extremity, proximally	a (<7 days)	W (working)
3	Pain + radiation to extremity, distally*	b (7 days–7 weeks)	I (idle)
4	Pain + radiation to upper/lower limb neurologic signs	c (>7 weeks)	
5	Presumptive compression of a spinal nerve root on a simple roentgenogram (ie, spinal instability or fracture)		
6	Compression of a spinal nerve root confirmed by Specific imaging techniques (ie, computerized axial tomography, myelography, or magnetic resonance imaging) Other diagnostic techniques (eg, electromyography, venography)		
7	Spinal stenosis		
8	Postsurgical status, 1–6 months after intervention		
9	Postsurgical status, >6 months after intervention 9.1 Asymptomatic 9.2 Symptomatic		
10	Chronic pain syndrome		W (working)
11	Other diagnoses		I (idle)

*Not applicable to the thoracic segment.

Fig. 4. A classification of activity-related spinal disorders (Spitzer et al. 1987, reprinted with permission).

meta-analyses, which are rarely possible today (Leboeuf-Yde and Lauritsen 1995).

Back pain must be clearly defined by symptoms (localization, type, intensity, frequency, and duration), consequences (functional limitations, work absenteeism, health services utilization, and costs), and clinical information (Leboeuf-Yde and Lauritsen 1995). Although it is impossible to develop a single disability measurement instrument (Mäkelä et al. 1993), scientific knowledge on back pain would benefit from the standard use of a few well-established questionnaires that allow comparison of results between studies and countries. A strong consensus is needed on definitions, classifications, and consequences of LBP, measures of frequency, and standard research methods. It would also be important to reach consensus on a minimum set of factors to control for in multivariate analyses.

One example is the classification of activity-related spinal disorders created by the Quebec Task Force on Spinal Disorders, which starts with the most frequent clinical entities and considers their stage of development (presented in Fig. 4) (Spitzer et al. 1987). A recent study supports the validity of this classification (Atlas et al. 1996). A standard classification, if widely used, would make an important contribution to research by allowing investigators to compare similar cases.

A second challenge we must address is the development of knowledge regarding the determinants of practice models and outcomes of health care interventions. Considering the wide variation in use of health services within and between countries, such information would constitute an important contribution toward the improvement of clinical management of LBP.

Finally, etiological studies on LBP must focus on specific factors and test specific models of interaction between the most important factors, and stop the repeated "fishing expeditions" or the testing of "laundry lists" of variables that provide partial answers to numerous questions (Skovron 1992). The best approach would rely on a new paradigm that transcends the traditional biomedical model to include psychosocial factors, which clearly have an important role in the natural history of the disease (Waddell 1987; Borkan and Cherkin 1996). Once again, given the scope of this challenge, joint efforts are indicated.

CONCLUSIONS

Clearly, we still have much to learn about low back pain. However, we should recognize the tremendous developments of the past 20 years, many of which have been collaborative efforts by investigators of different disciplines working in different countries. The future of back pain research, and hence the development of knowledge about this disease, lies in such collaborations. They appear to offer the best strategy to enhance our understanding of the extremely complex problem we still, despite extensive research efforts, call simply "low back pain."

REFERENCES

Abenhaim L, Suissa S. Importance and economic burden of occupational back pain: a study of 2,500 cases representative of Quebec. *J Occup Med* 1987; 29(8):670–674.

Abenhaim L, Suissa S, Rossignol M. Risk of recurrence of occupational back pain over three year follow up. *Br J Ind Med* 1988; 45(12):829–833.

Abenhaim L, Rossignol M, Gobeille D, et al. The prognostic consequences in the making of the initial medical diagnosis of work-related back injuries. *Spine* 1995; 20(7):791–795.

Adera T, Deyo RA, Donatelle RJ. Premature menopause and low back pain: a population-based study. *Ann Epidemiol* 1994; 4(5):416–422.

Åkerlind I, Hörnquist J, Bjurulf P. Psychological factors in the long-term prognosis of chronic low back pain patients. *J Clin Psychol* 1992; 48(5):596–605.

Akeson W, Murphy R. Low back pain. *Clin Orthop* 1977; 129:2–3.

Anderson JA. Epidemiological aspects of back pain. *J Soc Occup Med* 1986; 36(3):90–94.

Anderson ST, Charlesworth RW. Rheumatologic disease among Air Force recruits: a multimillion-dollar epidemic. *Semin Arthritis Rheum* 1993; 22(4):275–279.

Andersson GB. Epidemiologic aspects on low-back pain in industry. *Spine* 1981; 6(1):53–60.

Atlas SJ, Deyo RA, Patrick DL, et al. The Quebec Task Force classification for spinal disorders and the severity, treatment, and outcomes of sciatica and lumbar spinal stenosis. *Spine* 1996; 21(24):2885–2892.

Bacon NMK, Bacon SF, Atkinson JH, et al. Somatization symptoms in chronic low back pain patients. *Psychosom Med* 1994; 56:118–127.

Badley EM, Ibañez D. Socioeconomic risk factors and musculoskeletal disability. *J Rheumatol* 1994; 21(3):515–522.

Battie MC, Bigos SJ, Fisher LD, et al. Anthropometric and clinical measures as predictors of back pain complaints in industry: a prospective study. *J Spinal Disord* 1990; 3(3):195–204.

Battie MC, Hansson T, Bigos S, et al. B-scan ultrasonic measurement of the lumbar spinal canal as a predictor of industrial back pain complaints and extended work loss. *J Occup Med* 1993; 35(12):1250–1255.

Bergenudd H, Nilsson B. Back pain in middle age; occupational workload and psychologic factors: an epidemiologic survey. *Spine* 1988; 13(1):58–60.

Bergquist-Ullman M, Larsson U. Acute low back pain in industry: a controlled prospective study with special reference to therapy and confounding factors. *Acta Orthop Scand* 1977; (Suppl 170):1–117.

Biering-Sørensen F, Thomsen C. Medical, social and occupational history as risk indicators for low-back trouble in a general population. *Spine* 1986; 11(7):720–725.

Bigos S, Spengler D, Martin N, et al. Back injuries in industry: a retrospective study. III. Employee-related factors. *Spine* 1986; 11(3):252–256.

Bigos SJ, Battie MC, Spengler DM, et al. A prospective study of work perceptions and psychosocial factors affecting the report of back injury [erratum appears in *Spine* 1991; 16(6):688]. *Spine* 1991; 16(1):1–6.

Bigos SJ, Battie MC, Fisher LD, et al. A prospective evaluation of preemployment screening methods for acute industrial back pain. *Spine* 1992a; 17(8):922–926.

Bigos SJ, Battie MC, Spengler DM, et al. A longitudinal, prospective study of industrial back injury reporting. *Clin Orthop* 1992b; 279:21–34.

Bigos S, Bowyer O, Braen G, et al. *Acute Low Back Problems in Adults.* Clinical Practice Guideline No. 14. Rockville, MD: Agency for Health Care Policy and Research, Public Health Service, U.S. Department of Health and Human Services, 1994.

Blumer D, Heilbronn M. Chronic pain as a variant of depressive disease. *J Nerv Ment Dis* 1982; 170(7):381–406.

Bombardier C, Kerr MS, Shannon HS, Frank JW. A guide to interpreting epidemiologic studies on the etiology of back pain. *Spine* 1994; 19(Suppl 18):2047s–2056s.

Bongers PM, De Winter CR, Kompier MAJ, Hildebrandt VH. Psychosocial factors at work and musculoskeletal disease. *Scand J Work Environ Health* 1993; 19(5):297–312.

Borkan JM, Cherkin DC. An agenda for primary care research on low back pain. *Spine* 1996; 21(24):2880–2884.

Burdorf A. Exposure assessment of risk factors for disorders of the back in occupational epidemiology. *Scand J Work Environ Health* 1992; 18(1):1–9.

Burdorf A. Bias in risk estimates from variability of exposure to postural load on the back in occupational groups. *Scand J Work Environ Health* 1993; 19(1):50–54.

Burton AK, Tillotson M. Prediction of the clinical course of low-back trouble using multivariable models. *Spine* 1991; 16(1):7–14.

Burton AK, Tillotson KM, Troup JD. Prediction of low-back trouble frequency in a working population. *Spine* 1989; 14(9):939–946.

Burton AK, Symonds TL, Zinzen E, et al. Is ergonomic intervention alone sufficient to limit musculoskeletal problems in nurses? *Occup Med (Oxf)* 1997; 47(1):25–32.

Cassidy JD, Carroll LJ, Côté P. The Saskatchewan Health and Back Pain Survey: the prevalence of low back pain and related disability in Saskatchewan adults. *Spine* 1998; 23(17):1860–1867.

Cats-Baril WL, Frymoyer JW. Identifying patients at risk of becoming disabled because of low-back pain. The Vermont Rehabilitation Engineering Center predictive model. *Spine* 1991; 16(6):605–607.

Cherkin D, Deyo R, Wheeler K, Ciol M. Physician variation in diagnostic testing for low back pain: who you see is what you get. *Arthritis Rheum* 1994; 37(1):15–22.

Cherkin DC, Deyo RA, Street JH, Barlow W. Predicting poor outcomes for back pain seen in primary care using patients' own criteria. *Spine* 1996; 21(24):2900–2907.

Clinical Standards Advisory Group on Back Pain. *Back Pain.* London: HMSO, 1994.

Colvez A, Blanchet M. Disability trends in the United States population 1966–76: analyses of reported causes. *Am J Public Health* 1981; 71:464–471.

Coste J, Delecoeuillerie G, Cohen de Lara A, le Parc JM, Paolaggi JB. Clinical course and prognostic factors in acute low back pain: an inception cohort study in primary care practice. *BMJ* 1994; 308:577–580.

Croft PR, Rigby AS. Socioeconomic influences on back problems in the community in Britain. *J Epidemiol Community Health* 1994; 48(2):166–170.

Croft PR, Papageorgiou AC, Ferry S, et al. Psychologic distress and low back pain: evidence from a prospective study in the general population. *Spine* 1995; 20(24):2731–2737.

CSST. *Statistiques sur les affections vertébrales 1990–1993.* Quebec: Commission de la santé et de la sécurité du travail, 1994.

Cunningham LS, Kelsey JL. Epidemiology of musculoskeletal impairments and associated disability. *Am J Public Health* 1984; 74(6):574–579.

Cypress BK. Characteristics of physician visits for back symptoms: a national perspective. *Am J Public Health* 1983; 73(4):389–395.

Davis H. Increasing rates of cervical and lumbar spine surgery in the United States, 1979–1990. *Spine* 1994; 19(10):1117–1124.

Deyo RA. What can the history and physical examination tell us about low-back pain? *JAMA* 1992; 268(6):760–765.

Deyo RA. Practice variations, treatment fads, rising disability: do we need a new clinical research paradigm? *Spine* 1993; 18:2153–2162.

Deyo RA, Bass JE. Lifestyle and low-back pain. The influence of smoking and obesity. *Spine* 1989; 14(5):501–506.

Deyo RA, Tsui-Wu YJ. Descriptive epidemiology of low-back pain and its related medical care in the United States. *Spine* 1987; 12(3):264–268.

Deyo RA, Cherkin D, Conrad D, Volinn E. Cost, controversy, crisis: low back pain and the health of the public. *Annu Rev Public Health* 1991;12:141–156.

Dillane JB, Fry J, Kalton G. Acute back syndrome—a study from general practice. *BMJ* 1966; 2:82–84.

Dionne C, Koepsell TD, Von Korff M, et al. Formal education and back-related disability. In search of an explanation [erratum appears in *Spine* 1996; 21(10):1200]. *Spine* 1995; 20(24):2721–2730.

Dionne CE, Koepsell TD, Von Korff M, et al. Predicting long-term functional limitations among back pain patients in primary care settings. *J Clin Epidemiol* 1997; 50(1):31–43.

Dueker JA, Ritchie SM, Knox TJ, Rose SJ. Isokinetic trunk testing and employment. *J Occup Med* 1994; 36(1):42–48.

Dwyer AP. Backache and its prevention. *Clin Orthop* 1987; 222:35–43.

Engel CC, Von Korff M, Katon WJ. Back pain in primary care: predictors of high health-care costs. *Pain* 1996; 65(2–3):197–204.

Ernst E. Smoking, a cause of back trouble? *Br J Rheumatol* 1993; 32(3):239–242.

Fardon D, Pinkerton S, Balderston R, et al. Terms used for diagnosis by English speaking spine surgeons. *Spine* 1993; 18(2):274–277.

Frank JW, Brooker AS, DeMaio SE, et al. Disability resulting from occupational low back pain. Part II: What do we know about secondary prevention? A review of the scientific evidence on prevention after disability begins. *Spine* 1996; 21(24):2918–2929.

Frymoyer JW. Predicting disability from low back pain. *Clin Orthop* 1992; 279:101–109.

Frymoyer JW, Cats-Baril W. Predictors of low back pain disability. *Clin Orthop* 1987; 221:89–98.

Frymoyer JW, Nelson RM, Spangfort E, Waddell G. Clinical tests applicable to the study of chronic low-back disability. *Spine* 1991; 16(6):681–682.

Fulcher OH. The backache as a manifestation of nervous tension. *Georgetown Med Bull* 1962; 16(1):40–42.

Garg A, Owen B. Reducing back stress to nursing personnel: an ergonomic intervention in a nursing home. *Ergonomics* 1992; 35(11):1353–1375.

Gebhardt WA. Effectiveness of training to prevent job-related back pain: a meta-analysis. *Br J Clin Psychol* 1994; 33(Pt 4):571–574.

Gentry WD, Shows WD, Thomas M. Chronic low back pain: a psychological profile. *Psychosomatics* 1974; 15:174–177.

Gibson ES. The value of preplacement screening radiography of the low back. *Occup Med* 1988; 3(1):91–107.

Gilchrist IC. Psychiatric and social factors related to low-back pain in general practice. *Rheumatol Rehabil* 1976; 15(2):101–107.

Goertz MN. Prognostic indicators for acute low-back pain. *Spine* 1990; 15(12):1307–1310.

Guo HR, Tanaka S, Cameron LL, et al. Back pain among workers in the United States: national estimates and workers at high risk. *Am J Ind Med* 1995; 28(5):591–602.

Hadler N. Regional back pain. *N Engl J Med* 1986; 315:1090–1092.

Hadler NM. Backache and work incapacity in Japan. *J Occup Med* 1994; 36(10):1110–1114.

Hambly MF, Mooney V. Effect of smoking and pulsed electromagnetic fields on intradiscal PH in rabbits. *Spine* 1992; 17(6):S83–S85.

Harreby M, Kjer J, Hesselsøe G, Neergaard K. Epidemiological aspects and risk factors for low back pain in 38-year-old men and women: a 25-year prospective cohort study of 640 school children. *Eur Spine J* 1996; 5(5):312–318.

Harreby M, Hesselsøe G, Kjer J, Neergaard K. Low back pain and physical exercise in leisure time in 38-year-old men and women: a 25-year prospective cohort study of 640 school children. *Eur Spine J* 1997; 6:181–186.

Hart LG, Deyo RA, Cherkin DC. Physician office visits for low back pain: frequency, clinical evaluation, and treatment patterns from a U.S. national survey. *Spine* 1995; 20(1):11–19.

Heir T, Glomsaker P. Epidemiology of musculoskeletal injuries among Norwegian conscripts undergoing basic military training. *Scand J Med Sci Sports* 1996; 6(3):186–191.

Heistaro S, Vartiainen E, Heliövaara M, Puska P. Trends of back pain in Eastern Finland, 1972–1992, in relation to socioeconomic status and behavioral risk factors. *Am J Epidemiol* 1998; 147(7):671–682.

Heliövaara M, Mäkelä M, Knekt P, Impivaara O, Aromaa A. Determinants of sciatica and low-back pain. *Spine* 1991; 16(6):608–614.

Hillman M, Wright A, Rajaratnam G, Tennant A, Chamberlain MA. Prevalence of low back pain in the community: implications for service provision in Bradford, UK. *J Epidemiol Community Health* 1996; 50(3):347–352.

Himmelstein JS, Andersson GB. Low back pain: risk evaluation and preplacement screening. *Occup Med* 1988; 3(2):255–269.

Houtman I, Bongers P, Smulders P, Kompier M. Psychosocial stressors at work and musculoskeletal problems. *Scand J Work Environ Health* 1994; 20:139–145.

Hurwitz E, Morgenstern A. Correlates of back problems and back-related disability in the United States. *J Clin Epidemiol* 1997; 50(6):669–680.

Jayson MIV, R. M, Keegan A, Tomlinson I. A fibrinolytic defect in chronic back pain syndromes. *Lancet* 1984; November 24:1186–1187.

Karasek R, Theorell T. *Healthy Work: Stress, Productivity, and the Reconstruction of Working Life*. New York: Basic Books, 1990.

Kelsey JL, White AA. Epidemiology and impact of low-back pain. *Spine* 1980; 5(2):133–142.

Klenerman L, Slade P, Stanley M, et al. The prediction of chronicity in patients with an acute attack of low back pain in a general practice setting. *Spine* 1995; 20(4):478–484.

Kuwashima A, Aizawa Y, Nakamura K, Taniguchi S, Watanabe M. National survey on accidental low back pain in workplace. *Ind Health* 1997; 35(2):187–193.

Lancourt J, Kettelhut M. Predicting return to work for lower back pain patients receiving worker's compensation. *Spine* 1992; 17(6):629–640.

Lawrence R, Helmick C, Arnett F, et al. Estimates of the prevalence of arthritis and selected musculoskeletal disorders in the United States. *Arthritis Rheum* 1998; 41(5):778–799.

Leavitt S, Johnston T, Beyer R. The process of recovery: patterns in industrial back injury. Part 2: Predicting outcomes from early case data. *IMS Ind Med Surg* 1971; 40(9):7–15.

Leboeuf-Yde C, Lauritsen JM. The prevalence of low back pain in the literature: a structured review of 26 Nordic studies from 1954 to 1993. *Spine* 1995; 20(19):2112–2118.

Leboeuf-Yde C, Yashin A, Lauritzen T. Does smoking cause low back pain? Results from a population-based study. *J Manipulative Physiol Ther* 1996; 19(2):99–108.

Lee P, Helewa A, Smythe H, Bombardier C, Goldsmith C. Epidemiology of musculoskeletal disorders (complaints) and related disability in *Canada. J Rheumatol* 1985; 12:1169–1173.

Lee PWH, Chow SP, Lieh-Mak F, Chan KC, Wong S. Psychosocial factors influencing outcome in patients with low-back pain. *Spine* 1989; 14(8):838–843.

Leino P. Symptoms of stress predict musculoskeletal disorders. *J Epidemiol Community Health* 1989; 43:293–300.

Leino P, Magni G. Depressive and distress symptoms as predictors of low back pain, neck-shoulder pain, and other musculoskeletal morbidity: a 10-year follow-up of metal industry employees. *Pain* 1993; 53:89–94.

Leino PI, Berg MA, Puska P. Is back pain increasing? Results from national surveys in Finland during 1978/9–1992. *Scand J Rheumatol* 1994; 23(5):269–276.

Liberty International Canada. *Unfolding Change*. Liberty International, 1995.

Liira JP, Shannon HS, Chambers LW, Haines TA. Long-term back problems and physical work exposures in the 1990 Ontario Health Survey. *Am J Public Health* 1996; 86(3):382–387.

Linton SJ, Warg LE. Attributions (beliefs) and job satisfaction associated with back pain in an industrial setting. *Percept Mot Skills* 1993; 76(1):51–62.

Lloyd DC, Troup JD. Recurrent back pain and its prediction. *J Soc Occup Med* 1983; 33(2):66–74.

Main CJ, Wood PL, Hollis S, Spanswick CC, Waddell G. The Distress and Risk Assessment Method. A simple patient classification to identify distress and evaluate the risk of poor outcome. *Spine* 1992; 17(1):42–52.

Mäkelä M, Heliövaara M, Sievers K, Knekt P, Maatela J, Aromaa A. Musculoskeletal disorders as determinants of disability in Finns aged 30 years or more. *J Clin Epidemiol* 1993; 46(6):549–559.

Mannion AF, Dolan P, Adams MA. Psychological questionnaires: do "abnormal" scores precede or follow first-time low back pain? *Spine* 1996; 21(22):2603–2611.

McKinnon ME, Vickers MR, Ruddock VM, Townsend J, Meade TW. Community studies of the health service implications of low back pain. *Spine* 1997; 22(18):2161–2166.

Murphy KA, Cornish RD. Prediction of chronicity in acute low back pain. *Arch Phys Med Rehabil* 1984; 65:334–337.

Nachemson A. Work for all: for those with low back pain as well. *Clin Orthop* 1983(179):77–85.

Nelson RM. Standardized tests and measures for assessing low-back pain in the occupational setting. A developmental model. *Spine* 1991; 16(6):679–681.

Nordin M, Skovron ML, Hiebert R, et al. Early predictors of outcome. *Bull Hosp Jt Dis* 1996; 55(4):204–206.

Orvieto R, Rand N, Lev B, Wiener M, Nehama H. Low back pain and body mass index. *Mil Med* 1994; 159 (January):37–38.

Papageorgiou AC, Croft PR, Ferry S, Jayson MIV, Silman AJ. Estimating the prevalence of low back pain in the general population: evidence from the South Manchester Back Pain Survey. *Spine* 1995; 20(17):1889–1894.

Philips HC, Grant L. Acute back pain: a psychological analysis. *Behav Res Ther* 1991; 29(5):429–434.

Pietri-Taleb F, Riihimaki H, Viikari-Juntura E, Lindström K, Moneta GB. The role of psychological distress and personality in the incidence of sciatic pain among working men. *Am J Public Health* 1995; 85(4):541–545.

Punnett L, Fine LJ, Keyserling WM, Herrin GD, Chaffin DB. Back disorders and nonneutral trunk postures of automobile assembly workers. *Scand J Work Environ Health* 1991; 17(5):337–346.

Riihimaki H. Low-back pain, its origin and risk indicators. *Scand J Work Environ Health* 1991; 17(2):81–90.

Rossignol M, Suissa S, Abenhaim L. Working disability due to occupational back pain: three-year follow-up of 2,300 compensated workers in Quebec. *J Occup Med* 1988; 30(6):502–505.

Rossignol M, Suissa S, Abenhaim L. The evolution of compensated occupational spinal injuries. A three-year follow-up study. *Spine* 1992; 17(9):1043–1047.

Sargent MM. Psychosomatic backache. *New Engl J Med* 1946; 234(13):427–430.

Shi L. A cost-benefit analysis of a California county's back injury prevention program. *Public Health Rep* 1993; 108(2):204–211.

Silman AJ, Ferry S, Papageorgiou AC, Jayson MI, Croft PR. Number of children as a risk factor for low back pain in men and women. *Arthritis Rheum* 1995; 38(9):1232–1235.

Skovron ML. Epidemiology of low back pain. *Baillieres Clin Rheumatol* 1992; 6(3):559–573.

Skovron ML, Szpalski M, Nordin M, Melot C, Cukier D. Sociocultural factors and back pain: a population-based study in Belgian adults. *Spine* 1994; 19(2):129–137.

Snook SH. The costs of back pain in industry. *Occup Med* 1988; 3(1):1–5.

Soukka A, Alaranta H, Tallroth K, Heliövaara M. Leg-length inequality in people of working age. The association between mild inequality and low-back pain is questionable [see comments]. *Spine* 1991; 16(4):429–431.

Spengler DM, Bigos SJ, Martin NA, et al. Back injuries in industry: a retrospective study. I. Overview and cost analysis. *Spine* 1986; 11(3):241–245.

Spitzer WO. Low back pain in the workplace: attainable benefits not attained [editorial]. *Br J Ind Med* 1993; 50(5):385–388.

Spitzer WO, LeBlanc FE, Dupuis M, et al. Scientific approach to the assessment and management of activity-related spinal disorders: a monograph for clinicians. Report of the Task Force on Spinal Disorders. *Spine* 1987; 12(Suppl 7):S9–S59.

Steinberg GG. Epidemiology of low-back pain; In: Stanton-Hicks M, Boas R (Eds). *Chronic Low Back Pain*. New York: Raven Press, 1982.

Sternbach RA, Wolf SR, Murphy RW, Akeson WH. Traits of pain patients: the low-back "loser." *Psychosomatics* 1973; 14:226–229.

Svensson HO, Vedin A, Wilhelmsson C, Andersson GB. Low-back pain in relation to other diseases and cardiovascular risk factors. *Spine* 1983; 8(3):277–285.

Svensson HO, Andersson GBJ, Hagstad A, Jansson PO. The relationship of low-back pain to pregnancy and gynecologic factors. *Spine* 1990; 15(5):371–375.

Szpalski M, Nordin M, Skovron ML, Melot C, Cukier D. Health care utilization for low back pain in Belgium: influence of sociocultural factors and health beliefs. *Spine* 1995; 20(4):431–442.

Taylor VM, Deyo RA, Cherkin DC, Kreuter W. Low back pain hospitalization: recent United States trends and regional variations. *Spine* 1994; 19(11):1207–1213.

Troup JD. Causes, prediction and prevention of back pain at work. *Scand J Work Environ Health* 1984; 10(6 Spec No):419–428.

Troup J, Martin J, Lloyd D. Back pain in industry: a prospective study. *Spine* 1981; 6:61–69.

Vallförs B. Acute, subacute and chronic low-back pain: clinical symptoms, absenteeism and working environment. *Scand J Rehabil Med* 1985; (Suppl 11):1–98.

Videman T. Evaluation of the prevention of occupational low-back pain. *Spine* 1991; 16(6):685–686.

Viikari-Juntura E, Vuori J, Silverstein BA, et al. A life-long prospective study on the role of psychosocial factors in neck-shoulder and low-back pain. *Spine* 1991;16(9):1056–1061.

Volinn E, Van Koevering D, Loeser J. Back sprain in industry: the role of socioeconomic factors in chronicity. *Spine* 1991; 16(5):542–548.

Volinn E, Mayer J, Diehr P, et al. Small area analysis of surgery for low-back pain. *Spine* 1992; 17(5):575–581.

Von Korff M, Parker RD. The dynamics of the prevalence of chronic episodic disease. *J Chron Dis* 1980; 33:79–85.

Von Korff M, Saunders K. The course of back pain in primary care. *Spine* 1996; 21(24):2833–2839.

Von Korff M, Dworkin S, Le Resche L, Kruger A. An epidemiologic comparison of pain complaints. *Pain* 1988; 32:173–183.

Von Korff M, Ormel J, Keefe F, Dworkin S. Grading the severity of chronic pain. *Pain* 1992; 50:133–149.

Von Korff M, Deyo RA, Cherkin D, Barlow W. Back pain in primary care. Outcomes at 1 year. *Spine* 1993a; 18(7):855–862.

Von Korff M, Le Resche L, Dworkin SF. First onset of common pain symptoms: a prospective study of depression as a risk factor. *Pain* 1993b; 55(2):251–258.

Waddell G. A new clinical model for the treatment of low-back pain. *Spine* 1987; 12(7):632–644.

Waddell G. Low back disability: a syndrome of Western civilization. *Neurosurg Clin North Am* 1991; 2:719–738.

Waddell G. How patients react to low back pain. *Acta Orthop Scand* 1993; 64(Suppl 251):21–24.

Waddell G. Low back pain: a twentieth century health care enigma. *Spine* 1996; 21(24):2820–2825.

Walsh K, Cruddas M, Coggon D. Low back pain in eight areas of Britain. *J Epidemiol Community Health* 1992; 46(3):227–230.

Webster B, Snook S. The cost of compensable low back pain. *J Occup Med* 1990; 32:13–15.

Weinstein SM, Scheer SJ. Industrial rehabilitation medicine. 2. Assessment of the problem, pathology, and risk factors for disability. *Arch Phys Med Rehabil* 1992; 73(5-S):S360–S365.

Westrin CG, Hirsch C, Lindegård B. The personality of the back patient. *Clin Orthop* 1972(87):209–216.

White AA, Gordon SL. Synopsis: workshop on idiopathic low-back pain. *Spine* 1982; 7:141–149.

Correspondence to: Clermont E. Dionne, PhD, Department of Rehabilitation, Faculty of Medicine, Laval University, Sainte-Foy, Quebec, Canada G1K 7P4. Tel: 418-656-2131; Fax: 418-656-2535; email: clermont.dionne@erg.ulaval.ca.

Epidemiology of Pain, edited by
I.K. Crombie, IASP Press, Seattle, © 1999.

19

Knee Pain

Robert McCarney and Peter R. Croft

*Primary Care Sciences Research Centre, School of Postgraduate Medicine,
Keele University, Hartshill, Stoke-on-Trent, United Kingdom*

Joint pain is the most common regional pain category in older persons. In the Canadian community survey of pain by Crook and colleagues (1984), the prevalence of chronic pain, defined as pain lasting for 3 months or longer, increased with age. Data from another community pain survey (the American Nuprin Pain report) illustrate that in older persons chronic pain is due almost entirely to joint problems; all other regional pain syndromes are more common at younger ages and tend to peak in prevalence in middle age (Sternbach 1986). Musculoskeletal disorders are the most important cause of disability in older persons in developed countries, and as a public health problem that is likely to increase as the population ages, lower limb joint pain is of major importance. Please refer to Chapter 8 for an in-depth discussion of pain in older people.

In clinico-pathological terms, joint pain can be broadly separated into two categories: pain associated with disease of the joint itself and pain associated with primary injury or disease in the soft tissues surrounding the joint. Examples of joint pain appear elsewhere in this book (neck, shoulder, temporomandibular), but joint pain in the lower limb justifies a separate chapter for two reasons. First, conditions associated with lower limb joint pain are proportionally the most important musculoskeletal cause of restricted physical activity (disability) in older persons. Second, the most frequent of these conditions is osteoarthritis. The epidemiology of lower limb joint pain is inextricably linked with the epidemiology of osteoarthritis, and presents an opportunity to explore issues surrounding this important cause of pain. We have chosen knee pain as an example for this review.

Pain at the knee exemplifies the general principle alluded to above, namely that at older ages (usually and arbitrarily defined as 55 years or above), osteoarthritis in the joint is increasingly associated with knee symptoms, while at younger ages, acute injury to the soft tissues in and around the joint dominates the picture. In one population survey in the United Kingdom, knee pain was the second most common regional musculoskeletal pain after the back (Urwin et al. 1998).

OSTEOARTHRITIS

Osteoarthritis is a clinical syndrome of joint pain and stiffness, but is formally defined in pathological terms as a condition of subchondral bone stiffening ("subchondral" implies that the bony change occurs close to the joint), cartilage degeneration, and active new bone formation. It is an active process in which bone and cartilage disease is balanced by the body's attempts to shore up the damaged joint with the scaffolding of new bone. Radiographic changes are the traditional cornerstone of diagnosis because the presumptive pathological changes are reflected in the X-ray appearances of bony opacity, narrowing of the joint space, and osteophytes (the new bone "spurs"). The importance to the epidemiology of joint pain is that, even with this clearcut pathological story, the relationship of local pathology to pain is not simple.

In the National Health and Nutrition Examination Survey (NHANES I), a survey of a representative sample of the U.S. population (National Center for Health Statistics 1979), the subjects were asked about the presence of daily knee pain with a duration of at least 1 month during the previous year. The responders then had radiographs of the knees and the films

Table I
Prevalence of knee pain

Study Type	Disease Definition	Source of Sample	Sample Size	Age Range (y)	Duration of Symptoms	Type of Prevalence Estimate	Prevalence	Reference
Population survey, interview	Significant pain around knees on most days for ≥1 mo in past year	U.S. population: probability sample	6913	25–74	≥1 mo	1-y period	10.2%	National Center for Health Statistics 1979
Population survey, interview	Ever had pain in or around knee on most days for ≥1 mo	U.S. population: probability sample	1805	63–94	≥1 mo	Lifetime	16.1%	Felson et al. 1987
Population survey, interview	Current pain in right knee	Random population sample	2865	45+	Current	Point	12.9%	Claessens et al. 1990
Population survey, postal	Self-reported pain, swelling or stiffness in joint	U.K. representative local population sample	42826	16+	Current	Point	10.1%	Badley et al. 1992
Population survey, postal	Pain on most days for ≥1 mo in past year	U.K. representative local population sample	1694	55+	≥1 mo	1-y period	24.6%	McAlindon et al. 1992
Population survey, interview	Pain on most days of preceding month	Community random sample	105	85+	≥3 wk	1-mo period	23.8%	van Schaardenburg et al. 1994
Population survey, postal	Pain on most days for ≥1 mo in past year/ever	Community sample	452	19–92	≥1 mo	[a]1-y period; [b]lifetime	[a]15.4%; [b]23.1%	Lethbridge-Cejku et al. 1995
Population survey, postal	Pain on most days of preceding month; pain on most days for ≥1 mo in past year	U.K. representative local population sample	3322	40–79	[a]≥3 wk; [b]≥1 mo	[a]1-month period; [b]1-y period	[a]19.3%; [b]28.3%	O'Reilly et al. 1996
Population survey, postal	Pain for >24 h in past month, shaded on the knee area of a pain manikin	U.K. representative local population sample	2606	18–75	≥24 h	1-mo period	18%	McCarney 1998
Population survey, postal	Pain for >1 wk in past month	U.K. population sample, age and sex stratified	5752	16+	≥1 wk	1-mo period	19% (20% men; 19% women)	Urwin et al. 1998
Population survey, interview	Pain in past month	Random sample of all residents of Rotterdam, The Netherlands	2895	55+	No restriction	1-mo period	18.4% (12.6% men; 22.3% women)	Odding et al. 1998
Survey, interview	Painful knees in the past year	Random sample of secondary schoolchildren	446	13–17	No restriction	1-y period	30.5%	Fairbank et al. 1984

(continued)

Table I
Continued

Study Type	Disease Definition	Source of Sample	Sample Size	Age Range (y)	Duration of Symptoms	Type of Prevalence Estimate	Prevalence	Reference
Population survey, postal	Pain in knee for >1 mo in the past year	Birth cohort	574	55+	≥1 mo	One year period	10.1%	Bergenudd et al. 1989
Population survey, interview	Pain or swelling for at least 4 wk, ever	Saudi Arabia household area samples: one affluent, one poor	4232	15+	≥1 mo	Lifetime	3.1% in affluent area; 1.8% in poor area	Gibson et al. 1996
Population survey, interview/ exam	Pain on movement, tenderness, swelling, limitation and/or deformity	[a]North China, [b]South China population samples	[a]4192, [b]5057	20+	No restriction	Point	[a]24.0% men, 36.0% women; [b]1.8% men, 3.4% women	Wigley et al. 1994

were graded according to the severity of osteoarthritic changes in the joints. The more severe the changes, the higher the probability that knee pain had been reported. However only a minority of those with radiographic osteoarthritis reported pain, although the proportion increased with age. Other studies have found a similar dislocation between pain and radiological change. For example, from a U.K. study of women aged 55 years and over, it can be estimated that 50% of older persons with knee pain do not have radiographic osteoarthritis and 50% with radiographic changes do not have pain (McAlindon et al. 1992). However, this condition is still age-related: for each narrow age-group above 55 years, each step-up in age showed an increased probability of radiographic osteoarthritic change associated with pain.

The conclusion from such results is that knee pain can justifiably be studied in its own right and not just as a clinical indicator of osteoarthritis. Arguments made by authors such as Hadler (1992), in commentaries such as that of Creamer and Hochberg (1997) and others, and found elsewhere in this book in relation to other regional pain syndromes, justify this conclusion in other ways. Namely, the presence of a regional pathological cause for pain does not rule out other influences as important in the generation and persistence of pain.

PREVALENCE AND INCIDENCE OF KNEE PAIN

PERIOD PREVALENCE STUDIES OF KNEE PAIN

Several studies have investigated knee pain in open population samples. They have differed with respect to definition and population characteristics such as age. Given these variations, the results are surprisingly consistent (Table I). In particular, a group of five population studies that focused on knee pain in adults during 1-month or 12-month periods, suggest summary figures of 19% for the 1-month prevalence (O'Reilly et al. 1996; McCarney 1998; Odding et al. 1998; Urwin et al. 1998) and 25–28% for the 1-year prevalence (McAlindon et al. 1992; O'Reilly et al. 1996).

The U.S. national survey gives lower estimates, as it does for most musculoskeletal problems when compared with other surveys, which probably reflects the use of an interview subsample to determine the overall frequency (National Center for Health Statistics 1979).

Figures for "any pain in the last year" or for "knee pain ever" are more variable and more difficult to interpret. In particular "knee pain ever" is greatly influ-

Table II
Prevalence of chronic or disabling knee pain

Study Type	Disease Definition	Source of Sample	Sample Size	Age Range (y)	Duration of Symptoms	Type of Prevalence Estimate	Prevalence	Reference
Population survey, postal	Pain in knee (using pain manikin)	Random sample from population register	1609	25–74	≥3 mo	Point	13.4%	Andersson et al. 1993
Population survey, postal	Pain almost daily	Random sample from population register	1853	35–54	≥3 mo	Point	15.1%	Petersson et al. 1997
Population survey, interview	Pain at least several times per week	Sample of schoolchildren in two age groups	[a]383; [b]473	[a]9–10; [b]14–15	≥3 mo	Point	[a]3.9%; [b]18.8%	Vähäsarja 1995
Population survey, interview	Current pain in right knee plus function limitation	Community sample	371	45+	Current	Point	22.0%	Claessens et al. 1990
Population survey, postal	Pain on most days for at least 1 mo in past year, plus problem with daily living	Local representative population sample, U.K.	1694	55+	≥1 mo	1-y period	12.5%	McAlindon et al. 1992
Population survey, postal	Problems with knee joint for >6 wk in past 3 months, plus difficulty with everyday activities	Systematic random sample from population register, U.K.	16191	55+	≥ 6 wk	3-mo period	7.9%	Tennant et al. 1995
Population survey, two-phase postal	Current knee pain plus restricted activity	Local representative population sample, U.K.	279	18–74	Current	Point	15.7%	McCarney 1998

enced by age: a 60-year-old has a longer period during which pain might have occurred compared with a 16-year-old. In this context, the high 1-year prevalence of 30% for current knee pain in one study of children is worth noting (Fairbank et al. 1984).

PREVALENCE OF SIGNIFICANT KNEE PAIN

What defines "significant" pain for any person is, of course, subjective, but it is important to consider ways to measure severity because the prevalence figures for all knee pain easily reduce to "there's a lot of it about."

Two dimensions of significance that might sensibly categorize prevalence figures for knee pain are its duration and its impact on everyday life. Many of the population studies listed in Table I report on duration through a minimal definition of "knee pain on most days of the past month." Some studies concentrate on

patients who have chronic knee pain, defined as greater than 3 months' duration (Table II). The two random population sample studies shown in the table are consistent with a prevalence of approximately 14% for such chronic knee pain in adults, although neither investigation included the very elderly or very young adults. One study of persistent knee pain in 14–15-year-olds found a prevalence of 18% (Vähäsarja 1995).

More helpful are studies that add some measure of disability or handicap to the data on reported pain (Table II). If any restriction of everyday living is allowed in the definition, then figures suggest that 16% of all adults will be affected by such a problem in a 1-month period (i.e., most of those with pain have some associated disability); knee pain with significant impact on daily living in those over 55 years is estimated at approximately 10%, depending on the disability scale used and whether pain duration is included in the definition.

AGE AND GENDER

Knee pain and osteoarthritis are clearly age-related phenomena, and one of the strongest arguments for lower limb joint pain being more strongly linked with regional pathology (such as underlying osteoarthritis) than are other pain syndromes is that the age-related increase in pain prevalence continues into the oldest age bands, in parallel with the age-related radiographic changes. Knee pain is usually more common in women than men, which reflects the pattern for other pain syndromes and may be related to the consistently observed higher prevalence of radiographic changes in women. However, the sex ratio differs with age. Two recent studies that reported similar overall 1-month period prevalences of knee pain in adults (19%) reported a marked contrast in sex ratios. In the U.K. study (Urwin et al. 1998), the 1-month period prevalence of knee pain adjusted to the total population was 19% in women and 20% in men; in the Rotterdam (The Netherlands) study (Odding et al. 1998) the figures were 22.3% and 12.6% for women and men, respectively. The main difference between the two studies was that the U.K. investigation included all adults aged 16 and over, whereas the Dutch focused on those aged 55-plus. Within the U.K. study, knee pain prevalence under 45 years was higher in men, similar in the two genders between 45 and 64 years, and higher in women in the 65-plus age group. This higher prevalence in women in the older age groups again reflects the pattern seen with radiographic osteoarthritis of the knee.

SOCIAL CLASS

The U.S. national survey revealed that radiographic osteoarthritis of the knee was most frequent in black women, after adjustment for obesity, but reports of knee pain associated with radiological osteoarthritis did not differ according to social and ethnic group (Hochberg et al. 1989). In one U.K. population study, knee pain reported in a large general population survey showed a clear gradient across socioeconomic groups, with the more socially deprived groups having higher pain prevalence (Urwin et al. 1998).

GEOGRAPHY

Knee pain is ubiquitous. Studies from China, for example, suggest that knee pain is common; indeed, in one Chinese study knee pain was the most frequent site of pain complaints in those aged 70 years and over (Woo et al. 1994). Estimates from different studies vary widely (Wigley et al. 1994; Gibson et al. 1996), perhaps reflecting methodological differences rather than true variations in prevalence.

Few studies have investigated cross-cultural variations in radiographic knee osteoarthritis; Sun et al. (1997), in a wide-ranging review of population prevalence studies, highlighted the wide variation in population type and study design. However, structural knee osteoarthritis seems to be universal, and similar prevalences are reported from different populations. Zhang et al. (1995) found a prevalence of 9.6% in rural Chinese adults, and in Greenland the prevalence of moderate to severe radiographic changes in the knee was 8% in adults over 40 years (Andersen and Winckler 1979). This lack of geographic variation contrasts markedly with hip osteoarthritis, which shows clear variations, including lower rates of the radiographic disease in Asiatic and African populations. This variation between the pictures presented by knee and hip osteoarthritis may be due to different risk factor profiles; for example, squatting may protect against hip osteoarthritis but exacerbate structural changes in the knee.

The ubiquitous nature of knee pain and radiographic changes in the knee argues that knee problems affect all cultures. However, a person's evaluation of joint pain may vary with culture, a factor noted by Kellgren and Lawrence in their classical surveys of joint problems in different social and ethnic groups (Lawrence 1977). Pain prevalence in relation to radiographic change, for example, varied with geography and ethnicity.

INCIDENCE AND PREVALENCE OF KNEE PAIN IN YOUNGER ADULTS

Table II illustrates that knee pain is a frequently reported symptom in younger persons, among whom it is most likely to be associated with overuse and injury. Knee osteoarthritis does occur in young adults but is unusual. Most knee pain in young adults is not associated with clearcut pathology, but likely reflects overuse rather than mechanical derangement.

Several studies have attempted to chart the incidence of injury and overuse syndromes in groups of young persons considered to be at unusual risk of such problems, namely new recruits to the armed forces during their initial training period, and athletes. Knee injuries in young adults are the most common problem in hospital-based or primary care sports medicine clinics. Two American studies (Matheson 1988; Butcher et al. 1996) found that knee pain affects 25–40% of patients visiting such clinics.

The more severe problems, such as cruciate ligament and meniscal tears, account for a minority of knee pain in young adults, even among sports clinic patients, but these problems may have a greater impact on later structural osteoarthritis than do overuse syndromes. One general population study estimated an incidence of 0.6 per 1000 for meniscal injury "severe enough for meniscectomy to be considered" (Baker et al. 1985). This finding could explain a significant proportion of knee pain and osteoarthritis later in life, but the extent of the link is yet to be firmly established (see "Risk factors," below).

Table III summarizes some of the studies examining particular groups. It is difficult to judge their importance, given the opportunities for selection bias, but they are useful in highlighting the high proportion of injuries and painful overuse problems that involve the knee. They do not, however, provide data on the population occurrence of painful knee syndromes.

INCIDENCE STUDIES OF KNEE PAIN

Few studies have examined incidence of knee pain. Chief among the available studies is the Framingham cohort from the United States. Felson and colleagues (1995) found the cumulative incidence of radiographic osteoarthritis in knees previously free of such disease to be 15.6% over a 10-year period. The mean age of subjects was 70 years, and half had symptoms. Incident rates were 1.7 times higher in women than men. These findings are consistent with data from the Mayo Clinic studies (Wilson et al. 1990), which focused on patients seeking care for osteoarthritis at a hospital clinic. In this population cohort study from Rochester, Minnesota, USA, the incidence of symptomatic radiographic knee osteoarthritis referred to a hospital was 10 per 1000 per year in 60- to 79-year-olds. A study of a Health Maintenance Organization (HMO) population in the United States suggested an overall annual incidence of 2.4 per 1000 for first consultation with definite radiographic knee osteoarthritis and accompanying pain. The incidence rose to 10 per 1000 in women aged 70–89 years, again a figure similar to that derived from the Rochester study (Oliveria et al. 1995).

RISK FACTORS FOR KNEE PAIN

In general, there are three approaches to summarizing the risk factors for knee pain in the population: risks for radiographic osteoarthritis and soft tissue injury; risks for symptomatic osteoarthritis; and risks for knee pain. Table IV offers a summary comparing risks for radiographic osteoarthritis, symptomatic osteoarthritis, and knee pain in older persons (i.e., at ages when radiographic osteoarthritis also is likely).

RISK FACTORS FOR RADIOGRAPHIC KNEE OSTEOARTHRITIS AND SOFT TISSUE INJURY

Risk factors that influence the development of pathology can be studied for their relevance to knee pain. An extensive literature addressing the potential causes of radiographically defined knee osteoarthritis provides consistent evidence that overweight and weight gain are important causes of osteoarthritic change in the knees. A series of studies suggest a combination of loading and metabolic mechanisms. Mechanical stress on the joint has been identified as a risk for radiographic osteoarthritis in several studies, particularly as measured by occupational knee bending and kneeling, and by manual handling of heavy weights and regular climbing of steps and stairs. In younger adults, injury, including meniscal damage, and overuse syndromes affecting soft tissue structures are the predominant clinico-pathological correlates of knee pain. Sport and physical training are the major risk factors studied, and the knee is consistently the most common type of injury reported for a range of sports (Table III). Increasing evidence suggests that severe knee injuries at young ages predispose to osteoarthritic change later in life, although the influence of iatrogenesis may also be important given evidence that the operation of meniscectomy itself may predispose to later degenerative change (Roos et al. 1998).

RISK FACTORS FOR SYMPTOMATIC KNEE OSTEOARTHRITIS

The second group of studies adopts the case definition of "symptomatic" or "clinical" osteoarthritis. These terms imply that the studies are relevant to pain as well as to structural joint damage. However, these studies are still focused on structural osteoarthritic change, although they limit this focus to the subgroup with symptoms. The range of risk factors is similar to

Table III
Knee injury and overuse

Study Type	Study Group	Sample Size	Age (y)	Clinical Topic	Frequency Estimate	Comments	Reference
Case record review	Referrals to outpatient sports medicine clinic	[a]722; [b]685	[a]<50; [b]50+	Knee injuries	[a]40.7% of referrals; [b]29.5% of referrals		Matheson et al. 1988
Case record review	Referrals to sports medicine clinic	1857	7–92	Knee injuries	26.5% of visits		Butcher et al. 1996
Sample survey, interview	Male former elite athletes	117	45–68	Knee pain during 1 mo	45% soccer players; 17% shooters		Kujala et al. 1994
Prospective survey	Bicycle riders participating in a 339-mile recreational ride	1638	mean 39	Injuries and overuse syndromes	13.7 overuse syndromes per 100,000 person-miles	Knee pain most common problem. Increased risk for first-time riders	Dannenberg et al. 1996
Prospective survey, Germany	Professional football players			Injuries	15.7 injuries per 1000 player-hours	Knee pain most common problem	Baltzer and Ghadamgahi 1998
Prospective survey, Denmark	Soccer players	496	12–18	New injuries	3.7 injuries per 1000 player-hours	Knee pain most common problem	Schmidt-Olsen et al. 1991
Prospective survey, Norway	Service conscripts	6488		Injuries during initial training	13 injuries per 100 conscript months	Low back and overuse knee pain most common problems	Heir and Eide 1996

those described in studies based on radiographic change alone (Table IV), and it seems that painful osteoarthritis is a subset of radiographic osteoarthritis, defined by severity or health service use, rather than being a separate pain syndrome. The severity of pain, in both British and American prospective studies of patients with symptomatic knee osteoarthritis at baseline, was an independent predictor of the likelihood of progression of structural changes (Hochberg et al. 1989; Spector et al. 1994).

RISK FACTORS FOR KNEE PAIN

Despite the disparity between reported knee pain and radiographic changes of osteoarthritis in subjects over 50 years old, the presence of severe radiographic features of osteoarthritis is still a risk factor for pain. One U.K. population study found an odds ratio of 4.0 for the association between knee pain and advanced severe osteoarthritis seen on X-ray film after adjust-

ment for anxiety, depression, and quadriceps muscle strength (O'Reilly et al. 1998). Lesser degrees of radiographic change (which are more common in the older population than is severe osteoarthritis) were not associated with pain, however.

Studies of radiographic and clinical osteoarthritis have been dominated by the clinico-pathological or biomedical model. Far more than is the case for low back pain or facial pain, for example, knee pain has been treated as a symptom of local disease, and researchers have tended to argue that the best way to study causation is to obtain an unselected sample of subjects with evidence of local pathology. However, some studies have examined potential risks for knee pain that are independent of radiographic change. For example, the higher the educational level that had been reached by adults participating in the first American National Health and Nutrition Examination Survey (NHANES), the less likely they were to report knee pain occurring in a 1-year period (Hannan et al. 1992).

Table IV
a) Summary comparison of risk factors for radiological and symptomatic osteoarthritis (OA) and knee pain

Risk Factor	Knee Pain	Painful Knee OA	Radiological OA	Self-reported Knee Arthritis
Obesity, weight increase	Sobti 1997, Hartz 1986	Cooper 1994a, Felson 1992, Kohatsu 1990	Anderson 1988, Felson 1988, Hartz 1986, Cicuttini 1997, McAlindon 1996, Sowers 1996, Felson 1997, Cicuttini 1996, Spector 1994	Davis 1988, Manninen 1996
Occupational lifting, bending, squatting	Sobti 1997, Jensen 1996	Cooper 1994b, Kohatsu 1990, Jensen 1996, Vingard 1991	Felson 1991, Maetzel 1997, Jensen 1996, Anderson 1988	
Knee injury		Cooper 1994a, Kohatsu 1990,	Roos 1994, McAlindon 1996, Sowers 1996	Deacon 1997
Meniscectomy		Cooper 1994a, Wroble 1992	Roos 1994, Roos 1998	
Sport, elite	Deacon 1997, Spector 1996	Kujala 1994	Deacon 1997, Spector 1996	
Regular sport or physical activity			Imeokparia 1994 women only, Felson 1997	
No link to regular sport		Lane 1993	Hannan 1993	
Social class, education	Hannan 1992		Leigh 1994	

This finding persisted after adjustment for other socioeconomic factors and was independent of X-ray evidence of osteoarthritis. Educational attainment is an important indicator because it is "set" relatively early in life and thus cannot itself be influenced by the presence of illness and symptoms at older ages. Obesity appears to influence the onset of symptoms in those with radiographic change in addition to its influence on the structural change itself (Felson et al. 1992, 1997).

Other analyses of NHANES and a population study of a rural community in America have provided evidence that well-being is linked to knee pain, irrespective of the severity of radiographic change (Hochberg et al. 1989; Davis 1992; Jordan et al. 1997). In a Nottingham, U.K., population study, quadriceps weakness, anxiety, and depression were strong independent predictors of pain and pain severity, with radiographic osteoarthritis a weaker predictor of pain and not linked at all with pain severity (O'Reilly et al. 1998). Another U.K. population study has confirmed the link between knee pain and depression (McCarney 1998).

Can knee pain be treated as a regional pain syndrome, on a par with back pain, facial pain, and so on? Are the general influences on chronic pain (i.e., those risk factors common to the persistence of all regional pains regardless of their location) just as likely

to be found, and to the same extent, in connection with the knee as with other parts of the body? The theoretical answer must be "yes"; the psychosocial background, pain behavior, learning, attitudes, and employment context of persons suffering from knee or other osteoarthritic joint pain must surely be similar to factors influencing chronic pain at other sites. Some commentators are clear that the clinical evidence favors this interpretation (Hadler 1992; Creamer and Hochberg 1997).

However, the empirical answer at this stage must be more cautious. Studies of the psychosocial correlates of knee pain are remarkably scarce. The studies quoted above are cross-sectional, and the results may simply represent the impact of any chronic pain on psychological status and functioning. Furthermore, joint pain is unique among pain syndromes in its increasing frequency with age up to the very oldest in our population. Studies of the predictors of the outcome of surgery present evidence for nonspecific effects on knee problems. In one study, higher expectations of surgery, early return to activity, and a sense of "control" over the condition were all strong predictors of reduced dependency at 9 months postsurgery (Orbell et al. 1998). It may well be that the type of guidelines developed for the primary care management of low back pain, freed of the emphasis on regional pathology, will apply to knee pain in the future. This

Table IV
b) Commentary

Reference	Comments
Anderson and Felson 1988; Leigh and Fries 1994; Hartz et al. 1986; Hannan et al. 1992	Cross-sectional population health survey (NHANES). Hartz added evidence that obesity increased the likelihood of radiographic OA even in the absence of knee pain. Hannan identified an increased risk of knee pain in relation to education, independent of radiographic change.
Cicuttini et al. 1997	Cross-sectional radiographic population survey of middle-aged women.
Cooper et al. 1994a,b	Case-control community study.
Deacon et al. 1997	Retired elite Australian football players versus age-matched controls.
Hannan et al. 1993; Felson et al. 1991, 1992, 1997, 1998; McAlindon et al. 1996	Prospective population cohort; included follow-up of subjects free of radiographic OA (Framingham). McAlindon et al. added evidence that obesity and knee injury were risk factors for OA in both compartments of the knee. Hannan et al. found no link between knee OA and habitual physical activity. Felson et al. (1992) suggested that the onset of symptoms in the knee was related to weight increase or failure to lose weight.
Imeokparia et al. 1994	Retrospective case-control community study.
Jensen and Eenberg 1996	Systematic overview identified 19 controlled studies of knee disorders in relation to occupational activity. Consistent evidence that bursitis and OA are related to kneeling tasks; contrasting evidence for and against link between OA and heavy physical work.
Kohatsu and Schurman 1990	Retrospective case-control study, severe knee OA.
Kujala et al. 1994	National cohort of all hospital admissions in Finland; retrospective cohort analysis of elite athletes.
Lane et al. 1993	Prospective cohort of runners and age-matched controls.
Maetzel et al. 1997	Systematic overview identified 123 studies concerned with mechanical occupational exposure for OA: 17 had controls and were based on radiographic diagnosis; 7 were good quality, and confirmed occupational knee bending as a risk for knee OA in men.
Roos et al. 1994	Cross-sectional study, former soccer players versus controls.
Roos et al. 1998	Prospective cohort, post-meniscectomy, age- and sex-matched controls.
Sobti et al. 1997	Cohort of retired post office workers, surveyed for musculoskeletal symptoms.
Spector et al. 1994	Prospective community cohort of women with unilateral radiographic knee OA, increased risk of OA in contralateral knee compared with controls.
Spector et al. 1996	Retrospective cohort of female elite athletes in weight-bearing sports, with age-matched community controls. Radiographic knee OA increased, but pain reporting levels were similar.
Vingard et al. 1991	National cohort of hospital admissions in Sweden; retrospective cohort analysis in relation to census-based occupation. Farmers, construction workers, firemen, and female cleaners all had increased risk of future knee replacements.

possibility is strengthened when attention is turned to the impact and consequences of knee pain.

CONSEQUENCES OF KNEE PAIN

The important issues for patients with knee problems are the degree of pain and the extent of associated disability they experience in everyday living. Research has blossomed on the interactions among pain, restricted functioning, and local pathology of the knee. The main results are summarized in Table V.

In a population study, McAlindon and colleagues (1993) demonstrated that the degree of radiographic change in the knee was a weak predictor of disability;

much stronger influences were quadriceps strength and knee pain. Another group has suggested, based on a population study, that given some structural osteoarthritic damage in the knee, quadriceps weakness may be the key primary risk factor in predicting pain, disability, and the further progression of structural change (O'Reilly et al. 1998). The major prospective study of this issue followed 1416 subjects in the Framingham population cohort and found that dependence on other people for assistance in everyday activity was linked overall to the presence of radiographic knee osteoarthritis (OR = 1.3); even stronger was the link between dependency and symptomatic knee osteoarthritis (i.e., X-ray changes plus symptoms) (OR = 1.9). Most importantly, the odds of difficulty in walking after 10

Table V
Impact of knee pain on everyday function

Study Type	Functional Measure	Sample Size	Association with Knee Pain	Association with Radiographic OA	Commentary	Reference
Population cohort	Any dependency in home	1416	OR = 1.9	OR 1.3	Mild radiographic OA with no pain; no increased dependency	Guccione et al. 1990
Population survey and 10-y follow-up of subgroup	Difficulty walking, difficulty arising	367	RR = 2.8 (normal X-ray); RR = 4.0 (OA on X-ray)	RR = 2.1 (no knee pain); RR = 3.0 (knee pain)	Weaker links in men; psychological status also influenced pain reporting in those with radiographic disease.	Hochberg et al. 1989
Cross-sectional rural population survey	Difficulty in daily activity (HAQ)	1192	All 20 tasks affected in the presence of moderate to severe knee pain	No independent link after adjusting for knee pain severity	Knee pain strongest predictor of restricted activity	Jordan et al. 1997
Case-control population study	WOMAC, HAD, and quadriceps strength	300 with knee pain, 300 without knee pain; ages 40–79	Quads strength independently linked with pain; OR = 18.8 for weakest 10%. Depression OR = 2.4; link with disability	No association with disability after adjusting for depression and quads strength.	Depression and anxiety are also independently linked with disability, after adjusting for quads strength (OR = 8.3 for depression, 2.0 for anxiety; 5.0 for quadriceps strength)	O'Reilly et al. 1998
Population survey, interview	Difficulty in daily activity (HAQ)	2895, randomly sampled from ages 55+	OR = 2.9 men, 2.1 women, adjusted for hip pain, obesity, and X-ray OA	OR = 1.1 men, 1.4 women. For severe radiographic OA, OR = 2.7 men, 2.4 women	Knee pain accounted for 20% of locomotor disability in the presence of X-ray changes, whereas radiological severity accounted for <5%	Odding et al. 1998
Cross-sectional population survey	Quadriceps strength	462	RR = 0.7 per 4 kg quads strength	RR = 0.8 per 4 kg quads strength		Slemenda et al. 1997
Population cohort, year of birth 1914	Dependency	307 75–80-year olds followed for 5 y	Knee extension only marginally predictive of 5-y function	Not studied	Strongest predictors were level of physical activity and presence of two or more chronic diseases	Schroll et al. 1997
Population cohort of farmers, Finland	Social security benefits 10 years later	6647		Diagnosed clinical knee OA, 4–7-fold risk	Age, female gender, and body mass index also predictive	Manninen et al. 1996
Population samples of persons with and without knee pain	Difficulty in daily activity (HAQ)	159	OR = 1.7	No independent link after adjusting for pain and quads strength	Age and quadriceps strength also predictive	McAlindon et al. 1993

Abbreviations: HAD = Hospital Anxiety and Depression Index; HAQ = Health Assessment Questionnaire; OR = odds ratio; RR = relative risk; WOMAC = Western Ontario McMaster Osteoarthritis Index.

years follow-up were increased by the presence and severity of baseline pain, irrespective of the radiological severity, although the strongest link was with X-ray changes in conjunction with frequent pain (Guccione et al. 1990). In a rural population in America, the severity of knee pain was the strongest independent predictor of difficulty with lower limb tasks; controlling for the knee pain showed no independent link between X-ray change and difficulty with such tasks (Jordan et al. 1997). (Of course, this finding does not mean that structural osteoarthritis was not contributing to the mechanism of pain production, but pain per se seems to be a more important factor than X-ray change per se in the resulting lower limb disability.)

These findings have been confirmed in two more recent population studies from the United Kingdom and The Netherlands. In the Nottingham study of 40–79-year-olds, knee pain was an important predictor of disability; in addition, depression and quadriceps strength, but not radiographic change, predicted disability in both pain-positive and pain-negative subjects (O'Reilly et al. 1998). The Dutch adult population study showed a clear link between knee pain and disability but no overall association between radiographic change in the knee and disability (Odding et al. 1998). However, severe radiographic osteoarthritis was also associated with restricted daily activity independent of pain.

Another major factor in determining disability is co-morbidity, particularly at older ages. Some studies have suggested that chronic disease in other systems and current general physical activity may be a more important factor in determining subsequent lower limb disability in older age cohorts than are local factors such as knee pain and extensor strength (Schroll et al. 1997). The prevalence of reported disability is higher if three or more joint sites are reported to be painful, but in the population study by Urwin and colleagues (1998), isolated knee pain was also associated with a high degree of disability.

The complex interaction between pain, local muscle strength and general physical fitness is an important topic for future epidemiological research. For example, in one community-based study of 55–74-year-olds, with subsamples defined by pain, radiographic change, and disability, the overall health status of those with and without knee pain was identical unless mobility restriction or psychological distress were added factors (Hopman-Rock et al. 1997). In a cohort of Finnish farmers followed for 10 years, the

risk for claiming disability pensions was stronger for depression and upper limb problems than for knee osteoarthritis alone (Manninen et al. 1997).

In summary, a shift of attention toward functioning in everyday life as a crucial measure of the impact of lower limb disease has emphasized that knee pain and pain severity, whether directly or as markers of disease severity, play important roles that are distinct and separate from the extent of structural damage to the knee joint.

IMPLICATIONS FOR PREVENTION

Despite the shift in emphasis from the epidemiology of radiographic change to the epidemiology of pain severity, muscle strength, and disability, the implications for prevention and treatment should not necessarily be drawn directly from the results of such studies. It may be that tackling the structural disease by knee arthroplasty, for example, is a good treatment for pain, for weak extensors, and hence for disability; but this theory needs to be proven. What seems reasonably clear is that such tertiary prevention applies to the minority of older persons with severe degrees of radiographic change.

It may also be that tackling risk factors for structural disease is a good way to lower the incidence of later pain and disability. In this regard, obesity and weight gain stand out as major attributable risks for knee osteoarthritis, both radiographic and clinical. Cohort studies referenced in Table IV suggest that weight loss predicts improvement in both these parameters, but strong randomized trial evidence is lacking. Given the pessimistic results of targeted weight loss, the benefits of preventive programs will probably emerge only from primary societal changes that result in a downwards shift in weight distribution. Current trends in the opposite direction to this desirable goal suggest that knee pain prevalence may increase in the future.

There is better evidence that targeted secondary prevention to increase quadriceps strength in older persons is a useful intervention. However, the great potential once again lies in improving general physical activity and strength at younger ages (Sonn 1996); both knee pain and disability, as well as radiographic and clinical osteoarthritis, are likely to decline in frequency as a result. The public health potential is enormous, given that lower limb disability is the single most important cause of restricted mobility in older persons.

More research is needed, however, to define optimal programs that avoid the potentially deleterious effects of sport and physical activity on joints and on the musculoskeletal system in general. In particular, occupational activities that load the knee, and injuries to the joint and the soft tissues in children and younger adults, are major potential areas for preventive activity.

Finally, evidence is emerging that general principles of pain management are likely to be helpful in the tertiary prevention of chronic knee pain, regardless of whether structural change is present in the joint. However, empirical trials of such approaches remain to be carried out.

HEALTH CARE UTILIZATION

The proportion of adults under 55 years old who consult their family doctor with knee strains and sprains in the course of a year is estimated at 12 per 1000 registered population in the United Kingdom (Royal College of General Practitioners 1995). Also based on this same source, 10% of registered 65- to 74-year-olds consult their doctor about osteoarthritis in the course of one year, half of them with chronic problems. This figure rises to 14% of those over 85 years old, but is lower for those younger than 65. The knee is not identified separately in these figures, and such data refer to "osteoarthritis as diagnosed by the general practitioner," which is likely to be a mixture of "pain thought to be osteoarthritis" and radiographically confirmed osteoarthritis.

Parallel figures come from the Rotterdam study, which used radiographs, symptoms, and self-reported consultations to evaluate disability in a random population sample of persons over 55 years old (Odding et al. 1996). The proportion of this older community sample who reported current pain in the hip or knee for which they had consulted their general practitioner and which had been given a label of "arthritis, rheumatism, wear-and-tear, or aging" was 15%, with just under half (6.2% of the whole sample) also having X-ray evidence of knee osteoarthritis.

In a population study from the North of England (Tennant et al. 1995), most of those identified as having severe pain and disability related to the lower limb (8% of adults over 55 years) had been seen by a general practitioner within the previous year and been told at some time that they had arthritis. These figures are also compatible with the estimate of 4.8% of the Dutch population who consult their general practitioner about knee pain each year (Roland and Jamoulle 1997).

Although patients in HMOs represent only a proportion of all symptomatic problems that are investigated and followed in the American population, the annual incidence of symptomatic knee osteoarthritis in one such setting (quoted earlier) is comparable with the European data, namely 2.4 per 1000 of the population, rising to 10 per 1000 per year in 70- to 89-year-olds (Oliveria et al. 1995). It is assumed that these cases represent confirmed radiographic osteoarthritis and first presentations. Overall, osteoarthritis accounts for 46 million annual patient visits to doctors in America, and knee osteoarthritis is the most common initiator of such visits (Abyad and Boyer 1992).

In the Rotterdam disability study, most persons (65%) who stated that they had been diagnosed with arthritis by their general practitioner had been referred to a specialist (Odding et al. 1996). Four percent of this older population saw a specialist because of symptomatic knee osteoarthritis; 4.7% had visited a physiotherapist, which may reflect the wide availability of physiotherapy services to primary care practitioners in The Netherlands. Such figures will vary between different health care systems.

The most common form of knee joint replacement operation involves the whole knee (the total knee replacement or TKR). The Rochester population studies estimated the incidence of TKRs in a defined population as 0.6 per 1000 per year (Wilson et al. 1990). In those over 65 years, it was 4 per 1000 per year. More than 90% of these referrals were for osteoarthritis or rheumatoid arthritis. Such figures obviously reflect the level of health care provision at Rochester's Mayo Clinic, as well as the demand for such care, but their value is that they represent one estimate of "need" for TKR. The National Arthroplasty Registries in Sweden, Norway, and Finland indicate that by the 1990s about 70% of knee arthroplasties were being performed for osteoarthritis (Knutson et al. 1994; Paavolainen et al. 1994; Furnes et al. 1996). In Finland the annual incidence of knee arthroplasties was estimated from registry data at 0.3 per 1000 population (Paavolainen et al. 1994).

AREAS FOR FUTURE RESEARCH IN LOWER LIMB JOINT PAIN

This chapter has highlighted several potential areas of research activity. From the perspective of pain epidemiology, the interesting aspect of lower limb joint pain is that it has been researched from a much more obviously biomedical viewpoint in comparison to many other regional pain syndromes. The reasons seem straightforward (common joint pathology, distinct age profile, and radiographic changes associated with age). However, the challenge to pain epidemiologists is clear: to address the question of whether chronic joint pain in population samples shares similar characteristics to those of other regional pain syndromes, and to examine whether risk factors for chronicity of pain operate in a similar fashion in groups of patients who have radiographic changes of osteoarthritis as they do in other pain syndromes. Although cohort studies of osteoarthritis are difficult to conduct because of the slow and latent onset of the structural changes, further cohort studies of joint pain onset in groups of subjects with radiological evidence of osteoarthritis would allow a more rigorous study of risk factors for joint pain and joint pain progression than can be obtained from cross-sectional studies alone.

Some areas of research neglect are apparent. Foot and ankle pain is grossly under-researched as a regional pain syndrome, but is clearly a major source of disability in the elderly. Hip pain has not received the attention given to knee pain. The field of joint pain and osteoarthritis offers interesting potential as a model for epidemiological studies of the predictors of chronic pain and its relationship to regional pathology and disability.

REFERENCES

Abyad A, Boyer JT. Arthritis and aging. *Curr Opin Rheumatol* 1992; 4:153–159.

Andersen S, Winckler F. The epidemiology of primary osteoarthrosis of the knee in Greenland. *Arch Orthop Traum Surg* 1979; 93:91–94.

Anderson JJ, Felson DT. Factors associated with osteoarthritis of the knee in the first national Health and Nutrition Examination Survey (HANES I). Evidence for an association with overweight, race, and physical demands of work. *Am J Epidemiol* 1988; 128:179–189.

Andersson HI, Ejlertsson G, Leden I, Rosenberg C. Chronic pain in a geographically defined general population. *Clin J Pain* 1993; 9:174–182.

Badley EM, Tennant A. Changing profile of joint disorders with age: findings from a postal survey of the population of Calderdale, West Yorkshire, United Kingdom. *Ann Rheum Dis* 1992; 51:366–371.

Baker BE, Peckham AC, Pupparo F, Sanborn JC. Review of meniscal injury and associated sports. *Am J Sports Med* 1985; 13:1–4.

Baltzer AW, Ghadamgahi PD. American football injuries in the German Federal League: risk of injuries and pattern of injuries. *Unfallchirurgie* 1998; 24:60–65.

Bergenudd H, Nilsson B, Lindgarde F. Knee pain in middle age and its relationship to occupational workload and psychosocial factors. *Clin Orth* 1989; 245:210–215.

Butcher JD, Zukowski CW, Brannen SJ, et al. Patient profile, referral sources, and consultant utilization in a primary care sports medicine clinic. *J Family Prac* 1996; 43:556–560.

Cicuttini FM, Baker JR, Spector TD. The association of obesity with osteoarthritis of the hand and knee in women: a twin study. *J Rheumatol* 1996; 23:1221–1226.

Cicuttini FM, Spector T, Baker J. Risk factors for osteoarthritis in the tibiofemoral and patellofemoral joints of the knee. *J Rheumatol* 1997; 24:1164–1167.

Claessens AA, Schouten JS, Van den Ouweland FA, Valkenburg HA. Do clinical findings associate with radiographic osteoarthritis of the knee? *Ann Rheum Dis* 1990; 49(10):771–774.

Cooper C, McAlindon T, Snow S, et al. Mechanical and constitutional risk factors for symptomatic knee osteoarthritis: differences between medial tibiofemoral and patellofemoral disease. *J Rheumatol* 1994a; 21:307–313.

Cooper C, McAlindon T, Coggon D, Egger P, Dieppe P. Occupational activity and osteoarthritis of the knee. *Ann Rheum Dis* 1994b; 53:90–93.

Creamer P, Hochberg MC. Why does osteoarthritis of the knee hurt—sometimes? *Br J Rheumatol* 1997; 36:726–728.

Crook J, Rideout E, Browne G. The prevalence of pain complaints in a general population. *Pain* 1984; 18:299–314.

Dannenberg AL, Needle S, Mullady D, Kolodner KB. Predictors of injury among 1638 riders in a recreational long-distance bicycle tour: Cycle Across Maryland. *Am J Sports Med* 1996; 24:747–753.

Davis MA, Ettinger WH, Neuhaus JM. The role of metabolic factors and blood pressure in the association of obesity with osteoarthritis of the knee. *J Rheumatol* 1988; 15:1827–1832.

Davis MA, Ettinger W, Neuhaus JM, Barclay J, Degal M. Correlates of knee pain among US adults with and without radiographic knee osteoarthritis. *J Rheumatol* 1992; 19:1943–1949.

Deacon A, Bennell K, Kiss ZS, Crossley K, Brukner P. Osteoarthritis of the knee in retired, elite Australian Rules footballers. *Med J Aust* 1997; 166:187–190.

Fairbank JC, Pynsent PB, van Poortvliet JA, Phillips H. Mechanical factors in the incidence of knee pain in adolescents and young adults. *J Bone Joint Surg Br* 1984; 66:685–693.

Felson DT, Zhang Y, Anthony JM, Naimark A, Anderson JJ. Weight loss reduces the risk for symptomatic knee osteoarthritis in women. The Framingham Study. *Ann Int Med* 1992; 116:535–539.

Felson DT, Naimark A, Anderson J, et al. The prevalence of knee osteoarthritis in the elderly. The Framingham Osteoarthritis Study. *Arth Rheum* 1987; 30:914–918.

Felson DT, Hannan MT, Naimark A, et al. Occupational physical demands, knee bending, and knee osteoarthritis: results from the Framingham Study. *J Rheumatol* 1991; 18:1587–1592.

Felson DT, Zhang Y, Hannan MT, et al. The incidence and natural history of knee osteoarthritis in the elderly. The Framingham Osteoarthritis Study. *Arth Rheum* 1995. 38:1500–1505.

Felson DT, Zhang Y, Hannan MT, et al. Risk factors for incident radiographic knee osteoarthritis in the elderly: the Framingham Study. *Arth Rheum* 1997; 40:728–733.

Furnes A, Havelin LI, Engesaeter LB, Lie SA. Quality control of prosthetic replacements of knee, ankle, toe, shoulder, elbow and finger joints in Norway 1994. A report after the first year of registration of joint prostheses in the national registry. *Tidsskrift for Den Norske Laegeforening* 1996; 116:1777–1781.

Gibson T, Hameed K, Kadir M, et al. Knee pain amongst the poor and affluent in Pakistan. *Br J Rheumatol* 1996; 35:146–149.

Guccione AA, Felson DT, Anderson JJ. Defining arthritis and measuring functional status in elders: methodological issues in the study of disease and physical disability. *Am J Public Health* 1990; 80:945–949.

Hadler NM. Knee pain is the malady—not osteoarthritis. *Ann Int Med* 1992; 116:598–599.

Hannan MT, Anderson JJ, Pincus T, Felson DT. Educational attainment and osteoarthritis: differential associations with radiographic changes and symptom reporting. *J Clin Epidemiol* 1992; 45:139–147.

Hannan MT, Felson DT, Anderson JJ, Naimark A. Habitual physical activity is not associated with knee osteoarthritis: the Framingham Study. *J Rheumatol* 1993; 20:704–709.

Hartz AJ, Fischer ME, Bril G, et al. The association of obesity with joint pain and osteoarthritis in the HANES data. *J Chron Dis* 1986; 39:311–319.

Heir T, Eide G. Age, body composition, aerobic fitness and health condition as risk factors for musculoskeletal injuries in conscripts. *Scand J Med Sci Sports* 1996; 6:222–227.

Hochberg MC, Lawrence RC, Everett DF, Cornoni-Huntley J. Epidemiologic associations with pain in osteoarthritis of the knee: data from the National Health and Nutrition Examination Survey and the National Heath and Nutrition Examination. I. Epidemiologic follow-up survey. *Sem Arth Rheum* 1989; 18:(Suppl 2):4–9.

Hopman-Rock M, Odding E, Hofman A, Kraaimaat FW, Bijlsma JW. Differences in health status of older adults with pain in the hip or knee only and with additional mobility restricting conditions. *J Rheumatol* 1997; 24:2416–2423.

Imeokparia RL, Barrett JP, Arrieta MI, et al. Physical activity as a risk factor for osteoarthritis of the knee. *Ann Epidemiol* 1994; 4:221–230.

Jensen LK, Eenberg W. Occupation as a risk factor for knee disorders. *Scand J Work Environ Health* 1996; 22:165–175.

Jordan J, Luta G, Renner J, et al. Knee pain and knee osteoarthritis severity in self-reported task specific disability: the Johnston County Osteoarthritis Project. *J Rheumatol* 1997; 24(7):1344–1349.

Knutson K, Lewold S, Robertsson O, Lidgren L. The Swedish knee arthroplasty register. A nation-wide study of 30,003 knees 1976–1992. *Acta Orthop Scand* 1994; 65:375–386.

Kohatsu ND, Schurman DJ. Risk factors for the development of osteoarthrosis of the knee. *Clin Orthop* 1990; 261:242–246.

Kujala UM, Kaprio J, Sarna S. Osteoarthritis of weight bearing joints of lower limbs in former elite male athletes. *BMJ* 1994; 308:231–234.

Lane NE, Michel B, Bjorkengren A, et al. The risk of osteoarthritis with running and aging: a 5-year longitudinal study. *J Rheumatol* 1993; 20:461–468.

Lawrence JS. Rheumatism in populations. London: Wm Heinemann Medical, 1977.

Leigh JP, Fries JF. Correlations between education and arthritis in the 1971–1975, NHANES I. *Soc Sci Med* 1994; 38:575–583.

Lethbridge-Cejku M, Scott WW, Jr, Reichle R, et al. Association of radiographic features of osteoarthritis of the knee with knee pain: data from the Baltimore Longitudinal Study of Ageing. *Arth Care Res* 1995; 8:182–188.

Maetzel A, Mäkelä M, Hawker G, Bombardier C. Osteoarthritis of the hip and knee and mechanical occupational exposure—a systematic overview of the evidence. *J Rheumatol* 1997; 24:1599–1607.

Manninen P, Riihimaki H, Heliövaara M, Mäkelä P. Overweight, gender and knee osteoarthritis. *Int J Obesity* 1996; 20:595–597.

Manninen P, Heliövaara M, Riihimaki H, Mäkelä P. Does psychological distress predict disability? *Int J Epidemiol* 1997; 26:1063–1070.

Matheson GO, MacIntyre JG, Taunton JE, Clement DB, Lloyd-Smith R. Musculoskeletal injuries associated with physical activity in older adults. *Med Sci Sports Exercise* 1988; 21:379–385.

McAlindon TE, Cooper C, Kirwan JR, Dieppe PA. Knee pain and disability in the community. *Br J Rheumatol* 1992; 31:189–192.

McAlindon TE, Cooper C, Kirwan JR, Dieppe PA. Determinants of disability in osteoarthritis of the knee. *Ann Rheum Dis* 1993; 52:258–262.

McAlindon T, Zhang Y, Hannan M, et al. Are risk factors for patellofemoral and tibiofemoral knee osteoarthritis different? *J Rheumatol* 1996; 23:332–337.

McCarney RW. The epidemiology of knee pain in primary care: prevalence, health care utilisation and disability. MPhil Thesis, Keele University, UK, 1998.

National Center for Health Statistics. Basic data on arthritis of the knee, hip and sacroiliac joints in adults aged 25–74 years. (Series 11, no. 213). (DHEW publication no. PHS 79–1161).Washington, DC: US GPO, 1979.

Odding E, Valkenburg HA, Algra D, et al. The association of abnormalities on physical examination of the hip and knee with locomotor disability in the Rotterdam Study. *Br J Rheum* 1996; 35:884–890.

Odding E, Valkenburg HA, Algra D, et al. Associations of radiological osteoarthritis of the hip and knee with locomotor disability in the Rotterdam Study. *Ann Rheum Dis* 1998; 57:203–208.

Oliveria SA, Felson DT, Reed JI, Cirillo PA, Walker AM. Incidence of symptomatic hand, hip, and knee osteoarthritis among patients in a health maintenance organization. *Arthitis Rheum* 1995; 38:1134–1141.

Orbell S, Johnston M, Rowley D, Espley A, Davey P. Cognitive representations of illness and functional and affective adjustment following surgery for osteoarthritis. *Soc Sci Med* 1998; 47:93–102.

O'Reilly SC, Muir KR, Doherty M. Screening for pain in knee osteoarthritis: which question? *Ann Rheum Dis* 1996; 55:931–933.

O'Reilly SC, Jones A, Muir KR, Doherty M. Quadriceps weakness in knee osteoarthritis: the effect on pain and disability. *Ann Rheum Dis* 1998; 57:588–594.

Paavolainen P, Hamalainen M, Mustonen H, Slatis P. Registration of arthroplasties in Finland. A nationwide prospective project. *Acta Orthop Scand* 1994; (Suppl):24–30.

Petersson IF, Boegard T, Saxne T, Silman AJ, Svensson B. Radiographic osteoarthritis of the knee classified by the Ahlback and Kellgren & Lawrence systems for the tibiofemoral joint in people aged 35–54 years with chronic knee pain. *Ann Rheum Dis* 1997; 56:493–496.

Roos H, Lindberg H, Gardsell P, Lohmander LS, Wingstrand H. The prevalence of gonarthrosis and its relation to meniscectomy in former soccer players. *Am J Sports Med* 1994; 22:219–222.

Roos H, Lauren M, Adalberth T, et al. Knee osteoarthritis after meniscectomy: prevalence of radiographic changes after twenty-one years, compared with matched controls. *Arthitis Rheum* 1998; 41:687–693.

Roland M, Jamoulle M. "Doctor, my knee hurts...", the generalist's point of view. *Rev Med de Bruxelles* 1997; 18:294–300.

Royal College of General Practitioners. Morbidity statistics from general practice. 1991–92. London: HMSO, 1995.

Schmidt-Olsen S, Jorgensen U, Kaalund S, Sorensen J. Injuries among young soccer players. *Am J Sports Med* 1991; 19:273–275.

Schroll M, Avlund K, Davidsen M. Predictors of five-year functional ability in a longitudinal survey of men and women aged 75 to 80. The 1914 population in Glostrup, Denmark. *Aging* 1997; 9:143–152.

Slemenda C, Brandt KD, Heilman DK, et al. Quadriceps weakness and osteoarthritis of the knee. *Ann Int Med* 1997; 127:97–104.

Sobti A, Cooper C, Inskip H, Searle S, Coggon D. Occupational physical activity and long-term risk of musculoskeletal symptoms: a national survey of post office pensioners. *Am J Ind Med* 1997; 32:76–83.

Sonn U. Longitudinal studies of dependence in daily life activities among elderly persons. *Scand J Rehabil Med* (Suppl) 1996; 34:1–35.

Sowers MF, Hochberg M, Crabbe JP, et al. Association of bone mineral density and sex hormone levels with osteoarthritis of the hand and knee in premenopausal women. *Am J Epidemiol* 1996; 143:38–47.

Spector TD, Hart DJ, Doyle DV. Incidence and progression of osteoarthritis in women with unilateral knee disease in the general population: the effect of obesity. *Ann Rheum Dis* 1994; 53:565–568.

Spector TD, Harris PA, Hart DJ, et al. Risk of osteoarthritis associated with long-term weight-bearing sports: a radiologic survey of the hips and knees in female ex-athletes and population controls. *Arthritis Rheum* 1996; 39:988–995.

Sternbach RA. Survey of pain in the United States: the Nuprin Report. *Clin J Pain* 1986; 2:49–53.

Sun Y, Sturmer T, Gunther KP, Brenner H. Incidence and prevalence of cox- and gonarthrosis in the general population. *Z Orthop Ihre Grenzgeb* 1997; 135:184–192.

Tennant A, Fear J, Pickering A, et al. Prevalence of knee problems in the population aged 55 years and over: identifying the need for arthroplasty. *BMJ* 1995; 310:1291–1293.

Urwin M, Symmons D, Allison T, et al. Estimating the burden of musculoskeletal disorders in the community: the comparative prevalence of symptoms at different anatomical sites, and in relation to social deprivation. *Ann Rheum Dis* 1998; 57:649–655.

Vähäsarja V. Prevalence of chronic knee pain in children and adolescents in northern Finland. *Acta Paed* 1995; 84:803–805.

van Schaardenburg D, van den Brande KJS, Ligthart GJ, Breedveld FC, Hazes JMW. Musculoskeletal disorders and disability in persons aged 85 and over: a community survey. *Ann Rheum Dis* 1994; 53:807–811.

Vingard E, Alfredsson L, Goldie I, Hogstedt C. Occupation and osteoarthrosis of the hip and knee: a register-based cohort study. *Int J Epidemiol* 1991; 20:1025–1031.

Wigley RD, Zhang Nai-Zheng, Zeng Qing-Yu, et al. Rheumatic diseases in China: ILAR-China Study comparing the prevalence of rheumatic symptoms in Northern and Southern Rural Populations. *J Rheumatol* 1994; 21:1484–1490.

Wilson MG, Michet CJ Jr., Ilstrup DM, Melton LJ III. Idiopathic symptomatic osteoarthritis of the hip and knee: a population-based incidence study. *Mayo Clin Proc* 1990; 65:1214–1221.

Woo J, Ho SC, Lau J, Leung PC. Musculoskeletal complaints and associated consequences in elderly Chinese aged 70 years and over. *J Rheumatol* 1994; 21:1927–1931.

Wroble RR, Henderson RC, Campion ER, el-Khoury GY, Albright JP. Meniscectomy in children and adolescents. A long-term follow-up study. *Clin Orthop* 1992; 279:180–189.

Zhang N, Shi Q, Zhang X. An epidemiological study of knee osteoarthritis. *Chin J Int Med* 1995; 34:84–87.

Correspondence to: Peter R. Croft, MD, MRCGP, Primary Care Sciences Research Centre, School of Postgraduate Medicine, Keele University, Thornburrow Drive, Hartshill, Stoke-on-Trent, ST4 7QB, United Kingdom. Email: pma07@keele.ac.uk.

Index

Locators in *italic* refer to figures.
Locators followed by t refer to tables.

A